Bone and Cartilage Engineering

Ulrich Meyer · Hans Peter Wiesmann

Ulrich Meyer · Hans Peter Wiesmann

Bone and Cartilage Engineering

With 95 Figures and 55 Tables

With a Contribution by Thomas Meyer

Springer

Ulrich Meyer, Prof. Dr. Dr.
Heinrich-Heine-Universität Düsseldorf
Klinik für Kiefer-
und Plastische Gesichtschirurgie
Moorenstraße 5
40225 Düsseldorf
Germany

Hans Peter Wiesmann, Priv.-Doz. Dr.
Universitätsklinikum Münster
Klinik und- Poliklinik für Mund-,
Kiefer- und Gesichtschirurgie
Waldeyer Str. 30
48149 Münster
Germany

ISBN-10 3-540-25347-5 Springer-Verlag Berlin Heidelberg NewYork
ISBN-13 978-3-540-25347-1 Springer-Verlag Berlin Heidelberg NewYork

Library of Congress Control Number: 2005931758

Springer is a part of Springer Science+Business Media

springer.com

Printed in Germany

Editor: Gabriele Schröder, Heidelberg
Desk Editor: Irmela Bohn, Heidelberg
Production: LE-TEX, Jelonek, Schmidt & Vöckler GbR, Leipzig
Typsetting: Satz-Druck-Service, Leimen
Cover Design: Frido Steinen-Broo, EStudio Calamar, Spain

Printed on acid-free paper 24/3100/YL 5 4 3 2 1 0

Dedicated to
Janine and Andrea

Preface

Bone and cartilage tissue engineering is a multidisciplinary, young and emerging field in biotechnology, which is expected to change medical practice profoundly, regenerating skeletal tissues and organs instead of just repairing them. This new medical discipline holds the promise of improved treatment possibilities, enhanced quality of the patient's life and the ability to overcome, in the future, the need for major grafting procedures. It is expected that this biotechnology will also have a strong economical impact on clinical medicine. To fulfil these expectations several challenges concerning scientific, technological, clinical, ethical and also social issues need to be met. Basic research still requires the evaluation and elaboration of fundamental processes and procedures in multiple research fields. However, the first tissue engineered bone and cartilage products have already been introduced to the market, and many more are in the preclinical stage, and many companies are involved in this area.

Extracorporal bone and cartilage tissue engineering is a narrower definition of bone and cartilage reconstruction and regeneration by means of the implantation of a cell/scaffold complex. This kind of tissue engineering approach is a multidisciplinary subject bringing together various scientific fields, including material science, cell biology and clinical disciplines. The promising biotechnology, now introduced as a new clinical tool in the restoration of bone or joint defects, is expected to change treatment regimes and to contribute significantly to clinical medicine in future decades. Current limitations in tissue engineering seem most likely be overcome in the near future, suggesting that generating bone or cartilage tissue ex vivo will replace other therapies in routine clinical practice.

One of the reasons for the fast growth of tissue engineering is the large number of excellent research papers covering all aspects of bone and cartilage tissue engineering. Additionally, numerous high quality books are available describing in detail different aspects of bone and cartilage tissue engineering. Despite the fact that such literature is already available, we decided to write a book on bone and cartilage tissue engineering for two reasons. First, during the experimental and clinical work on tissue engineering carried out over more than 10 years in our clinic as well as in our biomineralisation and tissue engineering research group, we observed that many specialists from the different fields involved in tissue engineering had difficulties in overviewing the complexity of the field. We therefore intended to write a comprehensive book covering all aspects of bone and cartilage tissue engineering. Second, as tissue engineering brings together basic researchers, mainly having a biological, biophysical or material science oriented background, with clinically oriented physicians, we found that they differed in the language used. To overcome this problem, the demanding and complex aspects of tissue engineering were divided into the different aspects of tissue engineering on a level that provides extended information for specialist, but also gives usable access to non-specialists. The text of this book is therefore augmented by numerous tables, schematic illustrations and photographs in order to provide a better understanding of the information provided.

We hope this book will add further stimulus for all basic researchers and clinicians who are involved in investigating and applying tissue engineering and will contribute to making bone and cartilage tissue engineering an attractive and reliable alternative treatment option in reconstructive surgery.

Ulrich Meyer
Hans Peter Wiesman

Acknowledgements

This book would not have been possible without the help and support of a multitude of esteemed colleagues. First of all, we would like to thank Prof. Dr. Dr. Dr. hc U. Joos who created through his enormous clinical and scientific potential the logistic, scientific and personal environment as well as the enthusiasm to establish the Biomineralisation and Tissue Engineering Group in his clinic. The expertise and enthusiasm of the members of this group have set the basis for this book. In this respect, we are extremely grateful to Prof. Dr. H. J. Höhling. PD Dr. Dr. J. Kleinheinz, Dr. Dr. B. Kruse-Lösler, Dr. U. Plate, Dr. Th. Szuwart, Dr. R. Cankay, Prof. U. Stratmann, and PD Dr. A. Büchter, who shared our interst and enthusiasm in tissue engineering and inspired the research with their excellent studies. In this regard, we are also very grateful to the medical, scientific and laboratory staff of the Clinic for Cranio-, Maxillofacial Surgery in Münster. Additionally, the willingness and close cooperation with other departments has enabled us to perform complex and multidisciplinary research activities.

The outcome of this research was based on cooperation with a variety of commited colleagues (namely Prof. Dr. W. Schlegel, Department of Gynecology; Prof. Dr. K.-D. Richter, Department of Animal Studies; Prof. Dr. H. Arlinghaus, Prof. Dr. H. Kohl, Prof. Dr. L. Chi and Prof. Dr. H. Fuchs, Department of Physics; Prof. Dr. P. Bruckner, PD Dr. C. Runte and PD Dr. D. Dirksen, Institute of Biophysics, Prosthetic Department; PD Dr. T. Stamm, Orthodontic Department; Dr. E. Krefting and Prof. Dr. R. Reichelt, Department of Medical Physics and Biophysics; Dr. J. Libera, co.don AG, Teltow; Prof. Dr. Dr. D. Weingart, Katharienhospital, Stuttgart). We specially thank Dr. K. Reichenmiller of the Department of Conservative Dentistry, University Tübingen for many helpful discussions and for leaving the PCR images to us and we thank PD Dr. Meffert and Prof. Dr. Raschke of the Department of Reconstructive Surgery, who supported us with their scientific knowledge and who gave us the photographs on joint surgery. We thank Dr. Dr. J. Handschel and Prof. Dr. Dr. N.R. Kübler for their excellent scientific work in embryonic stem cell research at the University of Düsseldorf. Mister Sailer and Dipl.-Ing. N. Huda provided us with excellent schematic drawings. We are also very greatful to Dieter Sommer who supported us in the realisation of the book. Moreover we would like to express our gratitude to Springer, especially Ms. Irmela Bohn, for the professional accompaniment to this project.

We acknowledge with thanks the support of our work by a multitude of research grants over the last decade. Without the support of the German Research Foundation (DFG), the Federal Ministry of Education and Research (BMBF), grants from the University of Münster (IZKF, IMF) and grants given by biomedical companies it would not have been possible to extensively work on bone and cartilage enginnering.

Our most important advisor in the creation of this book was my brother Prof. Dr. Dr. Dr. T. Meyer. With his enormous scientific knowledge in clinical medicine, biochemistry and philosophy, his criticism and useful suggestions in the realisation of this book, as well as with his excellent chapter on ethical considerations in bone and cartilage tissue engineering, he markedly improved the quality of this book.

However, most of our gratitude goes to our families, our dear wives Janine and Andrea, as well as our children Johannes and Carla, who showed virtually endless patience and understanding for our research activities as well as for the writing of this book. Thus, they deserve the highest respect for the completion of this book.

Ulrich Meyer
Hans Peter Wiesmann

Contents

Introduction

1

With the advancement of the concept of regenerative medicine and in particular the field of tissue engineering, a completely new strategy of patient treatment can be expected, with the potential to change treatment regimes profoundly (Fodor, 2003). Tissue engineering aims at regenerating defective or lost tissues or organs, and signals a transition from the historically material-based approaches, in which mechanically stable, biocompatible materials were used, to focus on cell-based devices (Hunziker, 2002; Parikh, 2002). The new approach combines the biological properties of living cells and the physical properties of specially designed materials in order to create artificial organs (Orban et al., 2002). To rapidly restore full functionality in the case of lost organs, artificial tissues are created ex vivo and are implanted at the site of the lesion. Improved quality of life in the sense of accelerated healing and better treatment outcomes can be envisaged, ideally accompanied by overall lower treatment costs (Garfein et al., 2003). Tissue engineering is a rapidly growing discipline and research in this field is steadily increasing, indicated by the increasing number of publications in biological and material science journals as well as in medical journals (Fig. 1.1).

Whereas research effort in this field covers a broad area of biological and material science, clinical tissue engineering is still in its initial phase (Lavik and Langer, 2004). The first tissue-engineered product (cartilage) was approved for clinical use in 1996. Since then, developments in basic and clinical research have resulted in several commercialised products. Skeletal tissue engineering, especially cartilage tis-

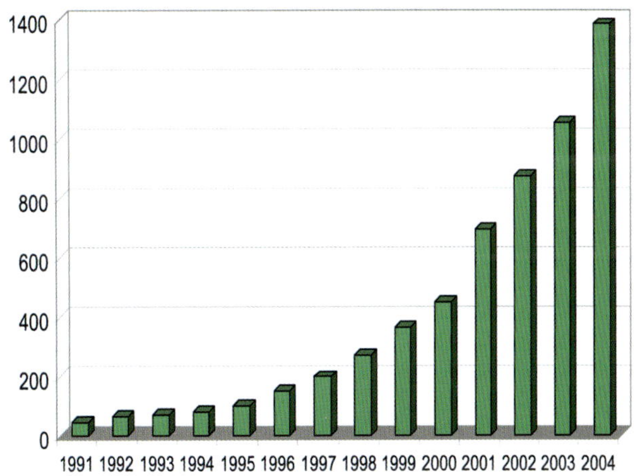

Fig. 1.1. Year upon year increase in the number of relevant publications

sue engineering with some bone engineering products on the market, is the leading field in extracorporal creation of human substitute tissues, followed by replacement of skin by tissue-engineered skin products (Lysaght and Reyes, 2001). The reason for the early introduction of these artificial tissue substitutes is the relative simplicity of these tissues. While they are on the way to gain acceptance in routine clinical practice, more advanced products such as multicellular systems and scaffold-free matrix systems are currently under development and may soon be in the pipeline (Lysaght and Reyes, 2001; Stock and Vacanti, 2001).

The economically most important skeletal tissue substitute is cartilage. Cartilage is present in the human body in loaded (mainly joints and intervertebral discs) and unloaded locations (e.g. ear and nose). As cartilage has only a limited capacity to regenerate itself, regeneration-supporting therapies are necessary in most clinical cases (Kaufman and Tobias, 2003). Lesions in cartilage are a significant problem in medical practice, with approximately one million patients treated annually, and approximately 250,000 knee arthroplasty procedures per year (Hunziker, 2002). It is well known that lesions that are confined to the articular cartilage alone have little or no capacity to heal. In general, the patients become symptomatic and a significant progression to osteoarthritis is possible (Lohmander, 2003). However, those lesions that penetrate the subchondral bone have access to the bone marrow space and chondroprogenitor cells and therefore have a limited repair capacity.

Most therapies are aimed at healing hyaline cartilage defects in loaded locations, whereas only a few cases are intended to regenerate non-loaded cartilage defects. Over the last decade autologous chondrocyte transplantation (ACT) has attracted much scientific and commercial interest. ACT and its several modifications are the most widespread applications of skeletal tissue engineering. The use of autologous chondrocytes was primarily performed in traumatically damaged knee joints (Vangsness et al., 2004). Based on new findings in cartilage tissue engineering, preclinical studies suggest expansion to joints other than the knee, to treat also non-traumatic cartilage defects (arthrosis, arthritis defects), and to repair complex tissue defects (osteochondral defects) by a combination of bone and cartilage products. It is assumed that the use of tissue-engineered cartilage products will gain further importance in the near future, developing a significant market size (Table 1.1). The expectation of a steadily increasing tissue-engineered cartilage market is based on the assumption of some restrictions on the current state of ACT being overcome in future research:

- The restriction of ACT to traumatic knee injuries
- The restriction of the recently limited health insurance reimbursement
- The required cooperation of patients (preferred non-loading period after transplantation).

New developments in cartilage tissue engineering (self-adhesion scaffold-free micromass tissue) promise simplification of surgical procedures and therefore open up new application fields in the cartilage repair market (Fig. 1.2).

Tissue-engineered cartilage products have recently been extended to three-dimensional constructs with the aim of regenerating or replacing intervertebral discs (O'Driscoll, 2001). The combination of chondrocytes and biomaterials in the form of spheres is in the preclinical testing stage and may be a therapeutic option in arthritic joints. All the ongoing developments open up the possibility of larger, eco-

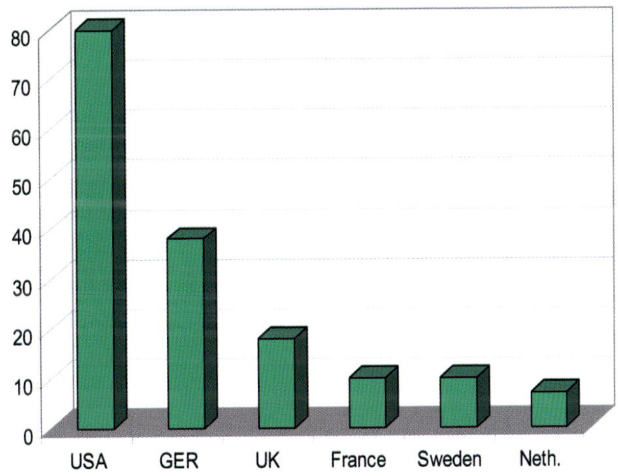

Fig. 1.2. Relevant applications by country

Table 1.1. Market for ACT procedures and companies involved

Country	ACT procedures/year	Calculated sales	Main companies
USA	2,000–3,000	€ 16–24 Mio	Genzyme Carticel
Germany	600	€ 3 Mio	Co.don Verigen ACI Chondrotransplant BioTissue
UK	300–850	€ 1.5–4.3 Mio	Verigen ACI
Italy	300–400	€ 1.5–2 Mio	Fidia Adv. Biomat.
Spain	40	€ 187,000	IsoTis
Total	3,240–4,850	€ 22.2–33.3 Mio	

nomically attractive market segments (Reddi, 1994). The promise of cartilage tissue engineering is mirrored by the number of core tissue engineering companies that are directly involved in cell-based tissue construction (Table 1.1).

In contrast to cartilage tissue engineering, commercial bone tissue engineering is at the beginning of clinical practice (Ripamonti and Tasker, 2000). Whereas many products claim to be tissue-engineered bone (biomaterial/growth factor products), most of them are not cell/biomaterial combinations and thus do not fully comply with the definition of tissue engineering used in this book (Calvert et al., 2003). Only a few companies are engaged in this area. The problems of commercial bone tissue engineering are based on:

- The established treatments in cases of small defects
- The need to reconstruct bone in acute cases (e.g. bone loss by accident)

- The required size and complexity of bone tissue substitutes (e.g. bone loss through ablative tumour surgery).

It is important to recognise that the worldwide market for bone replacement and repair strategies is estimated at about €300 million (Concord Corporate Finance Research). To date, synthetic bone materials, as well as xenogenic, allogenic or autologous materials are the preferred bone substitutes in clinical practice, but with improvements in tissue engineering technology the use of extracorporal grown bone tissue may cover a significant part of this market in the future (Hing, 2004; Salgado et al., 2004).

Tissue engineering is not a precisely defined term. Rather it is a multidisciplinary field of research, combining various aspects of medicine, biology, material science and engineering. Until recently, there were different definitions of tissue engineering, resulting in differences in what is meant by tissue engineering. Two main definitions of tissue engineering are in current use.

The US National Science Foundation defined tissue engineering as:

> The application of the principles and methods of engineering and the life sciences towards the fundamental understanding of structure/function relationship in normal and pathological mammalian tissues and the development of biological substitutes to restore, maintain or improve function.

The European Commission (Scientific Committee on Medical Products and Medical Devices; SCMPMD) preferred a narrower definition:

> Tissue engineering is the regeneration of biological tissue through the use of cells, with the aid of supporting structures and/or biomolecules.

The main difference between the two definitions is that the US definition includes the various approaches of in vivo tissue engineering strategies (biological and biophysical stimulation with or without supporting materials) as well as the use of pure cell therapies (autogenic, allogenic, xenogenic), whereas the EU regulations relate to the idea of extracorporal tissue engineering.

This book covers bone and cartilage tissue engineering as it relates to the EU definition. Whereas the main focus is set on generating bone or cartilage tissue ex vivo, the present book considers also borderline approaches (cell therapies), and overviews alternative tissue engineering strategies in the broader meaning (in vivo strategies). As the EU definition covers products that combine cells with degradable materials and, if used, biomolecules such as differentiation or growth factors, the different chapters of the book follow, in a methodical approach, the various aspects of extracorporal bone and cartilage engineering. Basic information on skeletal science, cell biology, and material science (as the main areas for cell/scaffold development) is given in detail initially. In order to better understand the prerequisites of bone and cartilage tissue engineering, the functional features of both tissues are presented, and special focus is given to the histological and ultra-structural appearance of both tissues. Additionally, the principle mechanisms balancing skeletal formation and turnover are described in order to identify possible targets that can be exploited in tissue engineering strategies. It is important to note, that repair, as distinct from regeneration, involves replacement of the damaged, defective or lost tissue with functional tissue that is not necessarily identical to the normal original tissue. As tissue engineering is aimed at generating the original tissue, the terms regeneration and repair are sometimes used in a broader and more common sense. The description of tissue function is followed by biotechnological issues such as cell/material interactions, use of bioreactors, biophysical stimulation of cells and recent ex vivo tissue micromass developments. The in vivo evaluation of bone and cartilage engineering, mainly through animal models, as well as clinical use are highlighted in the final parts of this book. Special emphasis is also given to regulatory and ethical issues in this new and emerging medical field. In consideration of all aspects of bone and cartilage tissue engineering and the overwhelming body of literature covering experimental and clinical studies, it must be noted that no common or consensus approach has been advised. This book therefore considers the most important aspects of each partial issue.

For the successful transfer of bone and cartilage tissue engineering to clinical practice it is important to have a clear and precise definition of clinical demands and of the problem being addressed (backward planning). Regardless of whether the application is focused on replacing or augmenting bone or cartilage tissue, the approach should start with identification of the individual clinical problem. The severity and location of the skeletal defect need to be precisely assessed before tissue engineering is planned. In particular, the complex anatomical nature of the skeletal defect to be substituted with extracorporally generated tissue constructs has to be taken into account (Fig. 1.3). This identification is the first step in defining the required properties of the extracorporally fabricated cellular hybrid material.

Fundamental aspects that should be considered in bone and cartilage tissue engineering include:

- The evaluation of the specific advantages of implanted cellular bone constructs over non-living materials
- Proven clinically applied models for skeletal tissue regeneration
- Mechanical properties of the implant materials
- Immunological reactions towards the cell/scaffold construct.

Whereas some of these aspects have been tested in preclinical and clinical studies, others have not or have only rarely been investigated in a standardised clinical setting. Therefore, when bone and cartilage tissue engineering is considered as an alternative surgical approach to the reconstruction of skeletal defects, experimental as well as clinical issues should be addressed in a comprehensive manner in order to improve the clinical outcome (for a review, see Rose and Oreffo, 2002).

Additionally, a functional definition of tissue may turn out to be more important than a biochemical or structural definition. Consequently, the focus has recently shifted towards functional tissue engineering to address issues that are relevant to the reconstruction of tissue that has a biomechanically relevant function (Reinholz et al., 2004).

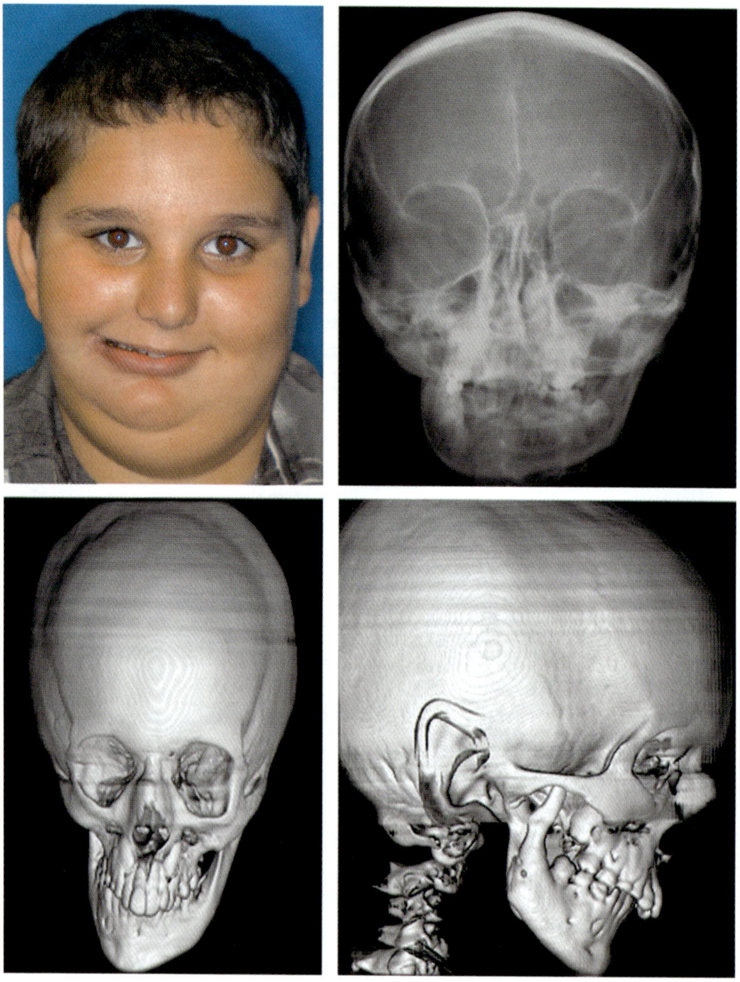

Fig. 1.3. The clinical problem, exemplified by a complex craniofacial malformation, encompassing a deficiency of mandibular bone and cartilage tissue

Bone and Cartilage 2

The first step in approaching bone and cartilage tissue engineering is the understanding of the structure and function of these tissues at the different hierarchial levels. The skeleton is a highly specialised form of connective tissue that is nature`s provision for an internal support system in all higher vertebrates. It is a complex living structure in which two main tissues are present: bone tissue and cartilage tissue. Cartilage and bone are specialised connective tissues that provide the body with mechanical support and protection. Both tissues have some common features in that they provide a unique combination of rigid, yet plastic, living tissue. Additionally, in endochondral ossification, one type of bone formation, cartilage models are converted to bone. In contrast to bone, where a variety of cell sources are responsible for the structural and functional integrity, cartilage tissue is a more uniform cellular tissue (Table 2.1). Human joints, as specialised parts of the skeleton, are composed of several different tissues (cartilage, calcified cartilage, bone) that interact in complex ways to allow joints to function. In addition to the structural properties, the skeleton actively participates in the body`s physiology (e.g. calcium homeostasis).

2.1 Bone Structure and Function

Bones are the principal support for the body. They provide a rigid structure for muscle attachment and constitute a system of levers that turn muscle contraction into purpouseful movements. Cartilage augments this function by providing flexible support. Bones are formed through two distinct developmental processes (Fig. 2.1). Endochondral ossification gives rise to long bones that comprise the appendicular skeleton, facial bones, vertebrae, and the lateral clavicles. Intramembranous ossification gives rise to the flat bones that comprise the cranium and medial clavicles.

Table 2.1. Cells of bone and cartilage tissue

Cortical bone	Cancellous bone	Cartilage
- Osteoblasts - Osteocytes - Lining cells - Osteoclasts - Endothelial cells - Fibroblasts	- Osteoblasts - Osteocytes - Lining cells - Osteoclasts - Endothelial cells - Fibroblasts - Marrow cells	- Chondrocytes

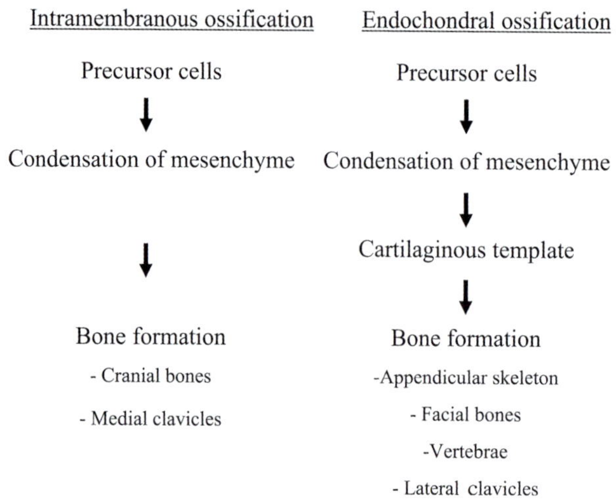

Fig. 2.1. Bone-forming pathways

Both types of ossification involve an initial condensation of mesenchyme and the eventual formation of calcified bone. However, intramembranous bone formation accomplishes this directly, whereas endochondral ossification incorporates an intermediate step in which a cartilaginous template regulates the growth and patterning of the developing skeletal element (Fig. 2.2).

Bone is composed of a variety of cell types and an organic matrix that is strengthened by matrix-associated calcium minerals (primarily calcium and phosphate in the form of hydroxyapatite). The organic matrix consists mainly of collagen (approximately 95%), the remaining organic component of 5% is composed of proteoglycans and numerous non-collagenous proteins. Morphologically there are two forms of bone, which impose different structural and functional properties: cortical and cancellous bone. Fig. 2.3 visualises the structure of cortical bone: densely packed collagen fibrils form concentric lamellae, fibrils in adjacent lamellae run in perpendicular planes towards the concentric lamellae. Blood vessels form a three-dimensional network, located in the centre of osteons and penetrating the cortical bone layer perpendicular to the osteons. Blood vessels are also present in the outer layer of cortical bone. The main cellular component of cortical bone is the osteocyte, a mature osteoblast surrounded by mineralised matrix. The osteocytes have the capacity not only to synthesise, but also to resorb bone matrix to a limited extent. Osteocytes occupy a space (lacuna) within the matrix and extend filopodial processes through canaculi to other osteocytes. The cells are connected to each other by gap junctions. The network of osteocytes is assumed to play a fundamental role in cell communication, important in functional adaption of bone to external stimuli.

Cancellous bone has a loosely organised porous structure (Fig. 2.4). The structure of the trabecular system is optimised to transfer the loads through the bone by a dynamic feedback between load perception of cells and their subsequent cellular reaction. The trabeculae are covered by osteoblasts and bone-/lining cells. Whereas osteoblasts actively secrete the components of the extracellular matrix in order to

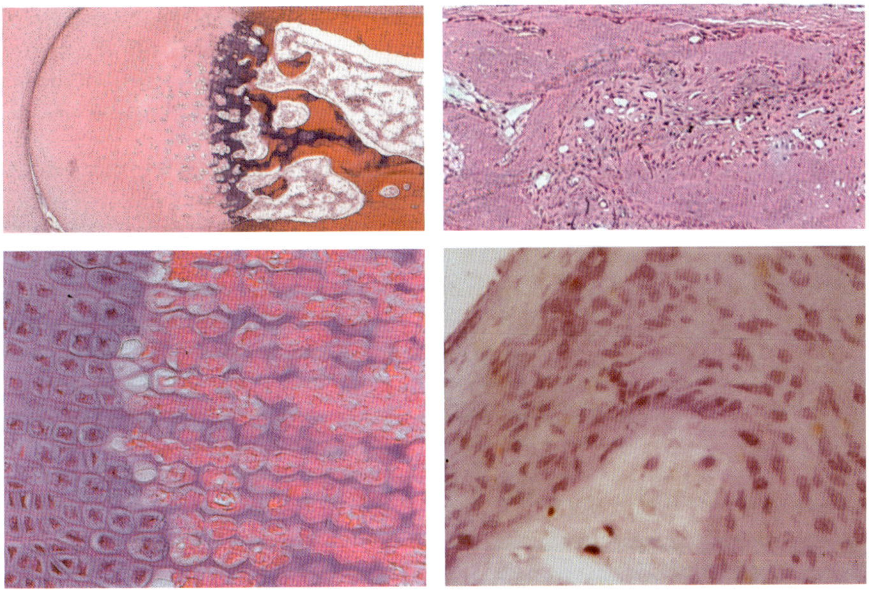

Fig. 2.2. Priciples of bone formation. *Top:* Overview. *Left:* Endochondral ossification of the epiphyseal growth plate. *Right:* Intermembraneous ossification of calvarian suture. *Bottom:* Detail aspect. *Left:* Endochondral ossification. *Right:* Intermembraneous ossification

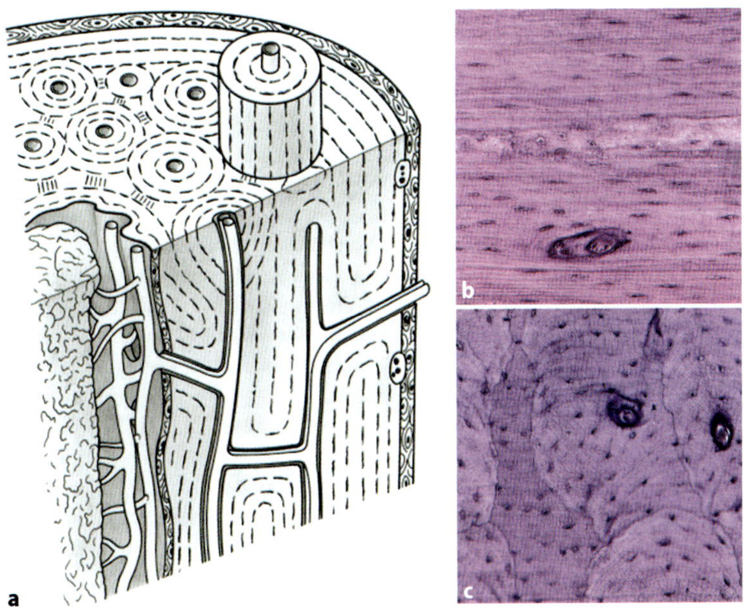

Fig. 2.3. Structure of cortical bone. **a** Schematic. **b** Longitudinal section. **c** Transversal section

build up bone tissue, bone-lining cells are in an inactive state. They cover surfaces where neither bone formation nor resorption is present. In contrast to the former cells, which originate from local osteoprogenitor cells, osteoclasts arise from the fusion of mononuclear precursors. They can be located in cortical as well as in cancellous bone. Their presence is indicative of bone resorption activities.

The difference between cortical and cancellous bone is not only structural but also functional. The differences in their histologic and ultrastructural appearance are related to their primary functions: the cortical part of bone provides mechanical and protective functions, whereas cancellous bone is more involved in metabolic functions (e.g. calcium homeostasis). Both aspects (structural and metabolic) are closely related to the features of the mineralised extracellular matrix. In order to engineer a bone-like tissue in vitro in an attempt to mimic the natural tissue structure (biomimetics), understanding of hard tissue formation and mineralisation processes in bone is fundamental. Additionally, as the ex vivo grown tissues interact with the host cells and the extracellular matrix at the implantation site, normal repair mechanisms have to be considered and even enhanced to accelerate the defect repair.

2.2 Matrix Mineralisation

The final fate of bone repair and regeneration is the establishment of a mineralised, mechanically competent tissue. Skeletal mineralisation itself is closely related to the features of the extracellular matrix of bone and cartilage. Collagens, as the major constituent of the extracellular matrix network, are of major importance in the formation of a mineralised and therefore mechanically competent matrix (Fig. 2.5). Concerning the composition and structural organisation of these collagen-rich matrices of the human mineralising tissues, they form a microenvironment that favours apatite nucleation (Fig. 2.6). In the different types of calcified tissues, such as bone and calcified cartilage, structurally different types of collagen exist, with collagen type I being the dominant matrix protein in bone. Ultrastructural investigations of collagen mineralisation in these different calcifying tissues have revealed principal similarities in general but also some differences from the stage of crystal nucleation to tissue maturation (Höhling et al., 1990). It has been found that the first bone mineralisation is connected with matrix vesicles (Anderson, 1967; Bonucci, 1967), which spreads over the border of the vesicle membrane and includes extra- and intra-collagenous mineralisation. Extra- and intra-collagenous mineralisation are complex processes, connected with different characteristic non-collagenous proteins outside and on the collagen surface. This complex process of collagen mineralisation, not yet fully clarified in detail, is still under intensive research (Fig. 2.7). Insight into these fundamental processes may help in generating a mineralised cellular construct ex vivo and may therefore be valuable in generating a mechanical competent bone-like tissue in the laboratory. As various matrix proteins are used as a backbone in tissue engineering (in the sense of coating materials with these proteins or using them as scaffold materials), knowledge of their structure and function is of special relevance. Additionally, some of these proteins can be used as a marker for bone versus cartilage tissue, since some of these proteins are found, exceptionally, in bone or cartilage tissue. The most important structural matrix proteins of bone and cartilage are therefore described in more detail.

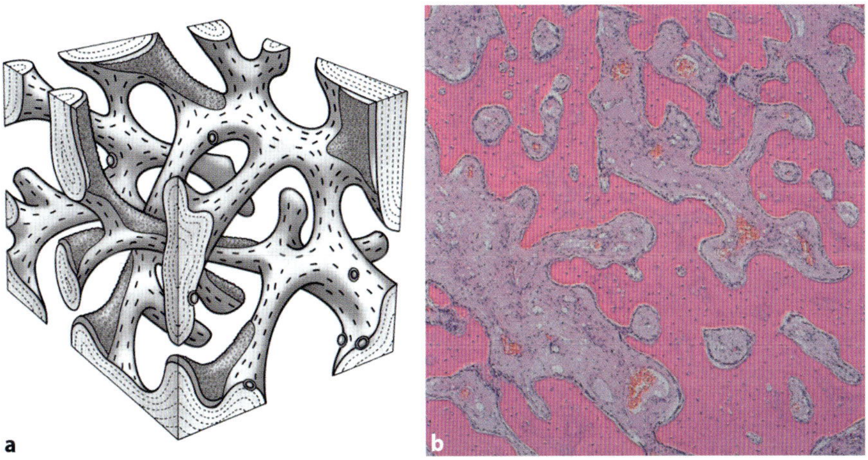

Fig. 2.4. Structure of cancellous bone. **a** Schematic. **b** Histological appearance

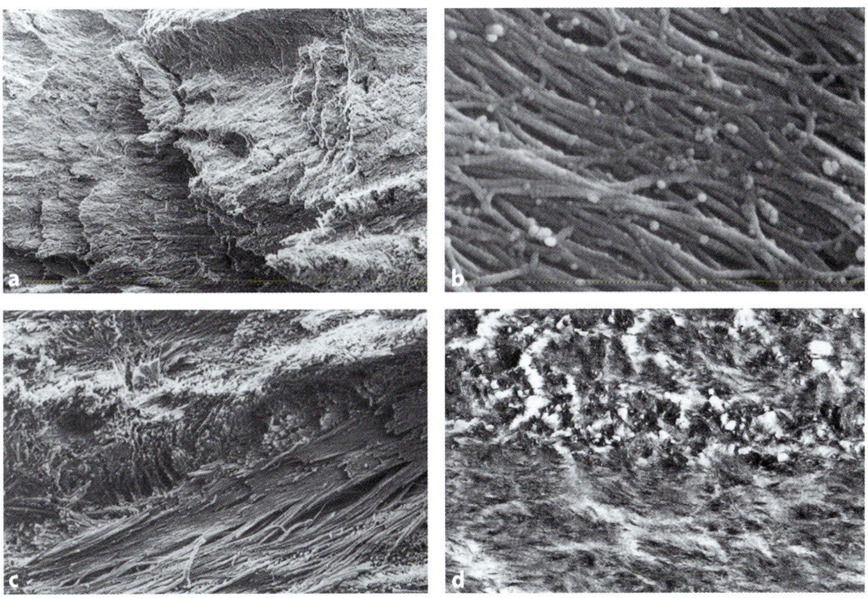

Fig. 2.5. **a** Scanning electron microscopy (SEM) image of freeze fractured full mineralized bone tissue. **b** SEM image of collagen fibres in bone. **c,d** Longitudinally and transversally oriented collagenous fibres in bone: c SEM of freeze-fractured specimen, d Transmission electron microscopy (TEM) image

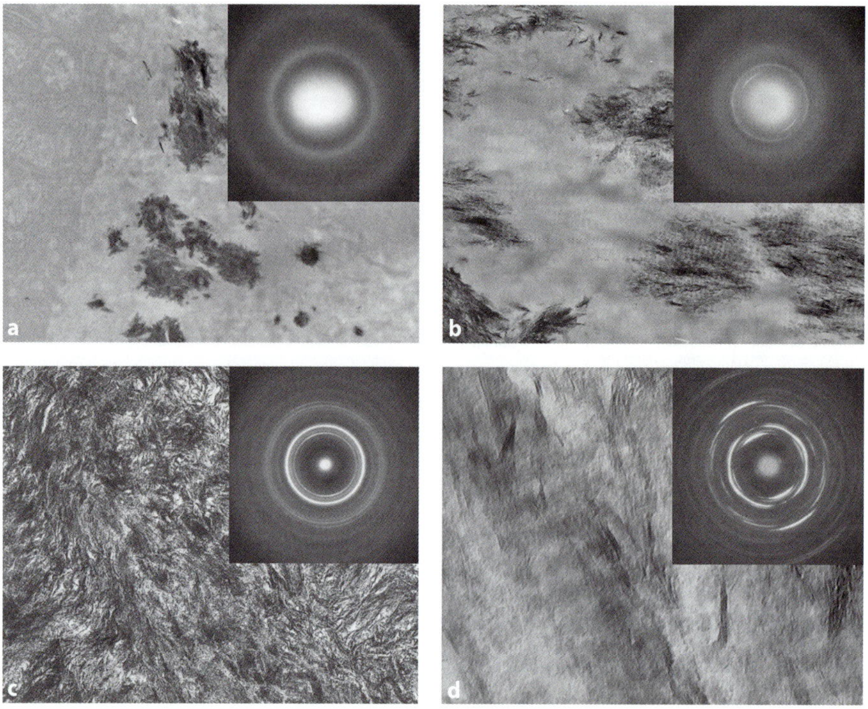

Fig. 2.6. Stages of mineral formation in bone as revealed by transmission electron microscopy (TEM) with electron diffraction analysis (EDA). **a** Early mineral formation of matrix vesicles. **b** early mineral formation at collagen fibres. **c** mature globular mineral formation. **d** mature collagen mineralization. The diffraction pattern of early mineral formation is diffuse; in contrast mature crystals represent a more clear-cut diffraction pattern. Further, in collagen mineralization the crystals are regular ordered and represent therefore a textured pattern

The collagens are the most abundant proteins in the human body, accounting for nearly 30% of all proteins. The different individual collagen types have been labelled with Roman numerals in the order of their discovery. These different collagen types provide the variety of structural units necessary to allow the connective tissue to adapt to the multitude of physiologic functions (Table 2.2).

The collagen types can be grouped according to variations in their structural features (Mayne and Brewton, 1993; Nielsen et al., 1994; Rehn and Pihlajaniemi, 1994; van der Rest and Garrone, 1991). The collagen types I to III, V and XI are banded, fibril-forming collagens, whereas the types IV, VI to X and XII to XIX are non-fibrillar. Additionally, the types IX, XII, XIV, XVI and XIX do not form supramolecular structures by their own, but are integrated in collagens of other types (Mayne and Brewton, 1993; Nielsen et al., 1994; Pan et al., 1992; Yamaguchi et al., 1992).

Collagen is the major constituent of the matrix of all mineralised tissues (except collagen-free enamel and otholites). The mineralising process of the different calcified tissues is characterised by a differentiated occurrence and distribution of the various types of collagen. Some proteins are present in bone and cartilage tissue,

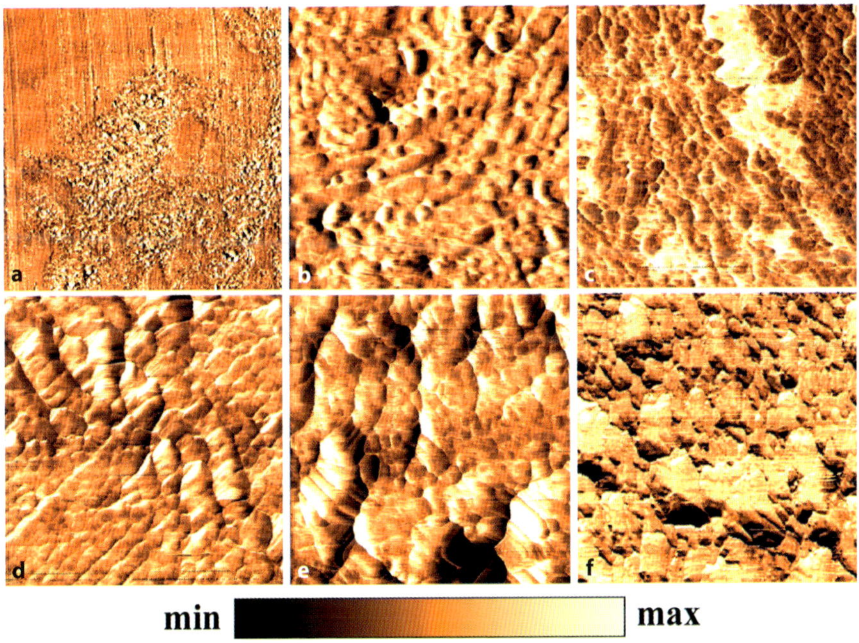

Fig. 2.7. Scanning force microscopy of intramembraneous bone formation. **a** Overview of mineralization front (image area 25×25 μm). **b** Non-mineralised collagen fibres (image area 2×2 μm). **c** Pre-osteocyte surrounded by osteoid (image area 5×5 μm). **d** Early and **e** late stages of mineralized collagen fibres (image area 2×2 μm). **f** Fully mineralized bone (image area 5×5 μm)

whereas others are solely found in one of the two tissues. Lane et al. (1986) developed an expression for the sequence of the appearance of collagen types I, II and III in bone healing. Different post-translational modifications distinguish the hard tissue collagen from the type I collagen of soft tissues, including different glycosylation and cross-linking patterns, and possibly differences in phosphorylation (Robey et al., 1992; Robey and Boskey, 1996). Collagen type I is present throughout mature bone and collagen type II in the mineralising cartilage of the epiphysial growth plate. Collagen types II, III and V have specific locations within fracture callus development. Chondrocytes and osteoblasts produce type II and III collagen during the early stages of callus formation. Osteoblasts secrete a matrix of type III collagen fibres along the periosteal surface, which serves as a substrate for cell migration. Type I collagen is secreted in trabeculae of developing bone within the fibrous tissue, whereas type II is formed during endochondral ossification stages in the stage of cartilage mineralisation. Hiltunen et al. (1993) using Northern blotting to evaluate the regulation of the collagens during bone healing confirmed the coexpression of type IX collagen with type II collagen and the coexpression of type X collagen with type I during the stages of endochondral ossification. In particular, collagen type X,found in the hypertrophic cartilage zone of endochondral ossification (Ayad et al., 1987), is suggested to be connected with the mineralisation process.

Table 2.2. Collagens of bone and cartilage tissue

Bone	Cartilage	Regenerate tissue
Major components - Collagen Type I - Collagen Type III - Collagen Type X	Major components - Collagen Type II - Collagen Type IX - Collagen Type XI	Major components - Collagen Type I - Collagen Type II - Collagen Type III
Minor components - Collagen Type V - Collagen Type VI - Collagen Type XIII - Collagen Type XIV	Minor components - Collagen Type III - Collagen Type VI - Collagen Type XII - Collagen Type XIII - Collagen Type XIV	Minor components - Collagen Type V - Collagen Type IX - Collagen Type X

Collagen Type I

- Triple-helical glycoprotein
- Molecular weight: 406 kDa
- Fibrillar molecule with 67 nm periodicity
- Major collagen of bone
- Fibrils stabilised by cross-links
- Provides tensile strength to the tissue
- Interacts with decorin and fibromodulin.

Collagen Type VI

- Glycoprotein
- Short collagenous central domain
- 5 nm diameter supramolecular structure
- 100 nm periodicity
- Type VI tetramers are stabilised by disulphide bonds
- No cross-linking by lysine/hydroxylysine-derived bonds
- Present in nearly all connective tissues
- Interacts in vitro with various extracellular macromolecules (type II and XIV collagen, hyaluronan, decorin, biglycan).

Collagen Type XIII

- Short chain, non-fibrillar collagen
- Homotrimeric molecule
- Molecular weight: 180 kDa
- Present in a variety of tissues
- Expressed in bone and cartilage tissue
- May act as a transmembrane protein of focal adhesion sites.

Collagen Type XIV

- Member of a subfamily of collagens (FACIT)
- Disulphide-bonded homotrimeric molecule
- Molecular weight: 607 kDa
- Present mainly in collagen type I rich tissues
- Found also in collagen type II containing tissues
- Expressed in bone and cartilage tissue
- Present in locations of elevated mechanical stress

Concerning the mineralising process in bone and calcified cartilage, it is suggested that not only the type of collagen but the fibrillar network with non-collagenous proteins gives rise to a structure configuration that is necessary for the process of mineralisation. The non-collagenous proteins found in mineralised matrices or cartilage are members of diverse types of molecules (Tables 2.3 and 2.4). The main groups are: glycosaminoglycan-containing molecules so-called proteoglycans, glycoproteins and gamma-carboxy glutamic acid-containing molecules (Robey, 1996). The distribution of these proteins in the collagen- containing mineralised tissues such as bone and calcifying cartilage shows an overlap.

Concerning the role of these non-collagenous proteins in the mineral formation of collagen-containing hard tissues, several aspects have to be considered. Whereas numerous studies indicate that collagen alone is not a direct nucleator of hydroxyapatite mineralisation, rather providing a template for mineral accumulation, nevertheless it becomes mineralised in a characteristic way (Robey et al., 1992; Robey

Table 2.3. Non-collagenous matrix proteins of bone

Glycoproteins	Gla proteins	Proteoglycans
– Ostepontin – Osteonectin – Bone sialoprotein – Alkaline phosphatase – Fibronectin – Vitronectin – Thrombospondin	– Osteocalcin – Matrix Gla protein – Protein S	– Decorin – Biglycan – Fibromodulin

Table 2.4. Non-collagenous matrix proteins of cartilage

Glycoproteins	Gla proteins	Proteoglycans
– Fibronectin – Vitronectin – Link protein – Chondroadherin – Prolargin – Thrombospondin – Cartilage matrix protein (except articular cartilage, intervertebral disc)	– Matrix Gla protein	– Aggrecan – Biglycan – Decorin – Epiphycan – Fibromodulin – Lumican

and Boskey, 1996). So it is obvious that it is not possible to build up a tissue like bone without collagen. Investigations of the knock-out mouse model have revealed that no or low amounts of collagen type I result in defective bone development (Robey, 1996). These findings support the hypothesis that collagen plays the major role in orienting the mineralisation process, producing a tissue structure with increased biomechanical properties, important for the ex vivo fabrication of a mechanically competent bone-like tissue. A multitude of other matrix proteins are morphologically, structurally and functionally connected to the collagen fibres. Complex interactions between collagen and the non-collagenous proteins (Meyer et al., 1999b) seem to facilitate crystal formation and subsequent crystal growth. Three different non-collagenous proteins are of special relevance in bone formation: osteocalcin, osteonectin, and bone sialoprotein.

Osteocalcin

- Member of the Gla protein family
- Molecular weight: 11 kDa
- Most abundant non-collagenous protein in bone
- Binds tightly to hydroxyapatite
- Regulates apatite crystal growth
- Synthesised specifically by osteoblasts.

Osteonectin

- Single chain polypeptide
- Molecular weight: 32 kDa
- Present in a number of tissues
- Expressed early in bone development
- High concentrations in sites of bone remodelling
- Binds to hydroxyapatite
- Involved in osteoblast adhesion.

Bone Sialoprotein

- Single polypeptide chain
- Molecular weight: 6×104 Da
- Comprises predominantly glutamic acid, aspartic acid and glycine
- Present in bone and mineralised connective tissue
- Deposited mainly at sites of de novo bone formation
- Promotes cell attachment via integrin binding
- Tightly connected to hydroxyapatite.

All three proteins are closely connected to hydroxyapatite. They do not only bind to hydroxyapatite but are also functionally involved in mineral formation. Osteocalcin is known to be involved in crystal growth, whereas the function of others (Osteonectin, Bone Sialoprotein) is not understood in detail. Despite their unknown role in the mineralising process, their localisation in the extracellular matrix of calcifying tissues is suggestive of important functional involvement in mineral formation (Butler and Ritchie, 1995).

2.3 Osteoblast Structure and Function

The osteoblast is defined as the critical cell type that forms bone tissue. Four maturation stages of osteoblast development can be distinguished: preosteoblasts, lining cells, osteoblasts and osteocytes (Fig. 2.8). The preosteoblast is considered as a precursor of osteoblasts and lining cells. Preosteoblasts share common phenotypical features of osteoblasts like alkaline-phosphatase activity, but they do not express all markers of mature osteoblasts (Aubin, 2001). Bone lining cells are, in contrast to osteoblasts, synthetically more inactive. The flat, thin and elongated cells cover bone surfaces where no significant remodelling takes place. A proportion of cells becomes embedded in bone; these cells, considered to represent the finally differentiated cell stage, are osteocytes (Figs 2.9 and 2.10). The mature osteoblast phenotype is characterised by the ability of the cells to sythesise a bone matrix that will finally mineralise (Fig. 2.11). Osteoblasts express various phenotypic markers such as high alkaline phosphatase (ALP) and synthesise collagenous and non-collagenous bone matrix proteins including osteocalcin (Aubin and Liu, 1996). Osteoblasts express receptors for various hormones including parathyroid hormonel (Dempster et al., 1993; 1995), 1α,25-dihydroxyvitamin D_3 [1α,25$(OH)_2D_3$] (Lian et al., 1999), estrogen (Turner et al., 1994; Boyce et al., 1999), and glucocorticoids (Delany et al., 1994; Ishida and Heersche, 1998), which are involved in the regulation of osteoblast differentiation. Osteoblast differentiation is also regulated by various local factors in a paracrine and/or an autocrine fashion (Aubin and Liu, 1996) to enable the cell to perform its main function: the synthesis of a mechanically competent hard tissue. Osteocytes are the most abundant cell type of bone. It is assumed that there are approximately 10 times as many osteocytes as osteoblasts in adult human bone (Parfitt, 1977). During the transition from osteoblasts to mature osteocytes the cells lose a number of osteoblastic characteristics, but acquire other, osteocyte-specific ones, including their typical morphology (for a review see Liu et al., 1977). Mature osteocytes are stellate shaped or dendritic cells enclosed within the lacuno–canalicu-

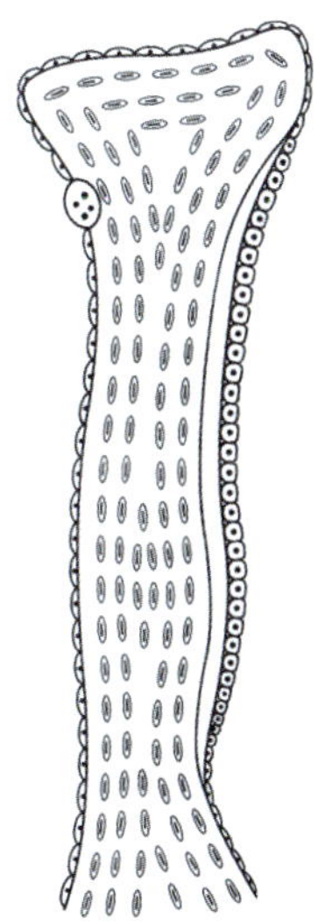

Fig. 2.8. Scheme of bone trabecula containing different osteoblastic cells

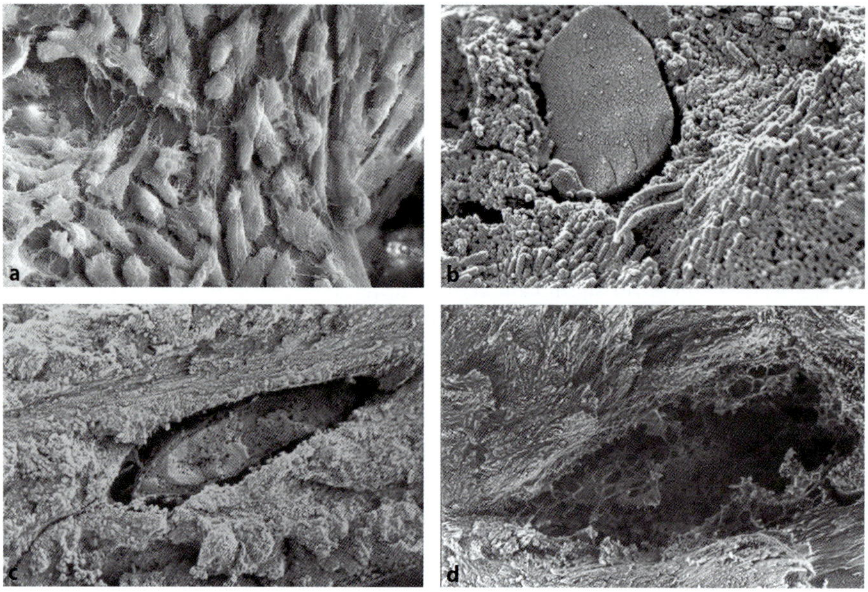

Fig. 2.9. Scanning electron microscopical (SEM) appearance of cancellous bone. **a** Osteoblast layer at the surface of bone trabecula. **b** Pre-osteocyte surrounded by extracellular matrix (freeze fractured specimen). **c** Mature osteocyte in mineralised bone matrix. d Pore containing osteocyte lacuna

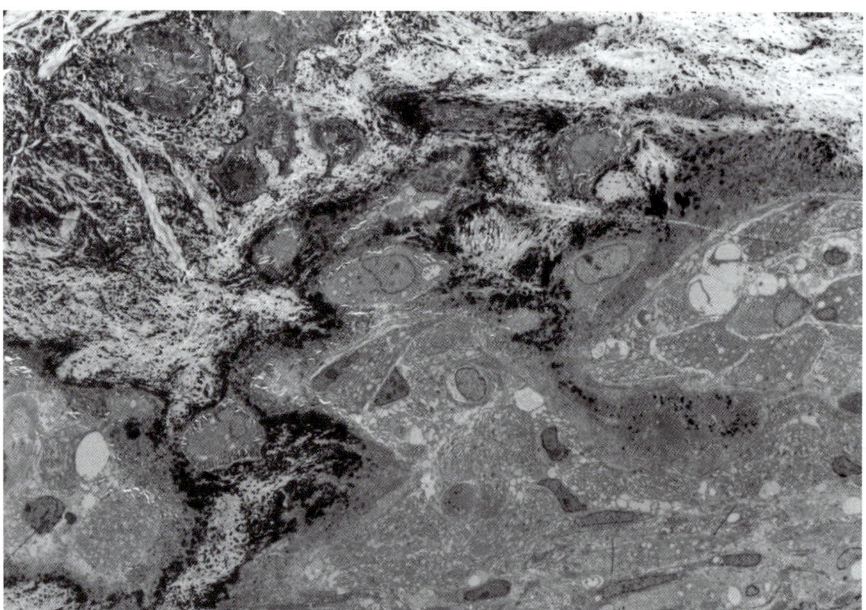

Fig. 2.10. Transmission microscopical appearance of mineralising area demonstrating the transition of osteoblasts to osteocytes

lar network of bone. Osteocytes are interconnected and connected with osteoblasts through cell contacts containing gap junctions (Aarden et al., 1994). Osteocytes have a main role in the blood-calcium homeostasis and in the functional adaptation of bones. Cells in all different stages of osteoblast development work together (and with other cells) in an interconnected fashion to dynamically regulate bone development, bone turnover and bone repair.

2.4 Osteoclast Structure and Function

In contrast to osteoblasts, osteoclasts are multinuclear cells derived from hematopoietic stem cells (Suda et al., 1992), thereby sharing common differentiation pathway of macrophages and dendritic cells (Fig. 2.12). The promyeloid precursor cell is able to differentiate into either an osteoclast, a macrophage or a dendritic cell. The differentiation pathway depends on whether the precursor cell is exposed to a receptor activator of various ligands (e.g. RANKL, OPGL, ODF) or colony-stimulating factors (M-CSF, GM-CSF) (Kong et al., 1999; Nutt et al., 1999; Rolink et al., 1999; Suda et al., 1999). The fact that bone marrow stromal cells and osteoblasts produce some of the above mentioned factors as membrane-bound and soluble substances is an indicater for the positive feedback mechanisms of osteoblasts on osteoclast formation (Lacey et al., 1998). Osteoprotegerin (OPG), as a counterpart of the above mentioned factors, strongly inhibits osteoclast formation in vitro and in vivo (Simonet et al., 1997). The inhibitory effect of OPG on osteoclast differentiation is due to the fact that it can prevent the binding of RANKL to its receptor, RANK (Hsu et al., 1999). Osteoclasts have a unique ability to dissolve mineral and degrade organic bone matrix (for a review see Väänänen et al., 2000). They are assumed to be also involved in the degradation process of foreign materials. After migration of the osteoclast to a resorption site, a specific membrane domain, the sealing zone, forms under the osteoclast. The plasma membrane attaches tightly to the bone matrix and seals the resorption site from its surroundings (Väänänen and Horton, 1995). Ultrastructural analysis indicates that osteoclasts contain in addition to the sealing zone, three other specialised membrane domains: a ruffled border, a functional secretory domain and a basolateral membrane. The ruffled border is a resorbing organelle. The fusion of intracellular acidic vesicles with the region of plasma membrane facing the bone (Blair et al., 1989; Väänänen et al, 1990) and the subsequent outside transport of the vesicle content leads to a lowering of the pH below the osteoclast. The low pH in the resorption lacuna is achieved by the action of proton pumps at the ruffled border membrane. The main physiological function of osteoclasts is to degrade mineralised bone matrix. This involves dissolution of hydroxyapatite minerals and proteolytic cleavage of the organic matrix. After dissolution of the mineral phase, proteolytic enzymes degrade the extracellular matrix. The organic degradation products are removed from the resorption lacuna through a special transcytotic pathway in order to liberate them into the extracellular space (Nesbitt and Horton, 1997; Salo et al., 1997).

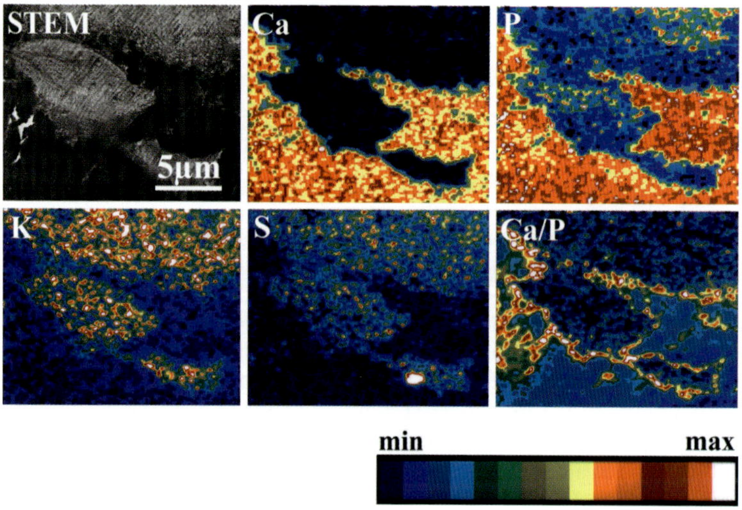

Fig. 2.11. Scanning transmission electron microscoy (STEM) image of bone mineral forming preosteocyte with energy dispersive X-ray analysis of element distribution for calcium (Ca), phosphorus (P), potassium (K), sulphorus (S) and the relation of calcium to phosphorus (Ca/P)

2.5 Bone Regeneration

Bone is one of the body´s tissues that have the ability to recapitulate specific aspects of their initial developmental processes and thereby undergo regeneration to a stage of repair, ad integrum under some circumstances. The repair of bone defects is one such regenerative process (Vortkamp et al., 1998; Ferguson et al., 1999). The postnatal tissue environment in which the regenerative processes of defect healing takes place is different in a number of specific respects from those present during embryological development, but the potential effects on the developmental process of defect healing are essential to our understanding of bone morphogenesis, and form the basis for bone tissue engineering approaches.

The instructive interactions between cells that are initiated within the bone repair and regeneration process must therefore occur between the newly formed tissue, the external soft tissues covering the defect site, and the adjacent cortical bone and bone marrow. Various sources of cells (periosteal cells, cortical cells, cells derived from the surrounding soft tissues, and marrow cells) and signals that set up these fields are responsible for the features of the repair tissue (Fig. 2.13). The primary tissue source of cells that form the repair tissue are believed to be from the periosteum (Nakahara et al., 1990a). Cells within the periosteum produce various morphogens starting from the onset of tissue disintegration (Bostrom et al., 1995), suggesting that these signal molecules act locally to recruit and induce skeletalgenic cells to proliferate and differentiate.

Other cells that contribute to repair tissue formation appear to be derived from the adjacent cortical and cancellous bone. It may be speculated that at least some of these cells are likely to have arisen from the proliferative expansion of committed

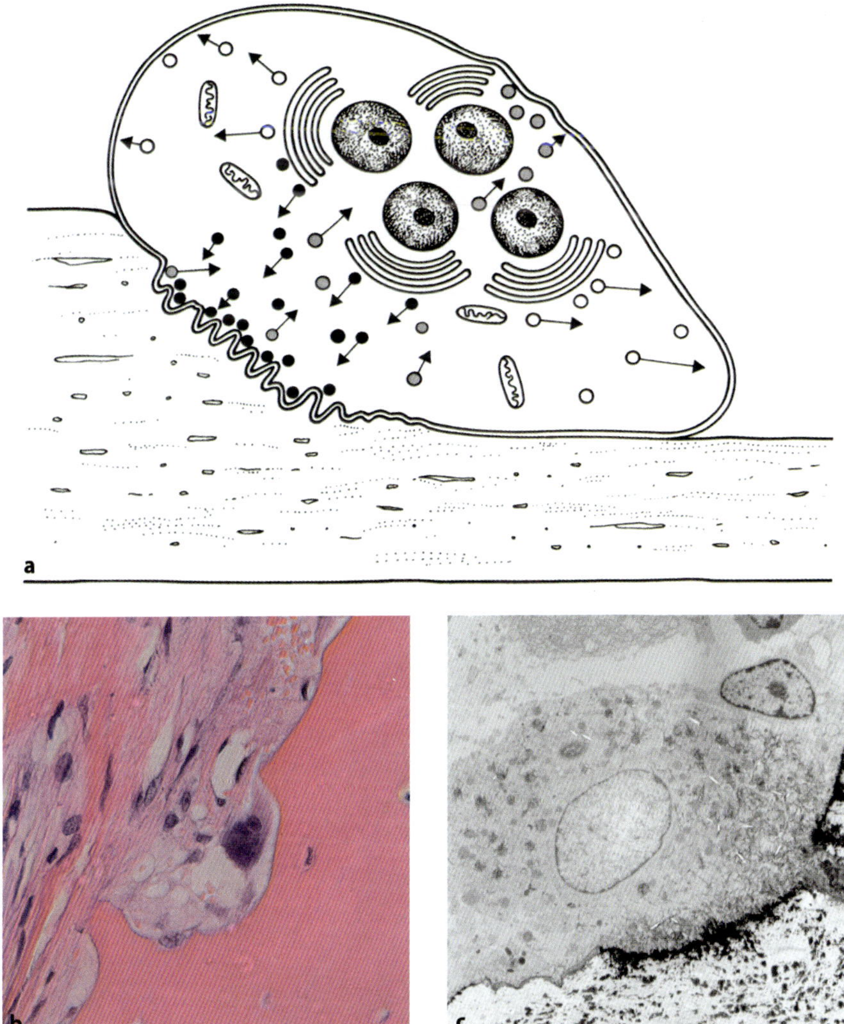

Fig. 2.12. **a** Schematic drawing of a resorbing osteclast, demonstrating the zonal structure at the resorption site. **b** Osteoclast located in a resorption lacuna. **c** TEM appearance of active bone resorption at the ruffled border of an osteoclast

skeletal precursors. Mesenchymal stem cells, assumed to be derived from either the surrounding muscle tissue or the marrow space, are the third source of cells that participate in the formation of new bone. Cells synthesise a network of collagenous and non-collagenous proteins. The regenerate tissue contains, in addition to collagen type I and II, mainly collagen types III, V, IX and X.

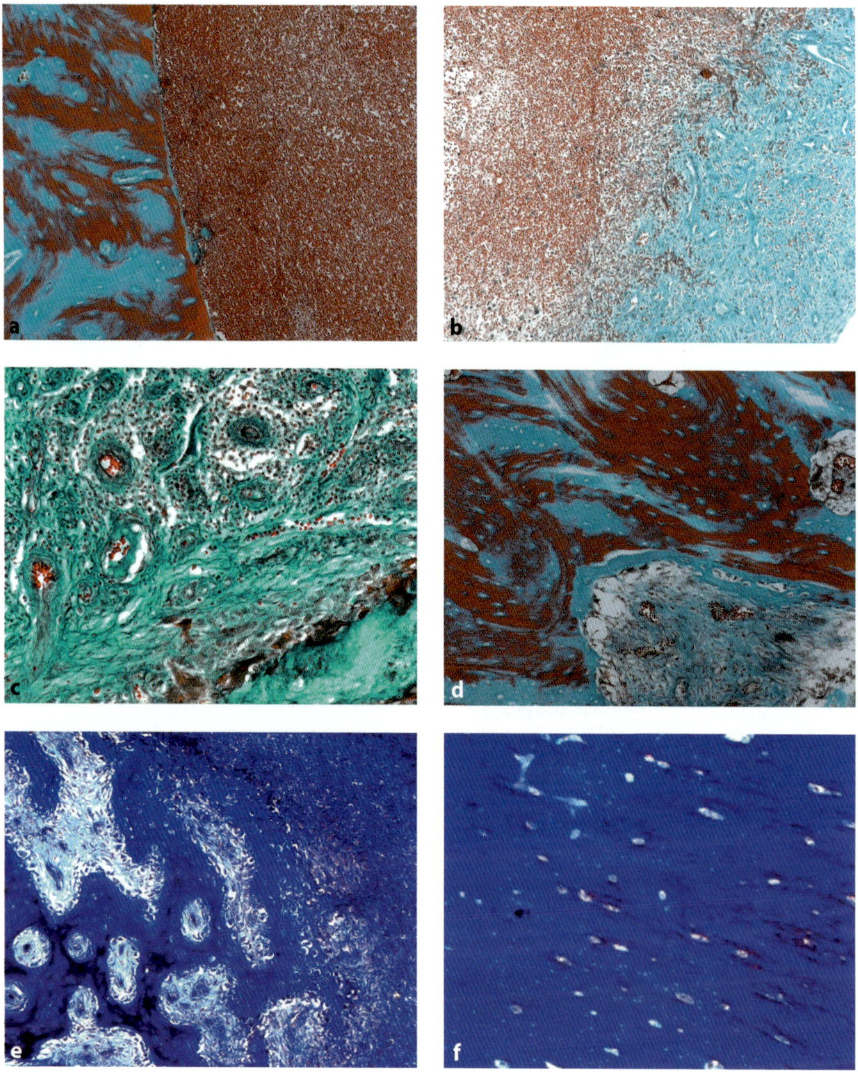

Fig. 2.13. Stages of bone repair. **a** Blood clot formation. **b** Substitution of blood cells by a matrix-rich repair tissue. **c** Invasion of blood vessels. **d** Organisation of predetermined osseous tissue. **e** Trabeculae formed by osteoblasts. **f** Final repair tissue

Collagen Type III

- Triple-helical glycoprotein
- Thin fibrillar molecule with 67-nm periodicity
- Fibrils stabilized by cross-links
- Molecular weight: 415 kDa
- Collagen present in small amounts in bone and cartilage

Collagen Type V

- Minor fibrillar collagen
- Thin fibrillar molecule with 67-nm periodicity
- Forms heterotypic fibrils with collagen type I or III
- Forms cross-type heterotrimers with type IX collagens
- Molecular weight: 421 kDa
- Interacts in vitro with various extracellular macromolecules (thrombospondin, decorin, biglycan)

Collagen Type X

- Short chain collagen
- Homodimer protein
- Molecular weight: 198 kDa
- Temporally and spatially regulated during fetal development
- Synthesised by hypertrophic chondrocytes
- Present in calcifying cartilage.

The mode of bone repair tissue critically depends on the defect size. Whereas non-critical size defects heal spontaneously, critical size defects will not completely fill with new bone tissue. As nutrition is another important parameter in determining the features of repair tissue formation, diffusion and vascularisation are two factors that influence to a great extent the outcome of histogenesis. Whereas the nature and origins of the initiating morphogenetic signals for the skeletogenic cells in the repair tissue are not completely determined, a multitude of signal factors have been identified (Table 2.5). Signals that initiate and maintain the bone-forming mechanisms are assumed to arise from the periosteum or bone marrow or are released from the

Table 2.5. Signals involved in bone repair

Molecules/Time	Initial	Early	Late	Remodelling
Cytokines				
Interleukines	x			
Interferone-γ	x	x	x	
TNF-α	x			
TNF-β	x			
RANKL	x		x	
OPG	x	x		
MCSF	x	x		
Morphogens				
TGF-β (1–3)	x	x	x	
BMP (2–7, 8)	x	x	x	
ILGF (1,2)		x	x	
GDF (1,5,9,10)	x	x	x	
Various				
VEGF	x	x	x	x
Ang. (1,2)		x	x	x
MMP (2,8,9,13)		x	x	x

injured bone matrix, many of these signals are part of the inflammatory processes (Einhorn et al., 1995; Barnes et al., 1999). The presence and time of appearance of these signal molecules are of special relevance, since such molecules can be used in tissue engineering approaches to improve tissue formation in vitro and in vivo (for reviews, see Lieberman et al., 2002; Gerstenfeld et al., 2003a; 2003b).

The role of inflammatory cytokines, morphogens, proteases, and angiogenic factors in directing the repair response has recently given rise to increased scientific interest, yet the role these molecules play in the regulation of bone remodelling are not completely determined (Gowen et al., 1983; Kimble et al., 1994; 1997; Barnes et al., 1999). Beneath interleucines, interferones and tumornecrosis factor alpha, members of the TGF-β superfamilie are assumed to be of major relevance in skeletalgenesis and bone repair (Joyce et al., 1990; Rosier et al., 1998). There is recent evidence that specific members of the transforming growth factor-β superfamily, including multiple BMPs, GDFs, and TGF-β1-3, act in combinations with other factors (e.g. metalloproteases) to promote the various stages of repair tissue formation (Cho et al., 2002).

Bone healing creates a demand on the surrounding tissues to increase blood flow so that induction of bone regeneration can occur within the larger sized defects. Ingrowth of vascular tissues into the developing tissue proceeds with the development of the new periosteal bone and occurs mainly from where the periosteal response originates. Thus, there is evidence that the interaction of the vascular elements and the initiation and propagation of the periosteal response are the primary driving mechanisms that enhance the new bone formation, especially in larger defects. It has also been suggested that periovascular mesenchymal cells that exist in blood vessel walls contribute to the initiation and maintenance of defect healing (Bouletreau et al., 2002a; 2002b). The influence of vessel- formation-dependent adequate blood flow on optimal bone healing has been well established (Glowacki, 1998; Rowe et al., 1999; Gerber and Ferrara, 2000; Einhorn and Lee, 2001). Furthermore, cartilage tissue formation (as an intermediate or final state of repair tissue) is assumed to require the coordination of both the molecular mechanisms that regulate the bone`s extracellular matrix remodelling capacity and the influencial processes of vascular cells (Vu et al., 1998). Thus, matrix degradation and angiogenesis are either correlated or concurrent processes during tissue formation. The formation of new vessels is assumed to be regulated by two separate pathways: a vascular endothelial growth factor (VEGF)-dependent pathway and an angiopoietin-dependent pathway (Suri et al., 1996). It seems that both sets of regulatory pathways regulate and modulate defect repair. The VEGF related family of molecules are essential endothelial-cell-specific mediators of neo-angiogenesis (Ferrara and Davis-Smyth, 1997), whereas angiopoietin 1 and 2 are molecules that directly control vascular growth. The latter molecules are assumed to act during the whole period of new bone tissue formation. They seem to be related to the formation of larger vessel structures and the development of co-lateral branches from existent vessels. Evidence from a multitude of experimental studies indicates that a high number of signal molecules are essential for skeletal regeneration and suggest that there seems to be an intimate relationship between them. The orchestrated action of the various sources of cells and signal molecules allow for the coordinated regulation of events that lead to bone repair. The final outcome of defect repair is initiated and modulated by these factors, but whether such a repair process will lead to a complete bone repair is dependent on a number of boundary conditions (defect size, tissue biomechanics, host conditions).

2.6 Cartilage Structure and Function

Adults have cartilage on their articular surface of long bones and in the trachea, bronchi, nose, ears, larynx, and intervertebral disks. Cartilage contains cells, fibres, and amorphous ground substance. It is dominated by the acellular elements and is devoid of blood vessels and nerves. Cartilage characteristics make it an excellent skeletal tissue for the fetus. Most adult bones existed as cartilaginous models during fetal life. Three types of cartilage can be destinguished: hyaline cartilage, elastic cartilage, and fibrocartilage. Hyaline cartilage is a bluish, opalescent tissue that is widely distributed and the most abundant type of cartilage present in the human body. Hyaline cartilage exists on the articular surface of bones, the ventral aspects of ribs, in the larynx, the trachea, and in the bronchial tree. Hyaline cartilage also exists at the epiphysal plates in the bones of fetuses and growing children. Elastic cartilage is present in the auricle of the external ear, the walls of the external auditory meatus, the eustachian tube, the epiglottis, and parts of the larynx. The main function of elastic cartilage is to ensure the patency of the lumina of tubes that are surrounded by this variety of cartilage. Fibrocartilage exists in the annulus fibrosus of intevertebral discs, the symphysis pubis, and the junctions between large tendons and articular cartilage in large joints. Intervertebral discs are specialised structures that consist of an outer layer of fibrocartilage (called annulus fibrosus) and an inner part of a special liquid connective tissue (nucleus pulposus). Despite the importance of all subsets of cartilage in maintaining the body`s function, articular cartilage has attracted the most scientific and economic interest in tissue engineering.

The primary bearing surface in a synovial joint is the articular cartilage (Fig. 2.14). Articular cartilage has a zonal assembly. In adults it is a comparatively acellular tissue, with cell volume averaging only approximately 2% of the total cartilage volume in human adults (Stockwell and Meachin, 1979). In contrast to the high cell volume during fetal life, the cartilage cell numbers decrease with age (Stockwell and Meachin, 1979), reaching its lowest point when the individual is 20 to 30 years. Chondrocytes are the most important cell source present in articular cartilage. All chondrocytes are surrounded by a narrow pericellular region. A territorial region surrounds this pericellular region which is present throughout the cartilage (Poole et al., 1982).

Cartilage has a zonal structure (Fig. 2.15).

Zonal Structure of Cartilage

- Superficial zone (SZ)
- Midzone (MZ)
- Deep zone (DZ)
- Calcified cartilage (CC)
- Subchondral bone plate (SBP)
- Subchondral trabecular bone (STB).

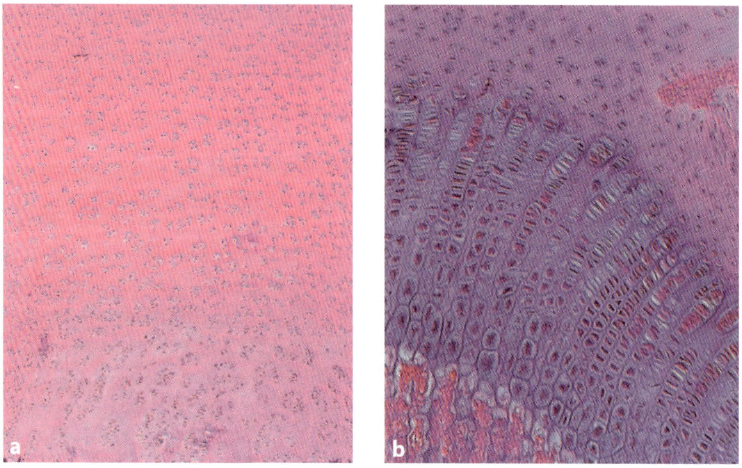

Fig. 2.14. Different cartilage structures. **a** Articular cartilage tissue. **b** Hypertrophic cartilage zone

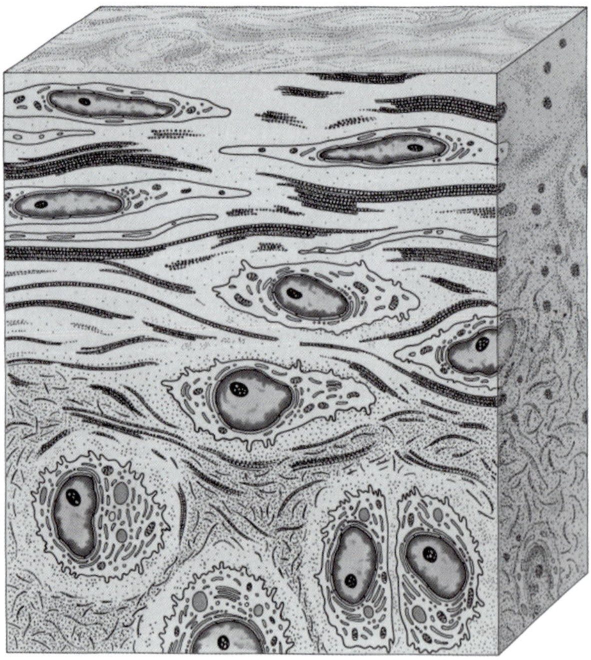

Fig. 2.15. Scheme of zonal structure of articular cartilage, showing a detailed aspect of the tissue structure from the deep zone (*bottom*) to the surface (*top*)

Cartilage is occupied by an extensive extracellular matrix that is synthesised by these cells. At its free (superficial) surface, which is contacted by synovial fluid, the chondrocytes are flattened and aligned parallel to the surface (for a review see Poole et al., 2001). Below the superficial zone is the midzone where cell density is lower. The ultrastructure of the midzone reveals morphologic features more typical of a hyaline cartilage with more rounded cells and an extensive extracellular matrix. Between this midzone and the layer of calcified cartilage is the deep zone. Below the articular cartilage, and separated from it, is a layer of calcified cartilage. The calcified cartilage is not very vascular normally, and the remodelling process is therefore not as effective as in vascularised locations. Cell density is lowest in this zone. Aggrecan content and fibril diameter are maximal in the deep zone, whereas collagen content is minimal. The chondrocytes in this calcified zone usually express the hypertrophic phenotype, reaching a stage of differentiation that can also be found in fracture repair. A unique feature of hypertrophic cells is the ability to synthesise type X collagen and to calcify the extracellular matrix. Below the calcified cartilage is the subchondral bone plate. The calcified interface provides excellent structural integration with the subchondral bone. Subchondral trabecular bone underlies the subchondral plate. The structure and appearance of subchondral bone is critically dependent on the load situation of the joint. Subchondral bone may change its density by remodelling, but may also thicken through direct apposition of bone to its distal surface through bone modelling. Subchondral trabecular bone is not homogeneous and is not isotropic in nature. The trabeculae are oriented in different directions, and the mechanical properties of this tissue zone are therefore different in different planes. The subchondral plate and the trabecular bone are, despite their similarities, differently organised, adapt to mechanical loads in different ways, and have quite different mechanical properties (Hunziker, 2002).

The extracellular matrix of hyaline cartilages is composed of differentially distributed collagen fibrils and non-collagenous proteins that form an extensive network. Many of the molecules play a structural role, whereas others may be involved in regulating cell function. Different types of collagen are present in cartilage. Type II and type IX collagen form the main part of the fibrils; type XI collagen is present within and on the surface of the fibril (Mendler et al., 1989).

Collagen Type II

- Triple-helical glycoprotein
- Fibrillar molecule with 67-nm periodicity
- Molecular weight: 425 kDa
- Predominant collagen of cartilage and intervertebral disc
- Provides tensile strength
- Enables the tissue to resist shearing forces
- Supports chondrocyte adhesion
- Induces phenotypic differentiation of cells.

Collagen Type IX

- Member of subfamily of collagens termed FACIT (termed fibril associated collagens with interupted triplehelices)
- Disulphide-bonded heterodimer
- Molecular weight: 222 kDa
- Present in cartilage and intervertebral disc
- Bridges collagen fibrils with other macromolecules
- Associates with the surface of type II collagen
- Participates in the formation of type II collagen

Collagen Type XI

- Minor fibrillar collagen
- Forms heterotypic fibrils with type II and IX collagens
- Molecular weight: 545 kDa
- Predominantly present in cartilaginous tissue
- Also expressed by non-chondrogenic tissues

The ground substance of articular cartilage contains also a large variety of non-collagenous proteins and polysaccharides. The molecules vary in their abundance and structure with anatomical site or the person's age. There are no common features of non-collagenous proteins with respect to their distribution, structure and function. Many of the molecules are proteoglycans, bearing glycosaminoglycan chains, whereas others are glycoproteins or even non-glycosylated proteins. Among the non-collagenous proteins, aggrecan is of major importance.

Aggrecan

- Large chondroitin sulphate proteoglycan
- Molecular weight: 205 kDa
- Comprises 87% chondroitin sulphate, 6% keratan sulphate
- 10% of cartilage dry weight
- No presence in bone
- Interacts with hyaluronan
- Large number of fixed negatively charged side groups
- Responsible for high osmotic pressure
- Pimary role to swell and hydrate collagen framework.

The high aggrecan content in the extracellular matrix of cartilage is responsible for the unique ability of the tissue to resist compression in a specialised way. Aggrecan belongs to the family of aggregating proteoglycans that form large, multimolecular complexes with hyaluronan (Gomes et al., 2004). All members of the aggrecan family have an amino-terminal globular domain, which is responsible for interaction with hyaluronan. The molecules' ability to interact with hyaluronan is the basis for an undisturbed articular cartilage function, as they provide the rheological properties necessary for resisting compression. The interaction of aggrecan with hyaluronan is stabilised by the presence of link proteins. Link protein of aggrecan can be lost from the cartilage matrix during periods of tissue degeneration, but such loss is most likely due to depolymerisation of hyaluronan and involves concomitant loss of aggrecan. The structure and content of aggrecan is altered in many cartilage diseases. Aggrecan itself has, in addition to the functional relation with hyaluronan, a high chondroitinsulfate and keratansulfate content.

Link Protein

- Glycoprotein
- Molecular weight: 45 kDa
- Binds to aggrecan and hyaluronan.

Matrix Gla Protein

- Glycoprotein
- Molecular weight: 12 kDa
- Present in bone and cartilage
- Acts as an inhibitor of calcification.

Additionally, human cartilage contains three dermatan sulfate proteoglycans (biglycan, decorin, and epiphycan) and two potential keratan sulfate proteoglycans (fibromodulin and lumican). The presence of the above mentioned extracellular matrix proteins in articular cartilage is important for normal articular cartilage function. The extracellular matrix of other cartilage types contains numerous other proteins (e.g. cartilage matrix protein) that are neither collagens nor proteoglycans (Nomura et al., 1989), and several of these are thought to play a structural role in the matrix. Of special relevance for cartilage tissue is hyaluronan and S-100.

Biglycan

- Small proteoglycan
- Predominant small proteoglycan of cartilage
- Contains two extended glycosaminoglycans
- Leucine-rich proteoglycan
- Relatively abundant in the mineral compartment of bone.

Fibromodulin

- Small chondroitin sulphate/dermatan sulphate proteoglycan
- Molecular weight: 42 kDa
- Found in a variety of tissues
- Abundant in cartilage
- Compromises 0.1–0.3% of cartilage wet weight
- Binds to type I and type II collagen in vitro
- Inhibits collagen fibrillogenesis in vitro.

Cartilage Matrix Protein

- Disulphide-bonded multimer
- Molecular weight: 54 kDa
- Amino acid sequence closely related to von Willebrand factor
- Major component of non-articular cartilage
- Presence especially in tracheal, nasal, and epiphyseal cartilage
- 5% wet weight of tracheal cartilage.

Hyaluronan

- High molecular mass polysaccharide
- Copolymer of glucoronic acid and N-acetylglucosamine
- Present in a number of tissues
- Synthesised in the plasma membrane of cells
- Catabolised preferentially at local sites

- High overall turnover rate
- Important role during tissue development and differentiation
- Important for water and plasma protein homeostasis.

Hyaluronan is a high molecular-mass polysaccharide found in the extracellular matrix, especially of connective tissue. It is synthesised by cells and then excreted into the intercellular space. One special feature of this polysaccharide is its high turnover rate in the tissue. Hyaluronan has diverse functions. It acts as a mediator of tissue development and cell differentiation and possesses also important functions in water homeostasis. Through this action hyaluronan plays an important role for the functional and structural integrity of connective tissues, with special respect to cartilage tissue. S100 protein is an acidic calcium-binding protein (molecular weight 21 kDa) found in high concentrations in glial and Schwann cells.

S100 protein

- Acidic calcium-binding protein
- Molecular weight: 21 kDa
- Present in various conformations
- Unknown function
- Modulates a wide range of cellular processes
- Used as a chondrocyte marker protein
- Distinguishes cartilage from bone tissue.

It exists in various forms depending on alpha or beta unit configuration. The protein was found to be also present in human chondrocytes (Stefansson et al., 1982). The protein has been detected in chondrocytes of the skull, vertebrae, ribs, sternum, larynx and long bones of the human fetus, and in the larynx and xiphoid process of the human adult. The exact functions of S100 proteins are not well known. As S100 proteins are mostly present intracellularly, the majority of the molecules function as intracellular calcium receptor proteins. In addition, it has been suggested that S100 proteins modulate a wide range of intracellular processes including inter-cell communication, cell structure, growth, energy metabolism, contraction and intracellular signal transduction. S-100 is often used as a marker protein for cartilage tissue, in order to distinguish this tissue from bone.

2.7 Chondrocyte Structure and Function

Chondrocytes are the constituent cells of cartilage, and through their function in endochondral ossification – the process by which most vertebrate bones are formed – play a central role in determining the rate of bone growth (Hunziker, 1994). A chondrocyte always generates from a mesenchymal cell, the prechondrogenic cell or chondrocyte precursor cell, which is – due to lack of specific markers – only defined by the expectation that its daughter cell will be a differentiated chondrocyte (for a review, see Behonick and Werb, 2003). Chondrocyte precursor cells are of general fibroblastic appearance and synthesise – like fibroblasts – type I and III collagen, fibronectin, and noncartilage-type proteoglycans (von der Mark and Conrad, 1979). Chondrocytes are either of mesodermal origin, such as chondrocytes from limb and vertebral cartilage, or of ectodermal origin, such as cranial cartilages, but never derived from endoderm. Stem cells with chondrogenic potential persist throughout adult life and can be induced to differentiate into chondrocytes during fracture callus formation, osteophyte formation, or as ectopic cartilage. Prechondrogenic cells arise in different parts of the embryo throughout all stages of development, starting with the chondrogenic differentiation of somite and limb bud mesenchyme in the very early embryo, and followed by the differentiation of neural crest cells into ocular, otic, and mandibular cartilage. Chondrogenic precursors follow a differentiation pathway mediated by a variety of signalling molecules including Indian hedgehog (Ihh), bone morphogenetic proteins (BMPs) and parathyroid hormone (PTH)-related peptide (PTHrP) (Jüppner, 2000; Katagiri and Takahashi, 2002). Chondrocytes impose two main features. They constitute the cellular aspect of chondral tissue and they play a central role in bone formation through the process of endochondral ossification. The process of endochondral ossification is an example of the close functional relationship between osteoblasts and chondrocytes. Endochondral ossification involves the replacement of an avascular cartilaginous template with a highly vascularised, mineralised tissue, and initiates during embryogenesis with the condensation of mesenchymal precursors at the future sites of skeletal elements (Poole, 1991). These mesenchymal condensations take on the shape of the skeletal elements for which they will serve as templates, and the precursor cells present in these dense cell masses then differentiate along an osteogenic pathway (ultimately producing osteoblasts, bone-depositing cells) or a chondrogenic pathway (ultimately producing chondrocytes, cartilage cells). Chondrocytes become organised according to their differentiation state, examplified by the process of long bone formation. Differentiation proceeds from the diaphysis of the bone anlage centripetal to the the epiphyses (Fig. 2.16). The formation of the epiphyseal growth plate is also reflective for a chondrocyte differentiation pathway. Differentiating chondrocytes within the growth plate are organised in the different layers. Whereas resting and actively proliferating chondrocytes are located proximal to the epiphysis, hypertrophic and apoptosing chondrocytes are located near the diaphysis. At each stage along this differentiation pathway, the chondrocytes express and secrete a distinct repertoire of collagens, proteoglycans and other matrix molecules (Karsenty and Wagner, 2002). Cells that differentiate along the chondrogenic pathway initiate a specific genetic program in which they express a number of characteristic ECM components including type II collagen, type IX collagen, and type XI collagen (Wagner and Karsenty, 2001). These cells progress through maturation to hypertrophy, when they express another cadre of ECM components including type X collagen (Wagner and Karsenty, 2001). Hypertrophic chondrocytes have the ability to secrete matrix vesicles containing enzymes that actively degrade and mineralise their surrounding matrix (Wuthier et al., 1985; Kirsch et al., 2000). As these cells undergo apoptosis the tissue space is then filled by blood vessels, osteogenic cells and mesenchymal precursors, finally leading to the formation of new trabecular bone (Horton, 1993; Wagner and Karsenty, 2001; Ortega et al., 2003).

Mature chondrocytes can be identified on the basis of common morphological features such as spherical cell shape with scalloped edges, an extensive rough endoplasmatic reticulum and Golgi apparatus, and an abundant extracellular matrix which stains metachromatically with toluidine blue or Giemsa dyes. At the ultrastructural level the chondrocytes (e.g. of hyaline cartilage) are surrounded by a net-

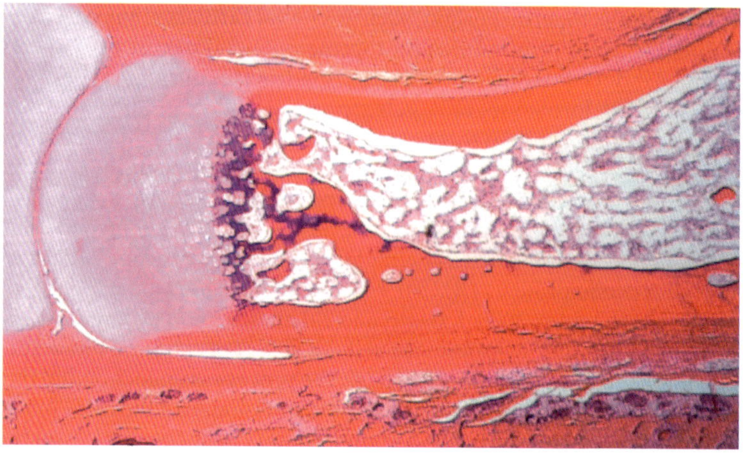

Fig. 2.16. Biomineral formation of long bone in the growth plate

work of unbanded, 20–70-nm collagen fibrils, in which proteoglycan granules are embedded. According to in vivo experiments, a shift in collagen expression may be observed throughout the process of chondrocyte development. Whereas chondrocyte precursor cells primarily express type III collagen, maturing chondrocytes shift to an expression of type II and then type X collagen (Reddi et al., 1977). In contrast, chondrocytes in the calcified cartilage region often contain thick, cross-banded collagen fibrils reminiscent of type I collagen fibrils. Recent studies indicate that the expression patterns of other ECM components including fibronectin, aggrecan and other proteoglycans, and the integrins are modulated during the process of endochondral ossification (Yu et al., 1991; Alini et al., 1992). Thus, the expression of matrix components by chondrocytes, in particular the distribution of the various collagen types, reflects their differentiation stage.

Evidence has accumulated that the expression of chondrogenic functions is strictly associated with the spherical cell shape, and a corresponding structure of the cytoskeleton, the expression of cartilage-specific genes, and the accumulation of a pericellular matrix (Gelse et al., 2003). However, the mechanism of such a control of gene functions by the cytoskeleton is not completely solved. It is assumed that the actin cytoskeleton of chondrocytes is stabilised through transmembrane connections to the extracellular protein matrix. Such transmembrane connections (demonstrated for fibronectin, which is linked to intracellular actin filaments by a specific membrane component called fibronexus) contain probably the fibronectin receptor and are associated with vinculin. The transfer of information from the pericellular region to the nucleus controls the features of chondrogenic differentiation (for a review, see Guilak et al., 1999). Chondrocytes are isolated within a voluminous extracellular matrix (ECM) that is neither vascularised nor innervated. As a result, nutrient/waste exchange occurs through diffusion and, consequently, under normal and pathological conditions, the cell is unique in its ability to exist in a low oxygen tension environment. Partly as a result of these properties, the tissue has a low reparative potential. In addition to cell characteristics, chondrocytes are (as indicated) recognised on the basis of their unique matrix components.

2.8 Cartilage Regeneration

Cartilage is a metabolically active tissue that under normal conditions is maintained in a relatively slow state of turnover by a sparse population of chondrocytes distributed throughout the tissue. Despite the activity of these cells, cartilage has a limited capacity for intrinsic repair, and even minor lesions or injuries may lead to progressive damage (and in the case of articular cartilage, lead to subsequent joint degeneration; Coutts et al., 2001; Roughley, 2001b; Burr, 2004). Isolated chondral or osteochondral lesions also may be a significant source of pain and loss of function, and will heal spontaneously only under some circumstances. The repair of cartilage is critically dependent on the extent of tissue destruction. Based on the extent of tissue damage, articular defects can be classified into three types:

- Mechanical disruption of articular cartilage, limited to articular cartilage
- Damage to the cells and matrices of articular cartilage and subchondral bone
- Mechanical disruption of articular cartilage and bone.

Each type of tissue damage initiates a distinct cell-driven repair response (Buckwalter et al., 1988a,b; Buckwalter, 1992). The ability of chondrocytes to sense changes in matrix composition and synthesise new molecules are the basis for repair processess (Buckwalter, 1997a/b; Martin and Buckwalter, 2000; Martin et al., 2002). The two features that are assumed to play main roles in the limited repair response of articular cartilage are the lack of blood supply and a lack of undifferentiated cells that can promote repair. Chondrocytes can repair defects ad integrum in circumstances where:

- The loss of matrix proteoglycans does not exceed what the cells can rapidly produce
- The fibrillar collagen meshwork remains intact
- Enough chondrocytes remain capable of responding to the matrix damage.

After superficial defects are present, chondrocytes proliferate and increase synthesis of matrix macromolecules adjacent to the defect borders (Fig. 2.17).

In most cases the newly synthesised matrix and proliferating cells do not completely fill the tissue defect. A rapid cessation in proliferation and matrix synthesis is the underlying reason for the limited capacity of articular cartilage for complete defect repair (Buckwalter et al., 1990; Buckwalter and Mow, 1991; Buckwalter and Mankin, 1997a,b). A permanent articular surface defect that can alter joint mechanical function and increase the risk of subsequent joint degeneration is the consequence of such limited repair capacity. The repair and remodelling of osteochondral defects differ from the events that follow injuries that cause only cell and matrix injury or disruption of the articular surface limited to articular cartilage (for a review see Buckwalter and Brown, 2004). The extent and outcome of the repair and remodelling responses is critically dependent on the disintegration of the subchondral tissue. Defects that extend into subchondral bone cause, in contrast to superficial defects, bleeding into the defect area. Soon after full thickness defects are present,

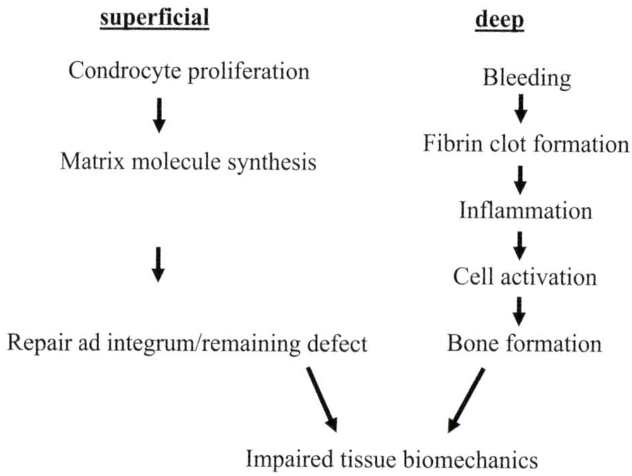

Fig. 2.17. Cartilage defect healing pathways

blood escaping from the damaged subchondral bone forms a hematoma that fills the injury site. Fibrin forms within the hematoma and platelets bind to fibrillar collagen, releasing together with the underlying bone various vasoactive mediators and growth factors: transforming growth factor-beta (TGFß), platelet-derived growth factor (PDGF), bone morphogenic proteins (BMPs), insulin-like growth factor I and II (IGF-I, IGF-II), and others. Release of these growth and differentiating factors modulate the features of repair tissue formation. This activation of the inflammatory response accelerates the defect healing process (Mitchell and Shepard, 1980; Buckwalter et al., 1990; Buckwalter and Mow, 1992). It is important to note that the various factors that control bone tissue repair are also directly involved in cartilage repair mechanisms. The occurrence of these signal molecules in both repair processes indicates also the close relationship between bone and cartilage formation. Cells, influenced by these factors, produce regions of hyaline-like cartilage in the chondral and bony portions of the defect. The repair tissue within the chondral region of osteochondral defects contains many chondrocyte-like cells in a matrix consisting of type II collagen and proteoglycans, some type I collagen and non-collagenous proteins. Cells located in deeper areas of the defect produce immature bone, fibrous tissue, and hyaline-like cartilage (Buckwalter et al., 2003). The final outcome of the repair tissue typically has a composition and structure intermediate between hyaline cartilage and fibrocartilage, imposing an impaired biomechanical competence. The newly formed tissue is, in structure and biomechanical competence, different from normal articular cartilage (Buckwalter and Mankin, 1997a; 1997b; Buckwalter et al., 1988a; 1998b; Buckwalter et al., 2001), imposing decreased stiffness and increased permeability. The altered cartilage structure may lead to increased loading of the macromolecular framework, resulting in a further structural damage to the joint. The increased loads exposed to the repair chondrocytes deteriorate even more the whole repair and regeneration process and compromise the ability of cells to restore the matrix (Buckwalter et al., 2003). In contrast, recent repair strategies focus on inducing a predetermined tissue response, for example by surgically creating a full thickness defect instead of repairing the superficial defect. Tissue engineering strategies have therefore to take into account what kind of tissue defect is present in order to build up a defect-specific ex vivo grown substitute.

2.9 Skeletal Biomechanics

Biomechanics is a critical issue in bone and cartilage tissue engineering. It is important for the in vitro development of tissues as well as for the in vivo fate of implanted cellular scaffold constructs. The biomechanical impact of skeletal tissue can be considered as a highly complex and dynamic process (Burger and Veldhuijzen, 1993). Physical and biological parameters affecting the success of regeneration and remodelling include the macro- and microscopical anatomy, the direction and amount of the applied forces, and the regenerative capacity of the tissues involved. Force transduction via adjacent structures (joints, ligaments, muscles, and soft tissue) influences the regeneration of the tissue by modulating the stress produced within the tissue environment. Skeletal biomechanics combines physical signals with biological reactions, thereby having a complex and dynamic interaction. To better understand the complex field of biomechanics, reaction to external forces can be conceptualised as:

- The reaction of loads to non-living compound materials (matrix/minerals) in a simplified way
- The reaction of cells towards the biophysical signals that are present in the micro-environment of the tissue.

The reaction of non-living skeletal parts (e.g. an explanted femur, acellular scaffold materials) to loads can be analysed at two levels. First, we can assess the material properties of bone and cartilage (or the replacement constructs) independent of its anatomical structure and geometry by performing standardised mechanical tests on uniform specimens (Turner et al., 1995). Second, by examining the mechanical behaviour of bone as an anatomical entity the contributions made by its structural properties can be assessed. Mechanically, these properties determine how bone (or bone substitute materials) responds to forces in a clinical setting.

Load is a commonly used and poorly defined term. It is not defined in terms of a physical determinable condition (Table 2.6). It is mostly used when a complex mechanically related state is meant. In contrast to load, various other terms are precisely defined. The internal resistance to an applied force is known as stress. Stress, defined as equal in magnitude but opposite in direction to the applied force, is distributed over the cross-sectional area of bone and cartilage. It is expressed in units of force per unit area: stress = δ = force/area. In loaded skeletal sites, mechanical forces are transduced through the soft tissue envelope. Due to the different material properties of bone, cartilage, and other tissues, the force/stress relationship is in most anatomical locations complex and therefore difficult to assess.

Most stress patterns are combinations of three stress types, namely tension, compression, and shear (Einhorn, 1996). Bending, for example, produces a combination of tensile forces on the convex side of a material and compression on the concave side. Torsion or twisting produces shear stresses along the entire length of a material, while tensile stress elongates it and compressive stress shortens it. In order to simplify the complex loading situation in distinct skeletal sites, tissue deformation

Table 2.6. Biomechanical parameters

Term	Definition	Units
- Load	Not precisely defined	-
- Force	Mass x acceleration	N
- Stress	Force/area	N/m^2
- Strain	Change in length/orig. length	%
- Young`s modulus	Stress/strain	N/m^2
- Resilience	Stored energy	$N \times m$

can be regarded as an axial elongation of the cell/matrix complex leading to the development of tensile stresses. The measurement of deformation (displacement of a defined point, measured in mm) normalised to the original length of the specimen is called strain (Fig. 2.18):

strain = E
= change in length/original length
= (deformed length–orig. length)/(orig. length)

Strain is dimensionless and expressed as a percentage change.

At low levels of stress there is a linear relationship between the stress applied and the resultant deformations in terms of strain (Curey, 1962). This proportionality is called the modulus of elasticity or Young´s modulus. It is a measure of the slope of the linear portion of the curve and is calculated by dividing the stress by the strain at any point along this portion of the curve. If the stress/strain area were to be gener-

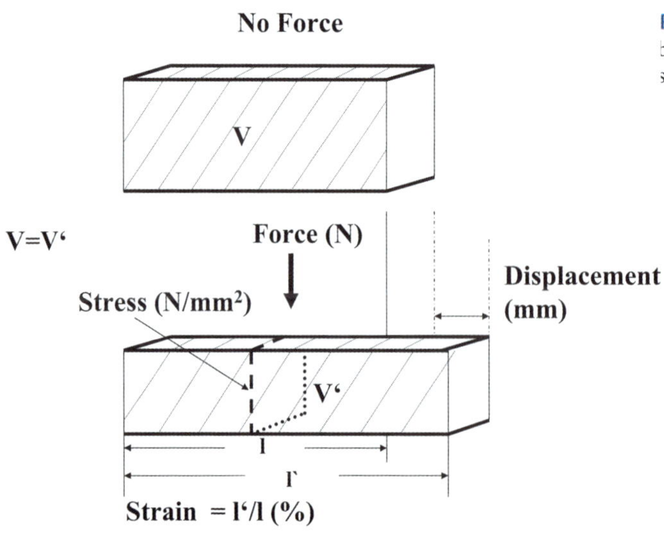

Fig. 2.18. Relationship between force, stress, strain, and volume

ated by testing a whole bone as opposed to a unifom specimen, this measurement of the linear slope would give the stiffness or rigidity of the bony or cartilagineous tissue. With respect to tissue engineering it is important to recognise that Young´s modulus is nearly stable in mature skeletal sites but varies in regenerate tissue during the ex vivo formation as well as after implantation due to the degradation and remodelling process. Thus, the modulus of elasticity of the ex vivo generated tissue construct can be expected not only to alter during the in vitro period but to a more profound extent, in the post-implantation period.

Energy put into deformation of an elastic material just prior to reaching the yield point can be recovered by removing the stress (Chamay, 1970). The energy recovered is known as resilience and is a measure of the ability of the material to store energy. Although this energy is not always recoverable in a useful form, it will not be lost as long as the material does not undergo permanent deformation.

Understanding the relation between load application and resultant tissue deformation is crucial for the outcome of tissue engineering approaches. It is obvious that the biomechanical behaviour of whole bones is more complex than those of its single components (cortical and cancellous bone, cartilage). A variety of powerful approaches have generated a comprehensive picture of how a tissue responds to load, but no in vitro measures are able to accurately predict the in vivo situation. In order to assess load-related tissue deformation in the in vivo setting, various approaches have been introduced (Table 2.7). Indirect measurements of deformations are measured by means of topographical sensors (Ahmad et al., 1982; Mosley et al., 1997) or strain gauges (Arendts and Sigolotto, 1989; 1990). Additionally, holographic interferometry has been performed to assess the impact of mechanical forces on tissue deformation (Ferre et al., 1985). One major disadvantage of all experimental studies using either strain gauges or holographic interferometry is the inability to determine strains at defined positions within the specimen. Biomechanical research using these methods is also limited to surface deformations and neither stresses nor dislocations within the tissue can be measured directly. Computer-aided simulation based on finite element analysis (FEA) has addressed the adequacy of mathematical models to relate mechanical factors such as load transfer to the biomechanical behaviour of bone and cartilage specimens. Various authors have reported that, given a high correlation between a calculated strain and stress state and the measured experimental data, various biomechanical parameters can be determined within deformed bone tissue (Meyer et al., 2000; Vollmer et al., 2000). Because of the complex challenges involved in measuring *in situ* loads and deformations of cartilage under realistic in vivo conditions, several investigators have used theoretical models of

Table 2.7. Determination of load-related biomechanics

Method	Method characteristics
– Holographic inferometry	Indirect, not quantifiable
– Topographic sensors	Direct, difficult measurements
– Pressure sensors	Direct, difficult to miniaturise
– Strain gauges	Direct, only usable at surfaces
– Finite element analyses	Indirect, complex possibilities
– Theoretical modelling	Indirect, difficult to perform

joint contact to predict load-related deformations in cartilage tissue (Blankevoort et al., 1991; Ateshian and Wang, 1995; Donzelli et al., 1999). Theoretical and experimental studies of cell–matrix interactions in cartilage, from macroscopic to microscopic levels (Mow et al., 1992; 1994; Guilak and Mow, 2000), constitute the basis for the calculation of biomechanical parameters that often cannot be measured. In combination with experimental measurements of cell-matrix interactions within cartilage tissue (Guilak, 1995; Guilak et al., 1995), theoretical models (e.g. FEA) may allow researchers to investigate hypotheses about the influence of various mechanical factors on the biology or biomechanics of cartilage. Whereas the accuracy of FEA in describing the biomechanical behaviour of non-living specimens has been demonstrated by various authors (Hart et al., 1992; Korioth and Verslius, 1997; Voo et al., 1996), it is unknown how exact the numerical methods mirror the real in vivo situation. In addition to the use of FEA in the prediction of load-related deformations, FEA methods have been used recently to model load situations in bioreactors (Meyer et al., 2005a) in an effort to enhance tissue formation by creating an optimal strain/stress environment.

In contrast to non-living specimens (explanted bone, cartilage, scaffolds), living tissue has a very different structure due to the high dynamics of tissue remodelling. Whereas a number of in vitro studies have investigated the relationship between the applied forces and the resulting tissue deformation, much less is known about the in vivo features of loaded bones and joints. Bone as well as cartilage undergoes deformation in a changing mechanical environment and reacts biologically when a force is applied (Aronson, 1992). If the skeletal sites are fixed so that they cannot move, or if equal and opposite forces are applied to them, deformations will occur, resulting in the generation of an internal resistance to the applied force (Brown and Ferguson, 1978). Because of the complex structure of both tissues (non-homogenous, non-isotropic tissue properties) and the technical problems involved, it is difficult to determine directly the force/tissue deformation relationship.

2.10 Bone Biomechanics

The purpose of bone is to provide structural strength corresponding to its mechanical usage (Fig. 2.19) (Brown and Ferguson, 1978). This means that bones provide enough strength to keep voluntary physical loads from causing pain or damage. Bone deformation through mechanical loads is a complex feature. It is dependent not only on the bone structure but on the action of various tissues (joints, muscles, ligaments, bones; Fig. 2.20). Recent research has suggested that bones display an extraordinary adaptive behaviour towards a changing mechanical environment, which is often regarded as phenotype plasticity (Aegerter and Kirkpatrick, 1973; Frost, 2000 a/b; Losos, 2001; Frost et al., 2002). Specific strain-dependent signals are thought to control this adaptive mode of bony tissue modelling (Meyer et al., 1997a). The adaptive mechanisms include basic multicellular units (BMUs) of bone remodelling. Effector cells within BMUs have been shown to function in an interdependent manner. While hormones may bring about as much as 10% of the postnatal changes in bone strength and mass, 40% are determined by mechanical effects. This has been shown by the loss of extremity bone mass in patients with paraplegia (more than 40%).

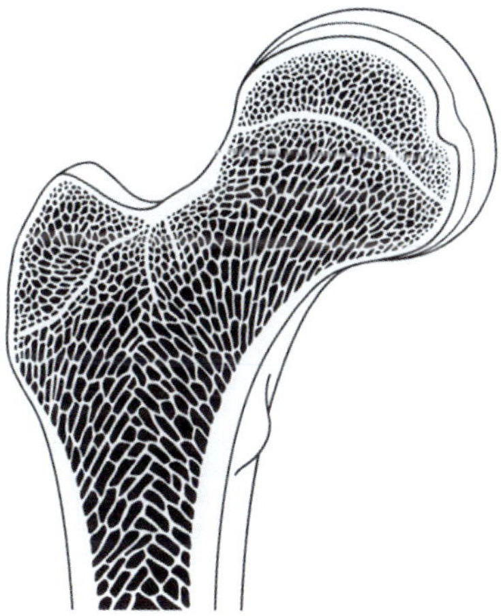

Fig. 2.19. Load-determined optimised bone structure, as exemplified by the femur bone

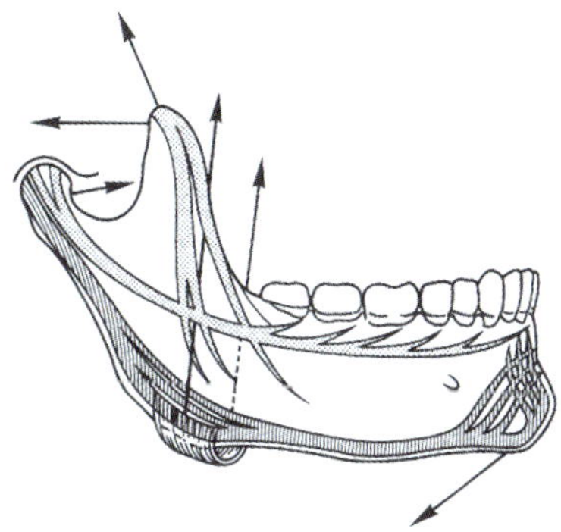

Fig. 2.20. Complex biomechanical behaviour of bone as exemplified by the mandible. Arrows indicate the main loading factors, applied by the mastication muscles. The load distribution leads to bone thickening at different bony locations (shadowed: mandibular basis, linea obliqua, alvelar bone)

Modelling occurs by separate formation and resorption drifts to reshape, thicken, and strengthen a bone or trabecula by moving its surfaces around in tissue space (Frost, 1964a,b; 1983; 1986; Takahashi, 1995). Remodelling also involves both resorption and formation of bone. Basic multicellular units turn bone over in small packets through a process in which an activating event causes some bone resorption, and bone formation follows (Frost, 1964b; Martin et al., 1998; Jee, 1999). This BMU-based remodelling operates in two modes: conservation mode and disuse mode (Fig. 2.21) (Frost and Schönau, 2000). A specific strain threshold range controls which of these two modes is active at any given time (Martin et al., 1998).

As load-related skeletal modelling and remodelling is a highly dynamic cellular process, tissue deformations in the sense of tensile strains are the leading stimuli for bone regeneration (Frost, 1992). It is generally suggested that forces leading to cellular deformation are signalled to the cellular genome through mechanotransduction mechanisms. Mechanotransduction, or the conversion of a biophysical force into a cellular response, is an essential mechanism in bone biology (Meyer et al., 1997b). It allows bone cells to respond to a changing mechanical environment. Mechanotransduction can be categorised in an idealised manner into (1) *mechanocoupling*,

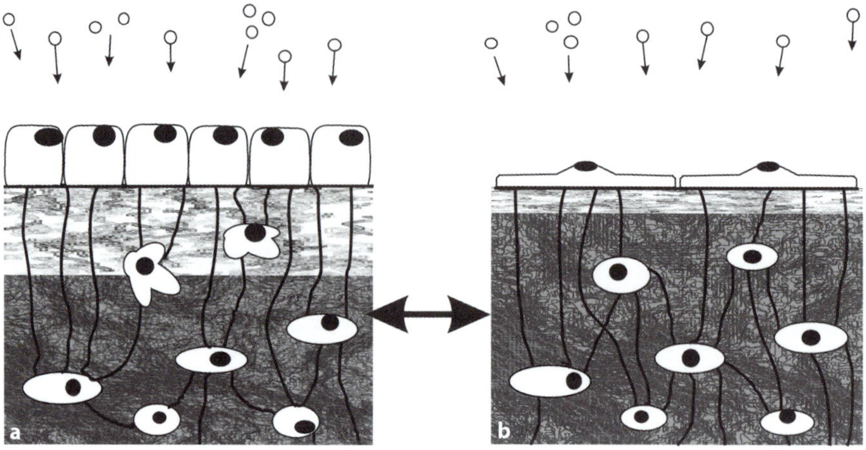

Fig. 2.21. Shematic drawing of (**a**) active bone formation in comparison to (**b**) resting bone state. Different external and autocrine factors regulate the state of bone formation. Active osteoblasts have a voluminous appearance, whereas resting cells are flattened at the bone surface. Synthetically active osteoblasts form a thick layer of newly deposited mineralising matrix. In contrast, in a resting bone state only a thin layer of osteoid is located underneath the lining cells

which means the transduction of mechanical force applied to the tissue into a local mechanical signal perceived by a bone cell; (2) *biochemical coupling*, the transduction of a local mechanical signal into biochemical signal cascades altering gene expression or protein activation; (3) *transmission of signals* from the sensor cells to effector cells, which actually form or remove bone; and ultimatively (4) *the effector cell response*. When loads are applied to bone, the tissue begins to deform causing local strains (typically reported in units of microstrain; 10,000 microstrain = 1% change in length). It is well known that osteoblasts and osteocytes act as the sensors of local bone strains and that they are appropriately located in the bone for this function. Various investigators have revealed that reactive loads give rise to relatively high strains at fundamental frequencies that extend from 1 to 10 Hz. It was found that peak strain magnitudes measured in a wide variety of species are remarkably similar, ranging from 2,000 to 3,500 microstrain. Lanyon and colleagues (1975) showed that, within a single period of loading, the remodelling process seemed to be saturated after only a few (<<50) loading cycles. Further strain repetitions then produced no extra effect.

There have been many suggestions for biophysical transduction mechanisms on a cellular level (Ando et al., 1988; Binderman et al., 1988; Jones et al., 1991; Takei et al., 1998).

Biophysical stimuli of cells

- Mechanical effects
- Electro-mechanical effects
- Thermic effects
- Radiation effects

- Pressure
- Pressure gradients
- Distortion
- Enhancement of molecular transport
- Energy dissipation.

Most studies have suggested that mechanical strain transduction might be directly related to mechanical deformation of ultrastructural organelles or proteins, thereby converting the mechanical information into a biochemical signal. Although hydrostatic compression has been proposed to be analogous to physiological strain and to re-create physiological strain effects, no significant distortion or compression of the fluid-filled cell can occur until very high pressures are attained (Bagi and Burger, 1989). Cell elongation seems to be the driving force for signal transduction. Studies of cell elongation in vitro have demonstrated that physiological loading of osteoblast-like cells induces the differentiation of osteoblasts, whereas hyperphysiological load tends to dedifferentiate cells towards a fibroblastic phenotype (Meyer et al., 2001c). It is assumed that the strain sensor is linked to the cytoskeleton, although other hypotheses have been suggested. If the strain sensor is located in the cytoskeleton, then deformations of this structure would tend not to be homogeneous because different compartments would have different mechanical properties and the weakest link would deform the most. In this model, elongation of bone cells appears to influence subsequent transcriptional events.

The functional biological environment of any bone tissue is thus derived from a dynamic interaction between various active basic multicellular units exposed to a biophysical microenvironment undergoing continuous load-related changes. Bone formation occurs through separate formation and resorption drifts to reshape, thicken, and strengthen a bone or trabecula by moving its surfaces around in tissue space (Frost, 1996). While the load-related bone modelling theory was long assumed to be applicable only to intact bones (Frost, 2000a), recent research has shown that this adaptive behaviour is also present in bone healing processes (Frost et al., 2002). As the oestrogen receptor was shown to be involved in the adaptive response of osteoblasts to mechanical strain (Damien et al., 1998), biophysical force transduction seems also to be closely connected with the hormonal regulation of bone turnover, indicative of the complex situation of the bone cell behaviour towards molecular-level signals. The evidence supporting the concept that biophysical signals are able to regulate bone cell behaviour positively is accepted, but the relation between defined biophysical forces and resultant effects on bone cell behaviour is to some extent contradictory. Whereas some investigations offered evidence that biophysical forces, including substrate deformation, hydrostatic pressure, fluid flow, or hypergravity, increase expression and/or synthesis of markers of bone cell differentiation (Harter et al., 1995; Owan et al., 1997; Yoshikawa et al., 1997; Kawashima et al., 1998; Matsuda et al., 1998; Meyer et al., 2001a), others failed to do so or even reported negative effects of biophysical stimuli on cell proliferation and differentiation (Hillsley and Frangos, 1994; Meazzini et al., 1998; Ozawa et al., 1990). This contradictory evidence can be assumed to be associated with the fact that various biophysical stimuli (physiological, non-physiological) were exerted on different bone cell lines (primary cells, altered cells) in the different experimental investigations.

When biomechanical effects are considered at the tissue level, it is important to recognise that mechanical and electrical effects are exerted simultaneously in bone (Spadaro, 1997). Mechanical and electrical interactions, being quite complex during the modelling and remodelling processes, integrate the action of several signals to form the final response. Tissue deformation as a key stimulus in bone physiology leads to a complex, non-uniform biophysical environment within bone tissue, consisting of fluid flow, direct mechanical strain, and electrokinetic effects on bone cells. At the tissue level, some researchers, assuming the differentiating tissue to be a continuous material, evaluated biophysical signals by characterising the stimulus in terms of engineering quantities. Based on the tissue material properties and approximations of tissue loading in the different experimental or clinical situation, these quantities were calculated throughout the tissue and were related to various patterns of tissue differentiation. The biophysical mechanisms underlying the tissue response were directly related to mechanical effects (Meyer et al., 1999a), electromechanical effects (Gross and Williams, 1982; Pienkowski and Pollack, 1983) or enhancement of molecular transport mechanisms (Piekarski and Munro, 1997). Pressure, distortion, pressure gradients, and energy dissipation are additional engineering-level quantities that were quantified and related to tissue responses by other authors (Einhorn, 1996).

Load-induced interstitial fluid flow has been suggested to provide a basic convergence feature between electrical and mechanical signals resulting from effecting the cellular level, thus triggering the subsequent hard tissue formation in adaptation (Chao and Inoue, 2003). Bone loading leads to a deformation of cells in the microenvironment of the tissue and simultaneously to a fluid-flow-related generation of electrical potentials. Pressure gradients from mechanical loading of bone tissue elongate cells and the mineralised matrix and move extracellular fluid radially outward. The fluid flow stream generates electrical potentials that exert effects on adjacent cells (Pienkowski and Pollack, 1983). Electric fields of a magnitude and frequency that would occur endogenously as a result of physiological bone load via piezoelectric effects, streaming potentials, or a combination of these (Fukada and Yasuda, 1957; Hastings and Mahmed, 1988), have been demonstrated to modulate bone formation in the craniofacial skeleton too (Marino et al., 1986). The sensitivity of the biophysical driven bone response was found to be much greater when the cells are part of a tissue than when they are evaluated as single entities. The bone tissue system integrates and amplifies a complex physical signal such as mechanical strain or functionally induced fluid flow by transmitting the signal from the signal-detecting cells to the change-effecting cells. Bone cells are functionally coupled both in vivo (Jeansonne et al., 1979) and in vitro (Schirrmacher et al., 1992) by gap junctions. Gap junctions, which are well suited to the integration and amplification of the response of bone cell networks to biophysical signals, are therefore important mediators of the effector response. The role of gap junctions in biophysical signal transduction at tissue level was examplified in the bone-cell response to electromagnetic fields (EMF). In contrast to single cells, the intercellular network was found to contribute to the ability of EMF's to stimulate alkaline phosphatase activity, a marker for osteoblastic differentiation, suggesting that gap junctions are involved in the enhancement of EMF-stimulated osteoblastic differentiation. Gap junctions were also demonstrated to contribute to bone-cell responsiveness to other biophysical signals such as cell deformation or fluid flow (Yellowley et al., 2000), indicating their special role in transmitting single cell signals into the tissue.

2.11 Cartilage Biomechanics

Cartilage biomechanics varies within the different subsets of cartilage. The development and maintenance of cartilage structure and mechanical characteristics are closely correlated to the effect of mechanical loading. The impact of load on cartilage structure and function is of outermost importance especially in hyaline articular cartilage. Physiologic joint loading maintains cartilage structure and function. In the context of tissue engineering, it is important to recognise that stresses in a cartilage defect or the surrounding tissue may be altered significantly from their normal mechanical environment, and therefore impair tissue integrity before and after cell/scaffold implantation. The histologic structure of articular cartilage is influenced by the local mechanical loading of chondrocytes in the different zones (for a review see Wong and Carter, 2003). In contrast to bone, where considerable quantitative information is available on the in vivo stresses and strains that are encountered under different conditions (Chuong and Fung, 1983; Biewener, 1993; Han and Fung, 1995; Korvick et al., 1996; Malaviya et al., 1998; Woo et al., 1999; Milgrom et al., 2000), for articular cartilage there are unique challenges with respect to the magnitude and rate of loading within the joint that make determinations of load parameters difficult. Cartilage can be considered as a compound material. It can be conceptualised as a mixture of fluid and solid constituents (despite the close interrelations of both components). Chondrocytes are directly attached to the ECM and can be considered part of the fluid continuum of cartilage tissue. The zonal structure of articular cartilage is essential to its ability to support physiologic joint forces. Patterns of stress, strain, and fluid flow created in the joint result in spatial and temporal alterations in chondrocyte function. The external forces are transmitted through the joint and the adjacent tissues resulting in the generation of pressure over the contact area of the two opposing cartilage surfaces (Fig. 2.22).

There is only limited information on the normal in vivo mechanical environment. Stresses in a normal joint are difficult to determine in vivo, but evidence from experimental studies indicate that normal stresses may range from 5 to 10 MPa in animals and human joints (Brown and Shaw, 1983; Ronskey et al., 1995; von Eisenhart et al., 1999). Pressure magnitudes in articular cartilage have been shown to exceed 18 MPa under distinct experimental conditions (Hodge et al., 1989). In areas of peak pressure most of the force is transmitted through a thin fluid film layer that is created between the solid matrices of the superficial cartilage layers on opposite areas of the joint (for a review see Wong and Carter, 2003). Loads tend to deform the cartilage tissue but these compressive loads and the subsequent tissue deformations are resisted by:

- Stresses in the solid phase
- The generation of fluid pressure
- The restriction of tissue deformation by the nearly impermeable subchondral bone and the surrounding adjacent cartilage surfaces.

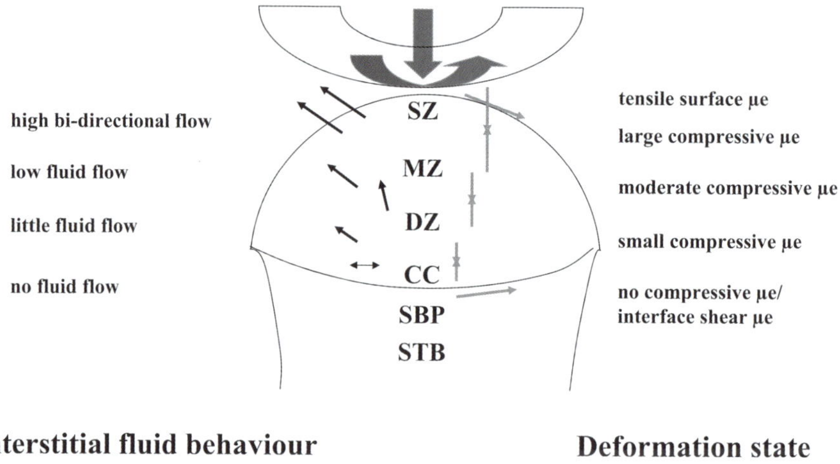

Fig. 2.22. Cartilage biomechanics

Intermittent loads (created by the normal movements of joints) transfer cyclic hydrostatic pressure in the interstitial fluid. In mature joints, cyclic loads produce cyclic hydrostatic fluid pressure through the entire cartilage thickness that is comparable in magnitude to the applied joint pressure. The pressure in the interstitial fluid component of cartilage transfers the loads to the surrounding tissues, by distributing the forces to the underlying bone tissues in an efficient manner (McCutchen, 1959; 1962; Maroudas and Bullough, 1968; Higginson and Snaith, 1979; Oloyede and Broom, 1993; Macirowski et al., 1994; Ateshian and Wang, 1995; Mow and Ateshian, 1997). The superficial zone of cartilage exsudes interstitial fluid and consolidates, forming an effective seal at the joint surface. In the radial zone of articular cartilage, fluid flow is lower then in the superficial zone, being restricted laterally by adjacent tissue, below by the subchondral bone layer, and above by the consolidated surface zone.

An outside directed fluid flow is therefore seen mainly in areas of the superficial layer just outside the contact area (Mow and Ateshian, 1997). Under these conditions compressive strains are substantial. The matrix of the superficial layer consolidates the cells in this region, leading to substantial compressive deformations (strains). The collagen network resists tensile and shear stresses and strains while the fluid component resists the high hydrostatic compressive stresses that are generated. Shear stresses created in cartilage are always associated with tensile strains in some direction. In addition to the load-related compressive strains, the rolling movement of opposite joint surfaces imposes cyclic tensile strains tangential to the surface of cartilage in the superficial area (Askew and Mow, 1978). In this thin zone, the collagen fibrils are oriented parallel to the articular surface. Stresses are inhomogenously distributed in the cartilage tissue. Peak compressive strains are present in superficial layers, whereas the strain environment decreases near the calcified cartilage layer. It is important to note that there is a contrasting effect of shear and pressure on chondrocyte function, indicative of the complex mechanobiology of cartilage.

It is important to recognise that chondrocytes (like bone cells) are not compressible and they do not provide any special structural resistance to loading. Because of the structural and compositional characteristics of articular cartilage and the intrinsic coupling between the mechanical and physiochemical properties of the tissue (Lai et al., 1991), it has been, in contrast to bone tissue, more difficult to achieve a complete understanding of the mechanical signal transduction pathways used by chondrocytes. Fundamental to this issue is an understanding of the mechanical environment of the chondrocytes within the articular cartilage ECM. For example, compressive loading of the cartilage in the extracellular matrix exposes the chondrocytes to spatially- and time-varying stress, strain, fluid flow and pressure, osmotic pressure, and electric fields (Maroudas, 1979; Frank and Grodzinsky, 1987; Lai et al., 1991). The relative contribution of each of these factors to the regulation of chondrocyte activity is an important consideration which is being studied by a number of investigators (Guilak et al., 1997). It was found that under loading conditions shapes, pressures, and chemical environments of chondrocytes are altered by deformations created in the ECM as well as by local fluid pressure and fluid flow. Chondrocytes in articular cartilage undergo large changes in shape and intercellular spacing as the ECM is deformed. The cells were found to recover their morphology upon removal of compression and to have a stiffness that was less than or equal to that of the surrounding tissues. Furthermore, collagen fibre orientation was shown to change with compression and recover upon removal of compression. New microscope techniqes allowed three-dimensional imaging of fluorescently labelled chondrocytes (Guilak et al., 1995) or subcellular structures (Guilak, 1995) within a tissue explant. Volumetric images of chondrocytes recorded decreases in cell height of 26, 19, and 20% and decreases in cell volume of 22, 16, and 17% of control values in different zones of an osteochondral explant, thereby differing from mechanically induced deformations of bone cells. In responding to mechanical signals the chondrocyte responds to the several different types of information using various signal transduction mechanisms (for a review see Guilak et al., 2001). It was demonstrated by in vivo and in vitro studies that chondrocytes are able (in a similar manner to bone cells) to detect an array of physical parameters (tissue pressure, deformation, fluid flow). The sum of cellular reactions in response to loading is a gene activation state of cell that determines the histomorphology of articular cartilage remodelling and repair (Carter et al., 1987; Carter and Wong, 1990; Smith et al., 1992; Holmvall et al., 1995; Knudson et al., 1996; Buschmann et al., 1995; von der Mark and Mollenhauer, 1997; Beaupre et al., 2000; Lee et al., 2000; Loeser, 2000; Mauck et al., 2000; Ragan et al., 2000; Reid et al., 2000; Davisson et al., 2002; Giannoni et al., 2003). The factors, pathways, and receptors of cell sensing and the response of cells concerning the effect on its external environment have not yet been identified, but as indicated for bone cells, chondrocytes respond to a number of external signals. The chondrocyte perceives its mechanical environment through complex biological and biophysical interactions with the cartilage ECM. This matrix consists of several distinct regions, termed the pericellular, territorial, and interterritorial matrices (Hunziker, 1992). The bulk of the tissue is made up of the interterritorial matrix, which consists primarily of water dissolved with small electrolytes (Na^+, Cl^-, Ca^{2+}, etc.). The transfer of information proceeds to some extent in a similar manner as described for bone cells from the cell membrane to the cell nucleus, interacting also with other signalling pathways. Current experimental studies in tissue engineering try not only to evaluate the complex mechanobiology that underlies load-related cartilage histogenesis, but use biophysical stimuli to promote cartilage-like tissue growth in specially designed bioreactors (Meyer et al., 2005a).

Principles of Bone and Cartilage Reconstruction

3

Bone and cartilage repair is the subject of intensive investigation in reconstructive surgery (for a review, see Schultz et al., 2000). Current approaches to skeletal reconstructive surgery use biomaterials, autografts or allografts, although restrictions on all these techniques exist. These restrictions include donor site morbidity and donor shortages for autografts (Damien and Parsons, 1991), immunological barriers for allografts, and the risk of transmitting infectious diseases. Numerous artificial tissue substitutes containing metals, ceramics, and polymers have been introduced to maintain skeletal function (Binderman and Fin, 1990). Each material has specific disadvantages, and none of these can perfectly substitute autografts in current clinical practice. The use of biomaterials is a common treatment option in clinical practice. One important reason for the priority of tissue grafts over non-living biomaterials is that they contain living cells and tissue-inducing substances, thereby possessing biological plasticity. Research is currently in progress to develop cell-containing hybrid materials and to create replacement tissues that remain interactive after implantation, imparting physiological functions as well as structure to the tissue or organ damaged by disease or trauma (Alsberg et al., 2001).

Bone and cartilage tissue engineering, as in most other tissue engineering areas, exploits living cells in a variety of ways to restore, maintain or enhance tissue functions (Langer and Vacanti, 1993; Lysaght and Reyes, 2001). There are three principal therapeutic strategies for treating diseased or lost tissue in patients: (1) in situ tissue regeneration; (2) implantation of freshly isolated or cultured cells; and (3) implantation of a bone-like or cartilage-like tissue assembled in vitro from cells and scaffolds. For in situ regeneration, new tissue formation is induced by specific scaffolds or external stimuli that are used to stimulate the body´s own cells and promote local tissue repair. Cellular implantation means that individual cells or small cellular aggregates from the patient or a donor are injected directly into the damaged or lost region with or without a degradable scaffold. For tissue implantation, a complete three-dimensional tissue is grown in vitro using autologous or donor cells within a scaffold, which has to be implanted once it has reached maturity (Loty et al., 2000; Schliephake et al., 2001; Meyer et al., 2004b). In this chapter we give some details on all of the above mentioned strategies and present alternatives to extracorporal approaches that are important in clinical decision making. Some of the techniques described here are clinically combined with extracorporal tissue engineering methods.

3.1 Bone Repair Strategies

The use of autologous bone in bone defect reconstruction can be considered to be the gold standard. There are two classical ways to repair bone defects by use of autologous cells: one utilises mechanisms of defect repair by enhancement of the local host cell population, while the other is based on transplantation of grafted bone (Fig. 3.1).

Augmentation of the host cell population can effectively be used to improve the healing of bone lesions. The ability to repair or reconstruct lost bone structure by this technique critically depends on the condition of the defect site. If the soft and hard tissues of the defect site are healthy, expansion of host cells is often successfully applied. In circumstances of impaired defect conditions such as wound infection and tissue necrosis or irritation, however, cellular augmentation of the local bone cell population will probably fail.

Membrane techniques can be used to improve defect healing by ingrowth of local host cells in the defect site (Fig. 3.2). This kind of defect repair procedure (guided bone regeneration, GBR) is mainly used in maxillofacial surgery to repair bony defects in the maxilla and mandible. The principle of GBR is to effectively separate bone tissue from the soft tissue ingrowth by a barrier (Lang et al., 1994). The application of the principle of guided bone regeneration (GBR) has proven to be successful in a number of controlled animal studies and clinical trials (Buser et al., 1996; Berglundh and Lindhe, 1997; Fiorellini et al., 1998). The healing pattern has been shown to involve all steps of de novo bone formation including blood clot formation, invasion by osteoprogenitor cells and their terminal differentiation into osteoblasts. Under these circumstances the extracellular matrix produced finally mineralises to form woven bone, and later is remodelled into lamellar bone (Hämmerle et al., 1998). The success of GBR depends critically on the defect size and geometry. Bone defects can be assumed to be repaired to a larger extent in cases where the defect is neighboured

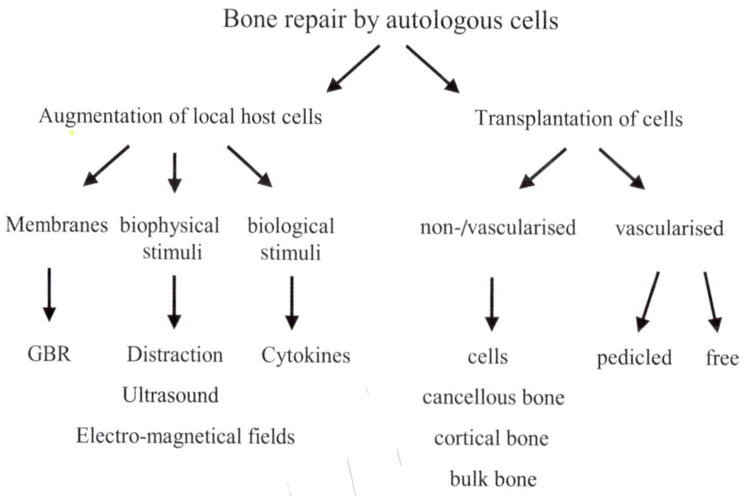

Fig. 3.1. Bone repair by autologous cells

by more than two bone walls. The main limitation of GBR is therefore the inability to reconstruct geometrically complex or large defect sites.

Biophysical effects, in particular mechanical loading and electromagnetic signals, are clearly important regulators of bone formation. Indeed, the regenerative capacity of bone tissue is largely due to the bone's capacity to recognise the functional environment required for the emergence and maintenance of a structurally intact bone tissue. Biophysical stimulation methods have therefore been introduced and have proved successful in clinical practice. Ultrasound application and electromagnetic field exposure are, besides distraction osteogenesis, considered to be a special form of mechanical stimulation, classical examples of biophysically driven approaches to influencing bone formation. Ample evidence from various prospective double-blinded, placebo-controlled clinical studies now documents the efficacy of mechanical and electrical stimulation (direct current, inductive coupling, capacitive coupling, and composite fields) and of mechanical stimulation (distraction osteogenesis, ultrasound stimulation, fracture activation) in enhancing bone repair

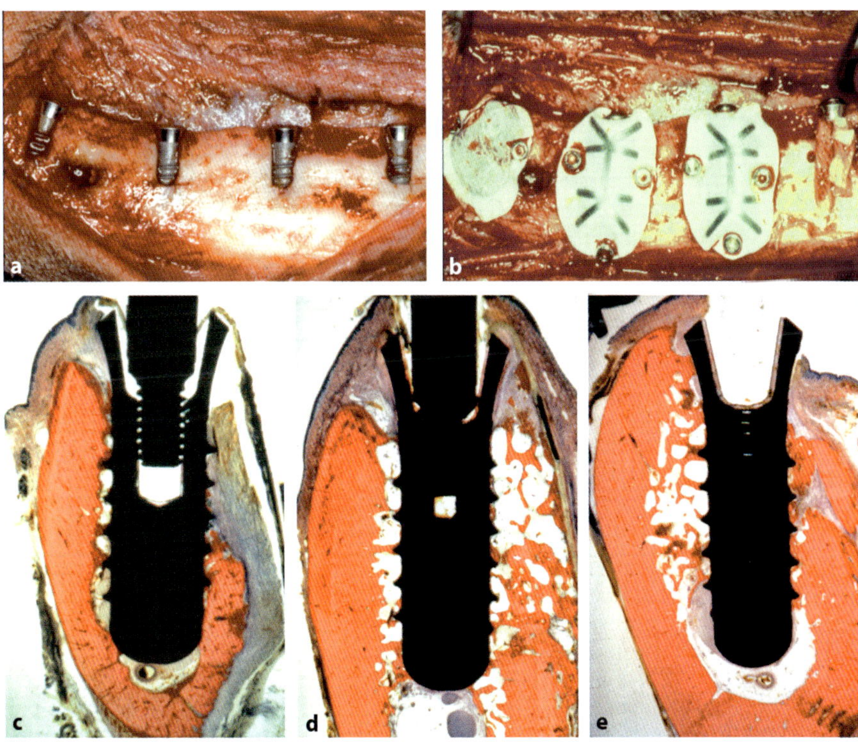

Fig. 3.2. Priciples of guided bone regeneration (GBR). **a** Implants are inserted in bone having a defect at the vestibular aspect of the alveolar crest. **b** Membranes are attached to the defect site, sealing the defect from tissue ingrowth of adjacent tissues. **c–e** Histology of bone regeneration. **c** Impaired bone regeneration without using a membrane. **d** New bone development by using the membrane technique. **e** Bone augmentation without the use of membranes led to an intermediate state of bone repair

(Brighton, 1998). Because of its clinical efficacy, biophysical stimulation is now one of several methods used to enhance bone formation in patients.

When applied to a patient, biophysical stimuli exert their effects at distinct skeletal sites. The response to ultrasound stimuli is altered by the anatomy of the application site. Ultrasound-related deformations through adjacent structures (joints, ligaments, muscles) have a major impact on the resultant biophysical signal at the desired effector site. Both patient-specific and technique-specific factors play an important role. When biophysical treatment strategies are considered, the specific forms of biophysical stimulation and their related dose effect and application timing must be carefully determined and validated. Despite limited knowledge concerning the biological effects of biophysical stimulation, it has long been the goal of many scientists and clinicians to find applicable clinical tools for using biophysical stimuli in the context of bone healing. In recent decades, different treatment strategies have been reported to be successful in animal experiments as well as in clinical trials. This has led researchers and clinicians to conduct a multitude of defined experiments to assess the effects of different biophysical stimuli in facilitating new bone formation (for a review, see Chao and Inoue, 2003) (Figs 3.3 and 3.4). Numerous investigations have been performed on electrical field exposure. When electrical stimuli are applied iatrogenically to a patient in order to enhance bone formation, one has to be aware that electrical stimuli exert their effects within the various hierarchical structures of the skeleton. The influence of external stimuli in skeletal regeneration can generally be addressed at organ, tissue, cellular, and molecular levels. Understanding the overall process of biophysical signalling requires an appreciation of these various levels of study and a knowledge of how one level relates to and influences the next. Electrical stimuli can be analysed as they act on whole bones. Additionally, the contributions of electrical effects made on multicellular systems can be evalu-

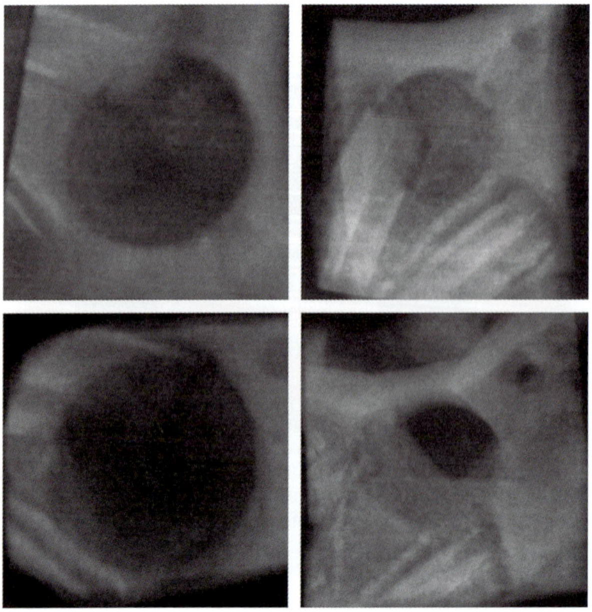

Fig. 3.3. X-ray images of bone defects with electrical stimulated bone regeneration *(top)* and without stimulation *(bottom)* after 1 *(left)* and 3 weeks *(right)*. Electrical stimulation improves biomineral formation in an in vivo setting of bone healing

ated by examining the tissue reaction towards the biophysical microenvironment. Thirdly, cellular and molecular reactions critically shape the tissue response. The key requirement of using the effects of such biophysical forces is therefore to define the precise cellular response to the stimulation signal in an in vitro environment and to use well-established animal and clinical models to quantify and optimise the therapeutic stimulation approaches. Whereas this seems to be achievable through research collaboration among different disciplines using complementary approaches, electrical stimulation is not a standardised or common treatment option to regenerate skeletal defects.

Distraction osteogenesis is frequently used to augment local bone in clinical settings (Meyer et al., 2004d) and is now an established bone reconstructive treatment option (Fig. 3.5). Histologically, distraction osteogenesis shares many of the features

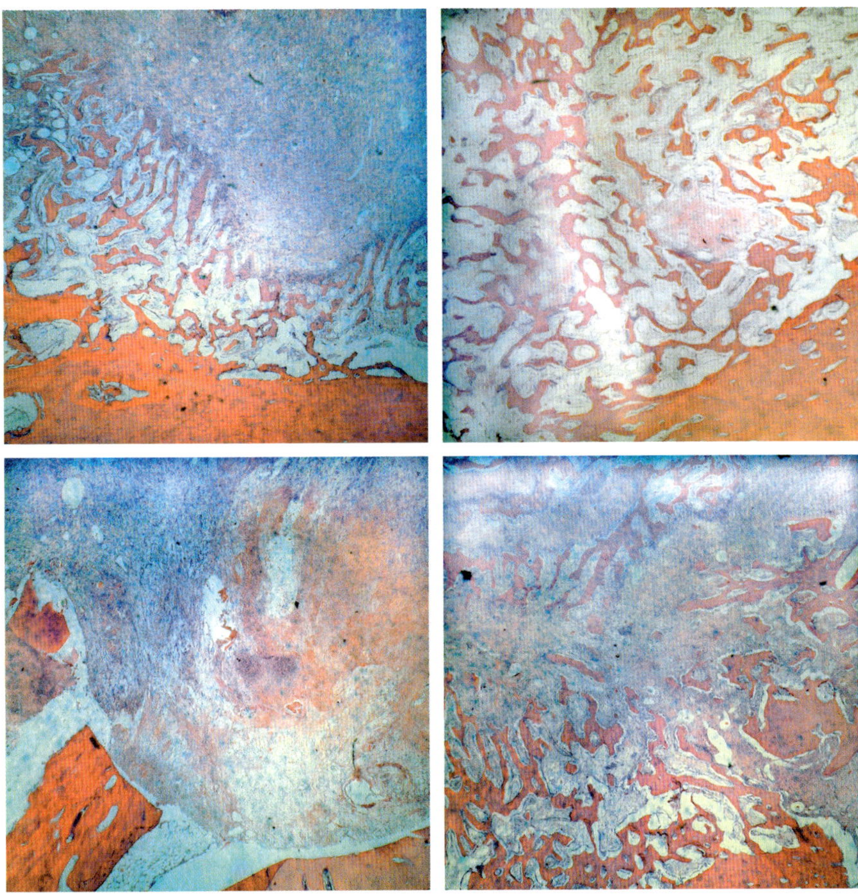

Fig. 3.4. Histology of bone defects with electrical stimulated bone regeneration (top) and without stimulation (*bottom*) after 1 (*left*) and 3 weeks (*right*). Critical size defects of mandibular bone were stimulated in rabbits by pulsed electric fields. Electric field application was able to enhance bone formation in critical size defects

of fetal tissue growth and neonatal limb development, as well as normal fracture gap healing (Ilizarov, 1992; Sato et al., 1999). Although the biomechanical, histological, and ultrastructural changes associated with distraction osteogenesis have been widely described, the molecular mechanisms governing the formation of new bone in the interfragmental gap of gradually distracted bone segments remain largely unclear. A growing body of evidence has emphasised the contribution of both local bone or bone precursor cells and neovascularity to bone formation during distraction (Choi et al., 2000). Recent studies have implicated a growing number of cytokines that are intimately involved in the regulation of bone synthesis and turnover during distraction procedures (Meyer et al., 2001b). The gene regulation of numerous cytokines (transforming growth factor-beta1, -beta2, -beta3, bone morphogenetic proteins, insulin-like growth factor-1, and fibroblast growth factor-2) and extracellular matrix proteins (osteonectin, osteopontin) during distraction osteogenesis have been best characterised and reviewed by Bouletreau et al. (2002a; 2002b). Refinements in the surgical procedure of bone distraction have significantly improved clinical outcomes (Meyer et al., 2004d). Distraction osteogenesis has therefore become a mainstay in bone tissue engineering and has significantly improved bone reconstructive procedures.

Biomolecules applied with or without a carrier have been suggested to augment the local bone cell population (Schliephake, 2002).

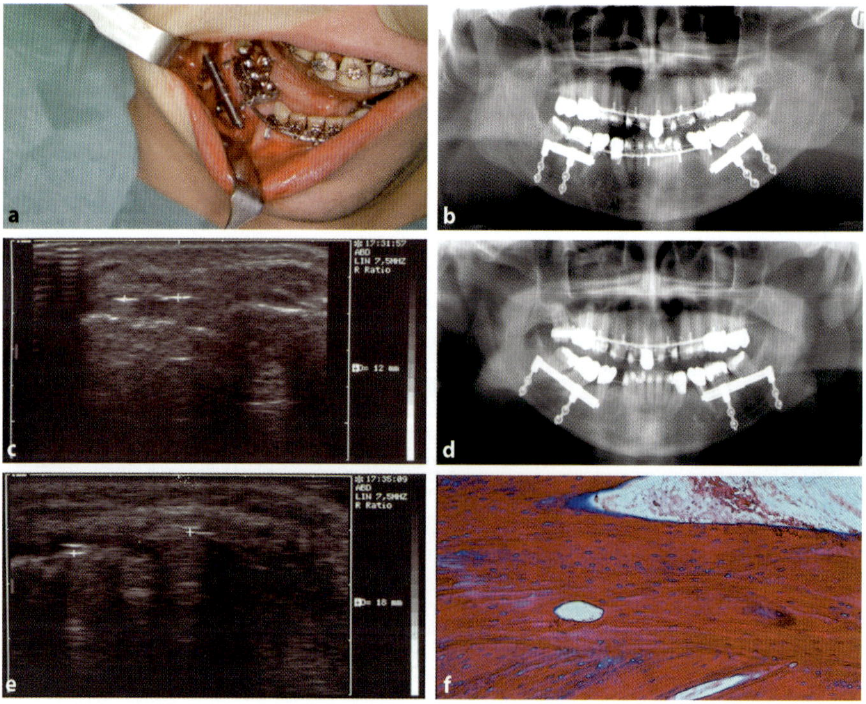

Fig. 3.5. Distraction osteogenesis. **a** Intraoperative view. **b** Radiograph and **c** ultrasound at the beginning of distraction. **d** Radiograph and **e** ultrasound at the end of distraction. **f** Histological appearance of the regenerated tissue

Biomolecules used to augment bone cell reaction

- Transforming growth factor beta (TGFß)
- Bone morphogenic proteins (BMPs)
- Insulin-like growth factors (IGFs)
- Platelet-derived growth factors (PDGFs)
- Fibroblast growth factors (FGFs).

It was suggested that bone reconstruction may be accomplished using various bioactive factors with varying potency and efficacy (Stevenson and Horowitz, 1992). Members of the TGF-ß superfamily and other growth factors, notably BMP, IGF, PDGF, and GDF are currently being tested for experimental use to engineer new bone. Evidence from a variety of studies indicates that exposure to osteoinductive growth factors can promote new bone formation (Hogan, 1996). Different healing environments require different types of bone tissue to be engineered. For example, a segmental long bone defect requires primarily cortical bone to be formed, whereas a maxillary alveolar crest augmentation requires primarily membranous (cancellous) bone. It is possible that different cascades of signalling molecules orchestrate these two healing processes. Alternatively, the same factors may be involved but have different outcomes because of the different mechanical environments or different host cell populations. It should be considered that different osteoinductive growth factors have a range of biological potencies and with increased efficacy comes increased cost and often increased risk. There are currently three strategies for delivery of osteoinductive growth factors, which are at various stages of development. The first strategy involves extracting and partially purifying a mixture of proteins from animal or human cortical bone, as described by Urist (1965) and Urist and Strates for BMPs (1971). The second strategy involves the use of recombinant proteins (e.g. rhBMPs), which was enabled by the cloning and sequencing of many of these genes (Wozney et al., 1988; Ozkaynak et al., 1990). The third and least developed strategy is that of gene therapy, which involves delivery of the DNA encoding a growth factor rather than delivery of the protein itself (Fang et al., 1996; Boden et al., 1998; Lieberman et al., 1998). It is also likely that there will not be one best strategy or one best growth factor and that success in the end may be determined by such factors as manufacturing cost and ease of use by the treating physicians or the flexibility to adapt to different bone tissue engineering environmental requirements. Regardless of the specific growth factor chosen, there are several common issues that, while unsolved, may place potential clinical limitations on all of the above strategies. These factors include dose, carrier, patient variability and confounding clinical factors.

Various donor sites allow the grafting of different types and amounts of bone. The use of autologous bone is accompanied by a grafting procedure and can be accompanied by donor site morbidity. Different surgical methods (Fig. 3.6) allow one to graft bone-forming tissue in the form of:

- Periosteal flaps
- Cancellous bone chips
- Cortical bone chips
- Bulk cortico-spongiosal grafts
- Vascularised bone.

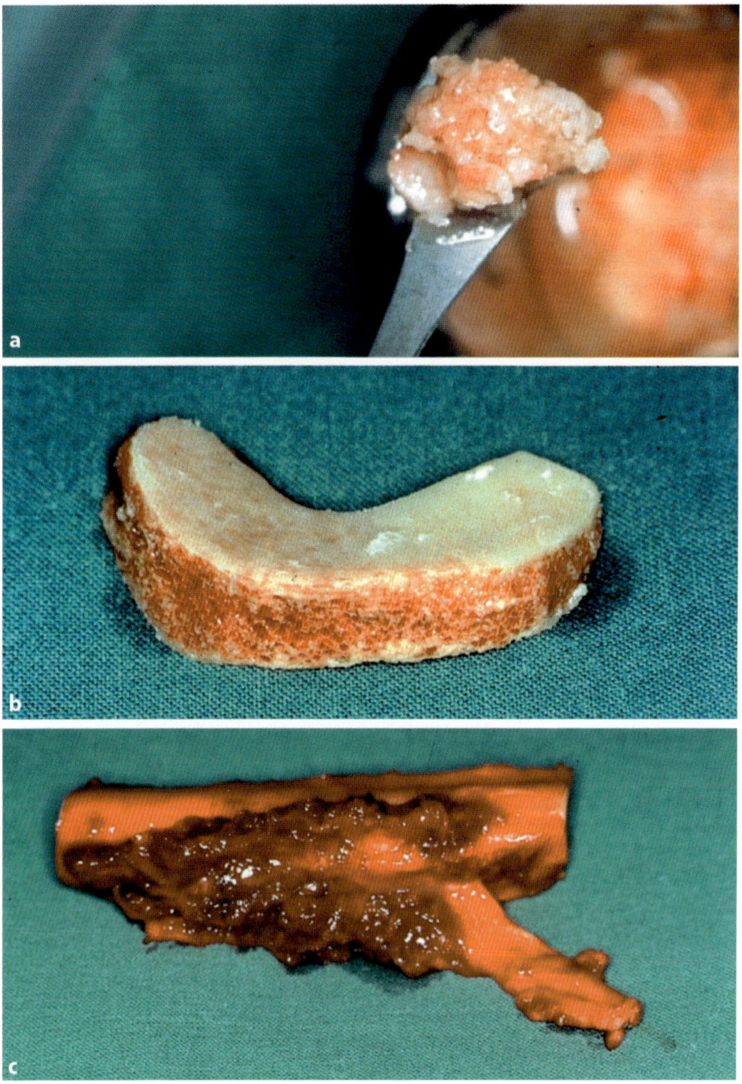

Fig. 3.6. Different methods for bone reconstruction. **a** Cancellous bone. **b** Cortical bone. **c** Microvascular fibular flap

Small bone defects can be treated with small bone grafts (periosteal flaps, cancellous or cortical bone chips) provided local conditions are appropriate for bone healing. Endochondral bone from the ilium, tibia or rib can be harvested as well as membranous bone from the facial skeleton. Animal studies indicate that membranous bone is less prone to resorption than endochondral bone (Zins and Whitaker, 1983). However, when the bone defect is large, bulk cortico-spongiosal grafts are necessary. Effective rigid fixation of the graft facilitates graft survival and hematomas should be avoided. Problems with conventional grafts include their susceptibility to infection, the unknown survival of transplanted cells and the unpredictable degree of resorption. The extent of resorption is dependent on the graft volume, the delay time before loading and the condition of the transplant bed.

A major improvement in bone reconstruction strategies was afforded by the use of vascularised bone tissue in combination with or without adjacent soft tissue (muscle, subdermal tissue, skin). The soft tissue of the flap can be used to obliterate the defect space to the desired extent, to prevent infection and to allow a better barrier against direct surface loads. Bone reconstruction by vascularised bone can be achieved through pedicled flaps or microvascular flaps. Several pedicled osteocutaneous or osteomuscular flaps have been established in clinical routine (Conley, 1972): sternocleidomastoid muscle combined with the clavicle (Siemssen et al., 1978), trapezius muscle with parts of the scapula (Demergasso and Piazza, 1979; Panje and Cutting, 1980; Guillamondegui and Larson, 1981), pectoralis muscle with part of a rib or sternum (Cuono and Ariyan, 1980; Green et al., 1981; Lam et al., 1984), latissimus dorsi osteomyocutaneous flap (Maruyama et al., 1985) and the temporalis muscle with calvarian bone (McCarthy and Zide, 1984; McCarthy et al., 1987; Rose and Norris, 1990). Free vascularised bone grafts provide the best possibility for reconstruction of large bone defects. Sufficient bone material with good quality cortico-cancellous bone can be harvested for use in reconstruction of large bone defects. A soft tissue paddle can be harvested together with the vascularised bone, as, for example, an osteocutaneous flap. The iliac crest (Taylor, 1982; Shenaq, 1988), the fibula (Taylor et al., 1975; Wei et al., 1986; 1994; Hidalgo, 1989) and the scapula (dos Santos, 1984; Swartz et al., 1986; Baker, 1989; Granick et al., 1990) are all well- /established donor sites from where a large amount of bone can be grafted (Frodel et al., 1993). This type of bone reconstruction combines the advantage of enlarging bone transplants while maintaining the nutritional needs of cells. In current clinical practice this technique overcomes the limitations of other approaches (free non-vascularised bone graft transfer, tissue engineered constructs) when large defects need to be reconstructed. The main disadvantage of free vascularised grafts is donor site morbidity, especially when large grafts are necessary.

3.2 Cartilage Repair Strategies

Most cartilage repair strategies have focused on healing articular cartilage, since this type of cartilage is the one most commonly diseased (Fig. 3.7), it is of special importance for an undisturbed joint function, and its disturbed function has a high socioeconomic impact. Various procedures have been introduced to induce the healing of histological and macroscopical lesions within mature articular cartilage in order to re-establish a structurally and functionally competent joint (Fig. 3.8).

Due to the multitude of pathogenical disturbances and based on the anatomy of cartilage joint, attempts to heal articular cartilage lesions span the whole range from symptomatic measures to extensive surgical interventions. There are two distinct goals for cartilage reconstruction. The first is the immediate need for clinical pain relief and restoration of joint function. The second goal is to prevent or at least delay the onset of arthritis. From a practical perspective, the current objective of articular cartilage repair is to delay joint replacement for a clinically significant

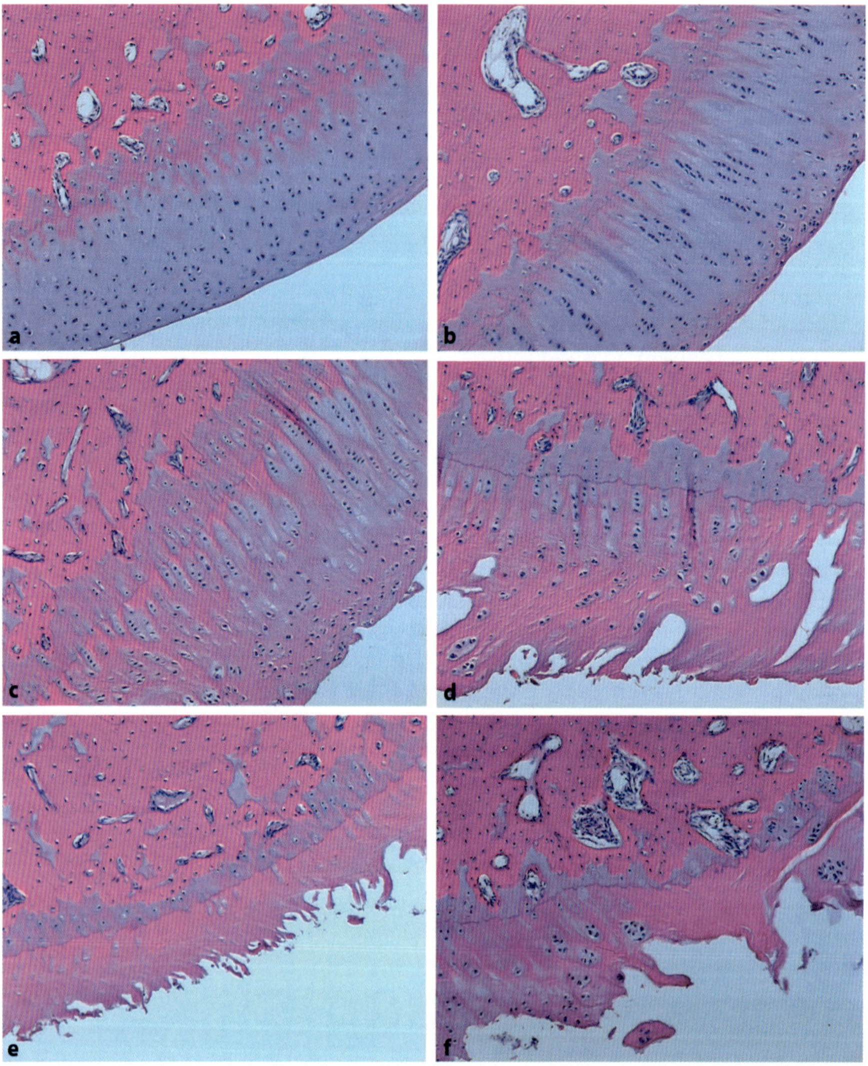

Fig. 3.7. Different states of chondroarthrosis. **a** Healthy cartilage layer. **b** Alteration of the superficial zone. **c** Destruction of the superficial zone accompanied by disturbance of deeper cartilage layers. **d** Destruction of cartilage down to the calcified cartilage layer. **e** Thinning of the cartilage layer. **f** Severe destruction of the basal cartilage zones

period (Reinholz et al., 2004). Besides non-surgical therapies that are based on the administration of drugs and biologicals, surgical options play a significant role, to provide pain relief, to restore joint functionality, and to prevent progression of joint destruction. In some instances drastic measures like total joint replacement by artificial materials are necessary to achieve clinical success. Most of the experimental and clinical attempts that have been made to restore articular cartilage structure aim at re-establishment of biomechanically competent tissue of an enduring nature. The

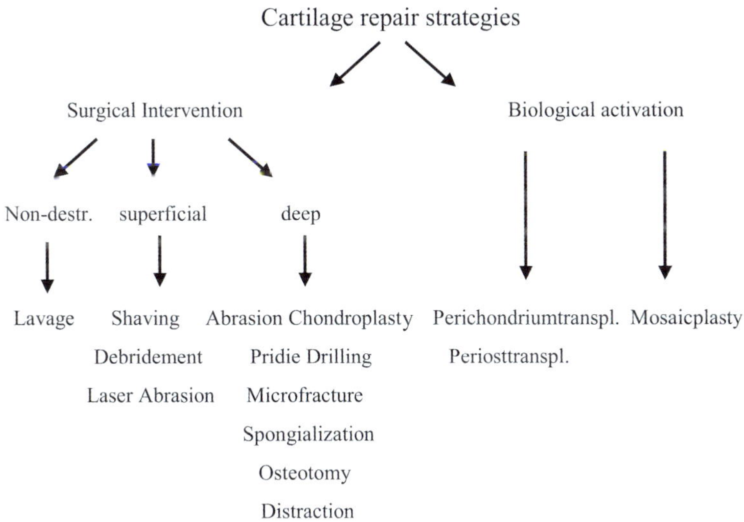

Fig. 3.8. Cartilage repair strategies

spontaneous repair response forms the basis and the rationale behind the surgical interventions. Unfortunately, when cartilage is damaged due to injury or disease, it has a limited capacity to heal (for a review, see Guilak et al., 2004). Articular defects larger than 2–4 mm in diameter rarely heal, even with continuous passive motion, due to the fact that adult articular cartilage contains no blood supply, neural network or lymphatic drainage. As a result, partial-thickness defects that do not reach the subchondral bone stimulate only a transient induction of cartilage repair (Reinholz et al., 2004). Since the physiological process of spontaneous repair is limited, new therapies are aimed at overcoming the biological restrictions on cartilage repair. As indicated in Chap. 2, different repair mechanisms are present in cartilage repair. It has been known for decades that large superficial lesions of cartilage tissue do not heal spontaneously. In contrast, once the bone and bone marrow spaces are involved, bleeding and hematoma formation start a repair cascade that leads to repair tissue formation. However, the resulting heterogenous repair tissue composition, which consists of a mixture of hyaline- and fibro-cartilage, contributes to an inferior biomechanical competence. Thus, histogenesis of the defect repair depends to a large extent on the defect size.

Therapeutical measures to improve joint structure and function without the use of biologically active substances can be conceptualised as methods to improve the condition of the joint fluids (lavage), to mechanically remove diseased or necrotic superficial chondral tissue (shaving, debridement, laser abrasion) and to gain access to the subchondral bone (abrasion chondroplasty, pridie drilling, microfracture techniques and spongialisation). The underlying reason for lavage or debridement is the removal of inflamed or diseased tissue, whereas gaining access to subchondral bone is aimed at initiating a spontaneous healing response. Arthroscopic lavage and debridement are often used to alleviate joint pain (Fig. 3.9). Lavage is mainly performed by arthroscopy. Through arthroscopy, debris may be removed from the joint space thereby alleviating pain. Both procedures routinely used to alleviate joint pain have been shown to be successful in treating early stages of osteoarthritis. It is important to consider, that both lavage and debridement do not induce repair of articular cartilage. A recent study has demonstrated that pain relief observed following debridement and lavage procedures may be no more than a placebo effect following surgery (Redman et al., 2005).

The provocation of bleeding from subchondral bone spaces and subsequent blood-clot formation has become a common therapy in cartilage surgery to induce spontaneous cartilage repair. Extensive surgical interventions like osteotomies or joint distractions are procedures for complex joint disturbances that exploit skeletal load transfers in cases of joint malposition. Despite the reported success rates, these invasive surgical options are reserved for severe joint diseases and are more beneficial if they are intended to correct malpositioning.

The use of cell-containing devices is performed by different measures. Transplants from either autologic or allogenic origin can be harvested in the form of perichondrial or periosteal tissue and as a bulk osteochondral part. Perichondrial or periosteal autotransplantation as a single procedure has been exploited in a variety of protocols elaborated for the treatment of articular cartilage defects. Other tissue engineering concepts such as autologous chondrocyte transplantation use a periosteal flap to cover the cell-filled defect in order to avoid the disappearance of injected cells. The basic biological principle behind the use of these transplants is the fact

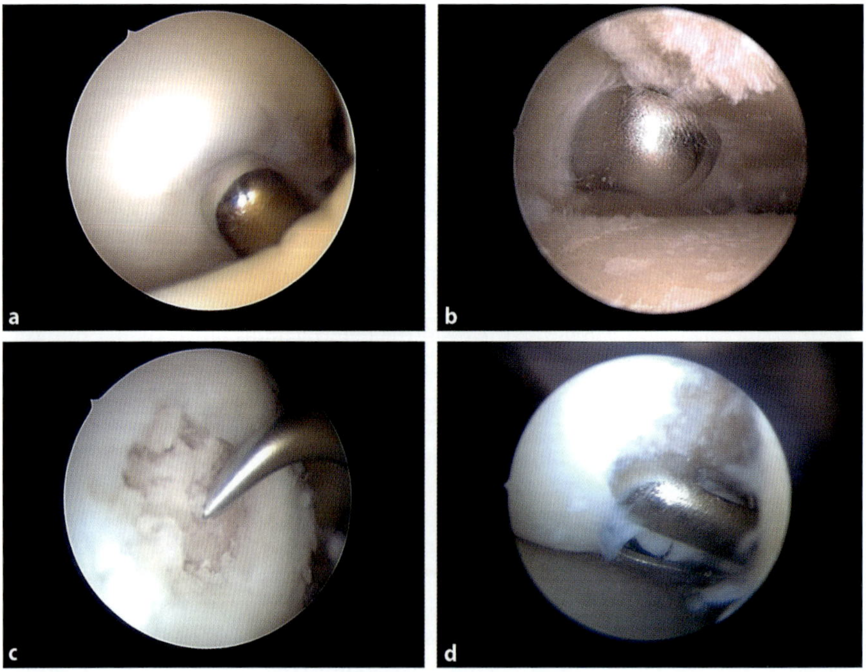

Fig. 3.9. Endoscopical images of cartilage defect treatment in different situations in human knee. **a** Lavage. **b**, **d** Debridement. **c** Microfracturing

that perichondrial as well as periosteal tissue contains cells that possess a life-long chondrogenic or osteogenic activity. A pool of precursor or adult-type stem cells are assumed to be present in these tissues that render self-renewable capacity and are able to induce tissue healing. Whereas experimental in vitro and in vivo studies have demonstrated cartilage tissue formation, complete defect filling was only seldom reported. In most cases, however, the use of this treatment strategy did not lead to a complete restitution of hyaline cartilage layer, because it is commonly accompanied by a long-term mechanical instability of the newly formed tissue.

Implantation of chondral or osteochondral tissue (mosaicplasty) is routinely used in joint and bone surgery to repair chondral or osteochondral defects (Fig. 3.10). Experimental studies revealed that graft material persisted for a short time, however, long-term effects have not been extensively evaluated. It was demonstrated by ret-

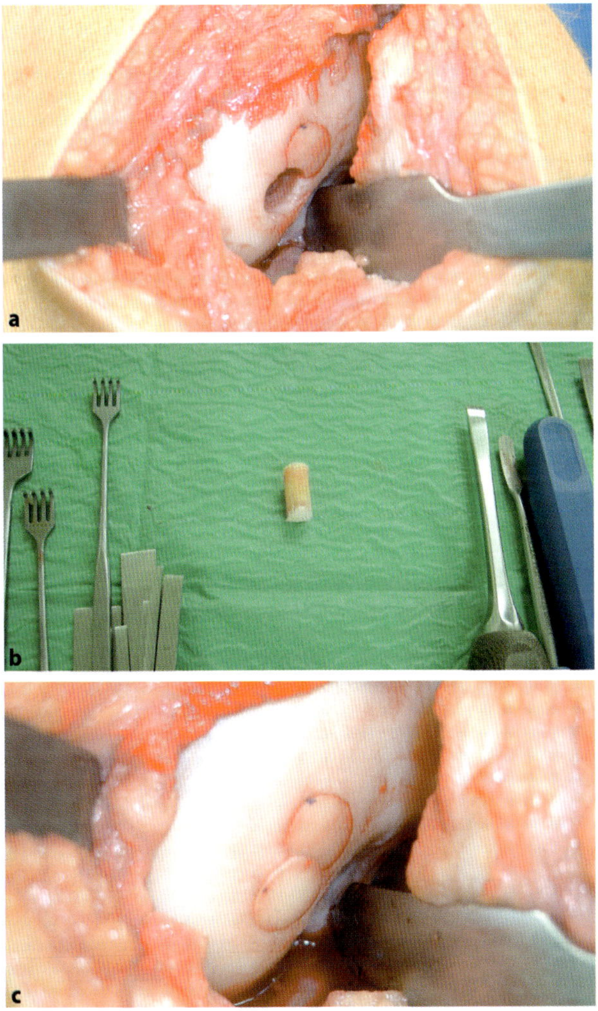

Fig. 3.10. Intraoperative views of a mosaic plasty procedure in the knee joint

rospective studies that clinical outcomes were acceptable in the sense of improved joint functionality and pain relief. Despite short-term clinical success, the use of autografts has a number of disadvantages. The donor site may experience severe morbidity since the explantation site will lose as much chondral or osteochondral tissue as the diseased implantation site will gain. Additionally, the surgical procedure to obtain the tissue is known to be accompanied by a loss of cells and matrix components at the transplant borders. Most important perhaps is the aspect that the translocation of tissue from a commonly used low-weight-bearing cartilage area to a weight-bearing-area (often accompanied by an incongruence between joint surfaces) may lead to overload- /induced degeneration of the transplant. The collateral damage to joint tissue and the problems inherent to this kind of tissue transfer are the main limitations on this autotransplantation technique.

The use of allogenic osteochondral grafts is another measure to substitute failed or lost cartilage tissue. The simplicity of filling cartilage defects with allogenic material retrieved from cadavers has made this therapy a common treatment option. In contrast to the relative ease of gaining grafts, immunologic barriers limit the use of allografts. Experimental investigations have revealed that allogenic tissue transplants survive longer under immunosuppression or when better histocompatibilty between the donor tissue and the host tissue is present. Immunologic reactions in humans have been reported not to be extensive, maybe based on the fact that cartilage is considered to occupy an immunologically privileged position within the joint. The kind of allogenic specimen preparation (fresh, cryopreserved, lyophilised) influences the clinical repair process. Fresh tissue possesses improved structural and mechanical competence as well as a longer life span compared to cryopreserved or lyophilised material, but transplantation of fresh tissue has an increased risk of transmitting diseases of the donor. Both, cryopreservation and lyophilisation techniques result in a limited biological activity and mechanical competence, since these techniques are prone to cause the death of chondrocytes. Despite these limitations, allogenic tissue transplantation is an established procedure, especially for patients with large osteochondral defects.

Autologous chondrocyte transplantation (ACT) is a recently established technique to treat cartilage defects. The use of single cells (chondrocytes multiplied in monolayers) for the restoration of tissue defects meets the US definition of tissue engineering but is not covered by the European definition, since this technique is devoid of a scaffold. Further developments of this technique (coating scaffolds with chondro-cytes, multilayer growth, scaffold-free chondrospheres) clearly fulfil the criteria of an ex vivo grown cartilage tissue. More details on this technique will be described in this and following chapters.

Articular chondrocytes are responsible for the unique features of articular cartilage; therefore, it seems rational to use committed chondrocytes to repair a cartilaginous defect. From arthroscopically harvested cartilage, chondrocytes can be isolated by enzymatic digestion and expanded in culture to 20–50 times the initial number of cells (Wei and Messner, 1999). Cells can be cultured in monolayers with serum supplementation in the culture media and during that time, the cells commence to dedifferentiate. The dedifferentiated chondrocytes share features of primitive mesenchymal cells and on implantation at high density the in vitro expanded primitive immature chondrocytes imitate prechondrogeneic cell condensation and cartilage formation (Brittberg, 1996; 1999). It was shown that in embryo-derived undifferentiated cells, a reduced rate of cell clustering and number of cell-to-cell contacts indicates a reduced number of cells that differentiate (Tacchetti et al., 1992). It was therefore suggested that there is a cascade of events, important in the early stages of chondrocyte differentiation, that consist of the acquisition of the ability to establish the cell to cell contacts, to form a permissive environment capable of starting the differentiation and to express differentiation markers. Furthermore, in an in vitro experiment with chondrocytes directly seeded to cartilage explants, the biosynthetic activity increased with the number of seeded chondrocytes, indicating how important the number of seeded cells is for the success of implantation (Chen et al., 1997). It was demonstrated that a high proportion of synthesised proteoglycan could be lost to the medium after cell seeding, which suggests that at least early in the culture an overlying membrane is important (Chen et al., 1997). In the clinical use of in vitro expanded autologous chondrocytes for cartilage repair the aim is to have an adequate number of expanded cells to implant and an overlying membrane to avoid cell and matrix loss. Brittberg et al. (1994) successfully reported autologous chondrocyte implantation using a monolayer culture system to treat cartilage defects. In this procedure, harvested autologous chondrocytes, expanded in a monolayer culture system, were transplanted to an osteochondral lesion, which was covered by a periosteal flap. This initial report had a high impact on cartilage surgery and was regarded as a breakthrough for cell-based cartilage repair strategies. The United States Food and Drug Administration approved in 1997 cell technology that uses the patient's own chondrocytes to repair cartilage injuries in the knee (Hauselmann et al., 1998). This was the first type of cell technology that was regulated by industry for use in expanding autologous cells for human transplantation. In the USA and Europe, cell processing in a monolayer culture is now being carried out on a commercial basis. An international autologous chondrocyte implantation study was initiated by Genzyme Tissue Repair to evaluate the clinical success of ACT. The study, monitored by a Registry Advisory Board and presenting 12 months of data on 249 patients and 24 months of data on 50 patients, revealed an overall significant improvement in patient and clinical scores from baseline scores through the ACT procedure (Mandelbaum et al., 1998).

In contrast to the clinical outcome rates, limited information is available on the histogenesis of cell-driven human repair tissue. Biopsy specimens from grafted areas in individuals obtained after autologous chondrocyte transplantation indicate that the ACT procedure helps to build up a tissue with hyaline and fibrocartilage-like features (Richardson et al., 1999; Peterson et al., 2000). Transarthroscopic biopsy specimens obtained from grafted areas demonstrated, in general, heterogeneity throughout the repair tissue (Richardson et al., 1999; Peterson et al., 2000). Although beneficial short- or middle-term clinical results were reported (Peterson et al., 2000; Minas, 2001), the ACT procedure has potential disadvantages, such as the risk of leakage of transplanted chondrocytes from the cartilage defects and an uneven distribution of chondrocytes in the transplanted site (Sohn et al., 2002). These limitations explain to some extent the finding of heterogenous tissue formation in the defect site. To overcome these limitations, further developments are focusing on the ex vivo growth of a three-dimensional cartilage-like tissue, which integrates intimately in the defect site after being implanted.

3.2.1 Flap Prefabrication

Flap prefabrication is one of the most exciting areas in reconstructive surgery because of its bridging role between conventional reconstructive surgery and tissue engineering (Tan et al., 2004). This new and exciting approach gained major public interest after Vacanti and colleagues fabricated a human ear on a mouse back (Cao et al., 1997). Using prefabrication technique, tissues such as bone or cartilage can be pre-assembled to form composite tissues that can fit even major defect sites. Prefabrication can expand the versatility of a graft. Existing organs can be transformed into a transplantable state, or completely new organs can be created. In its simple form, e.g. pre-lamination, a new tissue can be created by burying cartilage, bone, skin or mucosa underneath a fascia or in a muscle pouch, and later can be harvested as a composite tissue free flap to replace lost tissue (Alam et al., 2003; Jaquiery et al., 2004; Keser et al., 2004; Schultze-Mosgau et al., 2004; Staudenmaier et al., 2004; Tan et al., 2004; Terheyden et al., 2004; The Hoang et al., 2005; Top et al., 2005). Vascular induction is another approach in which new blood supply is generated in tissue to improve the survival of the transplanted construct. It was shown that bone chips wrapped in a vascular carrier such as muscular tissue became vascularised grafts (Fischer and Wood, 1987). The future of flap prefabrication can be envisioned to generate complex vascularised tissues in desired external shapes that mimic the defect to be replaced. The basis of such approaches may be the use of suitable vascular carriers, resorbable matrix components, attached cytokines, and incorporated cells. It was shown by various investigators that prefabrication can be started ex vivo and then transferred to the in vivo situation (Findlay et al., 2003), but can also be used solely in vivo. Warnke et al. (2004), for example, demonstrated the growth and transplantation of a custom vascularised bone graft in a man. The use of such complex tissue engineering strategies demonstrates the general feasibility of applying these therapies in humans, but problems with these therapy options have to be solved in detail before they can be used as routine treatment options.

3.3 Extracorporal Strategies

Extracorporal tissue engineering in the narrower (EU) definition of bone and cartilage engineering requires not only living cells, but additionally the interaction of three biological components: bone cells, the extracellular scaffolds, and in some instances, growth factors. To engineer living tissues in vitro, cultured cells are commonly grown on two-dimensional or three-dimensional bioactive degradable biomaterials that provide the physical and chemical basis to guide their proliferation and differentiation. In bioreactors outside the body the biomaterial is assembled as a complex three-dimensional construct. New approaches in extracorporal tissue engineering strategies are aimed at fabricating scaffold-free three-dimensional micro-tissue constructs. The technique of micro-tissue formation is described in detail in Chap. 9. Additionally, the use of biomolecules seems not to be dispensable since the cells themselves may be stimulated to synthesise some of the needed biomolecules in an autocrine fashion. The assembly of cells into tissue substitutes is a highly orchestrated set of events that requires time scales ranging from seconds to weeks, and dimensions ranging from 0.0001 to 10 cm. At the moment the techniques are moving from an experimental stage to the level of clinical application. In the following chapters we will consider bone and cartilage tissue engineering as a new approach to generating extracorporally, cell-containing artificial materials designed as substitutes and implants for reconstructive surgery. Cell/scaffold-based approaches for tissue engineering of bone and cartilage offer perspectives on future treatment concepts. The skeletal system contains a variety of different cell types: vascular cells, bone marrow cells, pre-osteoblasts, osteocytes, chondroblasts, chondrocytes and osteoclasts, all executing distinct cellular functions to allow the skeleton to work as a highly dynamic, load bearing organ. Whereas all these cells are necessary to build up a real skeleton, limited cell sources are regarded to be sufficient for engineering a bone-like or cartilage-like construct in vitro.

Cell Development, Cell Sources 4

4.1 Cell Development

The skeletal tissue contains various types of mesenchymal cells, such as osteoblasts, osteocytes, chondroblasts, chondrocytes, myoblasts, adipocytes and bone marrow stromal cells. Every cell of the skeletal system, responsible for the regulated synthesis and deposition of extracellular matrix, is necessary to build up a real substitute tissue. The orchestrated work of the different cell types enables the skeleton to perform its unique function. To extracorporally fabricate a bone- or cartilage-like tissue, different cell sources and different cell types are principally suited to tissue-like substitution. The different cell lineages are believed to originate from common progenitors (Taylor and Jones, 1979; Grigoriadis et al., 1988; Owen, 1988; Caplan, 1991; Yamaguchi and Kahn, 1991; Aubin and Liu, 1996; Pittenger et al., 1999) called pluripotent stem cells (Owen, 1988; Caplan, 1991; Pittenger et al., 1999). These progenitor cells acquire specific phenotypes depending on their maturation during differentiation. Stem cells and mesenchymal precursors arise in the embryo and at least some of these appear to persist in the adult organism, where they contribute to the replacement of lost cells in skeletal tissue remodelling and repair. In addition to haematopoietic stem cells, the bone marrow comprises a population of marrow stromal cells or mesenchymal stem cells (MSCs). Mesenchymal stem cells serve as the major reservoir for different classes of stem cells. Stromal cells have multilineage differentiation capacity, thereby generating progenitors with restricted developmental potential, such as fibroblasts, osteoblasts, chondrocytes and adipocyte progenitors (Caplan, 1991; Pittenger et al., 1999) (Fig. 4.1). Maturation of cells happens through stages of proliferation, commitment, progression and differentiation in the organism in order to generate the various tissues (Fig. 4.2). As described in Chap. 2, various hormones and cytokines regulate the fate of the cell during the differentiation process from progenitor cells to mature cells. Among these, members of the transforming growth factor family are the most potent inducers and stimulators of osteogenic and chondrogenic differentiation. For bone development, BMPs as classical examples, not only stimulate osteoprogenitors to differentiate into mature osteoblasts but also induce non-osteogenic cells to differentiate into osteoblast lineage cells (for a review, see Kale and Long, 2000). Other factors (dexamethasone, prostaglandines) also play important roles in the regulation of osteoblast differentiation in an orchestrated way. In this context, it is important to note that molecules of the TGF-β and BMP superfamily are also main regulators of differentiation of stem and precursor cells towards chondrocytes. This is an indication of the complex situation of cell differentiation induction.

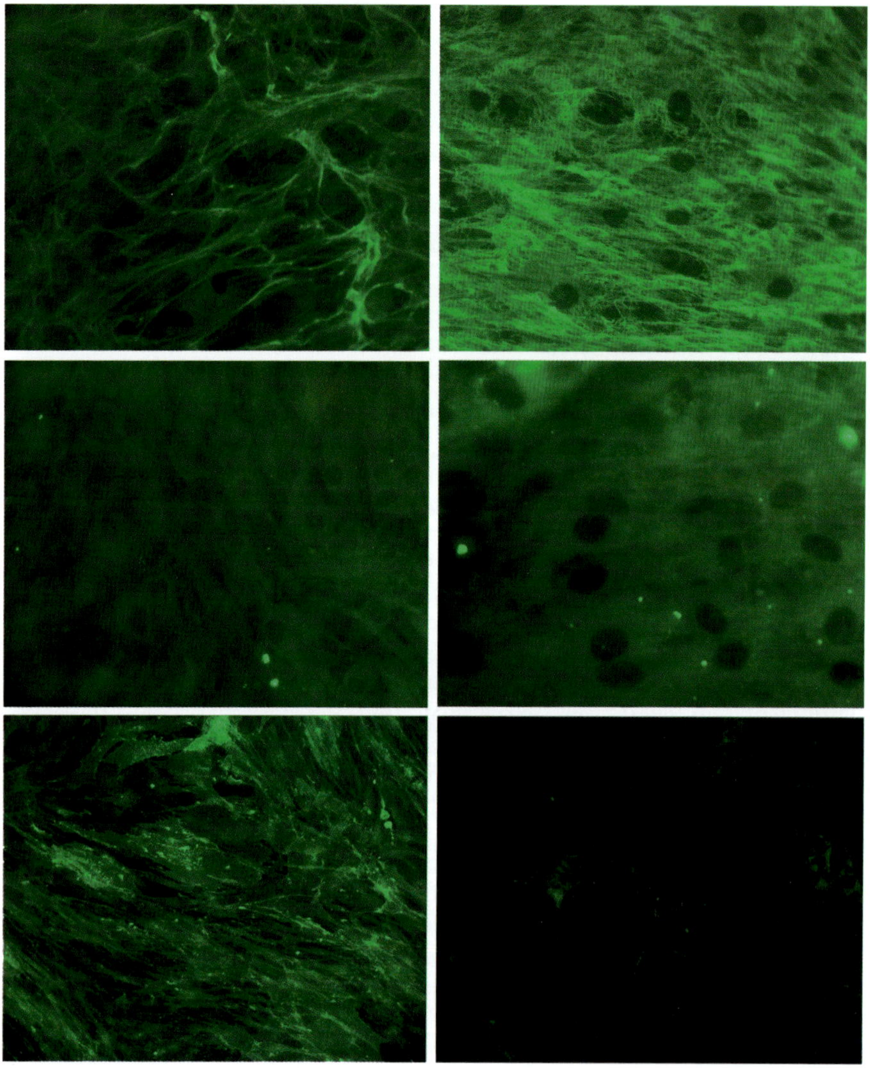

Fig. 4.1. Fluorescent staining of mesenchymal stem cells differentiated to osteoblasts, collagen type I (*top left*), fibronectin (*top right*), osteonectin (*midline left*), bone sialoprotein (*midline right*). For a significant characterisation of the osteoblast differentiation a combination of typical osteoblast and stem cell markers are necessary. For example, stem cells show a positive CD90 signal (*bottom left*) but differentiated osteoblast show no CD90 expression

4.2 Cell Sources

Principal sources of cells for tissue engineering include beneath xenogenic cells, autologous and allogeneic cells (Table 4.1). Each category can be subdivided according to whether the cells are stem cells (embryonic or adult) or whether the cells are in a more differentiated stage (Fig. 4.3). Various mature cell lines as well as multipo-

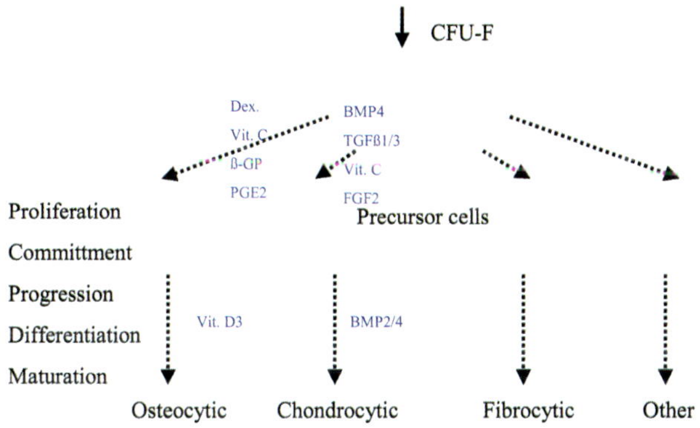

Fig. 4.2. Cell development pathways

Table 4.1. Principal cell sources used in tissue engineering studies

Experimental studies	Preclinical studies	Clinical studies
– Autologous – Allogeneic – Xenogeneic – Immortalised – Non-transformed clonal – Sarcoma	– Autologous – Allogeneic – Xenogeneic	– Autologous

tent mesenchymal progenitors have been successfully established (Yamaguchi et al., 2002) in bone and cartilage tissue engineering approaches. Additionally, other bone and cartilage cell lines like genetically altered cell lines (sarcoma cells, immortalised cells, non-transformed clonal cell lines) have been developed and used to evaluate basic aspects of in vitro cell behaviour in non-human settings.

The stem cell of skeletal tissue is a hypothetical concept with only circumstantial evidence for its existence, and indeed, there seems to be a hierarchy of stem cells each with variable self-renewal potentials (for a review, see Triffitt, 2002). Embryonic and adult stem cells can be distinguished. Embryonic stem cells reside in blastocysts. They were first isolated and grown in culture more than 20 years ago (Martin, 1981). The primitive stem cells renewing skeletal structures have been given a variety of names including connective tissue stem cells, osteogenic cells (Ham, 1969), stromal stem cells (Owen, 1988), stromal fibroblastic cells (Weinberg and Bell, 1986), and mesenchymal stem cells (Caplan, 1991). No nomenclature is entirely accurate based upon the developmental origins or differentiation capacities of these cells, but the latter term, although defective, appears to be in favour at the moment. Stem cells have the capacity for extensive replication without differentiation, and they possess, as mentioned, a multilineage developmental potential allowing them to give rise to not only bone and cartilage, but tendon, muscle, fat, and marrow stroma. This expansion of properties makes stem cells, whether derived from the hematopoetic system (HSCs) or marrow (MSCs), a very interesting source of cells for tissue engineering of bone and cartilage.

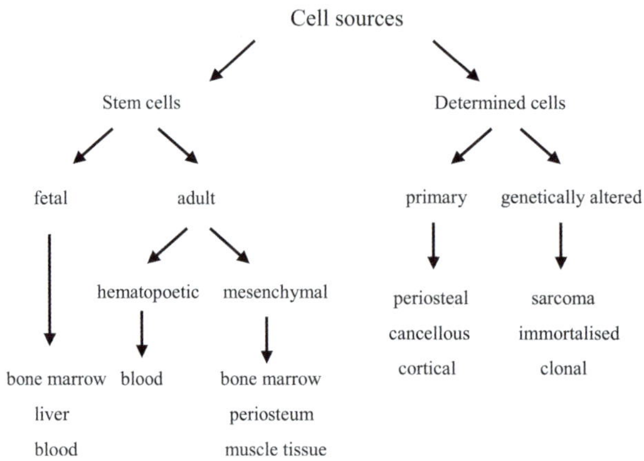

Fig. 4.3. Cell development pathways

Differentiated Phenotypes Derived from MSCs

- Fibroblast
- Osteoblast
- Chondrocyte
- Adipocyte
- Skeletal myocyte
- Cardiac myocyte
- Myofibroblast
- Endothelial cell
- Pericyte
- Tenocyte
- Thymic stromacell

MSCs are present in fetal tissue, post-natal bone marrow and also in the bone marrow of adults (Caplan, 1991). A number of markers are expressed on MSCs. Some of these have been used not only to characterise these cells but also to enrich MSCs from populations of adherent bone marrow stromal cells. However, none of these markers seem to be specific for MSCs. Although the bone marrow serves as the primary reservoir for MSCs, their presence has also been reported in a variety of other tissues (periosteum, muscle connective tissue (Nathanson, 1985; Nakahara et al., 1991), fetal bone marrow, liver, and blood (Campagnoli et al., 2001)). Transfer of these tissues (e.g. coverage of cartilage defects by periosteum) may act also through stem cell-induced repair mechanisms. Whereas MSCs have been identified in fetal blood (Campagnoli et al., 2001) and infrequently observed in umbilical cord blood (Erices et al., 2000; Gutierrez-Rodriguez et al., 2000; Mareschi et al., 2001), it is not definitively solved whether MSCs are present in steady state peripheral blood of adults or not, but the number of stem cells in peripheral blood is probably extremely low (Zvaifler et al., 2000).

A main problem in using adult stem cells in a given clinical situation is the difficulty in obtaining a significant number of stem cells to generate cell constructs of large size. Limitations of adult stem cell harvesting have therefore given rise to the use of fetal stem cells, particularly on fetal bone marrow cells (FBM). This cell source seems to be a promising source for tissue engineering approaches, since they have a significantly reduced immunogenity, compared to adult stem cells. In contrast to adult tissues, fetal tissues produce more abundant trophic substances and growth factors, which promote to a greater extent cell growth and differentiation. Research on fetal tissue transfer in animal models and in human experimental treatments have confirmed distinct advantages over adult tissues, including lowered immunogenicity and a higher percentage of primitive cells. Due to the lowered immunogenity, fetus-derived stem cells appear to remove, to some extent, the problems of tissue typing. As such cells also have a high capacity to differentiate into the complete repertoire of mesenchymal cell lineages, combined with the ability for rapid cellular growth, differentiation and re-assembly, fetal cells may become a more important subject in tissue engineering strategies. (Fig 4.4) Fetal stem cells have, beneath their enormous potential for biomedical and tissue engineering applications, some serious limitations. There is a lack of methods that enable tissue engineers to direct the differentiation of embryonic stem cells and to induce specific functions of the embryonic cell-generated tissue after transplantation (Wobus, 2001). Two other issues are of main concern (Wobus, 2001). (1) It must be assured that the cultivation and transplantation of such stem cells are not accompanied by a tumorigenic differentiation. As it was shown that undifferentiated ES cells give rise to teratomas and teratocarcinomas after implantation in animals, this potential misdevelopment constitutes a major problem for the clinical use of such cells. (2) It must be assured that the in vitro generation of cells does not lead to an immunological incompatibility towards the host tissue. Immunological incompatibilities can be avoided by using the somatic cell nuclear transfer methodology (SCNT) (Alison et al., 2002). However, nuclear cloning methods are often criticised for this potential risk. The main problem in employing fetal cells for use in tissue engineering is not only obtaining such cells, but perhaps more important, the clinical, legal and ethical issues involved in such treatment strategies, which are probably the most difficult barrier to overcome (see Chap. 12).

Many attemps have been undertaken to refine procedures for the propagation and differentiation of stem cells. Despite the various advantages of using tissue-de-

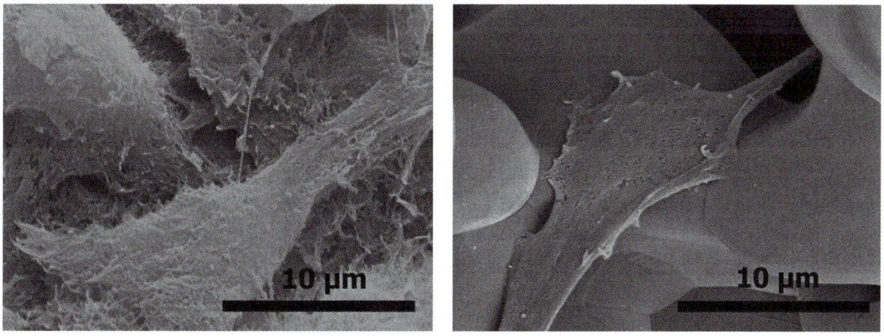

Fig. 4.4. Fetal stem cell-based tissue engineering. Fetal stem cell cultured under defined conditions on an artificial material display the phenotypic appearance of mature bone cells. a Scanning electron microscopical picture of osteoblasts at the surface of a bone trabecula. b SEM view of a murine fetal stem cell cultured on a PLA/PGA scaffold

Immortalisation of primary human chondrocytes has been done with SV40-TAg, HPV-16 E6/E7, and telomerase by retrovirally mediated transduction, and selection for neomycin resistance are described. It was observed that stable integration of an immortalising gene stabilises proliferative capacity, but not the differentiated chondrocyte phenotype.

Harvesting and Cultivation

5

In order to obtain well-defined ex vivo multiplied cells, it is important to consider the various aspects of cell-based tissue engineering strategies. These aspects include the techniques used to harvest cells, the methods used to isolate and enrich cells, the standard conditions used for cell cultivation, and the methods used to screen cell culture outcomes. The parameters differ dependent on the cell source used for the tissue engineering approach.

5.1 Marrow-derived Stem Cells

Bone/marrow-derived stem cells are commonly obtained through a marrow aspiration procedure. Common locations to harvest bone marrow are the iliac crest and the sternum. (Bruder et al., 1997; Jaiswal et al., 1997; Joyner et al., 1997; Meyer et al., 1998; Bianco et al, 2001). In the first attempts to create tissue-engineered bone, unfractioned fresh autologous or syngeneic bone marrow was used (Ohgushi and Caplan, 1999; Grundel et al., 1991; Wolff et al., 1994). Because bone marrow is known to contain osteogenic and chondrogenic precursor cells, its use was perceived to potentially facilitate bone and cartilage regeneration. Principally, mesenchymal stem cells (MSCs) were harvested for these investigations by marrow aspiration, expanded in culture, and then re-implanted. Studies using this protocol have indicated that mouse marrow fibroblastic cells, obtained through the aspiration procedure, implanted locally or injected systemically, homed to bony sites and persisted there, participating in the regenerative processes (Perka et al., 2000; Wiesmann et al., 2003). Various investigations have used different methods to selectively isolate and enrich MSCs (Jackson et al., 1981; Ogushi et al., 1989a; 1989b). Isolation of MSCs is commonly based on density gradient centrifugation and cell culture techniques. Various cell culture techniques have been developed to allow MSCs to be cultured and expanded in number without undergoing differentiation (Nakahara et al., 1990a; 1990b; Bruder et al., 1997). The phenotype of the cells appeared to be stable throughout the culture period without loss in osteogenic, chondrogenic or adipogenic potential (Bruder et al., 1997; Pittenger et al., 1999). It is important to note that presently no unique phenotype has been identified that permits the reproducible isolation of MSC precursors with predictable developmental potential. The isolation of stromal cells is mainly dependent on their ability to adhere to plastic as well as their selective expansion potential. Human bone marrow progenitor cells were shown to be isolated and enriched by using selective markers (Simmons and Torok-Storb, 1991; Stewart et al., 1999). As a number of markers are expressed on MSCs some of these have been used to selectively obtain subpopulations of more colonies are present. It seems that a proportion of the cultured cells remain multipotent and maintain multilineage potential into osteogenic, condrogenic, myogenic, endothelogenic, thymogenic and adipogenic lineages (Pittenger et al., 1999). These results indicate that even after isolation and enrichment strategies, some cells in culture retain multipotentiality.

As with differentiated cells, it is important to consider the basic cell culture conditions also for stem cell cultivation. In general, cell adhesion and cell differentiation is regulated by the conditions of the culture milieu. Cell adhesion is best, when cells are cultivated in a serum-containing media and when the surface of the culture dish is coated with proteins. In the absence of proteins, cells can hardly adhere to the surface as they have to synthesise the proteins to build up the proteinaceous interface (Fig. 5.1). Standard conditions for expansion of stem cells were established by a number of studies. These conditions include the cell density as well as the presence of serum (in most instances fetal bovine serum). As cell density is known to be a critical factor affecting the growth of cells, attempts to cultivate cells were done to enrich cells above a critical cell density. Additionally, cells can be grown directly – that is, unmanipulated after collection – or more often after density gradient separation. For clinical applications of stem cells used in extracorporal tissue engineering, it is imperative that in vitro culture protocols should be devoid of animal or human products, to avoid potential contamination with pathogens. By using defined standard conditions, it is possible to reduce the variability within the culture milieu, therefore providing also a more stringent level of quality control. A special problem of supplemented allogeneic animal or human proteins is the possibility that such proteins may enhance the antigenicity of cells upon transplantation. Ideally, the ideal culture milieu for stem cell differentiation in vitro should therefore be chemically defined, and either be serum-free, utilise synthetic serum replacements or use autologous serum (Wong and Tuan, 1993; Goldsborough et al., 1998). The possible supplementation of specific recom-

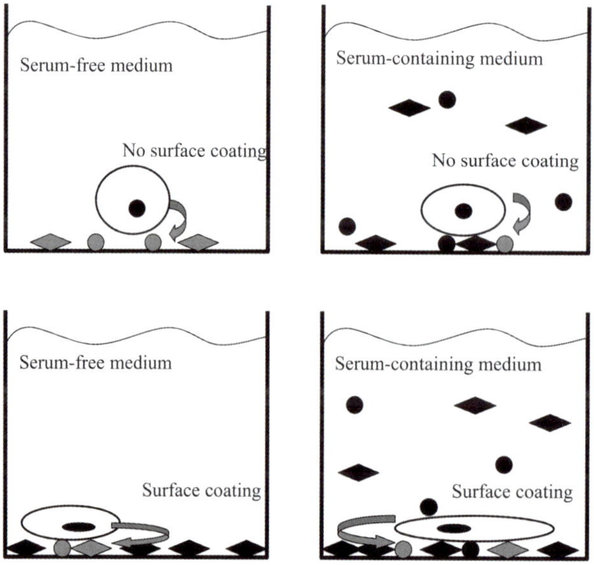

Fig. 5.1. Culture condition dependent cell attachment. *Top left*: Cell adhesion is impaired under serum-free culture conditions, especially when the substrate is not coated by adhesion proteins. Cell adhesion improves when a serum containing medium is in use (*top right*), or when the surface is coated prior sell seeding even in the absence of a serum containing medium (*bottom left*). Cell adhesion is best under conditions of surface coating in combination with the use of serum-containing medium (*bottom right*)

binant cytokines and growth factors may enhance the growth and differentiation of cells, especially when serum-free is in use. The major problems with culturing stem cells or more differentiated cells under serum-free conditions is that cells generally tend to have a lower mitotic index, become apoptotic, and display poor adhesion in the absence of serum compounds (Wong and Tuan, 1993). Serum supplementation is therefore usually required for in vitro culture of stem cells.

Autologous serum can be considered to be the ideal source of nutritional and stimulatory support of cells, when cells are used in immunocompetent animals or in clinical trials. For clinical applications, there are a number of reasons that serum should in future applications be completely eliminated from the in vitro culture milieu. The use of serum is accompanied by some disadvantages: the composition of serum is generally poorly defined. Serum batches possess a considerable degree of individual variation, even when obtained from the same patient. Additionally it is important to note that even serum is not completely physiological, since it is essentially a pathological fluid formed in response to blood clotting. Based on the individual patient situation, serum contains variable levels of growth and differentiation factors. The presence of these factors may therefore influence to an unknown extent the desired differentiation of stem cells into specific and well-defined lineages.

The development of chemically defined synthetic serum substitutes is therefore of special relevance. Commercially available synthetic serum substitutes (Wong and Tuan, 1993; Goldsborough et al., 1998) containing protein-based cytokines and growth factors or synthetic chemical compounds are currently under intensive investigation (Rogers et al., 1995; Schinstine and Iacovitti, 1997; Wobus et al., 1997; Liu et al., 2000; Buttery et al., 2001; Guan et al., 2001; Akita et al., 2002; Fukuda, 2002; Kim et al., 2002; Phillips et al., 2003; Rangappa et al., 2003). Such synthetic chemicals, possessing the advantage to be more stable compared to cell-based cytokines and growth factors, may improve not only the outcome of stem cell based tissue engineering approaches, but also strategies that use maturated cells.

Despite the success that has been obtained using bone-marrow-derived stem cells, one biological consideration limits its widespread application. Frequently, it is not feasible to obtain sufficient amounts of bone marrow with the requisite number of osteoprogenitor cells by marrow aspiration. In addition, the age-related decrease in bone marrow components, accompanied by a partial loss of precursor cells (Egrise et al., 1992; Quarto et al., 1995), is a frequent clinical limitation on obtaining sufficient numbers of stem cells. As mentioned before, the outcome of the in vitro use of bone marrow explants is critically dependent on the transfer of sufficient numbers of these progenitors. Therefore, the use of marrow-derived stem cells may be least applicable in those situations where it is most needed. It was in this respect shown that osteoprogenitors represent approximately 0.001% of the nucleated cells in healthy adult marrow (Haynesworth et al., 1992; Bruder et al., 1997), an indication of the practical problems obtaining pure stem cell sources by the cell culture strategies described. Therefore, improvements in all aspects of stem cell culture are necessary to further select, expand, and administer the progenitor marrow cell fraction in order to obtain clinically relevant numbers of osteogenic or chondrogenic stem cells.

5.2 Determined Bone Cells

It has long been known that the vast capacity for regeneration of bone is based on the presence of differentiated osteoblasts (Ashton et al., 1980). As the use of determined osteoblast-like cells does not raise (in contrast to the use of stem cells) legal issues and no problems of immune rejection, determined bone cells can be considered to be currently the most important cell source in bone tissue engineering. Therefore, in current clinical practice, differentiated autologous osteoblast-like cells are the most desirable cell source (Fig. 5.2). However, these cells may be insufficient to rebuild damaged bone tissue in a reasonable time. A considerable number of cell divisions is needed to bulk the tissue to its correct size. Former studies have regarded the propagation of adult mature cells in culture as a serious problem, because it was thought that most adult tissues contained only a minority of cells capable of effective expansion. However, in numerous recent investigations it has been shown that bone cells proliferate in culture without losing their viability. Various sources of determined bone cells can be used for cultivation. Committed osteoprogenitors, i.e. progenitor cells restricted to osteoblast development and bone formation, can be identified by functional assays of their differentiation capacity in vitro, such as the colony forming/units assay (CFU-O assay). A wide variety of systemic, local and positional factors regulate also proliferation and differentiation of determined cells, a sequence that is characterised by a series of cellular and molecular events distinguished by differential expression of osteoblast-associated genes, including those for specific transcription factors, cell cycle-related proteins, adhesion molecules and matrix proteins (for a review, see Yamaguchi et al., 2000). The mature osteoblast phenotype is in itself heterogeneous with subpopulations of osteoblasts expressing only subsets of the known osteoblast markers, including those for cytokine, hormones, and growth factor receptors, raising the intriguing possibility that only certain osteoblasts are competent to respond to regulatory agents at particular points in time.

Cultures containing determined osteoblastic or osteoblast-like cells have been established from different cell populations in the lineage of osteogenic cells (osteoprogenitor cells, lining cells, osteoblasts, and osteocytes) (for a review, see Hutmacher and Sittinger, 2003). They can be derived from several anatomical sites, using different explant procedures. Bone cell populations may be derived from the cortical or cancellous bone, bone marrow, periosteum, and in some instances from other tissues. Isolation of cells can be performed by a variety of techniques, including mechanical disruption, explant outgrowth, and enzyme digestion (Vacanti et al., 1995). Commonly used procedures to gain cells are digestive or outgrowth measures. Outgrowth of bone-like cells can be achieved through culturing of periosteum pieces or bone explants. Cells located within the periosteum and bone can differentiate into fibroblastic, osteogenic or reticular cells (Friedenstein, 1976; Nuttall et al., 1998; Triffitt and Oreffo, 1998; Dahir et al., 2000; Bianco et al., 2001) (Fig. 5.3). Periosteal-derived mesenchymal precursor cells generate progenitor cells committed to one or more cell lines with an apparent degree of plasticity and interconversion (Nakahara et al., 1992; Park et al., 1999; Bahrami et al., 2000; Schantz et al., 2002a; 2002b). In culture expanded periosteum cells were shown to retain the ability to heal a segmental bone defect after being reimplanted and induce osteogenic tissue when seeded into diffusion chambers (Ashton et al., 1980; Ohgushi et al., 1989a; 1989b; Nakahara

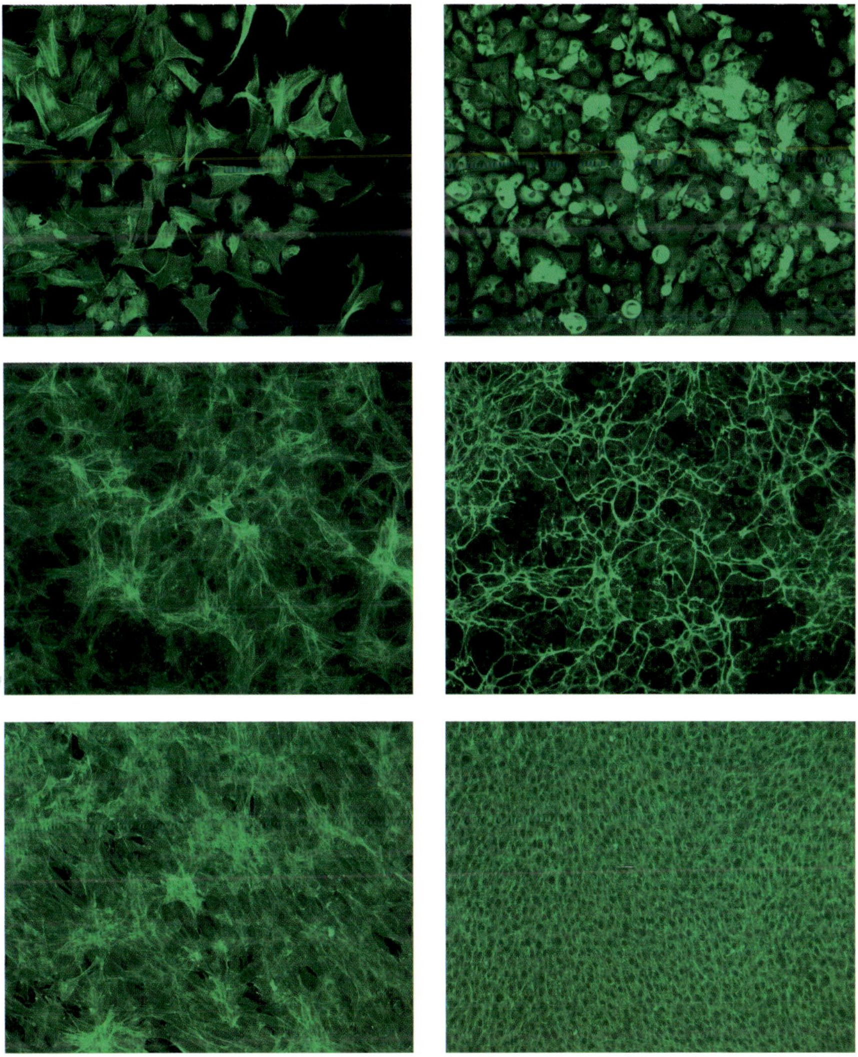

Fig. 5.2. Fluorescence microscopy of cell behaviour and extracellular matrix formation in osteoblast culture. During culture, subconfluent located cells (top left) proliferate over time (top right) in an attempt to form a confluent cell layer (bottom right). During the same time, a dense extracellular matrix formation can be observed between cells (midline, bottom left)

et al., 1990a). Outgrowth cultures of periosteum pieces favour the co-culture of different cell types (Osteoplasts and Osteolasts) /(Meyer et al., 1993b).

It remains controversial whether cortical or spongy bone, gained by different post-surgical processing techniques, is a better material of choice (Girdler and Hosseini, 1992; Chen et al. 1994; Schwipper et al. 1997) to outgrow cells in culture. It has been suggested that particulate culturing is superior to bone chip culturing (Marx et al. 1984; Shirota et al. 1996), based on the assumption that when particle

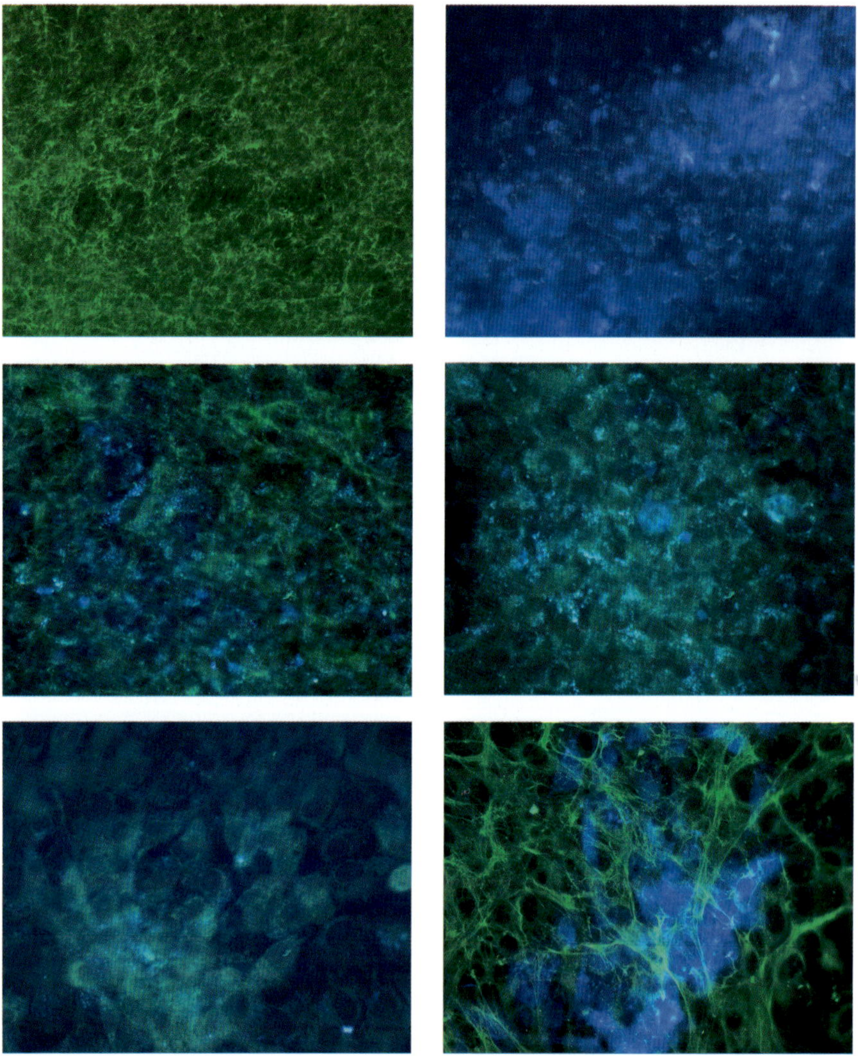

Fig. 5.3. Fluorescence microscopy of the mineral-matrix relationship in osteoblast culture. Mineral is deposited in direct contact to the extracellular matrix network. The green dye visualises the presence of immunostained proteins, blue colouring is indicative for the formation of hydroxyapatite. The colocalization approach gives insight into aspects of biomineral formation in osteoblast culture

size decreases, the absolute square measure of the surface of the tissue specimens in the culture dish increases. An increased absolute square measure of the transplant surface would increase the number of living cells released. Springer et al. (2004) demonstrated in an experimental study, that bone chips obtained from trabecular bone provided a higher cell number than those raised from cortical bone. Surprisingly, they found that processing of spongy bone graft in the bone mill (leading to bone particulates) results in lower absolute amounts of osteoblast-like cells, whereas use of the bone mill on cortical bone has much less impact on the number of cells counted. The authors speculated that the treatment of transplants with the bone mill or raising of transplants by rotating instruments should reduce the number of bone cells supplied, suggesting that a decreased particle size is disadvanageous when cell outgrowth methods are in use. Ecarot-Charrier and colleagues (1983) were the first to present a method for isolating osteoblasts from newborn mouse calvaria using digestive enzymes in solution. As it was demonstrated that isolated osteoblasts gained through this method retained their unique properties in culture, tissue digestion became a common method of cell harvesting for in vitro purposes.

Once such matured cells have been isolated from the tissue, there are also in such culture strategies a number of parameters that influence the expression of the osteoblastic phenotype in cell culture, most important the culture medium, culture time, number of passages and the presence of compounds. The presence of ascorbic acid, ß-glycerophosphate and dexamethasone influence the expression of the osteoblastic phenotype in a differentiated manner. β-Glycerophosphate for example induces phenotypic matrix maturation by enabling mineral formation in osteoblast-like cell cultures (Fig. 5.4). Dexamethasone, as an additional factor, is described as inducing cell differentiation but imposing a negative effect on cell proliferation, indicative of a reciprocal and functionally coupled relationship between proliferation and differentiation. Therefore, it is convenient to select suitable experimental conditions for cultivation. As with stem cell cultivation, the culture conditions should be well defined in order to standardise the ex vivo grown product.

Because endochondral bone formation and, frequently, fracture repair proceed through a cartilaginous intermediate, some investigators have suggested that the transplantation of committed chondrocytes would also ameliorate bone regeneration (Bahrami et al., 2000). Vacanti and colleagues (1995) compared the ability of periosteal progenitors and articular chondrocytes to effect bone repair. They showed that periosteal cells from newborn calves seeded on a scaffold and implanted in critical-sized calvarial defects generated new bone. Specimens examined at early times contained material that grossly and histologically appeared to be cartilage. The scaffold seeded with chondrocytes also formed cartilage. However, no endochondral ossification was observed, since the transplanted specimens remained in a cartilaginous state. Therefore, chondrocytes proved ineffective as a cell-based therapy for tissue engineering of bone. Because mature cartilage is thought to produce factors that inhibit angiogenesis, implants seeded with committed chondrocytes may prevent the endochondral cascade by preventing vascular invasion. Cells derived from cartilage seem to be committed to retaining their phenotype and, therefore, are unable to differentiate towards hypertrophic chondrocytes under the experimental conditions tested so far. In contrast, when precursor cells from the periosteum are provided, their primitive developmental state allows them to proceed through the entire chondrogenic lineage, ultimately becoming hypertrophic chondrocytes. The molecular basis for the difference in the phenotypic potential of these different cell types remains mysterious and is an area of intensive investigation.

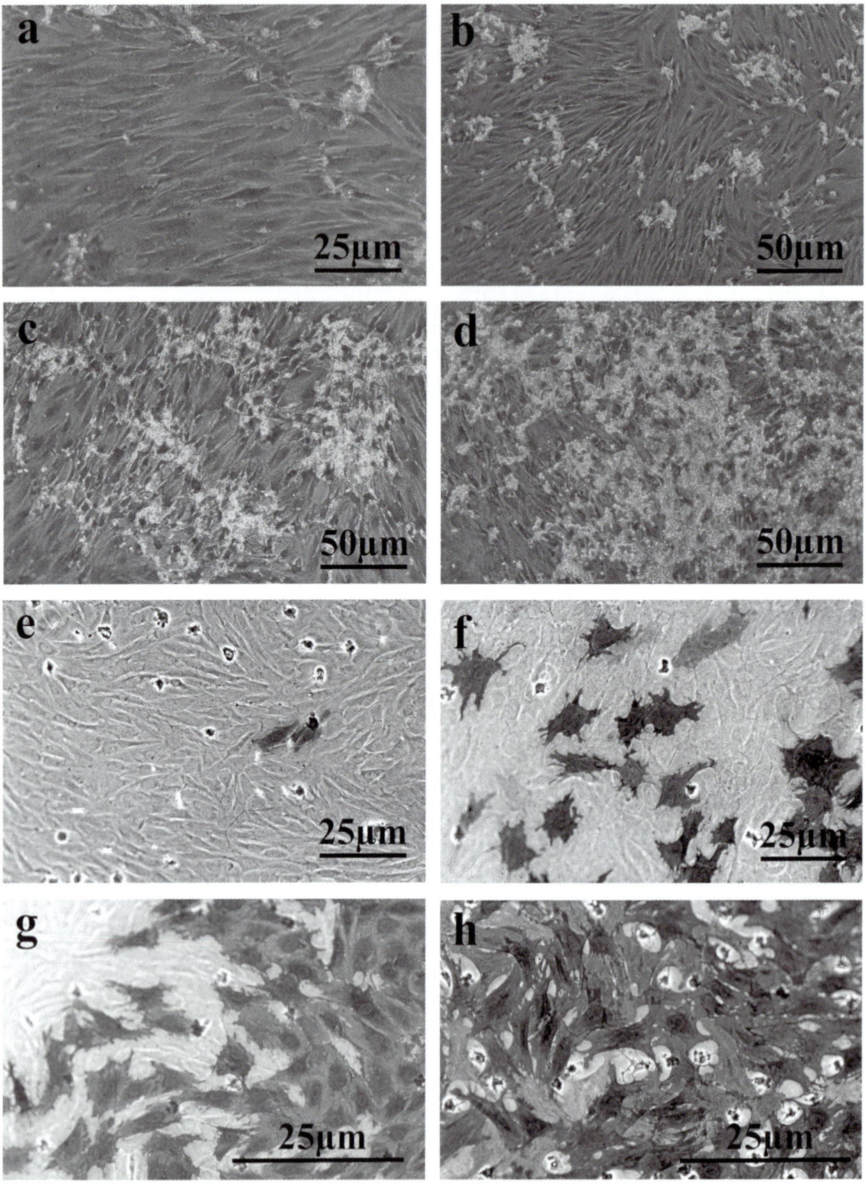

Fig. 5.4. Mineral formation and alkaline phosphatase (ALP) expression in osteoblast culture. **a–d** The amount of biomineral formation can be observed through the deposition of calcium phosphate-containing minerals *(bright areas)* after 1, 2, 3, and 4 weeks, respectively. **e–h** The extent of ALP expression *(dark areas)* correlates with the biomineral deposition after 1, 2, 3, and 4 weeks of culture

5.3 Determined Chondrogenic cells

Clinical cartilage engineering strategies have, to date, predominantly focused on the use of an unselected source of chondrocytes (Brittberg et al., 1994). In the ongoing search to improve cohondrocyte cell lines, the use of specific chondrocyte populations are now being considered to investigate whether an improved cartilaginous structure would be generated in vivo and in vitro by these specifically selected populations of determined chondrocytes (Redman et al., 2005). As distinct phenotypic and functional properties of chondrocytes across the zones of articular cartilage are present, it seems reasonable to search for the best source of chondrocyte subpopulations (Waldman et al., 2003). It was reported in this respect that a combination of mid- and deep-zone chondrocytes seems to be more suitable for the ex vivo generation of a hyaline-like cartilage tissue. Dowthwaite et al. (2004) recently reported on an isolation technique for chondrocytes that reside in the superficial zone of immature bovine articular cartilage. These cells, characterised as determined chondrogenic cells, were shown to allow appositional growth of the articular cartilage from the articular surface (Hayes et al., 2001). Therefore, when chondrocytes are aimed to generate a cartilage-like structure ex vivo, it seems to be reasonable not to gain full thickness cartilage implants but to use subpopulations of chondrocytes. Separation of cartilage zones after explantation and before cultivation with a selective subpopulation may therefore provide a tool to improve tissue engineering strategies using determined cells. Phenotypic plasticity was tested by a series of in ovo injections where colony-derived populations of these chondroprogenitors were engrafted into a variety of connective tissue lineages, thus confirming that this population of cells have properties akin to those of a progenitor cell. The high colony-forming ability and the capacity to successfully expand these progenitor populations in vitro (Dowthwaite et al., 2004) may further aid our knowledge of cartilage development and growth and may provide novel solutions in ex vivo cartilage tissue engineering strategies.

5.4 Osteoclasts

Osteoclasts may be used in bone tissue engineering strategies, since these cells play an important role in bone physiology and since a culture containing both cell lines would more closely mimic the in vivo bone situation. Osteoclasts are derived from mononuclear cells of hemopoietic bone marrow and peripheral blood. The potential to differentiate into mature osteoclasts in culture is maintained by a variety of cells (Hayashi et al., 1998; Chambers, 2000), including hematopoietic stem cells and colony-forming precursors cells, elicited by hematopoietic colony-stimulating factors, and their progeny in the colonies (Yamazaki et al., 2001). Moreover, well-differentiated cells, such as monocytes and even mature macrophages, are capable of differentiating into osteoclasts (Akagawa et al., 1996). As the differentiation pathway is common to that of macrophages and dendritic cells, factors can be used to selectively induce differentiation. A promyeloid precursor can differentiate into an osteoclast, a macrophage or a dendritic cell, depending on whether it is exposed to some osteoclast-inducing factors (RANKL, OPGL, ODF, M-CSF, GM-CSF). As some groups demonstrated that bone marrow stromal cells and osteoblasts produce membrane-bound and soluble RANKL/TRANCE/OPGL/ODF factors, an important positive regulator of osteoclast formation (Lacey et al., 1998) is a co-culture of osteoclasts with osteoblasts. Alternatively, culturing of osteoclasts can be performed by enrichment of osteoclast precursor cells from the peripheral blood or from bone marrow. Periosteum outgrowth techniques allow also the propagation of osteoclastic cells from monocytes located in the periosteum (Szulczewski et al., 1993). Recent research suggests that multinucleated osteoclasts can be cultivated by adding alveolar mononuclear cells to new-born rat calvaria osteoblasts in vitro.

5.5 Endothelial Cells

The additional use of vascular cells offers several theoretical advantages over approaches of extracorporal bone tissue engineering exploiting only bone cells as a single cell type. As a cell-based strategy, endothelial cell therapy promises to deliver at the same time both substrate (endothelial cells) and cytokines and growth factors. Endothelial progenitor cells as well as mature endothelial cells are capable of settling in areas of bone neovascularisation, thus exerting their effects in sites in need of new blood vessel growth (Asahara et al., 1999). As these cells are present in nearly all sites of the body, they exhibit no unfavourable side effects when transplanted autologously. The induction of angiogenesis as well as their participiation in new vessel formation makes them appealing components for bone tissue engineering. Endothelial cells promote synergistic vasculogenesis and bone formation. The action of endothelial cells on osteoblast function was demonstrated recently through various cell culture studies.

Endothelial progenitor cells were first described by Asahara et al. in 1997. Since then, significant progress has been made in defining the origin and lineage of these cells. A number of studies gave evidence that endothelial progenitors originate in the bone marrow and are then selectively recruited to sites of neovascularisation. Therefore, bone marrow cells as well as cells obtained from peripheral vessels are in use for tissue engineering approaches.

The relative ease of isolating and expanding mature endothelial cells (from explanted blood vessels) or endothelial progenitor cells (from bone marrow) makes them an attractive source of autologous vascular cells for the generation of a vascularised scaffold complex in vitro. Studies have demonstrated that endothelial cells form ring-like structures in two-dimensional cultures and tubules in three-dimensional extracellular matrices in vitro. It is assured that they are able to induce vascular invasion in the host tissue if implanted (Al-Khadi et al., 2001; Murayama et al., 2002). Studies with various cell lines indicated that patency rates were strongly correlated with the amount of host cells (smooth muscle cells and endothelial cells) incorporated into the graft (Jarrell et al., 1986; Weinberg and Bell, 1986; L´Heureux et al., 1998; Deutsch et al., 1999). Whereas most of these investigations were not intended to induce the formation of vascular matrices for tissue engineering, the findings are encouraging in light of recent work showing the potential of axial vessels to vascularise cellular scaffolds in vitro and in vivo (Chung et al., 2003).

By using osteoblast-like cells and endothelial cells it seems to be possible to create complex tissue-engineered vascularised bone constructs. In recent studies tissue-engineered bone constructs have been fabricated by combining autologous vascular cells and bone cells in a porous scaffold structure. Endothelial cells may accelerate the defect-healing process by improving cell nutrition in the scaffolds as well as at the defect site. It was shown that the success of grafts seeded with endothelial cells was significantly greater than that of non-seeded grafts (Kaushal et al., 2001). Vacanti and co-authors (1995) demonstrated early on in vivo studies that bone replacement materials could be effectively combined with autologous endothelial cells. An additional advantage of using endothelial cells is their potential for thrombus regression. As thrombosis is a serious problem in tissue engineering, prevention of microvascular failures is of major importance after a tissue-engineered bone construct is implanted in vivo. In the future, endothelial cells offer new perspectives to improve the ex vivo formation of a more mature bone construct, thereby accelerating the process of new blood vessel formation in vivo. With our recent understanding of the physiological roles of endothelial cells, the importance of vasculogenesis in extracorporal bone tissue engineering has come into focus, especially in light of the fact that cell survival balanced by nutrition is one of the main limiting steps in scaling up bone constructs for clinical use.

5.6 Co-cultures

Co-cultures of various cell lines (osteoblasts and osteoclasts, osteoblasts and endothelial cells as well as the co-culture of differentiated and stem cells) can be used to improve extracorporeal tissue engineering strategies (Richards et al., 2002; Yamaguchi et al., 2002). The major advantage of co-cultures of differentiated cells and stem cells for use in extracorporal tissue engineering strategies is that the pool of stem cells allows the renewing of cells and, via efficient signal transduction pathways, the induction of a differentiated cell population. As with pure differentiated cell co-culture systems, autocrine and paracrine factors secreted by one cell type readily interact with other cell types when different cell lines are in use. Hence, co-cultures provide a more physiological environment for cell regeneration in vitro that more closely resembles the in vivo conditions, especially in bone tissue engineering. However, recently it has been reported that under certain circumstances intimate physical contact between different cells during co-culture may lead to the fusion of different cell types, resulting in the formation of heterokaryons (Terada et al., 2002; Ying et al. 2002). Three different approaches for a co-culture of cells are possible:

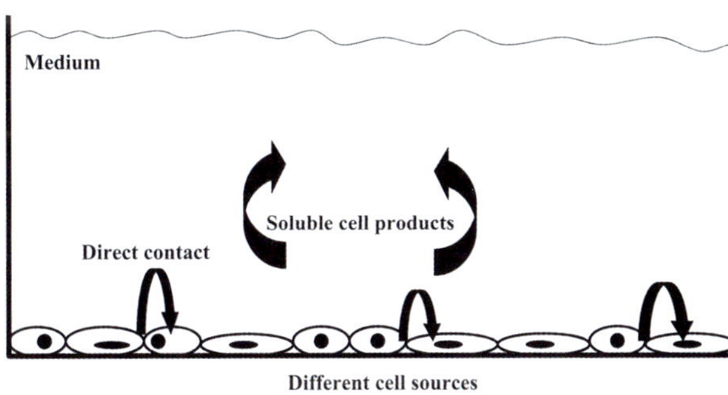

Fig. 5.5. Co-culture: two cell types in one chamber

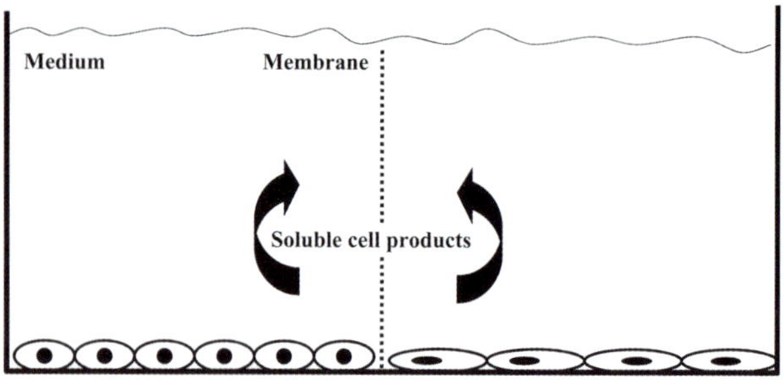

Fig. 5.6. Co-culture: two cell types in one chamber, separated by a permeable membrane

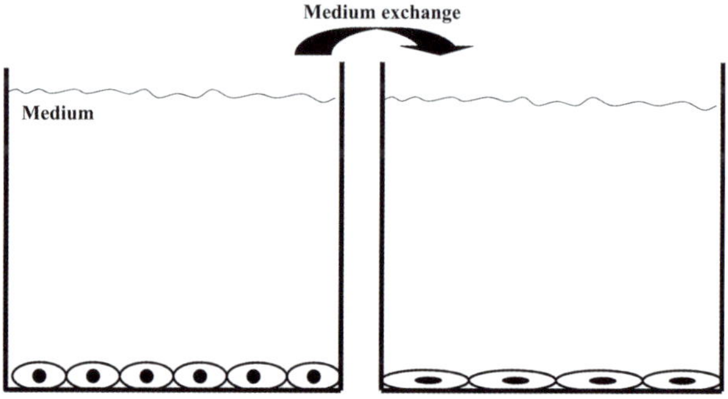

Fig. 5.7. Co-culture: different cell types are cultivated in different chapters followed by a medium exchange

first, the culture of two or more cell lines in one chamber (Fig. 5.5); second, the culture of two cells in one chamber, separated by a selectively permeable membrane (Fig. 5.6); and third, the exchange of medium secreted by cells (when cells are cultivated in different chambers) (Fig. 5.7). It is known that the last two approaches work through a culture media conditioned by one type of cells that contain various soluble factors, capable of inducing cell differentiation. As such factors are easy to transfer, a conditioned media seems to be desirable for cell scaffold maturation in vitro. The advantage of using cell-conditioned media or the separation of two different cell lines by a permeable membrane over pure co-culture techniques is that there is no risk of heterokaryon cell function. Additionally, filtering the conditioned media can significantly reduce the risk of contamination with a different cell type, and decreases the risk of disease transmission. The major disadvantage of using membranes or exchange medium, as opposed to conventional co-culture, is that there is no intimate physical contact and regulatory cross-talk between different cell types. The subsequent limitation of differentiating signal transduction between the various cells is also not close to the in vivo situation. Indeed, a number of studies have shown that, in some cases, conditioned media failed to elicit cell proliferation and differentiation, when compared to a pure co-culture (Rangappa et al., 2003).

5.6.1 Techniques of Cell Culture Evaluation

The success of cell culturing is monitored by both biochemical and morphological investigations (Figs 5.8–5.15). Biochemical criteria include all aspects from molecular features of the cell to the composition of the extracellular matrix (Table 5.1). Morphological aspects range from ultrastructural analysis of cells and matrix components to the spatial relationships of cells in a three-dimensional tissue construct (Table 5.2). Initially, biochemical assays used traditional methods of protein chemistry (e.g. immunostaining, electrophoresis and blot techniques) (Fig 5.8; Fig 5.9). More recently, the availability of genetic probes for many of the bones and cartilages proteins has made it easy to assess gene expression of multiple phenotypic markers (Fig 5.10). Advances in imaging and analytical techniques allow morphological insight into the creation of engineered tissue by using high resolution pictures (transmission electron microscopy, scanning electron microscopy, X-ray diffraction, atomic force microscopy) (for a review, see Manso et al., 2002). In addition, some of the new techniques enable combined biochemical and morphological analysis of probes (TOF-SIMS).

In addition, some of the new techniques enable combined biochemical and morphological analysis of probes (TOF-SIMS). Biomechanical features of cells in culture can be determined by special investigations. Cell adhesion strength, for example, can indirectly be assessed by cell detachment evaluations. The relative strength of cell adhesion can be determined by trypsination experiments (Fig. 5.11). The amount of adhered cells is an indicator for the number and strength of focal adhesions and can provide information concering the biology of cell–material interaction.

Generally, it is important to consider that the outcome of individual cell culture determinations is dependant on the chosen cell culture parameters. Characterisation of cells can be well performed by determination of the scope of synthesised extracellular matrix proteins (Fig. 5.12). The results of such immunostaining determinations are dependant not only on the preferred cell source but also on the chemicals used in the cell culture. The expression and the visualisation of synthesised matrix proteins, for example, differ in dependence of the preferred blocking system (Fig. 5.13) and serum batches (Fig. 5.14). One of the most influencing factors in cell differentiation is, as mentioned before, the spacial placement of cells. The phenotypical appearance as well as the differentiation capacity of chondrocytes differs significantly between culture of cells in a two- or three-dimensional cell culture system (Fig. 5.15), indicative for the complex reactivity of cells towards their cell culture microenvironment. Advancements in genetic analysis techniques allow the determination of cell differentiation not only at the protein level, but also at the level of gene expression (Fig. 5.11). Nowadays, the use of gene chips enables a comprehensive insight in gene activity of cells (Fig. 5.16, Table 5.3). The application of gene chip technology can therefore be expected to significantly improve the possibility to get a more detailed insight in cell behaviour, especially when the screening results of gene chip technology are confirmed by the PCR technique. Evaluation of cell-based tissue engineering strategies in vitro and in vivo can now be determined more precisely by gene analysis technology (Table 5.4, Appendix). In general it is mandatory, in order to compare results of different in vitro experiments, to consider the cell culture outcomes in light of the individual experimental setting and the chosen analytical techniques.

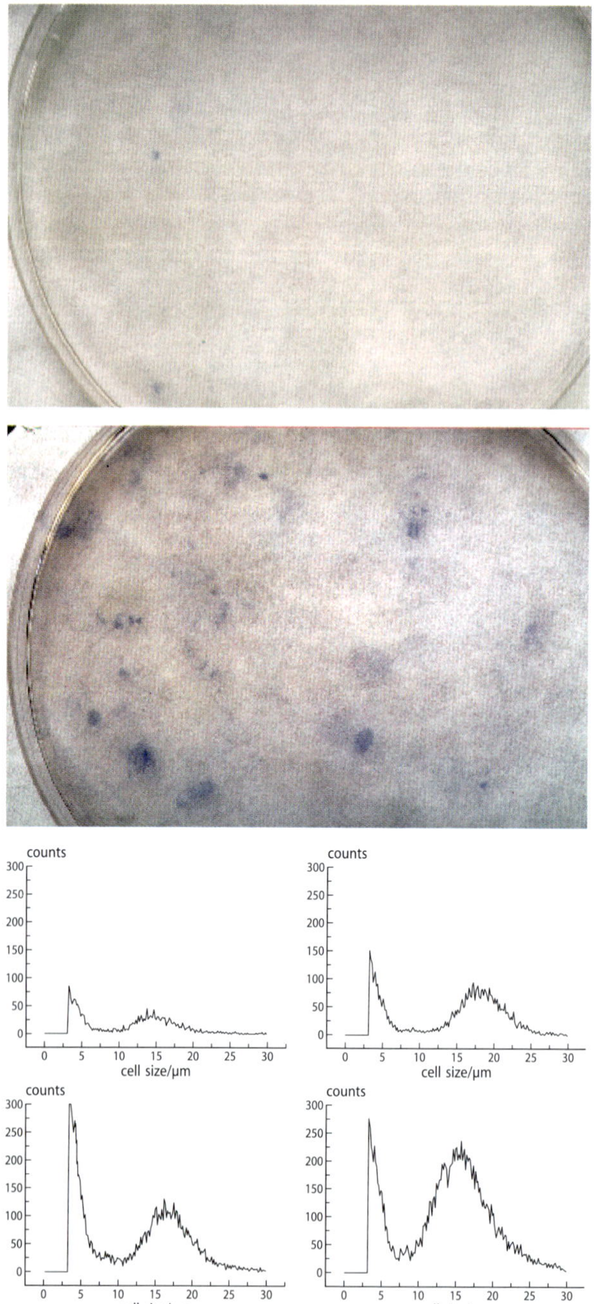

Fig. 5.8. Alkaline Phosphotase expression in petri dish and size distribution of osteoblasts in vitro. Alkaline phosphatase activity increases over time in culture. Additionally, the cell size increases during growth of cells in the culture dish (Coulter Counter measurements, graphics on right side). Both parameters are indicative of viable osteoblast-like cells

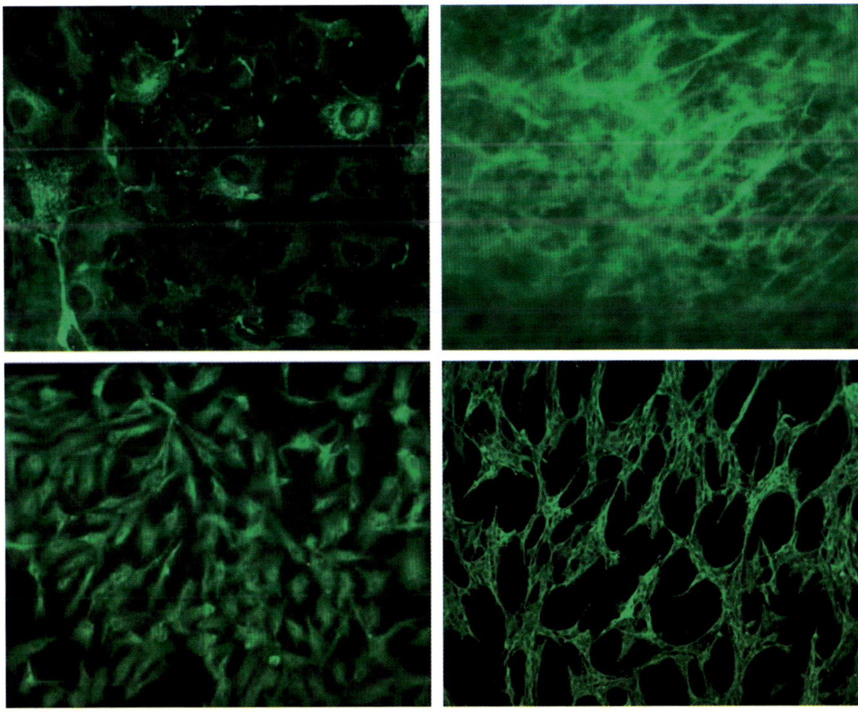

Fig. 5.9. Co-culture of osteoblasts and endothelial cells. Cells have no direct contact but can interact over the media. Top: collagen type I expression of osteoblasts in single (*left*) and in co-culture (*right*) after one week; bottom: actin expression of endothelial cells in single (*left*) and in co-culture (*right*) demonstrates ring format only in co-culture

Table 5.1. Biochemical evaluation methods

Method	Determination
Cell counter	Cell number, cell volume
Colorimetric assays	Cell viability, calcium-phosphate content
Fluorescence staining	Cytoskeletal proteins, Minerals
Immunostaining	Cell and matrix components
Gelectrophoresis	Proteins, non-proteinaceous components
HPLC	Proteins, non-proteinaceous components
Capillary electrophoresis	Proteins, non-proteinaceous components
Western-blot	Proteins
ELISA	Proteins, non-proteinaceous components
IRMA	Proteins, non-proteinaceous components
Radioimmunoassay	Proteins, non-proteinaceous components
DNA analysis (PCR)	DNA
Gene chips	Gene composition

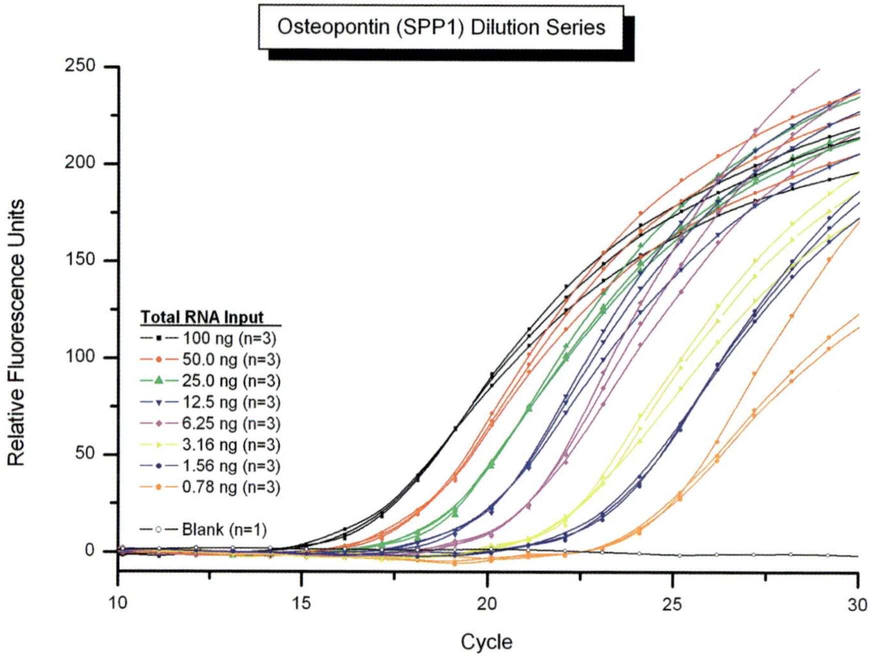

Fig. 5.10. Quantitative osteopontin detection by polymerase chain reaction (PCR). The quantitative analysis of gene expression by the PCR technology is a valuable tool in the determination of cell activity states in culture

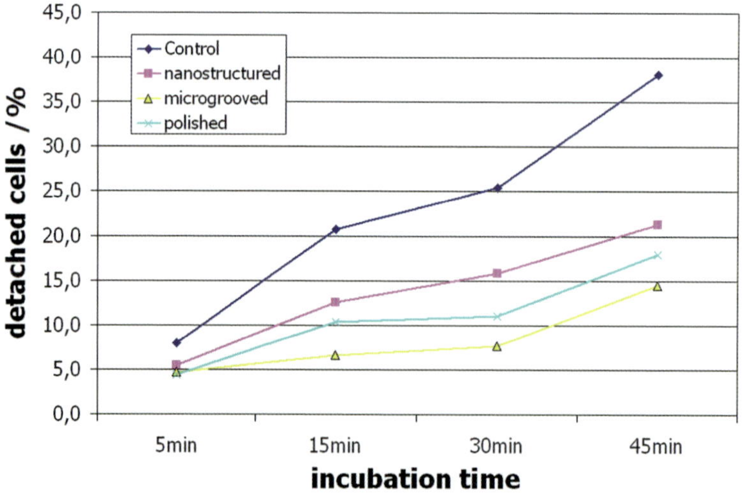

Fig. 5.11. Relative strength of cell adhesion at different surfaces can be determined by trypsinisation with diluted trypsin at different time points, plotting the percentage of detached cells versus trypsinisation time. Example shows cell attachment at a control compared with attachment at different surface nanostructures of titanium

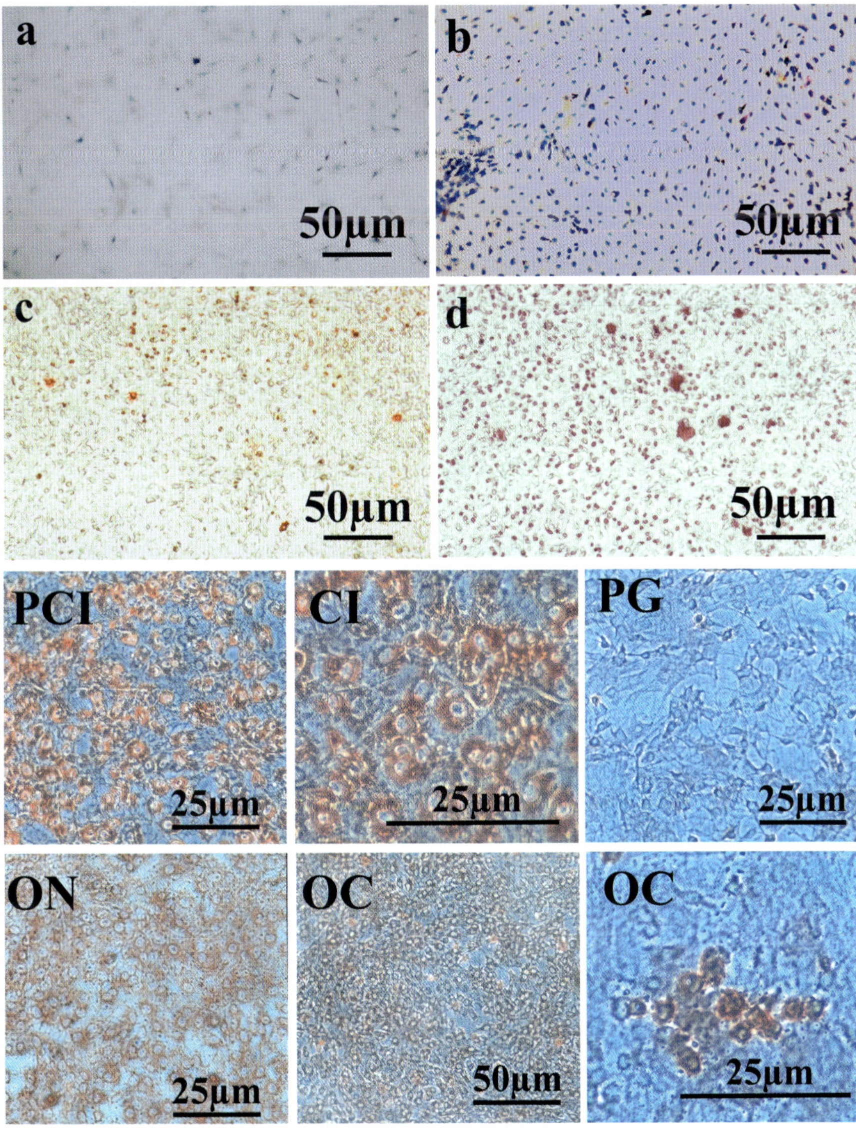

Fig. 5.12. Cell cultures can be well characterised by various staining procedures (*top,* **a–d**) and a comprehensive analysis of the array of proteins synthesised by cells (*bottom:* immunostaining). The presence of procollagen type I (PCI), collagen type I (CI), proteoglycans (PG), osteonectin (ON), and osteocalcin (OC) is indicative for a mature osteoblast cell culture

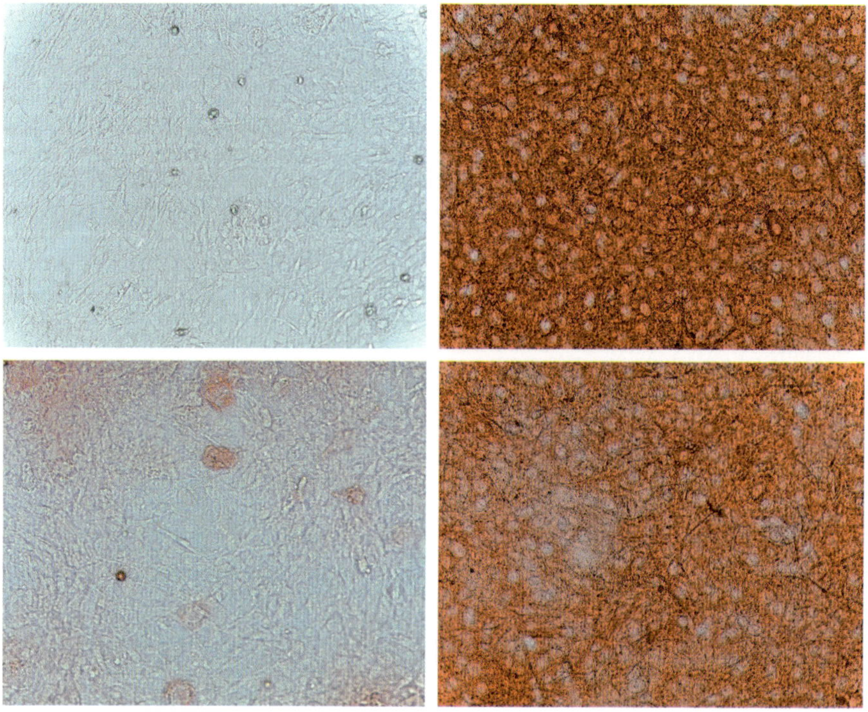

Fig. 5.13. Osteocalcin expression of osteoblasts. The extent of staining intensity depends on the used blocking systems, indicative for the difficulties to quantitatively compare results of different cell culture investigations. Defining the culture condition is a main requirement in cell biology research. *Left:* Candor blocking solution provides the correct osteocalcin expression in 1 day (*top, left*) and 7 days (*bottom, left*) and 14 days (*bottom, right*) in comparison to the overstaining by using a BSY blocking solution

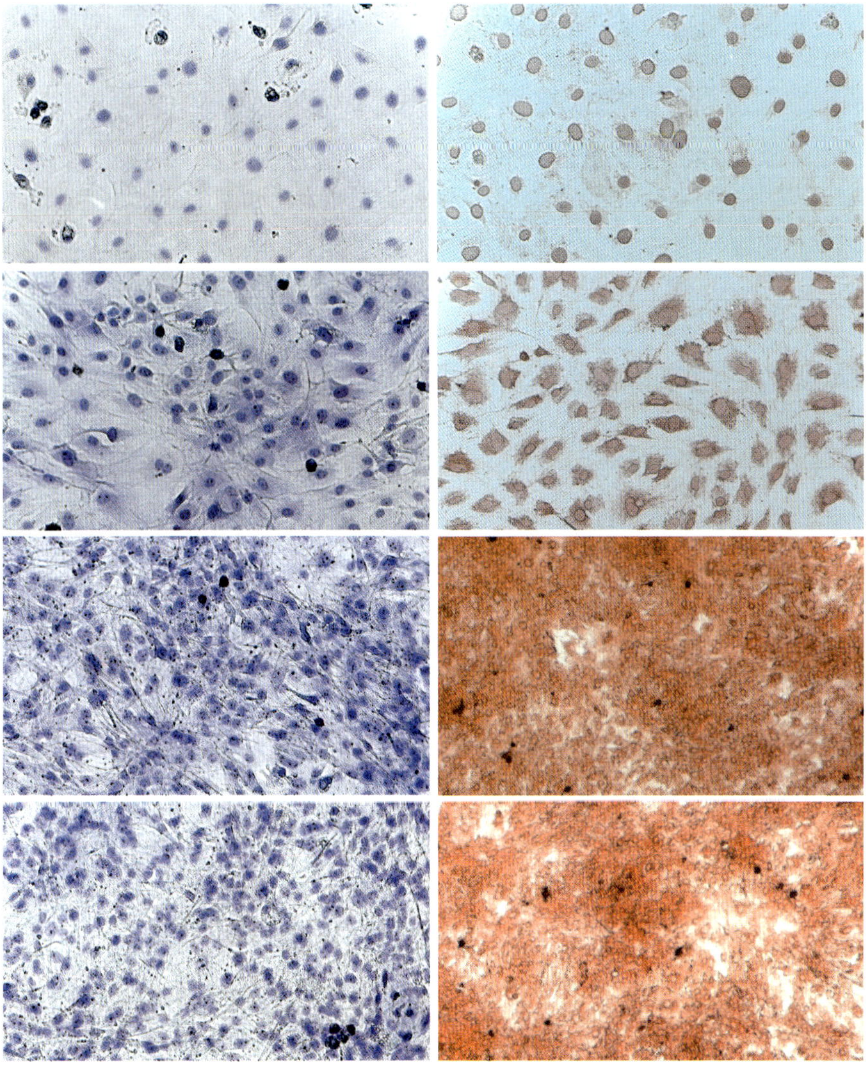

Fig. 5.14. Osteoblast monolayer culture. The outcome of cell cultures is dependent on different serum concentrations. Different serum concentrations lead to a significant difference in the growth and differentiation characteristics of cells during cell culture. 1. row: Richardson`s stain (*left*) and osteonectin expression (*right*) in serum-free culture; 2. row: Richardson`s stain (*left*) and osteonectin expression (*right*) in 2% serum culture; 3. row: Richardson`s stain (*left*) and osteonectin expression (*right*) in 10% serum culture; 4. row: Richardson`s stain (*left*) and osteonectin expression (*right*) in 15% serum culture show no prominent difference to 10% serum culture

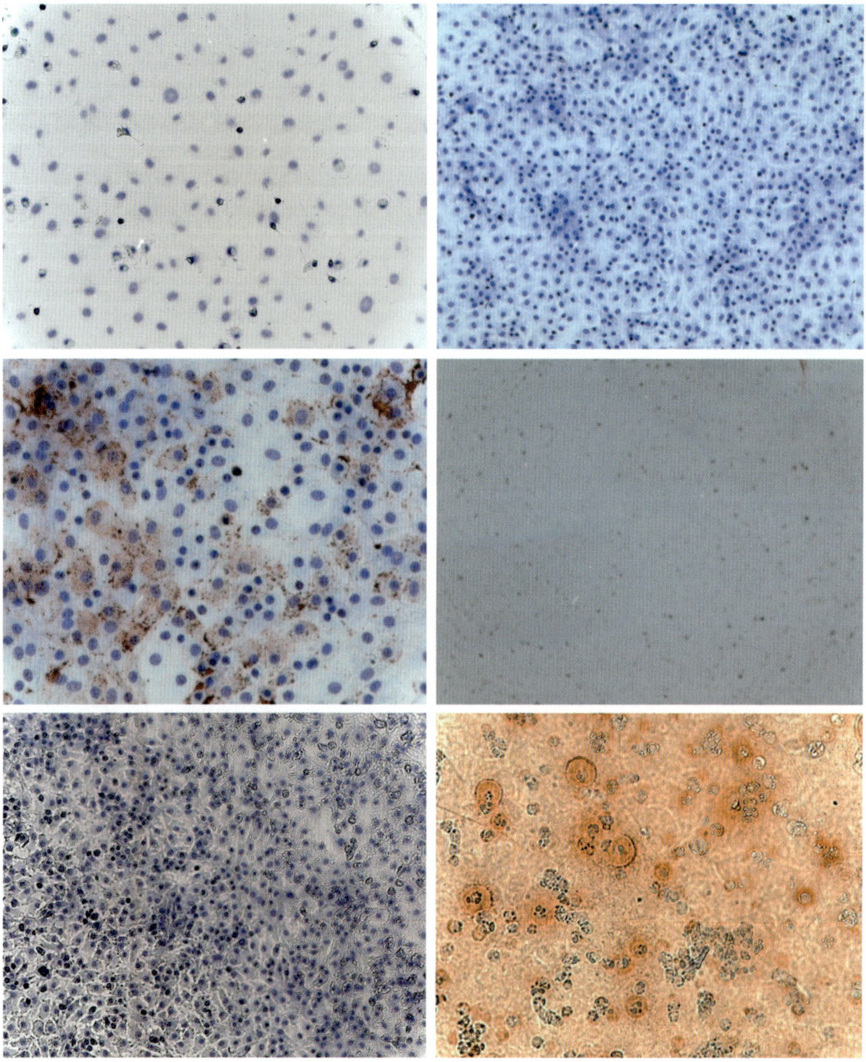

Fig. 5.15. Staining of chondrocytes in culture. The appearance of chondrocytes differs significant between cells cultured in a monolayer and in a three-dimensional gel system. *Top*: Monolayer culture with low (*left*) and high cell density (*right*); midline: collagen type I (*left*) and collagen type II (*right*) expression in monolayer culture; *bottom*: collagen type I (*left*) and collagen type II (*right*) expression in a three-dimensional gel culture. Chondrocyte differentiation is sensitive to the spacial environment. The different collagen expression of monolayer and gel culture represents the unequal cell differentiation

Table 5.2. Microscopical methods used in tissue engineering

Method	Resolution (nm)	Immuno-staining	Element analysis	Molecule analysis
Phase contrast microscopy	100	–	–	–
Conventional microscopy	100	+	–	–
Fluorescence microscopy	100	+	–	–
Scanning electron microscopy	10	+	+ (EDX)	–
Transmission electron microscopy	0.1	+	+ (EDX)	–
Atomic force microscopy	0.01	–	–	–
Laser SMS	10	–	+	–
ToF SIMS	10	–	+	–

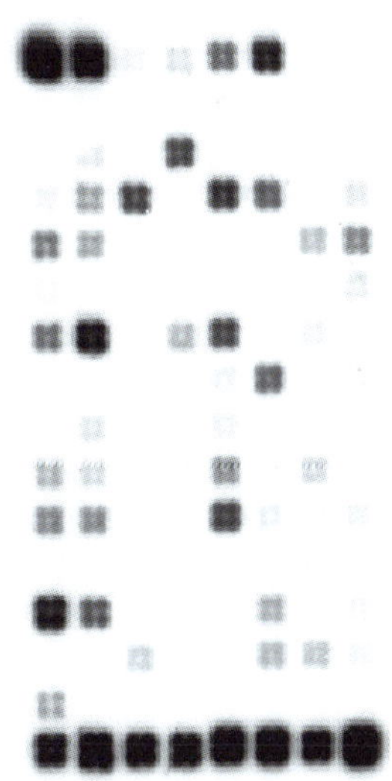

Fig. 5.16. View of staining pattern on an osteogenesis array gene chip (Super Array Bioscience Corporation, USA). Expression is measured on this array as intensity of the spots. Genes with higher expression are dark on the image

Table 5.3. Location of the different genes on the osteogenesis array gene chip (Fig. 5.16., Super Array Bioscience Corporation, USA)

Array Layout							
Gapdh	Ahsg	Akp2	Ambn	Anxa5	Bgn	Bmp1	Bmp2
1	2	3	4	5	6	7	8
Bmp3	Bmp4	Bmp5	Bmp6	Bmp7	Bmp8a	Bmp8b	Bmpr1a
9	10	11	12	13	14	15	16
Bmpr1b	Bmpr2	Calcr	Calcr	Cdh11	Col10a1	Col11a1	Col11a1
17	18	19	20	21	22	23	24
Col14a1	Col15a1	Col18a1	Col19a1	Col1a1	Col1a2	Col2a1	Col3a1
25	26	27	28	29	30	31	32
Col4a1	Col4a2	Col4a3	Col4a4	Col4a5	Col4a6	Col5a1	Col6a1
33	34	35	36	37	38	39	40
Col6a2	Col7a1	Col8a1	Col9a1	Col9a3	Comp	Csf2	Csf3
41	42	43	44	45	46	47	48
Ctsk	Dcn	Dmp1	Dspp	Egf	Enam	Fgf1	Fgf2
49	50	51	52	53	54	55	56
Fgf3	Fgfr1	Fgfr2	Fgfr3	Flt1	Fn1	Gdf10	Ibsp
57	58	59	60	61	62	63	64
Icam1	Igf1	Igf1r	Itga2	Itga2b	Itga3	Itgam	Itgav
65	66	67	68	69	70	71	72
Itgb1	Mglap	Mmp10	Mmp13	Mmp2	Mmp8	Mmp9	Msx1
73	74	75	76	77	78	79	80
Nfkb1	Pdgfa	Phex	Runx2	Scarb1	Ser- pinh1	Smad1	Smad2
81	82	83	84	85	86	87	88
Smad3	Smad4	Smad5	Smad6	Smad7	Smad9	Sost	Sox9
89	90	91	92	93	94	95	96
Sparc	Spp1	Tfip11	Tgfb1	Tgfb2	Tgfb3	Tgfbr1	Tgfbr2
97	98	99	100	101	102	103	104
Tgfbr3	Tnf	Tuft1	Twist1	Twist2	Vcam1	Vdr	Vegfa
105	106	107	108	109	110	111	112
Vegfb	Vegfc	PUC18	Blank	Blank	AS1R2	AS1R1	AS1
113	114	115	116	117	118	119	120
Rps27a	B2m	Hspcb	Hspcb	Ppia	Ppia	BAS2C	BAS2C
121	122	123	124	125	126	127	128

Table 5.4. Details on the proteins of the osteogenesis array gene chip (Fig. 5.16. and Table 5.3., Super Array Bioscience Corporation, USA).

Position	GeneBank	Symbol	Description	GO Term
1	NM_008084	Gapdh	Glyceraldehyde-3-phosphate dehydrogenase	Oxidoreductase activity; Mitochondrion; Glyceraldehyde-3-phosphate dehydrogenase (phosphorylating) activity; Glucose metabolism; Glycolysis; Glyceraldehyde-3-phosphate dehydrogenase activity
2	NM_013465	Ahsg	Alpha-2-HS-glycoprotein	Extracellular space; Ossification; Cysteine protease inhibitor activity
3	NM_007431	Akp	Alkaline phosphatase 2, liver	Hydrolase activity; Membrane; Extracellular space; Metabolism; Magnesium ion binding; Alkaline phosphatase activity
4	NM_009664	Ambn	Ameloblastin	Extracellular space; Odontogenesis (sensu Vertebrata); Ossification; Extracellular matrix organization and biogenesis; Extracellular matrix (sensu Metazoa); Structural constituent of tooth enamel; Extracellular matrix structural constituent conferring compression resistance
5	NM_009673	Anxa5	Annexin A5	Calcium ion binding; Blood coagulation; Calcium-dependent phospholipid binding
6	NM_007542	Bgn	Biglycan	Extracellular space; Extracellular matrix (sensu Metazoa)
7	NM_009755	Bmp1	Bone morphogenetic protein 1	Hydrolase activity; Calcium ion binding; Proteolysis and peptidolysis; Zinc ion binding; Organogenesis; Growth factor activity; Metalloendopeptidase activity; Cytokine activity; Metallopeptidase activity; Astacin activity
8	NM_007553	Bmp2	Bone morphogenetic protein 2	Protein binding; Extracellular space; Organogenesis; Growth factor activity; Cytokine activity; Transforming growth factor beta receptor signalling pathway; Embryonic development; BMP signalling pathway; Growth; Cardiac cell differentiation; Cell fate commitment; Epithelial to mesenchymal transition

Table 5.4. *Continued*

Position	GeneBank	Symbol	Description	GO Term
9	NM_173404	Bmp3	Bone morphogenetic protein 3	Growth factor activity; Cytokine activity; Transforming growth factor beta receptor signalling pathway
10	NM_007554	Bmp4	Bone morphogenetic protein 4	Protein binding; Extracellular space; Growth factor activity; Skeletal development; Angiogenesis; Cytokine activity; Heart development; Mesoderm cell fate determination; BMP signalling pathway; Growth; Eye morphogenesis (sensu Mammalia); Cell fate commitment; Metanephros development; Ureteric bud development; Forebrain development; Histogenesis
11	NM_007555	Bmp5	Bone morphogenetic protein 5	Protein binding; Extracellular space; Growth factor activity; Skeletal development; Cytokine activity; Transforming growth factor beta receptor signalling pathway; Growth; Pattern specification
12	NM_007556	Bmp6	Bone morphogenetic protein 6	Extracellular; Protein binding; Cell growth and/or maintenance; Extracellular space; Growth factor activity; Cell differentiation; Cytokine activity; BMP signalling pathway; Growth
13	NM_007557	Bmp7	Bone morphogenetic protein 7	Protein binding; Extracellular space; Organogenesis; Growth factor activity; Cytokine activity; BMP signalling pathway; Axon guidance; Growth; Pattern specification; Salivary gland morphogenesis
14	NM_007558	Bmp8a	Bone morphogenetic protein 8a	Development; Extracellular space; Growth factor activity; Cell differentiation; Spermatogenesis; Cytokine activity; Transforming growth factor beta receptor signalling pathway; Growth

Table 5.4. *Continued*

Position	GeneBank	Symbol	Description	GO Term
15	NM_007559	Bmp8b	Bone morphogenetic protein 8b	Extracellular space; Growth factor activity; Spermatogenesis; Cytokine activity; Transforming growth factor beta receptor signalling pathway; Growth
16	NM_009758	Bmpr1a	Bone morphogenetic protein receptor, type 1A	ATP binding; Transferase activity; Protein amino acid phosphorylation; Integral to membrane; Protein serine/threonine kinase activity; Protein-tyrosine kinase activity; Receptor activity; Membrane; Protein kinase activity; Extracellular space; Kinase activity; Cell differentiation; Transforming growth factor beta receptor signalling pathway; Transforming growth factor beta receptor activity; Transmembrane receptor protein serine/threonine kinase activity; Anterior/posterior pattern formation; Endoderm development; Ectoderm development; Mullerian duct regression; Dorsal/ventral axis specification; Mesendoderm development
17	NM_007560	Bmpr1b	Bone morphogenetic protein receptor, type 1B	ATP binding; Transferase activity; Protein amino acid phosphorylation; Integral to membrane; Protein serine/threonine kinase activity; Protein-tyrosine kinase activity; Receptor signalling protein serine/threonine kinase activity; Receptor activity; Membrane; Protein kinase activity; Kinase activity; Cell differentiation; Type I transforming growth factor beta receptor activity; Transmembrane receptor protein serine/threonine kinase signalling pathway; Transforming growth factor beta receptor signalling pathway; Transforming growth factor beta receptor activity; BMP signalling pathway; Transmembrane receptor protein serine/threonine kinase activity; Cartilage condensation; Eye morphogenesis

Table 5.4. *Continued*

Position	GeneBank	Symbol	Description	GO Term
18	NM_007561	Bmpr2	Bone morphogenic protein receptor, type II (serine/threonine kinase)	ATP binding; Transferase activity; Protein amino acid phosphorylation; Integral to membrane; Protein serine/threonine kinase activity; Protein-tyrosine kinase activity; Receptor activity; Membrane; Protein kinase activity; Extracellular space; Transforming growth factor beta receptor signalling pathway; Cell surface; Transforming growth factor beta receptor activity; Transmembrane receptor protein serine/threonine kinase activity
19	NM_007588	Calcr	Calcitonin receptor	Integral to membrane; G-protein coupled receptor protein signalling pathway; Receptor activity; Membrane; Extracellular space; G-protein coupled receptor activity; Calcitonin receptor activity
20	NM_007643	Cd36	CD36 antigen	Plasma membrane; Integral to membrane; Cell adhesion; Protein binding; Receptor activity; Membrane; Transport;
21	NM_009866	Cdh11	Cadherin 11	Plasma membrane; Integral to membrane; Calcium ion binding; Cell adhesion; Protein binding; Cytoplasm; Homophilic cell adhesion; Membrane
22	NM_009925	Col10a1	Procollagen, type X, alpha 1	Structural molecule activity; Cell adhesion; Cytoplasm; Extracellular space; Phosphate transport; Collagen; Extracellular matrix structural constituent conferring tensile strength; Extracellular matrix (sensu Metazoa)
23	NM_007729	Col11a1	Procollagen, type XI, alpha 1	Structural molecule activity; Cell adhesion; Cytoplasm; Extracellular matrix structural constituent; Phosphate transport; Collagen; Extracellular matrix structural constituent conferring tensile strength; Cartilage condensation; Proteoglycan metabolism; Extracellular matrix (sensu Metazoa); Collagen fibril organization;

Table 5.4. *Continued*

Position	GeneBank	Symbol	Description	GO Term
24	NM_007730	Col12a1	Procollagen, type XII, alpha 1	Structural molecule activity; Cell adhesion; Protein binding; Cytoplasm; Extracellular space; Phosphate transport; Collagen; Extracellular matrix structural constituent conferring tensile strength; Extracellular matrix (sensu Metazoa)
25	NM_181277	Col14a1	Procollagen, type XIV, alpha 1	Structural molecule activity; Cell adhesion; Protein binding; Cytoplasm; Phosphate transport; Collagen; Extracellular matrix structural constituent conferring tensile strength; Extracellular matrix (sensu Metazoa)
26	NM_009928	Col15a1	Procollagen, type XV	Structural molecule activity; Cell adhesion; Extracellular space; Collagen; Extracellular matrix structural constituent conferring tensile strength
27	NM_009929	Col18a1	Procollagen, type XVIII, alpha 1	Structural molecule activity; Cell adhesion; Protein binding; Cytoplasm; Positive regulation of cell proliferation; Development; Membrane; Extracellular space; Transmembrane receptor activity; Extracellular matrix structural constituent; Angiogenesis; Positive regulation of apoptosis; Phosphate transport; Collagen; Positive regulation of cell migration; Basement membrane; Extracellular matrix structural constituent conferring tensile strength; Extracellular matrix (sensu Metazoa); Endothelial cell morphogenesis
28	NM_007733	Col19a1	Procollagen, type XIX, alpha 1	Structural molecule activity; Extracellular space; Collagen; Myogenesis; Extracellular matrix organization and biogenesis

Table 5.4. *Continued*

Position	GeneBank	Symbol	Description	GO Term
40	NM_009933	Col6a1	Procollagen, type VI, alpha 1	Cell adhesion; Proteolysis and peptidolysis; Protein binding; Cytoplasm; Extracellular space; Extracellular matrix structural constituent; Phosphate transport; Collagen; Extracellular matrix structural constituent conferring tensile strength; Subtilase activity; Extracellular matrix (sensu Metazoa)
41	NM_146007	Col6a2	Procollagen, type VI, alpha 2	Cell adhesion; Protein binding; Cytoplasm; Extracellular space; Extracellular matrix structural constituent; Phosphate transport; Collagen; Extracellular matrix structural constituent conferring tensile strength; Extracellular matrix (sensu Metazoa)
42	NM_007738	Col7a1	Procollagen, type VII, alpha 1	Cell adhesion; Extracellular space; Collagen; Extracellular matrix structural constituent conferring tensile strength
43	NM_007739	Col8a1	Procollagen, type VIII, alpha 1	Cell adhesion; Protein binding; Cytoplasm; Extracellular space; Extracellular matrix structural constituent; Phosphate transport; Collagen; Extracellular matrix structural constituent conferring tensile strength; Extracellular matrix (sensu Metazoa)
44	NM_007740	Col9a1	Procollagen, type IX, alpha 1	Cell adhesion; Cytoplasm; Extracellular space; Extracellular matrix structural constituent; Phosphate transport; Collagen; Extracellular matrix structural constituent conferring tensile strength; Extracellular matrix (sensu Metazoa)

Table 5.4. *Continued*

Position	GeneBank	Symbol	Description	GO Term
45	NM_009936	Col9a3	Procollagen, type IX, alpha 3	Structural molecule activity; Cell adhesion; Protein binding; Extracellular space; Extracellular matrix structural constituent; Collagen; Extracellular matrix structural constituent conferring tensile strength; Extracellular matrix (sensu Metazoa); Collagen type IX
46	NM_016685	Comp	Cartilage oligomeric matrix protein	Calcium ion binding; Cell adhesion; Protein binding; Extracellular space; Extracellular region
47	NM_009969	Csf2	Colony stimulating factor 2 (granulocyte-macrophage)	Extracellular; Immune response; Extracellular space; Growth factor activity; Cytokine and chemokine mediated signalling pathway; Cytokine activity; Granulocyte macrophage colony-stimulating factor receptor binding; Dendritic cell differentiation
48	NM_009971	Csf3	Colony stimulating factor 3 (granulocyte)	Extracellular; Immune response; Extracellular space; Growth factor activity; Cytokine activity
49	NM_007802	Ctsk	Cathepsin K	Hydrolase activity; Proteolysis and peptidolysis; Cysteine-type peptidase activity; Extracellular space; Cysteine-type endopeptidase activity; Cathepsin K activity
50	NM_007833	Dcn	Decorin	Extracellular space; Extracellular matrix (sensu Metazoa)
51	NM_016779	Dmp1	Dentin matrix protein 1	Extracellular space; Ossification; Extracellular matrix organization and biogenesis; Extracellular matrix (sensu Metazoa)
52	NM_010080	Dspp	Dentin sialophosphoprotein	Extracellular space; Ossification; Extracellular matrix (sensu Metazoa)

Table 5.4. *Continued*

Position	GeneBank	Symbol	Description	GO Term
53	NM_010113	Egf	Epidermal growth factor	Integral to membrane; Calcium ion binding; Membrane; Extracellular space; Growth factor activity; Regulation of peptidyl-tyrosine phosphorylation;
54	NM_017468	Enam	Enamelin	Extracellular space; Ossification; Extracellular matrix (sensu Metazoa)
55	NM_010197	Fgf1	Fibroblast growth factor 1	Cell proliferation; Signal transduction; Regulation of cell cycle; Heparin binding; Growth factor activity; Angiogenesis; Fibroblast growth factor receptor bindin
56	NM_008006	Fgf2	Fibroblast growth factor 2	Cell proliferation; Signal transduction; Protein binding; Regulation of cell cycle; Extracellular space; Heparin binding; Growth factor activity; Angiogenesis; Positive regulation of cell differentiation; Regulation of retinal programmed cell death; Glial cell differentiation; Fibroblast growth factor receptor binding
57	NM_008007	Fgf3	Fibroblast growth factor 3	Cell proliferation; Signal transduction; Nucleus; Regulation of cell cycle; Extracellular space; Growth factor activity; Fibroblast growth factor receptor binding; Induction of an organ
58	NM_010206	Fgfrl	Fibroblast growth factor receptor 1	ATP binding; Transferase activity; Protein amino acid phosphorylation; Integral to membrane; Signal transduction; Protein serine/threonine kinase activity; Protein-tyrosine kinase activity; Receptor activity; Protein kinase activity; Extracellular space; Heparin binding; Kinase activity; Regulation of cell proliferation; Fibroblast growth factor receptor activity; Salivary gland morphogenesis; Brain development; Branching morphogenesis; Lung development; Induction of an organ; Inner ear morphogenesis

Table 5.4. *Continued*

Position	GeneBank	Symbol	Description	GO Term
59	NM_010207	Fgfr2	Fibroblast growth factor receptor 2	ATP binding; Transferase activity; Protein amino acid phosphorylation; Integral to membrane; Signal transduction; Nucleus; Protein binding; Protein serine/threonine kinase activity; Protein-tyrosine kinase activity; Positive regulation of cell proliferation; Receptor activity; Protein kinase activity; Extracellular space; Cell-cell signalling; Regulation of cell proliferation; Fibroblast growth factor receptor activity; Salivary gland morphogenesis; Bone mineralization
60	NM_008010	Fgfr3	Fibroblast growth factor receptor 3	ATP binding; Transferase activity; Protein amino acid phosphorylation; Integral to membrane; Signal transduction; Protein serine/threonine kinase activity; Protein-tyrosine kinase activity; Receptor activity; Protein kinase activity; Extracellular space; Kinase activity; Positive regulation of cell differentiation; Fibroblast growth factor receptor activity
61	NM_010228	Flt1	FMS-like tyrosine kinase 1	ATP binding; Transferase activity; Protein amino acid phosphorylation; Integral to membrane; Protein serine/threonine kinase activity; Protein-tyrosine kinase activity; Receptor activity; Transmembrane receptor protein tyrosine kinase activity; Membrane; Protein kinase activity; Extracellular space; Transmembrane receptor protein tyrosine kinase signalling pathway; Kinase activity; Vascular endothelial growth factor receptor activity; Angiogenesis; Patterning of blood vessels

Table 5.4. *Continued*

Position	GeneBank	Symbol	Description	GO Term
62	NM_010233	Fn1	Fibronectin 1	Cell adhesion; Extracellular; Protein binding; Oxidoreductase activity; Extracellular space; Heparin binding; Acute-phase response; Metabolism; Cell-substrate junction assembly; Wound healing; Extracellular matrix (sensu Metazoa)
63	NM_145741	Gdf10	Growth differentiation factor 10	Extracellular space; Growth factor activity; Cytokine activity
64	NM_008318	Ibsp	Integrin binding sialoprotein	Cell adhesion; Protein binding; Extracellular space; Integrin-mediated signalling pathway; Ossification; Extracellular region
65	NM_010493	Icam1	H1 histone family, member 0	Plasma membrane; Integral to membrane; Cell adhesion; Protein binding; Membrane; Cell-cell adhesion; Defence response
66	NM_010512	Igf1	Insulin-like growth factor 1	Extracellular; Anti-apoptosis; Organogenesis; Growth factor activity; Hormone activity; Physiological process; Neurogenesis; Glial cell differentiation; Insulin-like growth factor receptor signalling pathway
67	NM_010513	Igf1r	Insulin-like growth factor I receptor	ATP binding; Transferase activity; Protein amino acid phosphorylation; Integral to membrane; Protein binding; Protein serine/threonine kinase activity; Protein-tyrosine kinase activity; Receptor activity; Transmembrane receptor protein tyrosine kinase activity; Membrane; Protein kinase activity; Extracellular space; Epidermal growth factor receptor activity; Organogenesis; Transmembrane receptor protein tyrosine kinase signalling pathway; Insulin-like growth factor receptor signalling pathway; Brain development; Male sex determination

Table 5.4. *Continued*

Position	GeneBank	Symbol	Description	GO Term
68	NM_008396	Itga2	Integrin alpha 2	Integral to membrane; Cell adhesion; Protein binding; Receptor activity; Cell-matrix adhesion; Extracellular space; Integrin-mediated signalling pathway; Integrin complex; Magnesium ion binding
69	NM_010575	Itga2b	Integrin alpha 2b	Integral to membrane; Cell adhesion; Proteolysis and peptidolysis; Protein binding; Receptor activity; Cell-matrix adhesion; Extracellular space; Integrin-mediated signalling pathway; Integrin complex; External side of plasma membrane; Carboxypeptidase A activity
70	NM_013565	Itga3	Integrin alpha 3	Integral to membrane; Cell adhesion; Protein binding; Cell-matrix adhesion; Integrin-mediated signalling pathway; Integrin complex; Synaptosome; Basolateral plasma membrane; Memory; NOT fusion of sperm to egg plasma membrane; Neuronal migration
71	NM_008401	Itgam	Integrin alpha M	Integral to membrane; Cell adhesion; Protein binding; Receptor activity; Cell-matrix adhesion; Integrin-mediated signalling pathway; Integrin complex; Neutrophil chemotaxis; Cellular extravasation; External side of plasma membrane; Opsonin binding
72	NM_008402	Itgav	Integrin alpha V	Integral to membrane; Cell adhesion; Protein binding; Receptor activity; Cell-matrix adhesion; Integrin-mediated signalling pathway; Integrin complex; Angiogenesis; Blood vessel development
73	NM_010578	Itgb1	Integrin beta 1 (fibronectin receptor beta)	Plasma membrane; Integral to membrane; Cell adhesion; Protein binding; Oxidoreductase activity; Regulation of cell cycle; Receptor activity; Cell-matrix adhesion; G1/S transition of mitotic cell cycle; Extracellular space; Metabolism; Integrin-mediated signalling pathway; Integrin complex; Synaptosome

Table 5.4. *Continued*

Position	GeneBank	Symbol	Description	GO Term
74	NM_008597	Mglap	Matrix gamma-carboxyglutamate (gla) protein	Calcium ion binding; Development; Extracellular space; Cell differentiation; Extracellular region; Regulation of bone mineralization
75	NM_019471	Mmp10	Matrix metalloproteinase 10	Hydrolase activity; Extracellular; Proteolysis and peptidolysis; Zinc ion binding; Collagen catabolism; Extracellular space; Metalloendopeptidase activity; Metallopeptidase activity; Extracellular matrix (sensu Metazoa)
76	NM_008607	Mmp13	Matrix metalloproteinase 13	Hydrolase activity; Calcium ion binding; Proteolysis and peptidolysis; Zinc ion binding; Interstitial collagenase activity; Collagen catabolism; Extracellular space; Metalloendopeptidase activity; Metallopeptidase activity; Extracellular matrix (sensu Metazoa)
77	NM_008610	Mmp2	Matrix metalloproteinase 2	Hydrolase activity; Calcium ion binding; Proteolysis and peptidolysis; Zinc ion binding; Collagen catabolism; Extracellular matrix; Extracellular space; Gelatinase A activity; Metalloendopeptidase activity; Metallopeptidase activity; Extracellular matrix (sensu Metazoa)
78	NM_008611	Mmp8	Matrix metalloproteinase 8	Hydrolase activity; Calcium ion binding; Proteolysis and peptidolysis; Zinc ion binding; Collagen catabolism; Extracellular space; Metalloendopeptidase activity; Metallopeptidase activity; Extracellular matrix (sensu Metazoa)
79	NM_013599	Mmp9	Matrix metalloproteinase 9	Hydrolase activity; Proteolysis and peptidolysis; Zinc ion binding; Collagen catabolism; Extracellular space; Metalloendopeptidase activity; Metallopeptidase activity; Gelatinase B activity; Extracellular matrix (sensu Metazoa)

Table 5.4. *Continued*

Position	GeneBank	Symbol	Description	GO Term
80	NM_010835	Msx1	Homeo box, msh-like 1	DNA binding; Regulation of transcription, DNA-dependent; Nucleus; Transcription factor activity; Development; Transcription factor complex; Transcription; Forebrain development; Midbrain development
81	NM_008689	Nfkb1	Ubiquitin-conjugating enzyme E2D 3 (UBC4/5 homolog, yeast)	Signal transduction; DNA binding; Regulation of transcription, DNA-dependent; Nucleus; Protein binding; Apoptosis; Transcription factor activity; Lymph gland development; Specific transcriptional repressor activity; Negative regulation of interleukin-12 biosynthesis; Negative regulation of transcription, DNA-dependent
82	NM_008808	Pdgfa	Platelet derived growth factor, alpha	Cell proliferation; Cell growth and/or maintenance; Regulation of cell cycle; Membrane; Extracellular space; Organogenesis; Growth factor activity; Regulation of peptidyl-tyrosine phosphorylation; Actin cytoskeleton organization and biogenesis; Cell projection biogenesis;
83	NM_011077	Phex	Phosphate regulating gene with homologies to endopeptidases on the X chromosome	Hydrolase activity; Integral to membrane; Proteolysis and peptidolysis; Zinc ion binding; Membrane; Metallopeptidase activity; Neprilysin activity; Peptidase activity; Ossification

Table 5.4. *Continued*

Position	GeneBank	Symbol	Description	GO Term
84	NM_009820	Runx2	Runt related transcription factor 2	ATP binding; DNA binding; Regulation of transcription, DNA-dependent; Nucleus; Protein binding; Cytoplasm; Transcription factor activity; Skeletal development; Transcription; Odontogenesis (sensu Vertebrata); Chromatin binding; Regulation of fibroblast growth factor receptor signalling pathway; Positive regulation of transcription from RNA polymerase II promoter; Cell maturation; Osteoblast differentiation; Regulation of odontogenesis (sensu Vertebrata)
85	NM_016741	Scarb1	Scavenger receptor class B, member 1	Integral to membrane; Cell adhesion; Receptor activity; Membrane
86	NM_009825	Serpinh1	Serine (or cysteine) proteinase inhibitor, clade H, member 1	Response to heat; Extracellular space; Heat shock protein activity; Endoplasmic reticulum; Serine-type endopeptidase inhibitor activity
87	NM_008539	Smad1	MAD homolog 1 (Drosophila)	Regulation of transcription, DNA-dependent; Protein binding; Transcription factor activity; Regulation of transcription from Pol II promoter; RNA polymerase II transcription factor activity; Intracellular; Transcription factor complex; Organogenesis; MAPKKK cascade; BMP signalling pathway; Gametogenesis; Common-partner SMAD protein phosphorylation; SMAD protein heteromerization; Homeostasis

Table 5.4. *Continued*

Position	GeneBank	Symbol	Description	GO Term
88	NM_010754	Smad2	MAD homolog 2 (Drosophila)	Regulation of transcription, DNA-dependent; Nucleus; Protein binding; Intracellular; Transcription factor complex; Organogenesis; Transcription factor binding; Transforming growth factor beta receptor signalling pathway; Positive regulation of transcription from Pol II promoter; Cell fate commitment; Mesoderm formation; Anterior/posterior pattern formation; Common-partner SMAD protein phosphorylation; SMAD protein heteromerization; Paraxial mesoderm morphogenesis
89	NM_016769	Smad3	MAD homolog 3 (Drosophila)	Plasma membrane; Regulation of transcription, DNA-dependent; Nucleus; Protein binding; Transcription factor activity; Negative regulation of transcription from Pol II promoter; Transcription from Pol II promoter; Intracellular; Organogenesis; Transcription factor binding; Transforming growth factor beta receptor signalling pathway; Positive regulation of transcription from Pol II promoter; Mesoderm formation; Regulation of myogenesis; Common-partner SMAD protein phosphorylation; SMAD protein heteromerization; Paraxial mesoderm morphogenesis; Regulation of epithelial cell proliferation; Regulation of transforming growth factor beta receptor signalling pathway

Table 5.4. *Continued*

Position	GeneBank	Symbol	Description	GO Term
90	NM_008540	Smad4	MAD homolog 4 (Drosophila)	DNA binding; Regulation of transcription, DNA-dependent; Nucleus; Protein binding; Transcription factor activity; Regulation of transcription from Pol II promoter; Intracellular; Transcription factor complex; Organogenesis; Positive regulation of transcription from Pol II promoter; SMAD protein nuclear translocation; Common-partner SMAD protein phosphorylation;
91	NM_008541	Smad5	MAD homolog 5 (Drosophila)	Regulation of transcription, DNA-dependent; Protein binding; Intracellular; Organogenesis; Angiogenesis; Transforming growth factor beta receptor signalling pathway; BMP signalling pathway; Common-partner SMAD protein phosphorylation; SMAD protein heteromerization
92	NM_008542	Smad6	MAD homolog 6 (Drosophila)	Regulation of transcription, DNA-dependent; Intracellular; Common-partner SMAD protein phosphorylation
93	NM_008543	Smad7	MAD homolog 7 (Drosophila)	Regulation of transcription, DNA-dependent; Intracellular; Transforming growth factor beta receptor signalling pathway; Common-partner SMAD protein phosphorylation
94	NM_019483	Smad9	MAD homolog 9 (Drosophila)	Regulation of transcription, DNA-dependent; Protein binding; Intracellular
95	NM_024449	Sost	Sclerostin	Extracellular space; Ossification; Negative regulation of BMP signalling pathway

Table 5.4. *Continued*

Position	GeneBank	Symbol	Description	GO Term
96	NM_011448	Sox9	SRY-box containing gene 9	DNA binding; Regulation of transcription, DNA-dependent; Nucleus; Protein binding; Transcription factor activity; Transcription factor complex; Cell differentiation; Transcription; Heart development; Epithelial to mesenchymal transition; Cartilage condensation; Cell fate specification; Male gonad development; Positive regulation of transcription from RNA polymerase II promoter; Male germ-line sex determination
97	NM_009242	Sparc	Secreted acidic cysteine rich glycoprotein	Calcium ion binding; Extracellular space; Basement membrane; Extracellular matrix (sensu Metazoa)
98	NM_009263	Spp1	Secreted phosphoprotein 1	Cell adhesion; Protein binding; Extracellular space; Cytokine activity; Ossification
99	NM_018783	Tfip11	Tuftelin interacting protein 11	Nucleic acid binding; Nucleus; Cytoplasm, Intracellular; Ossification; Extracellular matrix (sensu Metazoa); Rhythmic process
100	NM_011577	Tgfb1	Transforming growth factor, beta 1	Protein amino acid phosphorylation; Cell proliferation; Protein binding; Negative regulation of cell proliferation; Regulation of cell cycle; Inflammatory response; Extracellular matrix; Extracellular space; Organogenesis; Growth factor activity; Skeletal development; Defence response; Regulation of cell proliferation; Necrosis; Transforming growth factor beta receptor signalling pathway; Transforming growth factor beta receptor binding; Cell growth; Lymph gland development; Growth; Myogenesis; Regulation of myogenesis; Regulation of protein-nucleus import

Table 5.4. *Continued*

Position	GeneBank	Symbol	Description	GO Term
101	NM_009367	Tgfb2	Transforming growth factor, beta 2	Cell proliferation; Regulation of cell cycle; Extracellular space; Growth factor activity; Transforming growth factor beta receptor binding; Cell growth; Growth; Extracellular matrix organization and biogenesis
102	NM_009368	Tgfb3	Transforming growth factor, beta 3	Cell proliferation; Negative regulation of cell proliferation; Regulation of cell cycle; Extracellular space; Organogenesis; Growth factor activity; Transforming growth factor beta receptor binding; Cell growth; Growth; Embryonic development (sensu Mammalia); Embryonic morphogenesis
103	NM_009370	Tgfbrl	Transforming growth factor, beta receptor I	ATP binding; Transferase activity; Protein amino acid phosphorylation; Integral to membrane; Protein binding; Protein serine/threonine kinase activity; Protein-tyrosine kinase activity; Receptor activity; Membrane; Protein kinase activity; Extracellular space; Kinase activity; Transforming growth factor beta receptor signalling pathway; Transforming growth factor beta receptor activity; Transmembrane receptor protein serine/threonine kinase activity

Table 5.4. *Continued*

Position	GeneBank	Symbol	Description	GO Term
104	NM_009371	Tgfbr2	Transforming growth factor, beta receptor II	ATP binding; Transferase activity; Protein amino acid phosphorylation; Integral to membrane; Protein serine/threonine kinase activity; Protein-tyrosine kinase activity; Receptor signalling protein serine/threonine kinase activity; Receptor activity; Membrane; Protein kinase activity; Kinase activity; Regulation of cell proliferation; Transmembrane receptor protein serine/threonine kinase signalling pathway; Transforming growth factor beta receptor activity; Cell fate commitment; Transmembrane receptor protein serine/threonine kinase activity
105	NM_011578	Tgfbr3	Similar to Ornithine decarboxylase (ODC)	Integral to membrane; Receptor activity; Extracellular space
106	NM_013693	Tnf	Tumour necrosis factor	Plasma membrane; Cell proliferation; Immune response; Cell growth and/or maintenance; Humoral immune response; Inflammatory response; Positive regulation of cell proliferation; Induction of apoptosis via death domain receptors; Signal transducer activity; Development; Positive regulation of I-kappaB kinase/NF-kappaB cascade; Integral to plasma membrane; Organogenesis; Tumour necrosis factor receptor binding; Defence response; Secretory granule; Regulation of cell proliferation; Cytokine and chemokine mediated signalling pathway; Cellular defence response; Lymph gland development; Cellular extravasation; Positive regulation of osteoclast differentiation; Programmed cell death, transformed cells; Regulation of osteoclast differentiation
107	NM_011656	Tuft1	Tuftelin 1	Ossification

Table 5.4. *Continued*

Position	GeneBank	Symbol	Description	GO Term
108	NM_011658	Twist1	Twist gene homolog 1 (Drosophila)	DNA binding; Regulation of transcription, DNA-dependent; Nucleus; Development; Cell differentiation; Embryonic limb morphogenesis; Neuronal migration; Hindlimb morphogenesis; Neural tube closure
109	NM_007855	Twist2	Twist homolog 2 (Drosophila)	DNA binding; Regulation of transcription, DNA-dependent; Nucleus; Transcription factor activity; Development; Transcription factor complex; Cell differentiation; Transcription; Transcriptional repressor activity; Regulation of transcription from RNA polymerase II promoter
110	NM_011693	Vcam1	Vascular cell adhesion molecule 1	Plasma membrane; Integral to membrane; Cell adhesion; Protein binding; Membrane; Cell-cell adhesion; Extracellular space
111	NM_009504	Vdr	Vitamin D receptor	DNA binding; Regulation of transcription, DNA-dependent; Nucleus; Protein binding; Transcription factor activity; Development; Receptor activity; Organogenesis; Skeletal development; Calcium ion homeostasis; Steroid hormone receptor activity; Transcription; Calcium ion transport; Ligand-dependent nuclear receptor activity; Transcription regulator activity; Negative regulation of transcription; Intestinal absorption
112	NM_009505	Vegfa	Vascular endothelial growth factor A	Cell proliferation; Cell growth and/or maintenance; Anti-apoptosis; Regulation of cell cycle; Mesoderm development; Membrane; Extracellular space; Heparin binding; Growth factor activity; Angiogenesis

Table 5.4. *Continued*

Position	GeneBank	Symbol	Description	GO Term
113	NM_011697	Vegfb	Vascular endothelial growth factor B	Cell proliferation; Cell growth and/or maintenance; Regulation of cell cycle; Membrane; Extracellular space; Heparin binding; Growth factor activity; Angiogenesis
114	NM_009506	Vegfc	Vascular endothelial growth factor C	Cell proliferation; Cell growth and/or maintenance; Regulation of cell cycle; Membrane; Extracellular space; Organogenesis; Growth factor activity; Angiogenesis; Morphogenesis of embryonic epithelium
115	L08752	PUC18	PUC18 Plasmid DNA	
116	SA_00005	AS1R2	Artificial Sequence 1 Related 2 (80% identity)(48/60)	
117	SA_00004	AS1R1	Artificial Sequence 1 Related 1 (90% identity)(54/60)	
118	SA_00003	AS1	Artificial Sequence 1	
119	NM_024277	Rps27a	Ribosomal protein S27a	Intracellular; Protein biosynthesis; Ribosome
120	NM_009735	B2m	Beta-2 microglobulin	Plasma membrane; Integral to plasma membrane; Extracellular space; Defence response; Cellular defence response; Antigen processing, endogenous antigen via MHC class I; MHC class I receptor activity; Antigen presentation, endogenous antigen

Table 5.4. *Continued*

Position	GeneBank	Symbol	Description	GO Term
121	NM_008302	Hspcb	Heat shock protein 1, beta	ATP binding; Protein binding; Mitochondrion; Response to heat; Protein folding; Unfolded protein binding; Response to unfolded protein; ATP binding; Protein binding; Mitochondrion; Response to heat; Protein folding; Unfolded protein binding; Response to unfolded protein
122	NM_008302	Hspcb	Heat shock protein 1, beta	ATP binding; Protein binding; Mitochondrion; Response to heat; Protein folding; Unfolded protein binding; Response to unfolded protein; ATP binding; Protein binding; Mitochondrion; Response to heat; Protein folding; Unfolded protein binding; Response to unfolded protein
123	NM_008907	Ppia	Peptidylprolyl isomerase A	Cytosol; Protein folding; Isomerase activity; Peptidyl-prolyl cis-trans isomerase activity; Cytosol; Protein folding; Isomerase activity; Peptidyl-prolyl cis-trans isomerase activity
124	NM_008907	Ppia	Peptidylprolyl isomerase A	Cytosol; Protein folding; Isomerase activity; Peptidyl-prolyl cis-trans isomerase activity; Cytosol; Protein folding; Isomerase activity; Peptidyl-prolyl cis-trans isomerase activity
125	SA_00007	BAS2C	Biotinylated Artificial Sequence 2 Complementary sequence	
126	SA_00007	BAS2C	Biotinylated Artificial Sequence 2 Complementary sequence	

Materials 6

Application of non-living biomaterials can be conceptualised as the use of materials to replace lost structures, augment existing structures or promote new tissue formation (Burg et al., 2000a; 2000b). Common degradable and non-degradable implant materials can be divided into synthetically produced metals and metallic alloys, ceramics, polymers, and composites or modified natural materials (Meyer et al., 2004a). Whereas non-resorbable materials like steel or titanium alloys are commonly used for prosthetic devices, resorbable substitute materials are currently being investigated for their utility in bone and cartilage replacement therapies. Whether or not a material is biodegradable, its surface properties will influence the initial cellular events at the cell–material interface. A major difference between degradable and non-degradable implants is that the surface adhesion towards osteoblasts or chondrocytes changes in degradable materials, while it remains constant in non-degradable implants. The clinical fate of implants, substitute materials and scaffolds used in tissue engineering strategies critically depends on the underlying material (Meyer et al., 2004b) and the mechanical properties of the material-based scaffold (Table 6.1). In the design process of cell-based implants and engineered bone and cartilage substitutes it is important to consider the cellular behaviour of the desired cell source towards the material (for a review, see Shin et al, 2003).

Four types of materials have been experimentally and/or clinically studied as bone and cartilage substitute materials or scaffold materials for applications in tissue engineering:

- Various groups of synthetic organic materials, including (1) biodegradable and bioresorbable polymers, which have been used for clinically established products, such as polyglycolide, optically active and racemic polylactides, polydioxanone,

Table 6.1. Mechanical properties of materials

	Young's modulus (GPa)	Strength (MPa) Compressive	Bending
Cortical bone	7–30	100–230	50–150
Cancellous bone	0.05–0.5	2–12	–
Cartilage	0.2–0.3	0.01–3	–
Synthetic HA	80–110	500–1000	115–200
PLGA 85/15	2	0.34	–
PLGA 75/25	2	0.34	–
A-W glass-ceramic	118	1080	220
Collagen tendon	1,5	0.14	–

and polycaprolactone; (2) polymers currently under clinical investigation, such as polyorthoester, polyanhydrides, and polyhydroxyalkanoate; and (3) entrepreneurial polymeric biomaterials, such as poly (lactic acid-co-lysine)
- Synthetic inorganic materials (e.g. hydroxyapatite, calcium/phosphate composites, glass ceramics)
- Organic materials of natural origin (e.g. collagen, fibrin, hyaluronic acid)
- Inorganic material of natural origin (e.g. coralline hydroxyapatite).

Several reports have been published on the physico-chemical properties and surface characteristics of these biodegradable and bioresorbable polymers (Hutmacher, 2000). It was found that features of the material surface are important for correct implantation and coverage by autochtonic cells.

A comprehensive overview of the materials used in bone and cartilage tissue engineering is given in this chapter. Additionally, surface properties of materials will be discussed, since material characteristics and surface properties of materials are closely related. The list of materials used for bone tissue engineering differs from that of cartilage engineering, in that organic materials are preferentially used for bone tissue engineering.

6.1 Synthetic Organic Materials

Various polymers are used extensively for the preparation of bone and cartilage scaffolds (Fig. 6.1). Most of them are fabricated on the basis of polyhydroxyacids, such as polylactides, polyglycolides, and their copolymers. Other synthetic materials include polyethylene oxide, polyvinyl alcohol, polyacrylic acid, and polypropylene

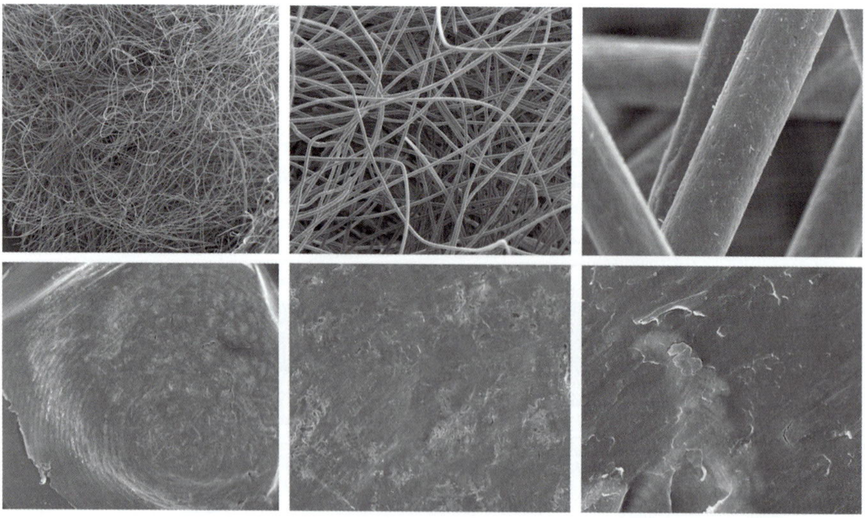

Fig. 6.1. Scanning electron microscopical view of hyaluronic acid-based biomaterials. The biomaterial can be processed as a fibre-based scaffold *(top row)* or as a bulk material. *From left to right:* detailed aspects of material structure and surface

furmarate-co-ethylene glycol. Scaffolds based on biodegradable polyhydroxyacids, such as poly-lactide-glycolide copolymers, have been widely used as materials for bone and cartilage tissue engineering, since these polymers support the attachment and proliferation of both cell types (Vacanti et al., 1991; Freed et al., 1993; 1994; Kim et al., 1994; Chu et al., 1995; Sittinger et al., 1996; Grande et al., 1997; Gugala and Gogolewski., 2000). Polylactic acid and polyglycolic acid (PLA/PGA) copolymers degrade primarily via chemical hydrolysis of the hydrolytically unstable ester bonds into lactic acid and glycolic acid, which are non-toxic and can be removed from the body by normal metabolic pathways (Athanasiou et al., 2001). Additionally, enzymatic degradation has been reported for those copolymers (Freed et al., 1993). It was found that the degradation behaviour of polyhydroxyacids depends on the polymer structure and surface properties (molecular weight, copolymer composition, crystallinity, overall material surface, etc.) and environmental conditions (medium exchange, temperature, polymer/host interaction, and pH) (Table 6.2). The degradation rate of polyhydroxyacids can be adjusted by changes of the PLA/PGA ratio, the molecular weight of each component, the crystallinity, and other factors in order to support the slow degradation rate. This degradation rate may be similar or slightly lower than the rate of tissue formation in the defect site (Burkart et al., 2001). It is important to note in this respect that the repair or remodelling turnover time of cartilage and bone differs significantly. Limited resistance of polyhydroxyacid materials to loading, as well as their limited deformability and elasticity are disadvantageous in their use for bone and cartilage tissue engineering strategies, especially if mechanical competence is required (Grad et al., 2003). Elastomeric polyurethanes are materials with enhanced molecular stability in vivo. Newly designed biodegradable polyurethanes were shown to degrade in vivo to non-toxic by-products (Gogolewski and Pennings, 1982; 1983; Gogolewski et al., 1983; 1987a; 1987b; Gogolewski and Galetti, 1986; Galetti et al., 1989; Elema et al., 1990; Klompmaker et al., 1991). Based on these findings, biodegradable polyurethanes have been used successfully as cancellous bone graft substitutes in animals (Gogolewski et al., 2001; 2002). However, very little attention has been paid to biodegradable polyurethanes as scaffolding materials for chondrocytes. To date, only hydroxybutyrate-co-valerate polyol-based polyurethane was used to culture rat chondrocytes (Saad et al., 1999).

Table 6.2. Properties of synthetic polymers

Polymer	Strength (GPa)	Degradationtime time (month)	Degradation products
Polyester (polyglycolic acid)	7.0	6–12	Glycolic acid
Polyester (poly(l)-lactic acid)	2.7	>>24	l-Lactic acid
Polyester (poly(d,l-lactic-co-glycolic) acid (85/15))	2.0	1–6	d,l-Lactic acid, glycolic acid
Polyester (polycaprolactone)	0.4	>>24	Caproic acid
Polyester (polydioxanone)		–	
Polyester (polypropylenefumarat)	2–30	–	Fumaric acid, propylene glycol

6.2 Synthetic Inorganic Materials

Various types of synthetic inorganic materials have been developed in skeletal replacement therapies (Table 6.4). These synthetic substrates, capable of supporting the natural process of bone remodelling, were mainly used in bone tissue engineering applications, which include the ex vivo generation of cell–scaffold complexes, in vivo resorbable bone cements, implantable coatings to enhance the bonding of natural bone to the implant, various forms of implantable prostheses and bone repair agents (Friedman et al., 1998; LeGeros, 2002; Ohgushi et al., 2003; Uemura et al., 2003). Synthetic inorganic materials are seldom used in cartilage tissue engineering strategies, since the matrix of cartilage does not contain crystalline inorganic materials (except for the calcified cartilage layer). Among the materials used as scaffolds for bone tissue engineering, calcium phosphate containing ceramics are most frequently exploited in bone replacement strategies (Fig. 6.2). These are: hydroxyapatite (HA) ($Ca_{10}(PO_4)_6(OH)_2$), β-tricalcium phosphate (TCP) ($Ca_3(PO_4)_2$) and hydroxyapatite/β-tricalcium phosphate bi-phase ceramics. Calcium phosphate materials have differing degrees of stoichiometry. Hydroxyapatite is the most widely used of a number of calcium–phosphorous (Ca–P) compounds, which are near the primary ionic component of natural bone. Pure hydroxyapatite has the stoichiometric Ca to P ratio of 1.67, lattice parameters: a axis = 0.94 nm and c axis = 0.69 nm, and the presence of only the OH and PO4 absorption bands in their infrared spectra. Other CaP materials also recommended for scaffolds in bone tissue engineering include octacalcium phosphate (Kamakura et al., 1999), whitlockite, or Mg-substituted tricalcium phosphates (Gatti et al.,1998), Zn-substituted tricalcium phosphate (Kawamura et al., 2000), carbonate-substituted apatites (Okazaki et al., 1998), and fluoride-substituted apatites (Monroe et al., 1971; Kazimiroff et al., 1996; Frondoza

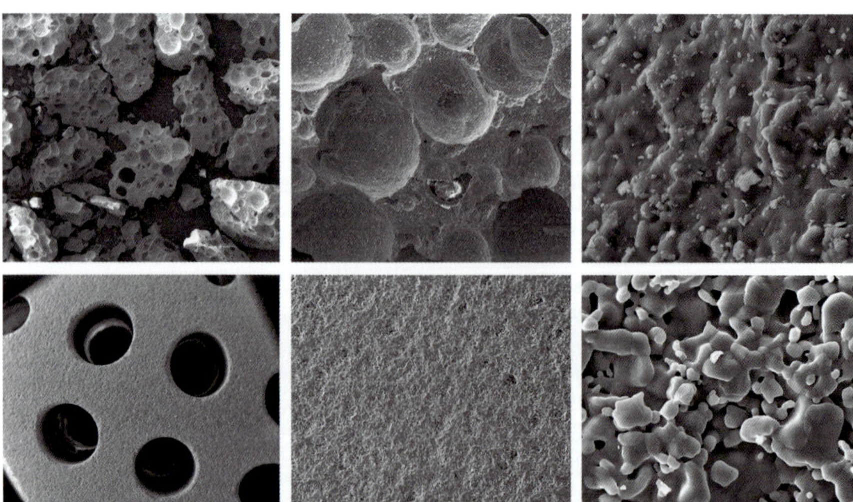

Fig. 6.2. Scanning electron microscopical view of two different tricalciumphosphate-based biomaterials *(top vs. bottom)*, showing different gross morphologies. *From left to right:* detailed aspects of material structure and surface

et al., 1998; Gatti et al.,1998). Substitution of single elements in the calcium phosphate or apatite structure affects the crystal and dissociation properties of CaP. Carbonate substitution for example causes not only the formation of smaller and more soluble apatite particles, but also better pH stability, whereas fluoride incorporation has the opposite effects upon material degradation while having no effect on the pH stability (Zapanta-LeGeros, 1965; Moreno et al., 1977; LeGeros, 1981; 1991; LeGeros et al., 1967; 1971; 1996). Magnesium incorporation in apatite is limited but causes reduction in crystallinity (smaller crystal size) and increases the extent of dissolution (LeGeros, 1981; 1991; LeGeros et al., 1989; 1995a; 1996). Magnesium or zinc substitution in different calcium materials also affects the properties (LeGeros, 1991; Okazaki and LeGeros, 1992; LeGeros et al., 1999).

Properties of ceramic materials can be manipulated by the fabrication process. Parameters like porosity, crystal size, composition, and dissolution properties determine to a great extent the fate of the material in the in vivo and in vitro situation (LeGeros, 1988; 1991; LeGeros et al., 1991). Due to their ionic, hydrophilic composition, ceramic materials have a particular affinity to bind proteins. They may therefore be suitable carriers for bioactive peptides or bone growth factors (Ohgushi and Caplan, 1999; Toquet et al., 1999; Reddi, 2000). However, it is important to note that although CaP biomaterials are osteoconductive they do not have osteoinductive properties meaning that they are unable to support de novo bone tissue generation at non-bony sites.

6.3 Natural Organic Materials

Naturally derived materials have frequently been exploited in tissue engineering applications because they are either components of or have macromolecular properties similar to the natural ECM (Table 6.3). For example, collagens, fibrin, hyaluronan or some proteoglycans are main proteins of hard tissue tissue ECM of vertebrates (Fig. 6.3). Additionally, non-mammalian molecules like alginate and chitosan are candidates for scaffold materials. Despite the fact that the latter materials are not present

Table 6.3. Naturally occurring and artificial polymeric scaffold materials

Natural		
- Collagen - Fibrin	- Hyaluronan	
Artificial		
- Gelatine	- Polylactic acid - Polyglycolic acid - Chitosan - Agarose - Alginate	- Polymethlymethacrylate - Polyethylene - Polytetrafluoroethylene - Polybutyric acid - Polycarbonate - Polyesterurethane
Protein-based	**Carbohydrate-based**	**Synthetic**

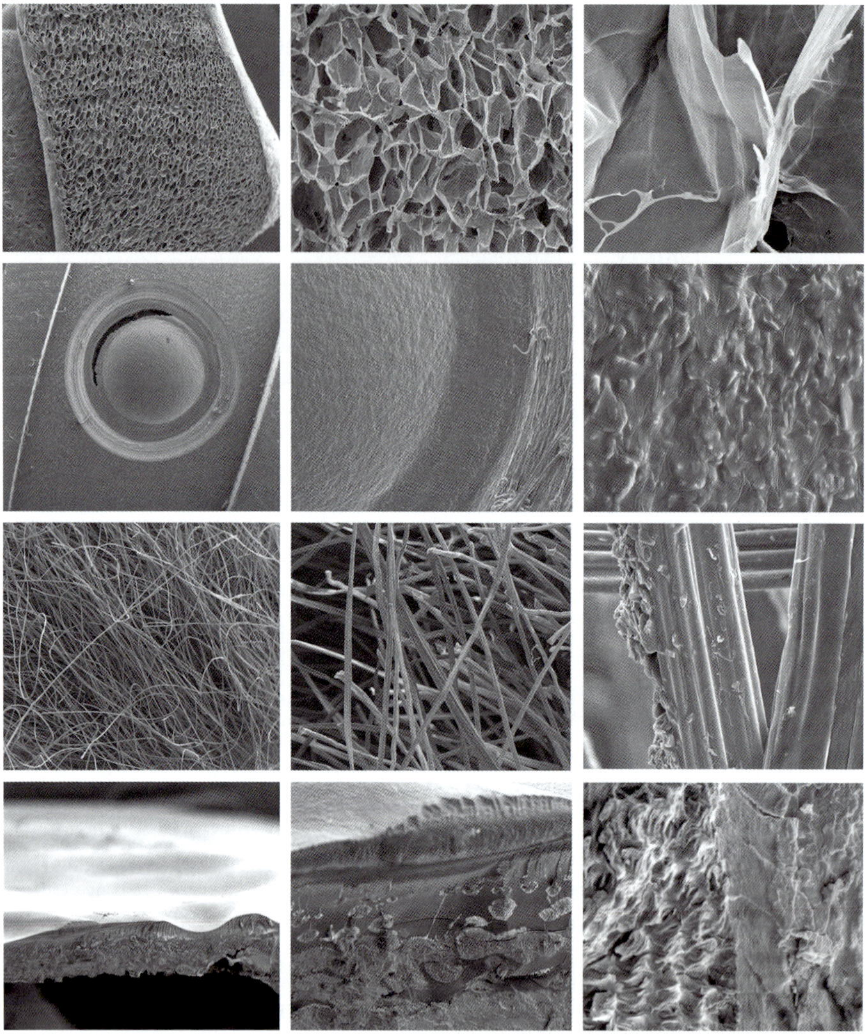

Fig. 6.3. Scanning electron microscopical view of differently structured biodegradable materials for bone and cartilage reconstruction. Materials can have a spongiosa-like *(top row)*, a bulk *(second row)*, a fibre-like *(third row)*, or a compound *(bottom row)* structure. *From left to right:* detailed aspects of material structure and surface

in human tissues, they have also been shown to interact in a favourable manner with the surface of implant devices and have been utilised as scaffold materials for bone and cartilage tissue engineering.

Collagens are attractive materials for bone and cartilage tissue engineering as this group of secreted proteins is present in skeletal tissues, where they constitute a main substrate of the ECM (Höhling et al., 1995; Sanchez et al., 2005; Wiesmann et al., 2005). Details of the ECM structure of bone and cartilage are described in detail in Chap. 2. Whereas collagen type I is the predominantly expressed collagen found in bone tissue, collagen type II is present in the ECM of cartilage. As ideal scaffold materials mimicking the real situation, collagen-based scaffolds for bone or cartilage should differ in their composition. The basic structure of all collagen is composed of three polypeptide chains, building up a three-stranded rope structure. The various types of collagen are naturally degraded by secreted collagenases. Thus, the degradation of collagen fibres is locally controlled by cells present in the engineered tissue and the balance between collagen synthesis and the activities of collagenases is expected to determine the turnover rate of the carrier. Moreover, it is important that collagen-based scaffolds usually do not provoke a foreign tissue response. From a biomaterials perspective it should be noted that the features of collagen scaffolds can be modified according to experimental or clinical needs. Collagen-based scaffolds can be created artificially and their mechanical properties altered to some extent by various chemical and physical techniques. Modification of collagen can be performed by incubation of collagen with chemical cross-linkers (i.e. glutaraldehyde, formaldehyde, carbodiimide), by physical treatments (i.e. UV irradiation, freeze-drying, heating), and by copolymerisation with other polymers (e.g polyhydroxyacids) (Knott and Bailey, 1998). Importantly, the mechanical strength of all collagen scaffolds is limited in clinical terms (since the e-modulus of collagen is much lower than that of bone), even when molecules are cross-linked. By using defined collagen types for scaffold production, cellular differentiation can be promoted (e.g. collagen type I for osteoblastic differentiation and collagen type II for chondrocytic differentiation).

During the last decade hyaluronan (HA) has received increased attention as a scaffold material for cartilage tissue engineering (Pavesio et al., 2003). Hyaluronan is the simplest glycosaminolglycan (GAG) and is found especially in cartilage tissue. Hydrogels of HA are formed by various chemical treatments (Hubbell, 2003). Additionally, HA has been combined with both collagen and alginate to form composite hydrogels. Similarly to collagens, HA is naturally degraded by secreted enzymes QVC, termed hyaluronidases, allowing tissue turnover by cells in the skeletal defect site.

Fibrin, associated with fibronectin, has been shown to support keratinocyte and fibroblast growth both in vitro and in vivo, and appears to enhance cellular motility in the wound (Marx, 2003). When used as a scaffold system for cultured mesenchymal cells, fibrin may provide some advantages over other natural materials (Hutmacher et al., 2001a). Fibrin glue works as an adhesive by emulating the exudative phase of wound healing. Early products were made with human fibrin concentrate and thrombin. When the two substances are mixed, the thrombin, in the presence of calcium, converts fibrinogen to fibrin. The resulting fibrin polymer has a stable structure that facilitates the growth of collagen-producing fibroblasts (Michel and Harmand, 1990). Further development has led to the addition of factor XIII, a fibrin-stabilising factor present in blood, or aprotinin, which is an antiplasmin protecting the fibrin polymer clot from premature fibrinolysis. Fibrin deposition depends on the relative rates of formation, degradation, and dissolution. Fibrin glue has also been shown to be a suitable delivery vehicle for exogenous growth factors that may in the future be used to accelerate wound healing.

Alginate has been used in a variety of tissue engineering applications, because it can be processed as a gel and has a low toxicity (Gutowska et al., 2001). Alginate as a polymer is composed of polymerised G and M monomers. Gels are formed when divalent cations cooperatively interact with blocks of monomers to form ionic bridges between different polymer chains. The cross-linking density and thus the mechanical competence and pore size of the ionically cross-linked gels can be adjusted by different techniques: by varying the M to G ratio or the molecular weight of the polymer chain as well as by covalently cross-linking alginate with adipic hydrazide or PEG (Thomas, 2000). Ionically cross-linked alginate hydrogels do not specifically degrade but undergo slow, uncontrolled dissolution.

Chitosan is sometimes used as a scaffold material in tissue engineering applications, because it is structurally similar to naturally occurring GAGs and is degradable by human enzymes (Yilmaz, 2004). It is a linear polysaccharide of (1–4)-linked D-glucosamine and *N*-acetyl-D-glucosamine residues. Dissolved chitosan can be fabricated as a gel by various methods (increasing the pH, extruding the solution into a non-solvent, glutaraldehyde cross-linking, UV irradiation, and thermal variations (Berger et al., 2004a; 2004b)). The crystallinity of chitosan, depending on the degree of N-deacetylation, influences the kinetics of degradation. Degradation of chitosan is experimentally performed through lysozym action. As the degradation rate of chitosan is inversely related to the degree of crystallinity (Berger et al., 2004a; 2004b), degradation kinetics can be adjusted by producing gels with different degrees of N-deacatylisation.

6.4 Natural Inorganic Materials

Hydroxyapatite of natural origin can be obtained from bone of various sources (LeGeros, 1992; LeGeros et al., 1995a; 1995b; 1995c; Valentini et al., 2000) or special species of marine corals (Holmes, 1979; LeGeros, 1988; 1991; 1992; Shors and Holmes, 1993) (Table 6.4). Naturally occurring hydroxyapatites are not pure but contain some of the minor and trace elements originally present in bone mineral or coral mineral. Bone-derived apatite contains different elements and ions (Mg, Na, CO3, trace elements) in varying concentrations that are important in bone physiology (LeGeros, 1981; 1991) (see Chap. 2). Coral-derived apatite or coralline hydroxy-

Table 6.4. Calcium phosphate biomaterials

Natural
- Freeze dried/banked human bones - Bovine bone derived (BioOssTM , EndoboneTM, TruboneTM) - Coral derived (InterporeTM, Pro-osteonTM)
Artificial – bulk
- Calcium hydroxyapatite (CalcititeTM , DurapatiteTM, OsteografTM, AlveografTM) - Beta-tricalcium phosphate (SynthografTM, AugmenTM) - Biphasic HA/TCP materials (OsteosyntTM)
Artificial – cement
- Ca-P cement (EndoboneTM)

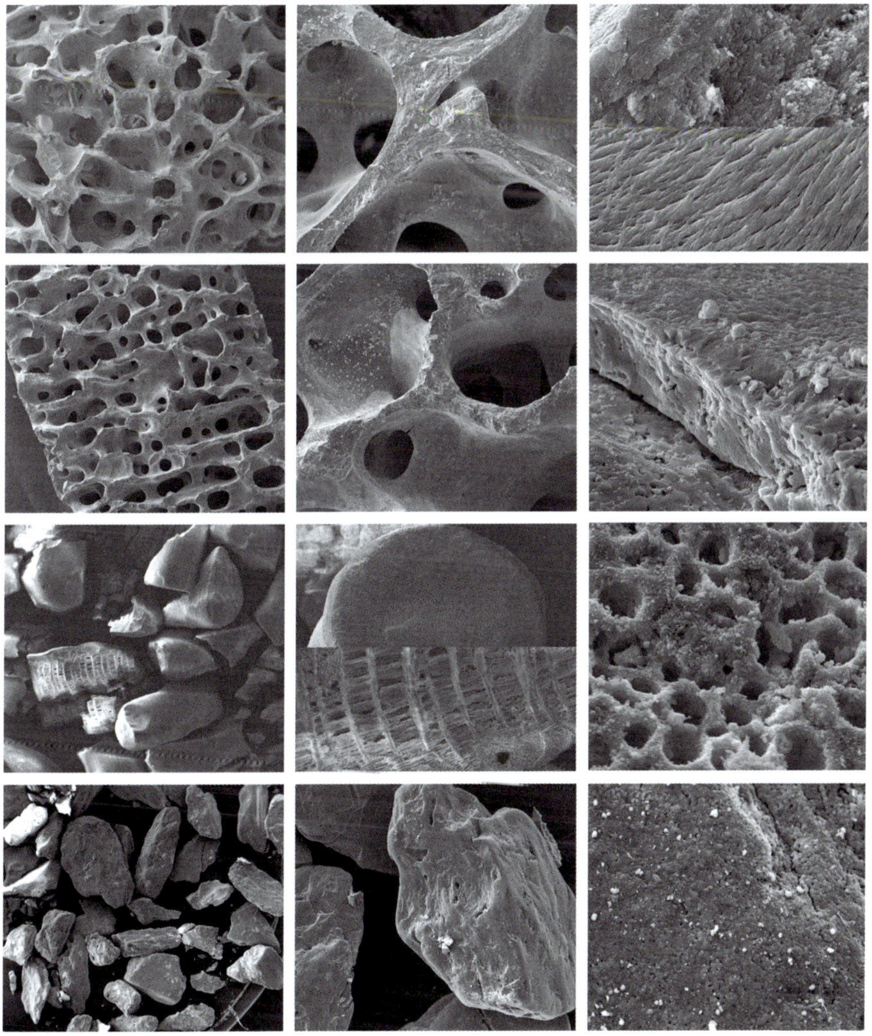

Fig. 6.4. Scanning electron microscopical view of different hydroxyapatite-based materials. Materials differ in particle size and shape, porosity, and surface microstructure. Hydroxyapatite-based biomaterials are commonly used for bone reconstruction approaches

apatite is similar in composition, with Mg and CO_3 (LeGeros, 1988; LeGeros et al., 1988; 1995[b]). Hydroxyapatite is used as a scaffold material in various forms. The composition and structure of HA depends on the method of preparation: (1) with organic matrix, unsintered; (2) without organic matrix, unsintered; or (3) without organic matrix and sintered. The difference between sintered and unsintered HA is that unsintered bone mineral consists of small crystals of bone apatite (carbonate hydroxyapatite), whereas sintered bone mineral consists of much larger apatite crystals without CO_3 when heated above 1000° C. The unsintered, material-containing organic matrix possesses a unique bone-like structure in the context of the three-dimensional macro- and microstructure. The naturally present hydroxyapatites have an interconnecting macroporosity that enables the ingrowth of cells into the scaffold structure both in vivo and in vitro. The degradation characteristics of hydroxyapatite as well as the cell reactions towards the material depend critically on the source of the material (Fig. 6.4).

Cell/Surface Interactions

7

Because cell/scaffold interactions take place at the material surface, the surface properties and the cell type covering the biomaterial surface have great impact on the generation of engineered tissues. A better understanding of bone and cartilage cell reactions towards artificial material surfaces is essential to optimise scaffold systems. Moreover, studies have to take into account the behaviour of osteoblasts and chondrocytes towards the biophysical constraints that will be present at the mechanically loaded scaffold material. To examine the cellular reactions towards the material surface it is therefore necessary to perform in vitro investigations of established cell culture systems on defined surface structures (Coelho and Fernandes, 2000).

In addition to the techniques applied to fabricate the gross scaffold structure, surfaces properties of the various materials are mainly defined by the basic processing technology. All scaffold material surfaces possess a complex, fabrication-dependent three-dimensional surface topography consisting of regular or non-regular micrometre- and nanometre-sized features. Surface properties are related both to molecular interactions and the surface topography (Barthlott and Neinhuis, 1997). Different surface properties have been proposed to influence the biological response.

Surface Factors Influencing Cell Responses

- Underlying material
- Element composition
- Element release
- Three-dimensional morphology
- Microtopography
- Nanotopography
- Wettability
- Zeta potential
- Biophysical constraints under function.

The surface topography and the physico-chemical surface characteristics are the most important parameters. Ion release from materials is an additional factor with possible impact on surrounding cells (Meyer et al., 1993a; Matsuoka et al., 1999). The relationship between the topographical and physico-chemical properties of materials and their effects on protein adsorption and consecutive cellular activity is complex and generally not understood. Although it is widely accepted that the topography and chemistry of the surface determine the biological reaction to the device, there is little information on how these factors interact in the production of biological responses on a molecular and cellular level. The lack of knowledge is based, to a great extent, on the difficulty in varying surface chemistry and topography independently, because the methods used to fabricate scaffold materials determine their surface topography, and particular methods of fabrication are often associated with specific materials. Therefore, it is difficult to compare in vitro findings at structured surfaces of different underlying materials. Hydroxyapatite coatings of underlying materials are, for example, often fabricated by plasma spraying or magnetron sputtering, and these techniques produce surface topographies that differ from those resulting from manufacturing polymer surfaces. Thus, interpretation of the separate effects of chemistry and topography on bone and cartilage cell responses is often limited by the inability to fabricate a defined surface. Only a few studies have been performed to investigate the relationship between surface topography and surface chemistry. In one of these studies a direct relationship was found, for example, between roughness and surface energy of polymethylmetacrylate (PMMA) materials (Combe et al., 2004). In this systematic study of PMMA material surfaces with various degrees of surface roughness it was demonstrated that the apolar component of surface energy increased significantly with roughness although the basic component decreased. The complex and sometimes undetermined interrelations between topographical and physio-chemical properties of materials make the predictions of cellular in vitro behaviour difficult, especially in light of the consideration that both parameters influence protein and cell adherence at the same time (Scotchford et al., 2003). It is therefore important to conceptualise and to some extent simplify basic reactions of bone and cartilage cells towards material surfaces.

The process of cell interaction with materials is highly dynamic and depends on various parameters influencing cell responses (Anselme, 2000). It is a step-by-step process from the initial contact to cell migration and propagation (Table 7.1). The whole interaction can be divided into different subcellular and cellular events. Protein adsorption is believed to be the first event that takes place after contact of body fluids with implants and is influenced by the physico-chemical characteristics of the material. It is followed by the attachment phase of cells which occurs rapidly (Boyan et al., 1996). The adhesion phase occurs over longer periods and involves various biological molecules (extracellular matrix proteins, cell membrane proteins, and cytoskeleton proteins) which interact together to induce the subsequent cell response in terms of migration and differentiation. The outcome of the long-term cell reaction is further influenced by the biophysical (mechanical and electrical) environment that constitutes the material/cell interface under functional conditions. Mineral forma-

Table 7.1. Cell/surface interaction

Step	Influencing factors	Time
- Fluid adhesion	Wettability	Seconds
- Protein adhesion	pH, ionic composition, temperature, fucntional groups	Seconds-minutes
- Cell attachment	van der Waal`s forces	Minutes-hours
- Cell adhesion	Matrix and membrane proteins, cytoskeleton proteins	Hours
- Cell spreading	Matrix and membrane proteins, cytoskeleton proteins	Hours

tion at the material surface should be the ultimate stage of a bone-like cell reaction (Davies et al., 1990).

7.1 Protein Adsorption

Cells do not interact with a naked material either in vitro or in vivo. At each step, the material is conditioned by the biological fluid components (Elwing, 1998). The pH as well as the ionic composition of the solution, the temperature and the functional protein groups are the factors determining protein adsorption. Protein adsorption is believed to be a very early event that takes place after initial contact of body fluids with artificial surfaces. Subsequently, the protein-covered artificial substrates guide the attachment of cells. It is important to note that the changing protein composition does not only result from the interaction between absorbed proteins and surface structures but also from the protein`s potential to flexibly change its structure. The globular structure of protein molecules is usually essential for their biological function. Some of the bone proteins have chemotactic or adhesive properties, notably because they contain an Arg–Gly–Asp (RGD) sequence, which is specific to the fixation of cell membrane receptors like integrins (fibronectin, osteopontin, bone sialoprotein, thrombospondin, type I collagen, vitronectin). Various experiments have demonstrated the importance of isolated RGD sequence-containing peptides in promoting adhesion of bone and cartilage cells (Moursi et al., 1997; Meyer et al., 1998). In order to confirm the spectrum of proteins involved in enhanced human bone and cartilage cell adhesion, experiments consisting of cell cultures on dishes coated with extracellular matrix proteins have been performed. Human osteoblasts were shown in in vitro studies to strongly adhere to RGD-containing proteins such as fibronectin (as compared with type I and type IV collagen) and vitronectin but weakly to laminin and type V collagen. These RGD sequence-containing extracellular proteins (vitronectin, fibronectin) can act as binding elements between artificial surfaces and skeletal cells, exerting strong effects on cell adhesion, matrix maturation, and mineralisation (Rezania and Healy, 2000). Serum depletion of vitronection, with or without fibronectin, greatly reduced cell attachment and spreading on patterned surfaces. The role of fibronectin adsorption in cell adhesion has also been established (Zhang et al., 1993). Changes in the fibronectin conformation affect the fibronectin cell binding domain conformations and then affect fibronectin affinity with its osteoblast surface receptor (Zhang et al., 1993; Globus et al., 1998). Different studies highlight the fact that fibronectin attached to a surface has the ability to strengthen osteoblast and chondrocyte attachment and to stimulate cell growth (Moursi et al., 1997; Meyer et al., 1998).

7.2 Cell adhesion

The firm attachment of anchorage-dependent mesenchymal cells like osteoblasts to synthetic surfaces is a prerequisite to subsequent transcriptional and translational events (Baier et al., 1984) (Fig. 7.1). Physico-chemical interactions between cells and materials including ionic forces, van der Waals forces, and other forces that govern this attachment process. The attachment of osteoblasts and chondrocytes to sur-

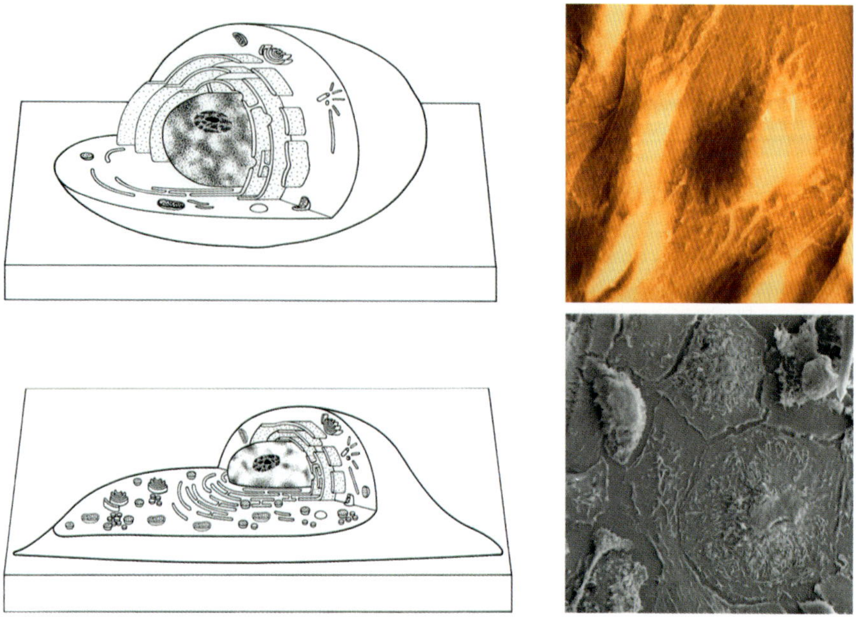

Fig. 7.1. Cell attachment, AFM and SEM images of cell at different attachment stages

faces has profound effects on the subsequent cell adhesion, followed by proliferation, migration and phenotypic differentiation. If cells are added to a medium in culture, various steps can be distinguished by a typical morphology: floating cells have a spherical shape, whereas in the subsequent contact phase cells tend to spread out and become more and more flattened (Fig. 7.2). Mesenchymal cells adhere to artificial substrates through adhesion molecules (Meyer et al., 1997b). Cells adhere to substrates through distinct contact sites, which are classified depending on the distance of the cell from the substrate and the presence of certain adhesion proteins, as focal contacts, close contacts and extracellular matrix contacts (Chen and Singer, 1982). Focal contacts are tenacious adhesion sites that remain attached to the substratum even when cells are forcibly detached, indicating their function as anchorage structures (Balaban et al., 2001). Focal contacts are closed junctions where the distance between the substrate surface and the cell membrane is between 10 and 15 nm (Fig. 7.3). The external faces of focal contacts present specific receptor proteins such as integrins. Integrins are the group of adhesion molecules responsible for the cell-substrate connection. Cell adhesion to extracellular matrix ligands through integrin receptors plays a central role in tissue formation and maintenance by anchoring cells and triggers signals that direct cell proliferation and differentiation (Zhang et al., 1993). Integrin receptors act at the interface between the intra- (cytoskeleton) and extra-cellular (matrix proteins) space. On the internal face, proteins like talin, paxillin, vinculin, tensin mediate interactions between actin filaments and membrane receptor proteins of osteoblasts and chondrocytes (Geiger et al., 1980). These cytoskeletal proteins are assumed to be important intracellular structures responsible for the intracellular part of cell attachment and for signal transduction (Jones

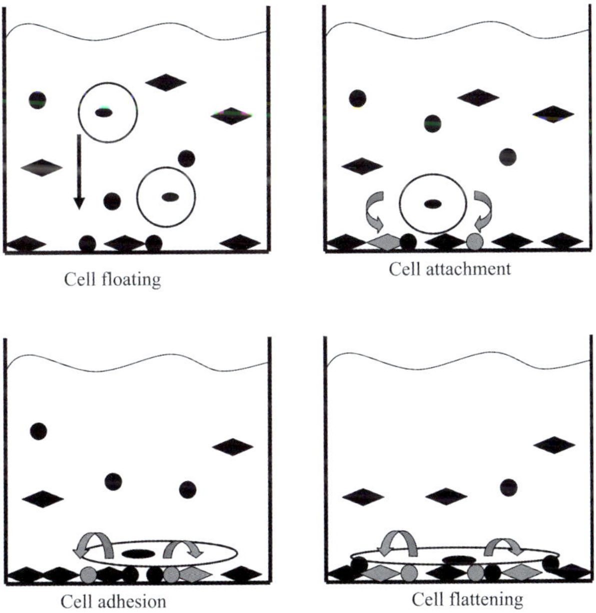

Fig. 7.2. Stages of cell/surface interaction

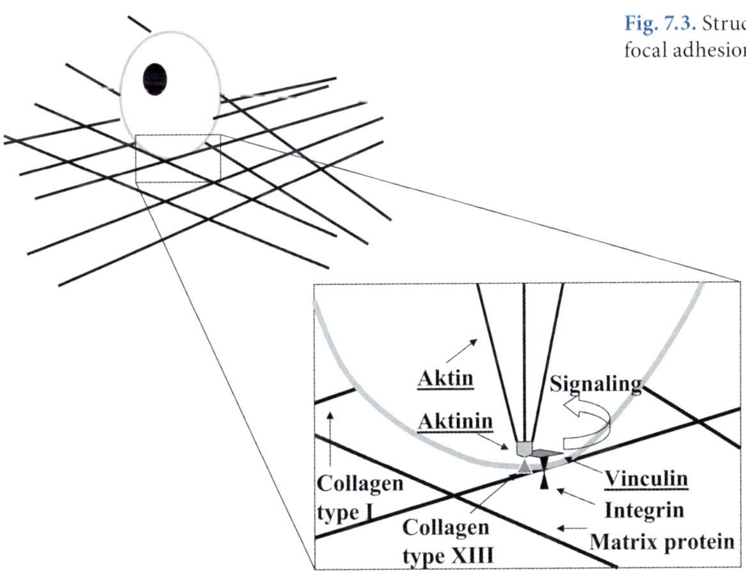

Fig. 7.3. Structure of focal adhesion site

et al., 1995). There is much structural and functional insight into the cytoskeleton, particularly on the nature of focal adhesion sites but there are only a few reports on the intracellular molecular mechanisms involved in substrate-dependent signalling in osteoblasts and chondrocytes (Krause et al., 2000).

It has been shown by different investigators, that tissue responses at material surfaces are regulated by the integrin-mediated cell adhesion (Liu et al., 2001; Kay et al., 2002; Price et al., 2003a; 2003b). Studies by Meyer et al. (1998) and Zinger et al. (2004) revealed that the osteoblast attachment process on structured surfaces is concomitant with the reassembly of vinculin from the cytoplasm into streak-like focal contacts clustered on the ventral side of cells. The kinetic of vinculin reassembly was shown to be dependent on surface protein coatings. While the reassembly of vinculin in focal contacts is a result of the integrin binding to extracellular matrix proteins, it appears to affect the subsequent cell behaviour in the sense of proliferation and differentiation on artificial substrates. The focal adhesion structure in osteoblasts may therefore represent a signalling complex involved in special situations like exposure to structured artificial surfaces (Curtis et al., 2001; Liu et al., 2001). Some authors have demonstrated that osteoblast adhesion to titanium showed similarities to osteoblast adhesion to fibronectin. Mitogen activated protein kinase, focal adhesion kinase and other factors are involved and activated in this signalling process (Krause et al., 2000). The composition of extracellular matrix proteins also plays an important role in chondrocyte adhesion, thereby imposing differentiation effects on chondrocytes. The expression of the ECM molecule fibronectin for example is upregulated at the onset of chondrogenesis. Fibronectin mediates the adhesion of chondrocytes and at the same time the formation of mesenchymal condensations by binding to cell-surface receptors (Widelitz et al., 1993). Although a precise mechanism for the initiation of cell differentiation through attachment has definitely not been solved, it is likely that fibronectin marks locations where cell condensations will form. It is hypothesised that focal contacts should be of a certain length to promote adhesion and that maximum contact of the cell with the substrate will be favourable. Other studies suggest, however, that cell-flattening or spreading is not always compatible with mesenchymal cell differentiation, particularly in the case of chondrogenesis (Boyan et al., 1996).

After attachment, cells tend to spread out and migrate over the material surface (Fig. 7.4). As extracorporal tissue formation should mimic the original tissue, coverage of cells on material surfaces requires sufficient numbers of differentiated cells with high biosynthetic activity. Both cell proliferation and migration require a dynamic interaction between the cell and the material surface (Anselme, 2000). Cells commence to develop a protrusion of their leading edge to form a lamellipodium. After formation and fixation of the lamellipodium, the cell exploits adhesive interactions to generate the traction and energies required for cell movement. The cytoskeleton and the protein layer at the material surface are mainly involved in this dynamic interaction (Pockwinse et al., 1992). The last step of the migratory cycle is the release of adhesions at the rear of the cell followed by its detachment and retraction. Smoother surfaces tend to spread the cells out more, forming a greater numbers of focal contacts (Jayaraman et al., 2004). In general, cells with a low motility form strong focal adhesions while motile cells form less adhesive structures, and an intermediate level of attachment force induces a maximal migration rate. Also, a high migration rate is associated with a lower level of cell differentiation. Migration tests on biomaterials with surface grooves have demonstrated that cell migration was faster in the direction of the grooves (Lenhert et al., 2005). No in vitro study so far has revealed surface-related multifold or order-of-magnitude changes in proliferation rates or cell numbers on ordered material surfaces.

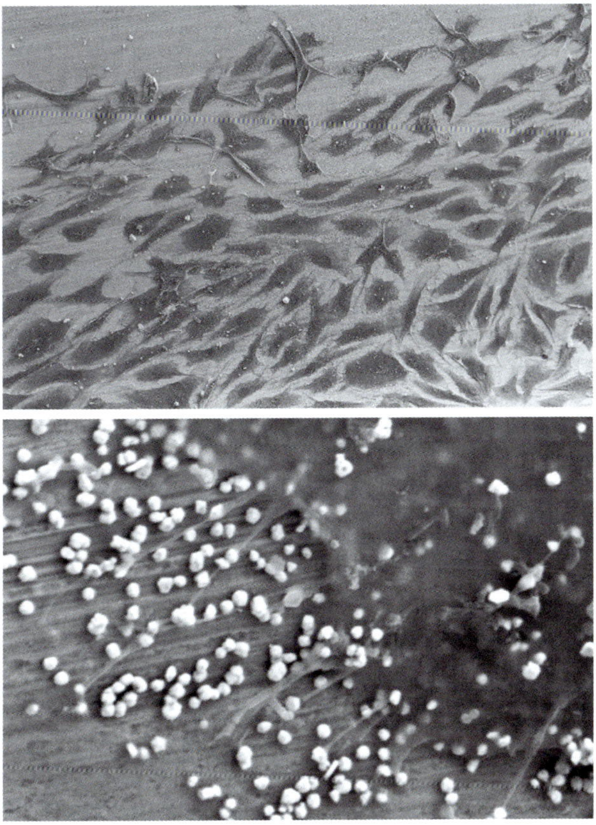

Fig. 7.4. Structure of focal adhesion site

7.3 Surface Topography

One of the most important parameter affecting mesenchymal cell reactivity is the three-dimensional morphology of the substrate. The three-dimensional morphology can be conceptualised as the size, the shape and the surface texture of the material. Various studies such as (Dalby et al., 2000) have demonstrated that bone and cartilage cells are sensitive to the gross morphology of a material. The investigation of material size and shape effects on cell reactions remains difficult. Recent research indicates that the size of a material alone can determine whether the material will elicit either an osteoblastic or a fibroblastic cell reaction in culture. When particles of calcium phosphates were tested in vitro, osteoblasts showed a cell reaction dependent on the particle shape and size (Midy et al., 2001).

When examining the behaviour of osteoblast- and chondrocyte-like cells on surfaces with different roughnesses, controversial findings were reported. In recent studies it was shown that the application of microgrooves to a surface can direct not only cellular morphology but also the deposition of a mineralised matrix by osteoblast-like cells (Matsuzaka et al., 2000). It was found in various studies that a lower percentage of cells attached to rougher surfaces (Bowers et al., 1992; Lange et al.,

2002; Jayaraman et al., 2004). However, recent investigations of the behaviour of primary osteoblasts on titanium surfaces reported that cell proliferation and differentiation is improved on smooth surfaces (Jayaraman et al., 2004), while other authors (Martin et al., 1995) demonstrated that osteoblast proliferation and differentiation was more pronounced on rough surfaces. The difference in osteoblastic phenotype towards different surface topographies may partly be based on the different cell lines used for surface testing, as some authors used primary (Jayaraman et al., 2004) and others osteosarcoma cell lines (Martin et al.,1995). More importantly, it is difficult to compare the in vitro findings on osteoblast behaviour on surfaces with different topographies because there is no consensus concerning the proper representation of surface topography (Cooper, 2000). Material surfaces are categorised either as rough or smooth, a difference that has segregated for example machined material surfaces from others. Defining a surface by its manufacturing process may be misleading. Whereas MacDonald and colleagues (2004) concisely defined topographic measurement methods which have to be applied to evaluate material surfaces, only a few in vitro studies determined accurately the three-dimensional configuration of both the magnitude and complexity of the surface roughness. It can be concluded that in order to compare skeletal cell reactions on surfaces with different topologies a more appropriate and meaningful description of the various surface topographies is needed.

In addition to the microtopography, cells use the nanotopography of the substrate for orientation and migration (Dalby et al., 2000; Wang et al., 2000; Curtis and Wilkinson, 2001). The critical influence of substratum topography on cells is reviewed by Curtis and Wilkinson (1997). Most of the earlier studies addressed the effects of surface features with dimensions of 0.5 μm and greater. The relevance of these studies for engineering bone and cartilage substitutes is questionable since in vivo adhesion structures (e.g. cell membranes, basement membranes) are comprised of much smaller, nanometre-scale features. Despite the apparent importance of substratum topography, relatively little is known about the cellular effects of topographical features at nanometre-scale dimensions (Webster et al., 2000). It was concluded that in order to fully understand the role of substrate topography in the regulation of cell behaviour, smaller and denser surfaces must be evaluated. Much work has been carried out on the reaction of cells to disordered nanotopography, however, cellular reactions to regular and ordered topographical microstructures have only recently been investigated. Wojciak-Stothard et al. (1999) for example described the reaction of macrophage-like cells to disordered nanosized steps. These authors showed that symmetrical groove structures enhanced cell adhesion, whereas irregular topography seemed to have little effect on adhesion, compared with planar surfaces. Whereas it is generally accepted that various cell types such as osteoblasts align themselves along defined substrate morphologies inscribed on culture surfaces (Domke et al., 2000), a process known as contact guidance, the relation between ordered nanotopography and cell behaviour is, to a great extent, unknown. Cell alignment, for example, has been shown to be inversely influenced by the spacing of culture plate grooves. In contrast, cell alignment was found to be influenced directly by the depth of grooves, with depth having increasing importance as the grooves become deeper. Recent investigations on ordered nano-structured surfaces, fabricated according to the method described by Gleiche et al. (2000), reveal that structured nanophase surfaces lead to a predictable osteoblast orientation and migration on these surfaces (Lenhert et al., 2005), a prerequisite to reach a defined cell colonisation during directed tissue formation. The mechanism of such alignment has been explained in terms of contacts between the plasme membrane and the surface topography of focal adhesions. Cells have also been found in recent investigations to preferentially migrate in the direction of alignment. Osteoblasts were quantitatively observed to align on grooves on highly defined large-scale nano-structured surfaces (Lenhert et al., 2004). Deep grooves showed a stronger alignment than shallow grooves. Cells that were aligned with the grooves appeared more elongated than those not aligned. It was suggested that cell orientation may have profound effects on the subsequent cell responses. And indeed, numerous studies have demonstrated that cell shape and orientation are related to gene expression, and changes in cell shape that follow cell adhesion on material surfaces by altered extracellular matrix contacts are associated with changes in the differentiated phenotype of cells. These alterations in cell shape are associated with cytoskeletal changes that may affect much of a cell's metabolism (Martines et al., 2004).

Chondrocytes were also demonstrated to be sensitive to subtle differences in surface roughness as well as surface chemistry (Boyan et al., 1996). Studies comparing chondrocyte response to TiO_2 of differing crystallinities show that cells can discriminate between surfaces as well as osteoblasts. Boyan and colleagues (1996) were able to demonstrate that osteoblasts and chondrocytes discriminated differences in titanium surfaces that varied in average surface roughness from 5 to 18 μm. It was demonstrated by Boyan et al. (1996) that the response to surface roughness is dependent on cell maturation state for both cell lines. They suggested thst cell maturation state may be a more important variable then the type of mesenchymal cell or the species of cell from which it is derived. This is an intriguing concept in terms of tissue regeneration, where the first cells that interact with a material are likely to be relatively undifferentiated mesenchymal cells rather than fully differentiated cells.

7.4 Surface Chemistry

As stated earlier, cells are also sensitive to differences in the physico-chemical properties of materials. The chemistry of the outermost functional groups of a surface clearly affects cell responses, although the exact mechanisms are not fully understood (Schwartz and Boyan, 1994). Anisotropic topographies, such as topographical grooves, chemically patterned stripes, or the curved surface of a fibre are known to exert morphological as well as regulatory impact on cells, indicative of the complex environmental influence on cells. Important physico-chemical characteristics of surfaces are the zeta potential and the interfacial tension.

The zeta potential is defined as the difference in potentials between the surface of a tightly bound layer and a diffuse layer, which is the electro-neutral region of the solution. It can be assumed that the potential is partly the property of the density and nature of the fixed charges on the material surface. It was found that osteoblasts are most likely influenced by properties of the surface charge (Möller et al., 1994). The zeta potential as an electrical parameter may be an important factor that determines, at least in part, the biocompatibility of materials. Electro-kinetic studies including measurements of zeta potentials have been performed and it was hypothesised by Ducheyne (1988) that the zeta potential of calcium phosphate ceramics is directly maintained under suitable culture conditions, some cells form bone-like nodules in cell culture (Wiesmann et al., 2003). Baksh and coauthors (1998) reported on mineral formation at the surfaces of calcium polyphosphate. In their in vitro study they found the formation of cement lines by rat marrow cells that were quite different to the cement lines they have seen in vivo. It is therefore not solved whether these mineralisation processes are culture artefacts or not. There is growing evidence that some cell populations appear capable of finally differentiating in vitro. Due to the finding that in cell culture matrix-vesicle mediated mineralisation is not followed by collagen mineralisation (Wiesmann et al., 2003; Lenhert et al., 2005) (Fig. 7.5), bone-like extracellular mineral formation on artificial surfaces has not been demonstrated up to now. This should be considered as a general problem of bone-like

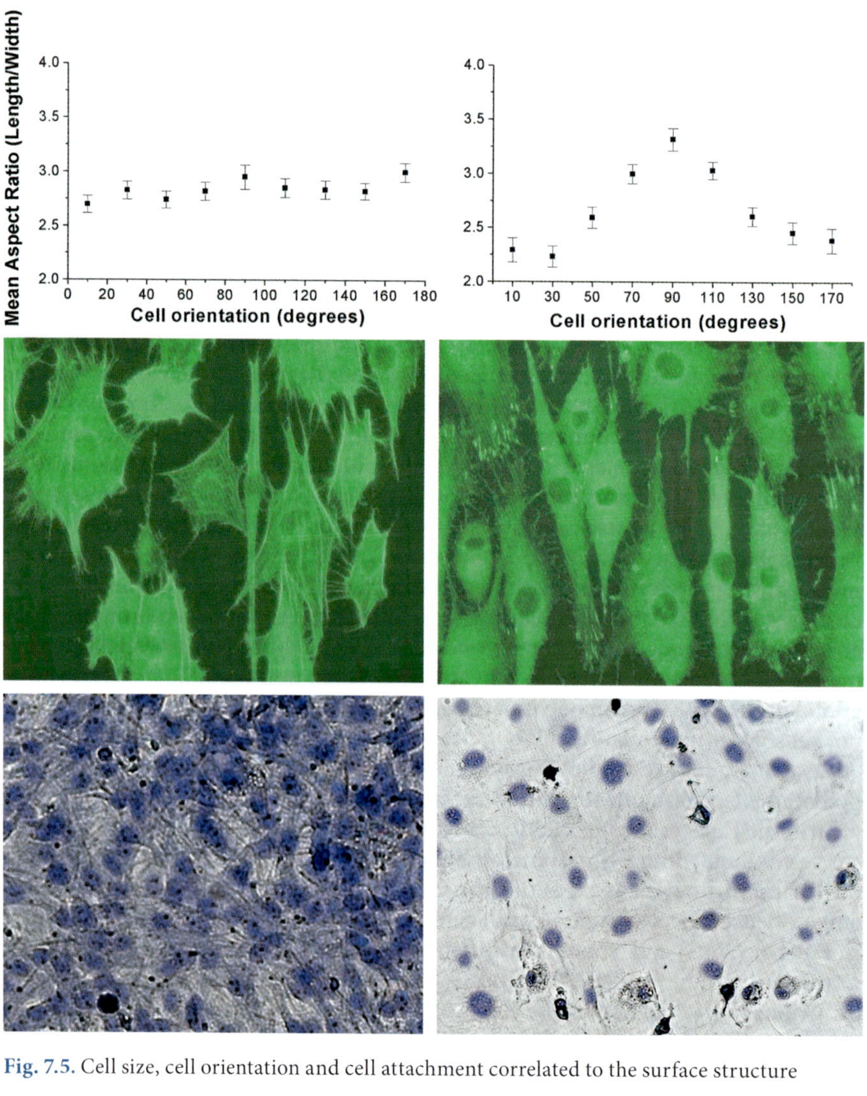

Fig. 7.5. Cell size, cell orientation and cell attachment correlated to the surface structure

structure formation on material surfaces in vitro (Wiesmann et al., 2004). The presence of initial calcified structures on material surfaces, either precipitated from the extracellular fluid or induced by cellular activity (Weis et al., 2002), is supposed to improve the subsequent osteoblast activity on these materials.

7.6 Functional Aspects of Biomaterial/Cell Interactions

Bone-derived cells are not only influenced by the material itself but also by the biophysical constraints of the material surface under investigation. Applying non-destructive physiological or hyperphysiological mechanical constraints to cultured bone-derived cells permits insight into mechanisms affecting the synthesis of adhesion proteins, cell growth and cell differentiation (Büchter et al., 2004). The mechanisms underlying the cell response to loaded material surfaces include direct or indirect mechanical effects (Frost, 2000a), electromechanical effects (Pienkowski and Pollack, 1983), or enhancement of molecular transport mechanisms (Piekarski and Munro, 1977). Load transfer to material surfaces leads to deformation of cells in the microenvironment of the tissue and concomitantly to the generation of electrical potentials. The complexity of the biophysical surface environment stresses the need for an investigation in a more physiological setting. As the influence of the biophysical environment on bone and cartilage tissue is described in more detail in Chaps 2 and 8, we refer the reader to these two chapters.

7.7 Surface Structuring

Tissue engineering and related biomolecular engineering strategies are aimed at increasing the biocompatibility of cell scaffold complexes by creating materials with defined surface structures (Jung et al., 2001). There are extensive technical challenges to generate scaffolds with desired macroscopic scaffold structures and at the same time defined micro- or nano-surface structures. However, it is doubtful whether in vitro evaluations are predictive of or correlate with the biocompatibility and outcome in vivo. This is because the in vivo effects of surface topography and chemistry on the nature of the adherent cell population, its cellular diversity, and the clinical relevance have not been fully elucidated for any of the scaffold materials. Most information concerning these items has been assessed by studying implant healing at titanium implants (one of the most commonly used and to some extent best investigated artificial materials, reviewed by Cooper, 2000). The investigation of non-degradable material surfaces is of relevance, since it gives baseline information about the relationship between surface structure and cell or tissue response. It is important to recognise that the influence of surface features on cell or tissue behaviour is much more complex at degradable material surfaces, because the degradation process itself alters the properties of the material surface over time. It was concluded from investigations of titanium surfaces that it is difficult to precisely state how surface topography and chemistry affects the bone-material interface, but the sum of the in vitro and in vivo findings are indicative that a structured titanium implant surface topography beyond a machined state improves the bone-to-implant contact and the mechanical properties of the interface. Up until recently it was unknown whether this finding can be attributed to a biologically more active surface state due to the altered topographies or whether it is based on an enhanced micro-mechanical interlock of materials after bone ingrowth in rough surfaces. Growing clinical evidence for increased bone-to-material contact at altered titanium implants supports previous observations made in preclinical studies that have demonstrated high bone-to-implant contact formation in humans. This seems to indicate that modified topography and chemistry of surfaces may impart favourable osteoconductive behaviour. In the absence of controlled comparative clinical trials, the existing experimental data support the use of implants with increased surface topography. However, it remains unsolved whether the improved mechanical properties can be attributed to the enhanced overall surface or to biologically optimised cell adhesion on rough surfaces (Hallgren et al., 2001; Schliephake et al., 2003). In contrast to bone implants, cartilage reactions towards rough surfaces is less well studied since most of the in vivo research on tissue reactions towards rough surfaces has been performed in dental implantology.

Based on the current knowledge of basic cell reactions on structured degradable or non-degradable materials, several means are currently being developed for biomaterial improvement. Despite the uncertainties and the complexity involved in cell reactions towards degradable materials, the question remains, what kind of surface structure may faciliate bone and cartilage cell ingrowth at degradable surfaces. Patterned material surfaces, surface alteration of materials by selectively absorbed adhesion peptides, coating of surfaces with proteins or growth factors, and imprintig surfaces with plasmids coding for clinically desired gene products are current approaches to activate scaffold surfaces (Garcia and Keselowsky, 2002).

7.8 Surface Patterning

Fabrication of patterned surface topographies seems to be a promising refinement in tissue engineering (Scotchford et al., 2003). Patterned arrays of single or multiple cell types in culture faciliate the ex vivo generation of bone- or cartilage- like tissues. Until a few years ago, this research was restricted to microtopographies due to the high costs of producing controlled nanotopography. New advancements are, as mentioned, starting to make controlled nanotopography available in quantities required for in vitro and in vivo research. Recent progress in material processing techniques allows higher quality and improved nanotopography surfaces with defined features to be produced (Curtis and Wilkinson, 2001). By applying these techniques the formation of chemically homogeneous and structurally controlled patterned surfaces at the nanotopography scale becomes feasible. A number of studies have begun to assess the response of various cellular phenotypes to nanotopography surfaces (Curtis and Wilkinson, 1999). A review of these studies indicates that different cell phenotypes have different levels of sensitivity towards alteration in nanotopography (Curtis et al., 2001; Dalby et al., 2002). For example, osteoblasts and macrophages can react to features (grooves and ridges) having dimensions as low as 10 nm, i.e. in the range of the diameter of a single collagen fibre. No statistically significant difference between osteoblast adherence to the range of nanotopographies (the resulting titanium dioxide surfaces were covered with 111 ± 5 nm high and 159 ± 9 nm wide hemispherical protrusions) was observed in a study by Rice et al. (2003). The in vivo effects of nanotopographies with respect to bone healing have been examined only in a limited number of studies. Hallgren and colleagues (2001) investigated the influence of various surface patterns on the integration of implants in rabbit bone. Using a photolithography technique a specific surface pattern containing microgrooves was produced on screw flanks of threaded titanium oral implants. The evaluation of bone healing at these implants revealed no statistically significant differences in the histomorphometric or biomechanical results between the patterned and control implants.

Creating topographic variations from the mean surface plane at a microscale level can be achieved by different manufacturing techniques (Cooper, 2000). Materials containing surfaces with defined biophysical properties can now be produced by using various nanotechniques, such as microcontact printing (Kumar et al., 1994; Evans et al., 1995; Xia and Whitesides, 1997), micromachining (Abott et al., 1992), photolithography (Calvert, 1993), and vapour deposition (Gau et al., 1999). The latter methods have been successfully applied to fabricate surfaces with nanoscale features, however it proved to be difficult to directly control the topographical and physicochemical features even with these advanced methods. Chemistry with extremely small amounts of material has become possible using liquid-guiding channels of submicrometre dimensions (Delamarche et al., 1997). A new strategy (Wittmann and Smith, 1991) for introducing defined nanoscale surfaces with anisotropic texture is based on the use of the intrinsic material properties of stretched ultrathin polymer coatings. It was recently shown by Gleiche et al. (2000) that ordered nanostructures can be extended over macroscopic distances by Langmuir Blodgett transfer and that the extent of the ordered surface is only restricted by the substrate size. Such surfaces can now be produced with high speed and reliability (Gleiche et al., 2000). These surfaces may be fabricated with selective adsorption and molecular recognition capabilities (Böltau et al., 1998), and controlled anisotropy in the surface properties (Wagner et al., 1996). It was demonstrated by Price et al. (2003a) that skeletal cells react differently towards nanosurfaces, with osteoblasts being more sensitive towards nanoscale features than other cells (chondrocytes, fibroblasts, smooth muscle cells).

7.9 Peptide Adhesion

Based on our knowledge that protein adsorption on surfaces influences the cellular adhesion behaviour, selective surface coating with adhesion proteins enhances osteoblast and chondrocyte attachment on artificial surfaces (Zhang et al., 2002). Materials containing surface-bound proteins in order to improve the subsequent cell attachment process have been clinically tested (Schaffner, 1998, Ruitz-Hitzky, 2003). As it is known that surface chemistry and topography influences the adherence of proteins at the material surface, much work was carried out to selectively bind protein on patterned surfaces (Sarikaya et al., 2003). In recent years, considerable attention has been given to the behaviour of protein-containing fluids spreading on surfaces at the nanofeature level.(Erikson et al., 1997) Gleiche et al. (2000) showed non-linear behaviour of interfacial forces on phospholipid strips localised at a glass/water interface. The different wetting of the hydrophilic channels and the hydrophobic stripes was used to deposit proteins along the channels, for example, by either an anisotropic wetting/dewetting process (determined by the surface structure, Biebuyck and Whitesides, 1994; Gau et al., 1999) or by using capillary (capillary filling, Kim et al., 1995; Xia and Whitesides, 1998) and electrostatic forces. The technique of molecular imprinting creates specific protein recognition sites in polymers by using template molecules (Mosbach and Ramstrom, 1996). Molecular recognition is attributed to binding sites that complement molecules in size, shape and chemical functionality (Cram, 1988). Whereas attempts to imprint defined proteins have met with only limited success, Shi et al. (1999) reported in a recent study on a new method for imprinting surfaces with specific protein recognition sites.

Nanotechniques are new options with impact on the functional behaviour of adsorbed macromolecules (Sutherland et al., 2001). Recently developed biomolecular strategies involve the incorporation of short adhesive peptides onto material surfaces in order to produce biofunctional surfaces (Cutler and Garcia, 2003). The identification of recognition sequences, such as RGD or fibronectin (FN) fragments, that mediate cell adhesion has stimulated the development of adhesive surfaces. Model FN mimetic surfaces were engineered for example by Cutler and Garcia (2003) through immobilising a recombinant fragment of FN encompassing the RGD binding domains onto material surfaces. Osteoblasts adhered to these functionalised surfaces over a range of ligand densities via interactions with integrins. Furthermore, adherent cells spread and assembled focal adhesions containing vinculin and talin. As previously mentioned, RGD peptides are important in promoting osteoblast and chondrocyte adhesion (Huang et al., 2003). In vivo studies on bone healing around RGD peptide-containing surfaces demonstrated inconsistent results. Schliephake (2002) analysed the effect of the organic coating of titanium implants on peri-implant bone formation and bone/implant contact. Differences between RGD-coated surfaces and control surfaces were not detected, however, enhanced bone/implant contact from 1 to 3 months post-operatively was found only in the group of RGD-coated implants. The results of Schliephake (2002) are, therefore, at least partially in line with those of Ferris et al., who showed enhanced bone formation on RGD peptide-coated implants after 2 and 4 weeks in rat femurs, with significantly increased thickness of bone deposition around small titanium rods (Ferris et al., 1999). Both studies provide only evidence that coating of titanium implants with RGD peptides has the potential to support bone formation at surfaces with imprinted proteins.

7.10 Protein Coatings

A challenging approach in biomolecular engineering is the coating of surfaces with extracellular matrix proteins or growth factors. Some of these proteins are currently being tested for their ability to promote bone and cartilage regeneration. The local ECM microenvironment may then determine whether a cell will differentiate along the chondrogenic or osteogenic pathway (Fig. 7.6). Among the extracellular matrix proteins, collagen is the most abundant extracellular protein of bone and a main candidate for surface coatings (Nagai et al., 2002; Schliephake 2002; Rammelt et al., 2004), followed by bone sialoprotein coatings (O`Toole et al., 2004). Various growth and differentiation factors, notably members of the transforming growth factor family (TGF-, BMP-2, BMP-7) are now being studied as material coatings in order to improve bone and cartilage healing (Kandziora et al., 2002; Schmidmaier et al.,

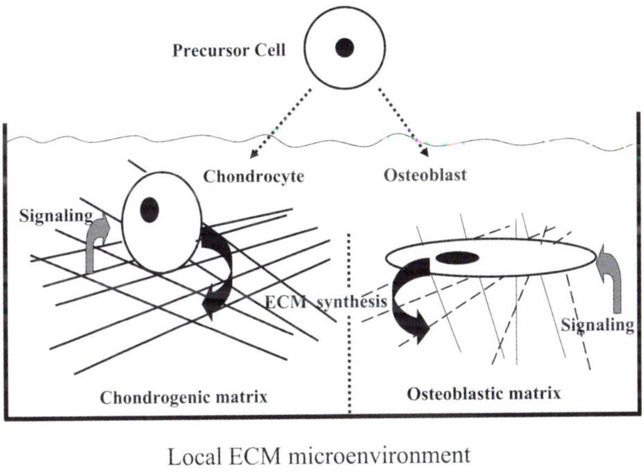

Fig. 7.6. Cell/ECM interaction

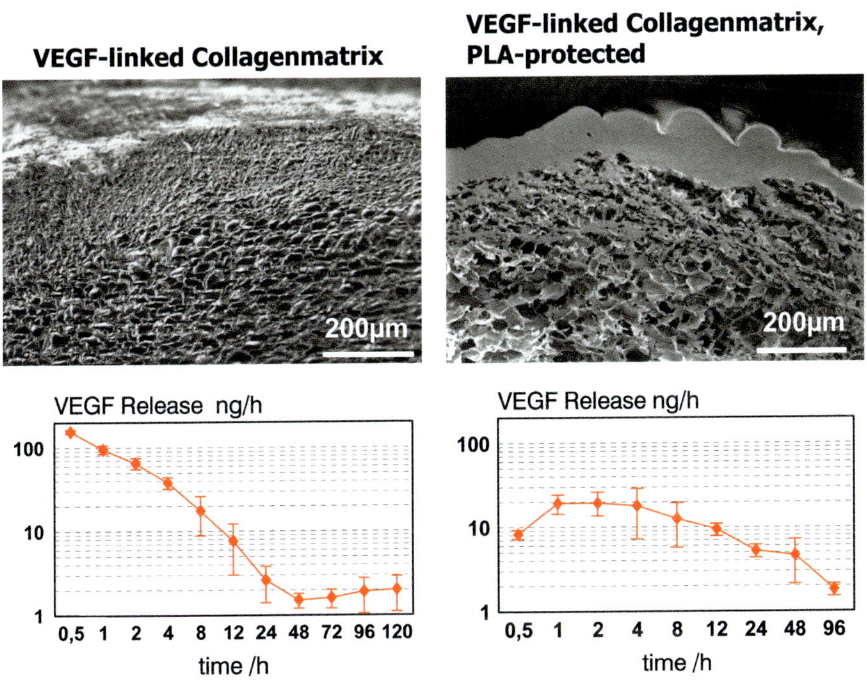

Fig. 7.7. Scanning electron microscopical view (top) and release kinetics (bottom) of VEGF coated collagen matrices. Release of VEGF can be modulated by embedding the collagen matrix in a PLA capsule

2002; Hartwig et al., 2003; Esenwein et al., 2003). Materials or scaffolds coated with growth factors have shown experimentally that they retain their biological activity (Liu et al., 2004)(Fig 7.7., Fig. 7.8.), but it was up until recently unknown whether these proteins improve tissue healing in vitro and in vivo. Coating of material sur-

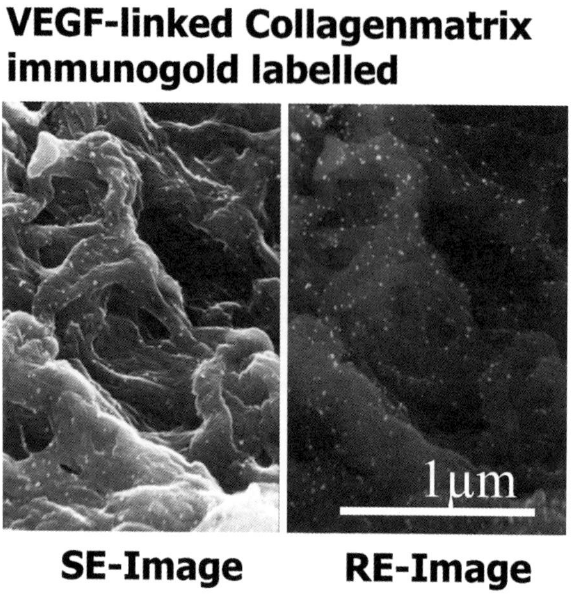

Fig. 7.8. Immunogold-labelled detection of VEGF attached to a collagen matrix by scanning electron microscopy (*left:* scanning mode, *right:* backscattered mode)

faces with plasmids encoding human genes is a future perspective (Thorwarth et al., 2004) in an effort to improve biomaterial surfaces, but biological, legal and ethical aspects have to be solved before this approach can be used in clinical trials.

Bioreactors and Cell Stimulation 8

8.1 Bioreactors

The current challenge for bone and cartilage tissue engineering is to raise research-scale products to a level of reproducible tissue substitute fabrication that is clinically effective by the use of bioreactors (Salgado et al., 2004). Various types of bioreactors have been tested for their utility in skeletal tissue engineering (Martin et al., 2004). Bioreactors can be considered as devices in which biological and/or biochemical processes are performed under controlled conditions (e.g. pH, temperature, pressure, oxygen supply, nutrient supply, and waste removal). Most bioreactors were initially developed to test biomaterials (Meyer et al., 1993b), but some were also constructed to allow extracorporal bone and cartilage tissue fabrication. The ex vivo generation of large three-dimensional tissues requires the development of new devices which can meet the physico-chemical requirements of large cell masses commonly coaxed with a scaffold (Griffith and Naughton, 2002). The main aspects of bioreactor development and usage are the following:

- Nutrition of cells in the scaffold
- Control over environmental conditions
- Long-term culture
- Biophysical and biological stimulation of cell/scaffold constructs
- On-line evaluation of biological parameters
- Automation of bioprocesses.

The control of these various aspects of bioreactor technology is necessary to improve the ex vivo development of tissues and to reduce manufacturing costs in order to facilitate clinical use. Cell seeding on scaffolds – that is, short-term coaxing of cells with a scaffold – and long-term cell ingrowth of cells in scaffolds are the two principle ways to generate a three-dimensional cell/scaffold complex. An alternative and recently established method of generating three-dimensional tissues is the use of scaffold-free micromass technology in bioreactors, described in more detail in Chap. 9. The design and performance of bioreactors is of special relevance to bone and cartilage tissue engineering. As both tissues are stimulated by mechanical forces, but react to the microenvironment very differently (e.g. O_2 tension), bioreactors with defined properties are desirable to optimise the ex vivo growth of the desired cell/scaffold constructs (Malda et al., 2003). It is therefore important to consider the in vivo situation of the different cell sources in skeletal tissues. The survival of cells in vivo as well as in bioreactors depends on the response of the paticular cells to the environment. A higher oxygen tension, for example, is needed for osteoblastic differentiation, whereas prolonged hypoxia favours formation of cartilage or fibrous tissue (Malda et al., 2003). Experimental findings have revealed that at least some connective tissue progenitors in bone and bone marrow are prone to survive in hypoxic conditions. Experimental data have shown that many stem and progenitor cells, including connective tissue progenitors in bone, exhibit a remarkable tolerance to, and are even stimulated by, hypoxia, not unlike endothelial cells. In metabolically active tissues such as trabecular bone and bone marrow, the distance that, for example, oxygen must diffuse between a capillary lumen and a cell membrane is almost never more than 40 to 200 μm. This diffusion distance is critical in maintaining the balance between oxygen delivery to a bone cell and consumption of oxygen by cells, both in native tissues and in extracorporal engineered tissue. The adjustment of oxygen tension in bioreactors is therefore a critical aspect of bioreactor design.

The simplest and most widely used bioreactor for bone and cartilage tissue engineering today is the culture dish (Fig. 8.1). It provides an environment that is easy

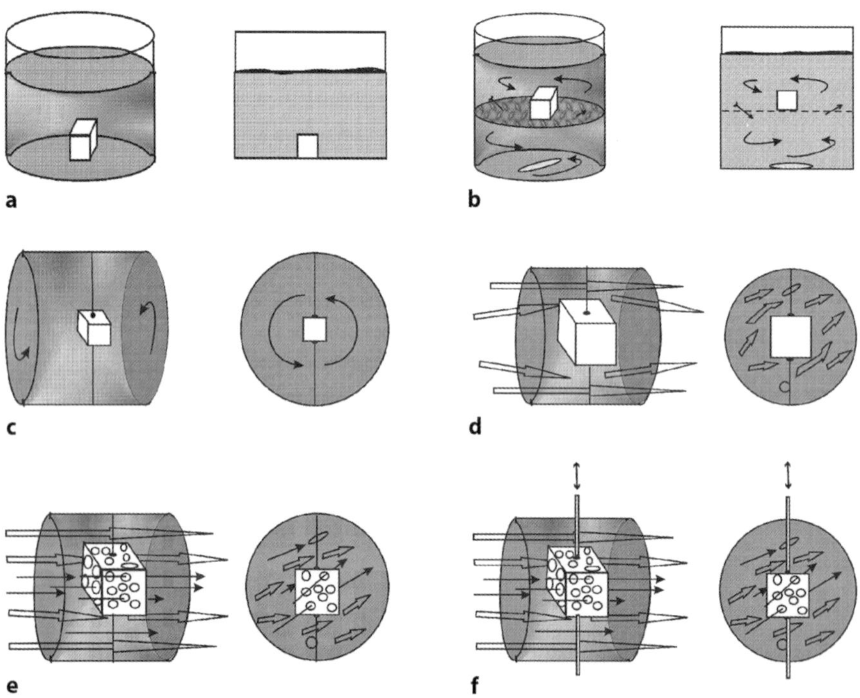

Fig. 8.1. Different principles of bioreactor systems. **a** Petri dish as a simple biorector system. **b** Stirring the medium improves cell nutrition. **c** Rotating bioreactor. **d** Rotating bioreactor with laminar flow as a more complex biophysical bioreactor system. **e** A porous scaffold improves the nutrition of cells located within that scaffold. **f** Mechanical loading of the bioreactor system described in (**e**) leads to the most complex bioreactor

to handle and economical to manufacture. Additionally, flasks are also commonly used bioreactors today (Langer and Vacanti, 1993), but both types of bioreactor are of limited value, especially when a three-dimensional bone construct has to be fabricated. The cultivation of cell monolayers to multiply the initial cell numbers has various advantages. Cells in monolayer culture are not generally nutrient-limited. Passive diffusion is more than adequate to supply the cell layers but the supply of oxygen and soluble nutrients becomes critical when the diffusion distance becomes wider than 100–200 μm. Cell cultivation in monolayers allows rapid multiplication of cells. This major advantage is accompanied by limitations on creating a three-dimensional construct.

In all settings in which cells are desired to grow in multiple layers or in which cells are located in scaffolds (Fig. 8.2), access to substrate as well as signalling molecules, growth factors, and nutrients (oxygen, glucose, amino acids and proteins) and clearance from metabolic products of metabolism (CO_2, lactate, and urea) are critical for cell survival (Vunjak-Novakovic, 2003). The diffusion of these substrates in and out of the cell-containing microenvironment is a prerequisite to scale up cell/material devices to tissue-like products. The transport of the various substrates can be mediated by inducing fluid flow in the cell-containing culture dishes or flasks, thereby creating more complex (e.g. multilayer) cell–scaffold constructs (Fig. 8.1).

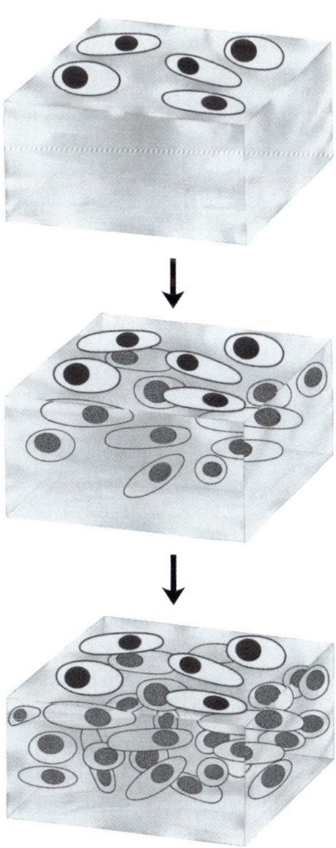

Fig. 8.2. Cell invasion in hydrogel

The pressure gradients driving this fluid flow can be induced by various techniques. The nutrient supply of cells can be, in part, improved by stirring the culture medium. As one of the most basic bioreactors, the stirred flask induces mixing of oxygen and nutrients throughout the medium and reduces the concentration boundary layer at the construct surface. Cell growth in a spinner flask therefore provides continuous exposure of the cells to various nutrients by convection. Convection is of special relevance in skeletal tissue engineering since cells are embedded in a dense extracellular matrix, which plays a regulatory role in enhancing the transport of large molecules (e.g. proteins and growth factors). However, in tissues like cartilage, passive diffusion along concentration gradients is another mechanism for mass transport, particularly for small molecules. Importantly, the turbulent flow generated within stirred-flask bioreactors leads to unpredictable flow effects in different regions of the multilayered cell/scaffold complex, which complicates the standardised evaluation of nutrient-dependent cell effects.

When cells are located in a more complex, scaled-up scaffold, the medium that delivers oxygen and other nutrients is commonly confined to the outer surfaces or the pores of the scaffold, even when the medium is stirred. As one moves deeper into the bulk scaffold material, each cell competes for oxygen, nutrients and signal molecules with other cells located in the same microenvironment. When complex cell/scaffold constructs (e.g. by co-culturing osteoblasts and endothelial cells) are fabricated, cells compete with the various cell sources that are located within a scaffold. More complex bioreactor systems thus need to be developed to improve cell survival in scaled-up scaffolds. Factors influencing and regulating cell viability in elaborated bioreactors include, besides the structure of the scaffold, the following:

- Oxygen concentration
- Oxygen need and consumption of cells
- Nutrient concentration
- Metabolite removal
- Medium/cell volume ratio
- Overall cell/scaffold construct size
- Material porosity
- Diffusion through the biomaterial
- Fluid flow within the site.

Each of these factors has a dramatic impact on the growth and survival of the tissue substitute, and when controlled can be used as major positive modulators. Providing such scaled-up three-dimensional tissues with nutrients is of major importance, since cells are aimed not to colonise the surface of scaffolds but should also be located within the scaffold in a viable state. In complex systems nutrients may therefore often be actively delivered by direct perfusion (Curtis and Riehle, 2001). A dynamic laminar flow environment is a desirable and efficient way to reduce diffusional limitations of nutrients and metabolites. If laminar flow can be adjusted in an ideal fashion, cells may, in addition to gaining sufficient nutrition, be stimulated through optimised levels of shear. The efficacy of laminar flow bioreactors for the generation of tissue equivalents has been demonstrated using chondrocytes and osteoblasts (Risbud and Sittinger, 2002). After a long period of cultivation under laminar flow, cartilaginous constructs can adopt biochemical and biomechanical properties superior to those of static or stirred-flask cultures, and approaching those of native cartilage (Darling and Athanasiou, 2003). Advances in bioreactor design are therefore closely related to improvements of scaffold design that are aimed to increase the nutrition of cells in complex constructs by combining laminar flow with tubular structures located in the scaffold. Bioreactors that perfuse medium either through or around semi-permeable tubes have been used successfully to enhance the metabolic function of cells by increasing the mass transport of nutrients and oxygen in central parts of cell/scaffold complexes. This concept has been extended to engineered tissues by perfusing culture medium not only at the surface but also directly through prefabricated interconnecting tubes and pores of scaffolds, thereby reducing mass transfer limitations, especially in the central parts of scaffolds. Direct perfusion bioreactors have been shown to enhance growth, differentiation and deposition of mineralised matrix by bone cells, and cartilage-like matrix synthesis by chondrocytes. It is obvious that the effects of medium perfusion depend to a great extent on the flow rate in the microenvironment of the cells. Therefore, in optimising a perfusion bioreactor for skeletal tissue engineering, one must carefully address the balance between the extent of nutrient supply, the transport of metabolites to and away from cells, and the fluid-induced shear stress effects on cells located at the surface and in the porous structures of the scaffold (Ratcliffe and Niklason, 2002).

Based on experimental data, oxygen is demonstrated to be a main limiting factor in cell survival in bioreactors containing scaled-up artificial tissues. As few cells tolerate diffusion distances greater than 200 μm, materials should be limited in their bulk size (especially in the case of bone tissue engineering) (Muschler et al., 2004). It was shown that osteoblasts seeded on porous scaffolds in vitro form a viable tissue that is no thicker than 0.2 mm. Similar observations were reported for different cell types cultured in three-dimensional scaffolds under diffusion conditions. Deposition of mineralised matrix by stromal osteoblasts cultured into poly(DL-lactic-co-glycolic acid) foams reached a maximum penetration depth of 240 μm from the top surface. Cartilage is, in contrast to bone and most other tissues, exceptional, since chondrocytes retain viability or may even be stimulated by low oxygen concentration. It must be stressed that, as with osteoblasts, chondrocyte function is not only dependent on the oxygen concentration present, but also on various other nutrients. It was shown that below a distinct level of nutritional supply chondrocyte function is disturbed. For example, glycosaminoglycan deposition by chondrocytes cultured on poly(glycolic acid) meshes was found to be poor in the central parts of three-dimensional constructs. Stirring-induced fluid flow in the flask was accompanied by an increase in the synthesis of glucosaminoglycans and fragments thereof, indicative of an improved chondrocyte function through enhanced delivery of metabolites.

In light of the importance of optimised cell nutrition, it is important to have some means of measuring/assessing levels of oxygen and other nutritive factors of cells located in the scaffold structure (Fig. 8.3). One way to optimise the nutrient supply in cell/scaffold constructs and to determine the diffusion-related flow conditions in deep structures of bulk materials is by mathematical modelling. Computational tools have recently become available to calculate parameters such as flow fields, shear stresses and mass transport in scaffold-

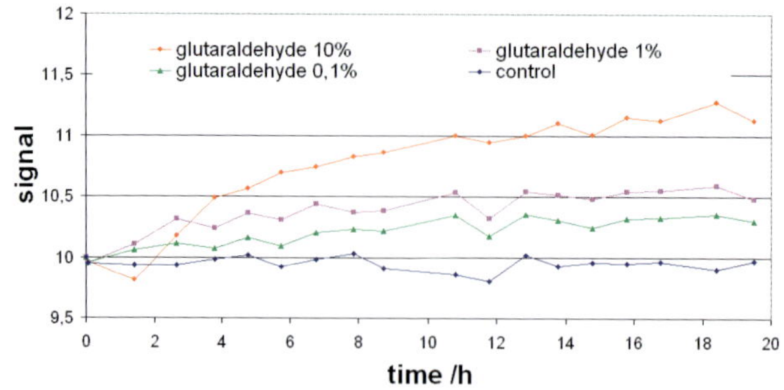

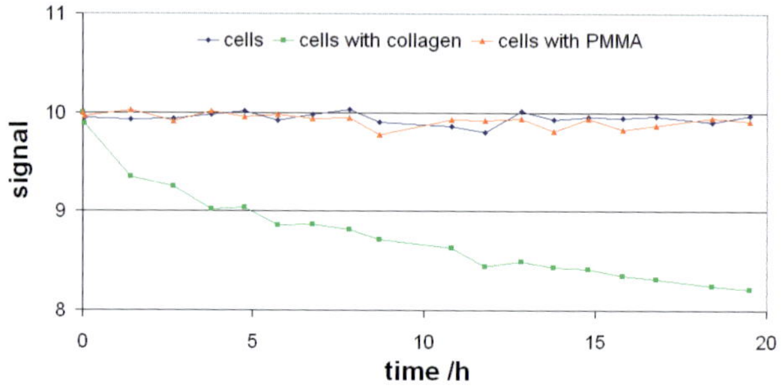

Fig. 8.3. Measurement of cell oxygen consumption is a sufficient tool for characterisation of cell promotion or impaired cell activity by biomaterials in vitro

containing bioreactors. These models have also been used to determine the relationship between mass transport and cell viability. Mathematical modelling enables researchers, for example, to calculate the momentum and oxygen transport within concentric cylinder bioreactors for cartilage tissue engineering and to design and characterise a scaled-up version. Theoretical modelling was also used to explore the relationships between cell density, diffusion distance, and cell viability within a cell/scaffold construct under a given nutrient supply. Muschler et al. (2004) presented a system of differential equations that can be used to calculate the relationship between cell density, diffusion distance, and cell viability in materials. Modelling of these parameters was performed to estimate when conditions of hypoxia will appear. It was calculated that increasing the scaffold dimension by a factor of 5 will decrease the maximum concentration of cells that can be delivered by oxygen by a factor of 25. This theoretical assumption confirms the finding that flat or porous scaffold structures work better than bulk materials. A combined approach of using both mathematical models (calculating flow and diffusion conditions) seems to be promising in order to most closely reflect the real in vivo situation for oxygen supply and consumption in complex scaffold systems.

The complexity of cell nutrition modelling is even greater when considering that not only oxygen tension but also the delivery, consumption and removal of nutrients and metabolic products are critical for cell survival. Since diffusion of oxygen is relatively slow in some of the biomaterials, while oxygen consumption is high, and the transport of other nutrients (e.g. glucose and amino acids) to and away from cells is more favourable in some biomaterials than in others, modelling of complex systems is difficult. Little, therefore, is known about the balance between diffusion, consumption and removal of nutrients and waste products on the one hand, and cell

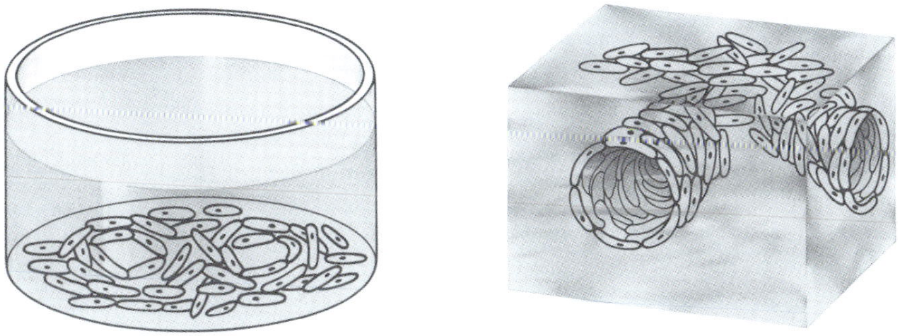

Fig. 8.4 . Schematic drawing of endothelial cell behaviour in cell monolayer and 3D culture

proliferation on the other. As this complexity is difficult to overcome by mathematical modelling, experimental data are necessary to gain a more detailed insight into nutrition-related cell reactions.

A totally different approach to improve the nutrition of cells is to enforce the formation of a vascular-like tissue in bioreactors (Fig. 8.4). Neovascularisation may be reached by the use of a co-culture system of bone cells and endothelial cells. However, since this approach introduces a new level of complexity, the technical challenges are significant. Aspects of ex vivo vascular formation are described in more detail in Chap. 13.

From a technical point of view, bioreactors can be classified according to their design properties. Bioreactors, connected to ports and filters for gas exchange, can be regarded as more open systems compared to conventional dishes and flasks. However, the fact that the culture dish requires individual manual handling for medium exchange, cell seeding, etc., ultimately limits its usefulness when large cell numbers are required. Closed bioreactor systems offer major advantages for manufacturing, since sterility can be assured and viability of the tissue product maintained. Closed and automated bioreactors should contain state-of-the-art systems for monitoring and adjusting physico-chemical as well as mechanical parameters. For reproducibility and standardisation, the culture conditions (e.g. temperature, pH, nutrient and oxygen supply) should be adjustable. An improvement in bioreactor design would be the addition of devices which allow online evaluation of the cell/scaffold maturation. The introduction of non-destructive analysis tools to monitor material parameters (e-modulus, degradation), biological parameters (cell number, cell differentiation) and metabolic parameters (pH, oxygen concentration, nutrient concentration) is helpful in adjusting culture conditions towards tissue needs. Advanced techniques (oxygen measurements, substrate monitoring, flow determination, fluorescence microscopy, micro-computerised tomography) aimed to predict the development of the tissue construct over time, have now been introduced in the manufacture of skeletal tissue-engineered products.

8.2 Mechanical Stimulation in Bioreactors

The skeletal system is continuously subjected to mechanical forces imposed by muscular contractions, body movement and various other external loadings. Similarly, externally applied mechanical forces in ex vivo generated bone tissue may elicit effects on osteoblast and chondrocyte proliferation, cell orientation, gene activity and other features of cellular activity (Cheng et al., 1996). It has been shown that mechanical forces applied from outside or organised from within a scaffold are beneficial (Schmelzeisen et al., 2003). Engineering bone and cartilage substitutes in vitro has been developed towards advanced bioreactor systems that mimic not only the three-dimensional morphology (Lee et al., 1996) but also the mechanical situation of bones (Cheng et al., 1997) or joints. Various studies have demonstrated the validity of this principle, particularly in the context of musculoskeletal tissue engineering (Hung et al., 2004). Despite numerous proof-of-principle studies showing that mechanical conditioning can improve the structural and functional properties of engineered bone and cartilage tissue, little is known about the specific mechanical parameters or regimes of application (i.e. magnitude, frequency, duration and mode of load application) that provide an optimal stimulation for bone or cartilage tissue (Butler et al., 2000). Most studies on the effects of load on osteoblasts were performed in monolayer cultures. Investigations of load-related chondrocyte reactions were done preferentially in explant cultures. In the context of bioreactor design for mechanically supported bone and cartilage tissues some aspects have to be considered here:

- Tissues at different stages of development or skeletal sites might require different regimes of mechanical conditioning.
- Cell deformations resulting from mechanical loading inside a bulk material may differ from deformations of surface-bound cells (Casser-Bette et al., 1990).
- The physiological strain environment of bone cells is much lower than that of other types of cells and they are correspondingly far more sensitive to mechanical deformations than most other cell types (e.g. chondrocytes).

In this highly complex field, a comprehensive understanding can only be achieved through experimental and theoretical investigations at different structural levels (monolayers, multiple layers, three-dimensional constructs). As load transfer through the scaffold and the substrate surface to cells (Rubin and Lanyon, 1987) exhibiting small deformations will have profound effects on cell behaviour, creating load devices in bioreactors has to take this aspect into account. Precise control over deformation at the various levels of hierarchy is most important. Bioreactors for mechanically supporting skeletal tissues have been custom-designed to provide defined deformations. Measuring strain and stresses in culture dishes and bioreactors can be done experimentally as well as theoretically (Fig. 8.5), however limitations on both approaches exist. Different authors have developed experimental systems aimed at applying defined mechanical loads on cells in culture (Granet et al., 1998; Hung et al., 2004). Some techniques used biaxial strain devices in an effort to apply homogeneous, isotropic strain to cells cultured in a monolayer, and used finite element analysis to predict the appropriate geometry for a uniform strain field. The accuracy of the strain field calculations was experimentally confirmed (Bottlang

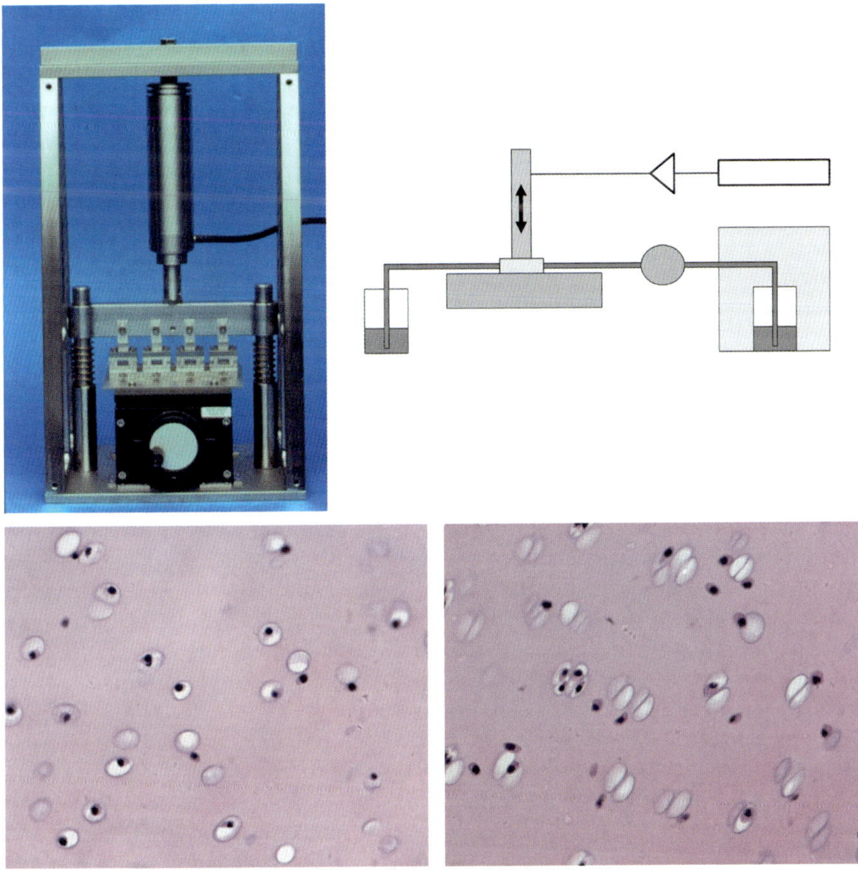

Fig. 8.5. Bioreactor for mechanical stimulation of cartilage or bone. Four tissue chambers can be loaded by a piezo-electric driven lever arm. Homogenuous strain fields can be applied. Use of the bioractor to stimulate explanted cartilage tissue (*bottom*). Histology of cartilage after mechanical loading: non-stimulated (*left*) and stimulated (*right*) cartilage

et al., 1997). However, it is not possible to measure the loading of cells in a three-dimensional space with the cell culture system used. Pressure application through lever-arm connected stamps is a common method to apply loads to three-dimensional tissue specimens. Although the stamp movement with subsequent deformation of the scaffold may be applied with high precision, determination of strain and stress fields within a specimen is much more complex than with biaxial systems. Assessment of the stress and strain fields by finite element analysis (FEA) is a commonly used approach, since other experimental measures are not able to determine load-related deformations in the microenvironment of a cell-containing scaffold, but the accuracy of FEA is limited by some simplifications. The matrix structure is, in most approaches, considered to be a homogenous incompressible structure, whereas in reality the cell-containing scaffold is generally more complex. Another limitation is that bioreactor and scaffold parameters are implemented on a simplified database.

Despite these simplifications, calculated strain fields seem to reflect real deformations in the tissue chamber. At least, the calculated magnitude that is biologically relevant allows one to discriminate between no, physiological and hyperphysiological load (Winston et al., 1989). Jones et al. (2003) developed an advanced loading device for application of specific compressive strains to tissue cylinders, which can be used to measure the resulting deformations. The device allows one to load the specimen at frequencies between 0.1 Hz and 50 Hz and amplitudes over 7,000 μstrain. This system combines accurate measurements of mechanical loading in real time with exact assessment of visco-elastic properties and may be useful in both, bone and cartilage tissue engineering applications.

Other investigators embedded osteoblast-like cells in gels that were subjected to cyclical tension forces and found that cell orientation and gene activity were altered as a result of cyclical mechanical loading. The most effective frequency of this loading lay around 1 Hz (Buschmann et al., 1995; Jones et al., 1995; Meyer et al., 2004c). Most in vitro studies indicate that mechanical stress is able to stimulate the proliferation of osteoblasts (Stein and Lian, 1993; Buschmann et al., 1995; Brown, 2000). The optimal strain magnitude in vivo and in vitro was found to be in the range from 1000 to 3000 μstrain (Meyer et al., 2004c). Mechanical stimulation was shown to result in an altered expression of bone-specific proteins, such as alkaline phosphatase, osteopontin, and osteocalcin. Concerning load-related cell effects in bioreactors, it is important to note, that the effects on protein synthesis (e.g. alkaline phosphatase, osteocalcin, or collagen expression) vary depending on the techniques used for loading (Masi et al., 1992; Krishnan et al., 2004). Some authors reported improved bone cell behaviour when cells were cultured under fluid flow-induced mechanical loads in spinner flasks. The underlying reason is assumed to be the existence of forces in the spinner flask exposing cells to physiological strains (Toma et al., 1997; Pavalko et al., 1998; Ogata, 2000). The sensitivity of osteoblasts to fluid shear stress is well established for cell cultures within flow chambers (Hillsley and Frangos, 1994). Rotating wall vessel reactors, originally designed to simulate a microgravity environment, were introduced and assessed for their relevance to skeletal tissue engineering. Rotating wall vessels have been tested mainly in cartilage and bone tissue engineering (Botchwey et al., 2001). This type of bioreactor rotates at a definable and controlled rate (Schwarz et al., 1992). By defining the centrifugal forces in these bioreactors, cells can be mechanically stimulated. Recent investigations showed that bone cells seeded on polymer constructs and grown in rotating bioreactors displayed minimal differentiation towards the osteoblastic phenotype. A low alkaline phosphatase activity compared to the static controls, a decreased extracellular matrix protein synthesis in the medium during long-term cultivation, and a reduced calcium deposition were found. These findings contradict earlier reports on the beneficial effects on osteoblastic cells cultured in rotating wall vessels (Botchwey et al., 2001). The underlying causes of the low inductive properties of some of the rotating wall vessel bioreactors in skeletal tissue formation are not understood, but non-physiological forces may be responsible for the experimental findings. The mechanisms whereby mechanical stimulation leads to cell proliferation and expression of tissue-specific genes reflect the in vivo situation of load-induced osteoblast behaviour (Duncan and Turner, 1995). In general, all bioreactor systems that expose cell/polymer constructs to biophysical stimuli not exceeding a physiologically tolerable range may support the differentiation of precursor cells towards the mature phenotype and enhance the function of mature cell types (Fig. 8.5). The sum of experimental data confirm that engineered skeletal tissue provides a good example that mimicking the native mechanical environment of cells can be beneficial for the ex vivo fabrication of bone or cartilage tissues (Meyer et al., 2004c). Under conditions of optimised periodic strains, the mechanical properties of engineered tissues appeared to improve significantly. In addition, the synthesis of matrix proteins and collagen, both being components of the secreted cell environment, can be enhanced by dynamic loading. Scaffold deformation on a physiological scale appears therefore to improve extracorporeal cell/scaffold maturation in bioreactors.

It is important to consider that, whereas the physiological microstrain environment for bone cells is well defined (Frost, 2000b), less is known about the physiological load environment of cartilage (Freed and Vunjak-Novakovic, 1997). What is generally accepted is that an important issue for cartilage bioprocessing relates to the development of bioreactors that produce a mechanically favourable load environment. Many bioreactors were introduced to load cartilage explants by external forcers, but only a few were developed to provide a uniform and quantifiable mechanical environment to promote chondrocyte proliferation and matrix growth under well-defined and controllable conditions. In contrast to bone tissue engineering, where porous scaffold structures are frequently in use, cartilage tissue engineering is commonly performed in bulk scaffold materials. Some of the scaffold matrices are in a gel-like condition. It was shown by some authors that more uniform cartilage tissue production is obtained in mechanically stimulated tissue cylinders, an effect attributed to the homogeneous hydrodynamic and favourable mass transport kinetics in the bioreactor (Martin et al., 2000). Load-related cartilage tissue maturation was reached by cartilage culturing in various bioreactor types, including spinner flasks, rotating wall vessel bioreactors and perfusion flow bioreactors. The observations and experience from various laboratories suggest that cartilage tissue should be dynamically loaded in order to support chondrocyte proliferation and differentiation (Buschmann et al., 1995; Freed and Vunjak-Novakovic, 1997; Martin et al., 2000). The application of micro-movements in extracorporal tissue chambers is therefore commonly considered as a promising approach in facilitating skeletal tissue engineering.

In addition to external mechanical stimulation as one strategy to promote tissue formation, another approach is the development of mechano-active scaffolds with optimised inherent physical properties (Yang et al., 2002b).

8.3 Biomagnetic and Bioelectric Stimulation in Bioreactors

Based on the discovery of piezoelectric potentials in bone tissue in the late 1960s, it was assumed that osteoblast physiology is influenced by electric fields (Domen et al., 2000). Many experiments have suggested that indeed electric fields modify the behaviour of bone cells. The effects of electromagnetic fields on bone cell behaviour have been the focus of many studies, however, cellular mechanisms of the action are not understood. Electromagnetic effects at biomaterial surfaces were considered to be an influencing factor in cell behaviour, since material-specific effects work through electrical changes at the surface. Within the scope of their in vitro studies, many investigators reported on osteoblast-like primary cultures, giving detailed de-

9 Scaffold Structure and Fabrication

9.1 Scaffold Structure

Whereas the properties of the material surface directly influence the behaviour at the single cell level, the three-dimensional scaffold structure plays a critical role in orchestration of tissue formation both in vitro and in vivo. Whereas the microstructure of the material refers to characteristics of a material at the nanoscale or microscale level (mainly used to characterise material surfaces, see Chap. 7), scaffold architecture defines the structure of the material in space at the tissue-length scale. Scaffolds do not only provide the structural basis that is available for cells to form a three-dimensional tissue-like construct in vitro, but also determine the features of mass transport (diffusion and convection). The scaffold architecture affects both single cell parameters (e.g. cell viability, cell migration, cell differentiation), and the composition of the generated tissue substitute.

Scaffolds can be grouped into different categories: underlying material, macrostructure (spacial geometry), micro-structure (bulk versus porous), mechanical properties, and degradation characteristics (Hutmacher, 2001).

Scaffold Characteristics

- Scaffold composition
- External geometry
- Macrostructure
- Microstructure
- Interconnectivity
- Surface/volume ratio
- Mechanical competence
- Degradation characteristics
- Chemical properties.

Whereas micro- and nano-properties are, to a great extent, related to the material surface and are described in detail in Chap. 7, micro- and macro-properties are also critical for tissue development. Scaffolds serve as space-holders for cells and allow ingrowth of surrounding tissues into the reconstruction site after transplantation. Thus, they provide structures that facilitate the three-dimensional proliferation, differentiation, and orientation of cells in order to enable a tissue-like construct growth ex vivo. Scaffolds facilitate the transfer of loads to surrounding tissues and ideally allow the reconstruction site to be mechanically competent directly after insertion. Scaffolds also provide a space in which tissue development and maturation towards complex multicellular systems can occur (Tsang and Bhatia, 2004). (Fig. 9.1) Two classical ways are in use to fabricate cell-containing scaffolds. One commonly used method is to coat cells with the scaffold by seeding cells on the scaffold. This approach is simple and fast, since cells attach to the scaffold within the first 24 hours. In contrast to the second method (to cultivate and maturate cells within a scaffold in a bioreactor), this approach is limited by the inhomogeneous distribution of cells. Various techniques to coat cells with scaffolds are in use. Static cell seeding techniques are the most commonly used methods, and involve placement of the scaffold in a bioreactor followed by adding a cell suspension to allow the adhesion of cells. (Fig. 9.2) However, the resulting cell distribution in the scaffold is random, and de-

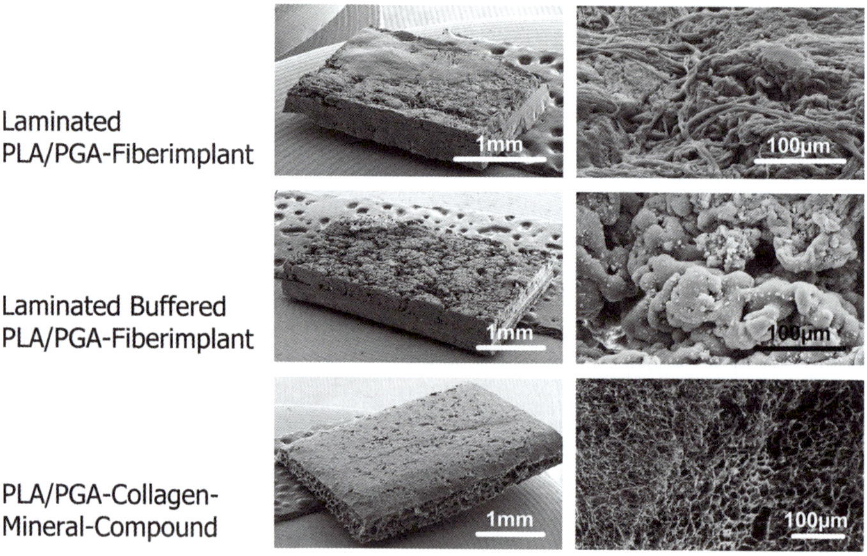

Fig. 9.1. Scanning electron microscopical view of different scaffolds (*left*: overview, *right*: detail), fabricated by conventional polymer fabrication technique. Polymer scaffolds can be altered by inclusion of buffer systems or mineral compounds in order to optimise their properties.

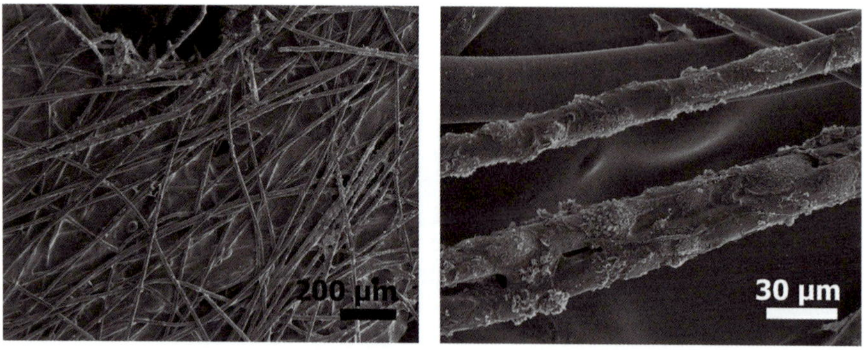

Fig. 9.2. Scanning electron microscopical view of cell/scaffold construct. Seeding of osteoblasts to a fiber scaffold lead to an adhesion of cells at the fiber surface without filling the space between fibers.

pendent on the gross scaffold structure, but in general with the majority of cells attached only to the outer surfaces. Wetting techniques applied to scaffolds prior to cell seeding allow for displacement of air-filled pores with water and facilitate penetration by the cell suspension into these pores. In contrast to simple seeding techniques, cells can also be coated with scaffolds by injection or by applying a vacuum to ensure penetration of the cell suspension. Using these techniques cells can be placed more homogenously throughout the three-dimensional space. However, uniformity is lost under static culture conditions because of nutrient and oxygen diffusion limitations within the scaffold. When cells are seeded on scaffolds, high cell densities are necessary to achieve uniform tissue regeneration. The effects of cell seeding density on cartilage formation indicates that high numbers of cells are required to obtain mature tissue formation (Vunjak-Novakovic et al., 1998; 1999; Burg et al., 2000a; Holy et al., 2000).

The second approach to coating cells with scaffolds is long-term culture of cells with scaffolds. (Fig. 9.3) Using this technique, cells have to proliferate, migrate and differentiate during culture with the scaffold. This longer-lasting method has the main advantage that cells are not restricted to the outer surface of the scaffold but may grow deep into scaffold structures. As bone and cartilage differs significantly in tissue composition at the different levels (cellular level, supracellular level, tissue level), optimal scaffold properties can be assumed to be different for scaffolds used for bone and scaffold used for cartilage tissue engineering (Wiesmann et al., 2004). Reviewing the literature reveals that bio-organic scaffold materials (e.g. collagen, fibrin, hyaluronan, alginate, chitosan) and polymer materials (e.g. polyhydroxy acids) are commonly used for both (cartilage and bone) tissue engineering strategies (Agrawal and Ray, 2001), whereas organic materials (hydroxyapatite, tricalcium phosphates) are preferably used in bone tissue engineering. Independent of the underlying material, various basic scaffold characteristics can be distinguished:

- *Scaffold composition*: Scaffold materials can be distinguished by the chemical composition. Pure non-organic materials can de distinguished from composite materials (containing also organic materials) and solely organic materials. Materials can also be grouped into solid or gel-like conditions (hydrogels, for example, contain a water content greater than 30% by weight).
- *Macrostructure*: The macrostructure reflects the external geometry and gross internal structure of the scaffold. A three-dimensional scaffold that is congruent to the external geometry of the tissue to be replaced is required for scaffold placement and fixation in the clinical situation. Direct contact between the defect borders and the scaffold will enhance the interaction between the ex vivo generated construct and the host site. An optimal internal scaffold structure will promote tissue formation by mimicking the native environment.
- *Porosity and pore interconnectivity*: Scaffolds are constituted of either bulk materials or they have a pore or tube geometry. Pores or tubes can be introduced in scaffold in an isolated fashion or they can be interconnected. An advantage of an interconnected porous or tubular system is the improved nutritional supply (by diffusion, convection or directed fluid flow) in deeper scaffold areas, thereby enabling cells to survive in these regions. A high interconnectivity of pores or tubes facilitates a hydrodynamic microenvironment with minimal diffusion constraints, but at the same time will reduce the mechanical strength. As spongiosal

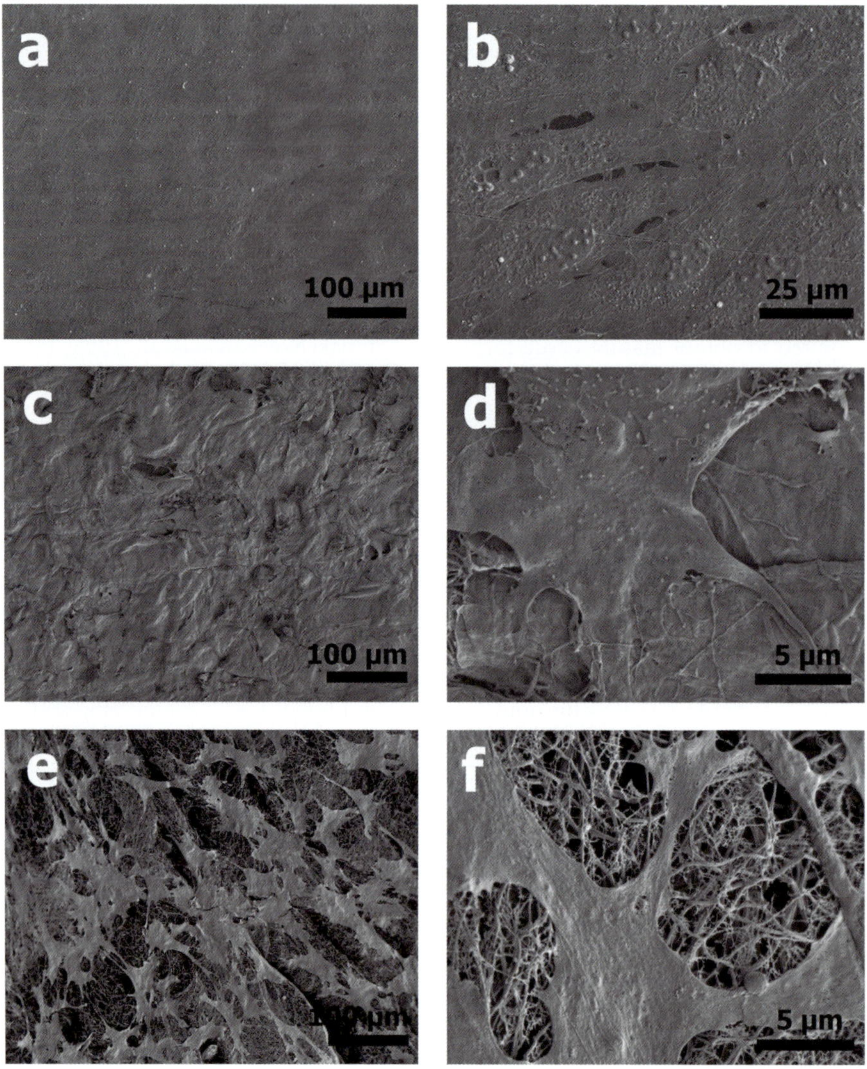

Fig. 9.3. Scanning electron microscopical view of osteoblasts cultured on a petri dish (top row), a collagen matrix (middle row), and a fibrin matrix (bottom row). Cells with an osteoblastic appearance cover the surface of scaffolds.

bone tissue has a porous structure these scaffold features seem to be advantageous, especially in the context of ex vivo bone tissue engineering.

- *Pore size/tube diameter*: Tissue generation ex vivo and regeneration in vivo may be achieved using scaffolds with optimal hollow structures (tube/pore combinations). The size of these hollow structures does not only improve the fluid flow through the scaffold but may also allow vascular ingrowth (in vitro and after transplantation in vivo) and therefore improve the outcome of tissue engineering

Table 9.1. Parameters affecting scaffold degradation

Material	Scaffold	In vitro	In vivo
– Composition – Structure – Configuration – Molecular weight – Molecular orientation – Cross-links – Chain motility	– Size – Mass – Porosity – Surface/volume ratio – Shape – Surface topography – Surface chemistry	– Medium – pH – Fluid flow – Biomechanics – Temperature – Cell sources – Cell number – Cell activity – Ionic strength	– Defect site – Species – Inflammation – Immunology – Biomechanics – Tissue turnover – Enzymes – Vascularisation

treatments. From a conceptual point of view, cartilage tissue as a non-vascular tissue, does not benefit from porous scaffolds, whereas bone formation critically depends on vascularisation. As researchers have suggested the need for pore sizes ranging from 200 to 500 μm for vascular ingrowth, scaffolds containing tubular structures of such diameters seem to be beneficial in bone tissue engineering applications.

- *Surface/volume ratio*: A high overall material surface area to volume ratio is beneficial, allowing large numbers of cells to attach and migrate into porous scaffolds. Since pore diameter and internal surface area are related linearly, a compromise between surface gain and mechanical stability has to be found depending on the application of the scaffold.
- *Mechanical properties*: Scaffolds should ideally have sufficient mechanical strength during in vitro culturing to resist the physiological mechanical environment in the regenerating load-bearing tissues (cartilage, bone) at the desired implantation site.
- *Degradation characteristics*: The ideal scaffold degradation must be adjusted appropriately such that it parallels the rate of new tissue formation and at the same time retains sufficient structural integrity until the newly grown tissue has replaced the scaffold supporting function (for a review see Lu et al., 2001). Additionally, degradation of the scaffold should not be accompanied by a lowering of the physiological pH in the in vitro environment or at the defect site. Moreover, during the degradation process there should be no release of toxic degradation products. Multiple parameters determine the degradationrate of a scaffold in the in vitro and in vivo situation (Table 9.1), (Fig. 9.4)
- *Chemical properties*: A scaffold should ideally be used as a carrier for proteins. The proteins, bound to the scaffold material, should be biologically active and they should be released in a predetermined fashion. (Fig. 7.7)

9.2 Scaffold Fabrication

A major technical challenge in scaffold production is to maintain accurate control over the desired macrostructural (e.g. external geometry, spatial composition, mechanical strength, density, porosity), microstructural (e.g. pore size, pore interconnectivity, degradation characteristics), and nanostructural (e.g. surface topography

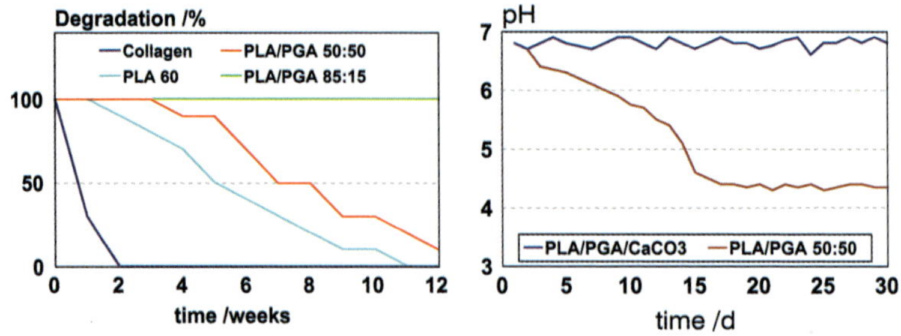

Fig. 9.4. Scaffold characteristics can be adjusted by chemical modification techniques. The degradation kinetics of polyesters can be adjusted by a defined co-polymerisation of different polymers (e.g. PLA and PGA). Additionally, a pH stability during scaffold degradation can be reached through an inclusion of a carbonate buffer system in the scaffold.

or physico-chemical surface characteristics) properties at the same time. Ideally, the processing technique used to fabricate the scaffolds should also allow use of various underlying materials. Besides the fabrication techniques that largely define the scaffold macro- and microstructure, there is a variety of natural or synthetic scaffolding materials to consider. It is important to note, that each underlying material possesses different processing requirements and varying degrees of processability to form scaffolds. The design of complex scaffolds composed of different materials adds a further step in complexity in scaffold fabrication. Various engineering parameters (technical procedure, fabrication accuracy, automation) determine the result of scaffold production.

- *Technical procedure*: The processing technique should not change the chemical and biophysical properties of the scaffold nor cause any damage to the material structure.
- *Fabrication accuracy*: The fabrication process should create spatially accurate three-dimensional scaffolds at the macro- and microscale level.
- *Automation*: The applied technique should be automated in order to ease the production process, reduce interbatch inconsistency, ideally reduce fabrication time, and at the same time be cost effective.

As mentioned earlier, the scaffold fabrication technique applied is primarily determined by the underlying material. It is obvious that naturally occurring non-organic materials are commonly processed by different methods to, for example, synthetic organic materials. Additionally, naturally occurring non-organic materials are generated by arrays of techniques different from those for synthetic organic materials. Fabrication of non-organic materials is performed by techniques commonly used in ceramic technology, whereas a wide range of techniques have been developed to process synthetic and natural (organic) polymer materials into scaffold structures (Peter et al., 1998a; 1998b). Conventional polymer fabrication techniques can be distinguished from the newly introduced solid-free form fabrication techniques (SFF) (Sachlos and Czernuszka, 2003) (Table 9.2). Conventional fabrication techniques are defined as processes that create scaffolds having a bulk or porous (interconnected or non-interconnected) structure that lacks any long-range channelling microstructure (Yang et al., 2002a; 2002b). (Fig. 9.1) Solid-free form fabrication, in contrast, uses

Table 9.2. Scaffold fabrication techniques

Conventional	Rapid prototyping
– Solvent casting/particulate leaching – Phase inversion/particulate leaching – Fibre meshing/bonding – Melt moulding – Gas foaming – Membrane lamination – Hydrocarbon templating – Freeze drying – Emulsion freeze drying – Solution casting	– Fused deposition modelling – Three-dimensional printing – Three-dimensional plotting – Selective laser sintering – Laminated object manufacture – Stereolithography – Multiphase jet solidification

layer manufacturing processes to form scaffolds directly from computer-generated models, thereby enabling the introduction of hollow or tubular structures in scaffolds. Additionally, SFF enables one to create the external geometry of the scaffold with high precision (Yang et al., 2001). Conventional scaffold fabrication is often used in scaffold fabrication for bone and cartilage tissue engineering. Commonly used techniques are: solvent casting/particulate leaching, phase inversion/particulate leaching, fibre meshing/bonding, melt moulding, gas foaming/high pressure processing, membrane lamination, hydrocarbon templating, freeze drying, emulsion freeze drying, solution casting, and combinations of these techniques. The principles and technical procedures of these techniques can be found in various reviews (Hutmacher, 2001; Nishimura et al., 2003; Liu and Ma, 2004). A wide variety of scaffolds has been successfully applied to engineer bone and cartilage tissue ex vivo and investigated for their success in animal experimental and clinical situations. In order to understand the advantages and limitations of each processing method, a brief description is given of the technical aspects involved.

Solvent casting/particulate leaching is a commonly used and widely investigated method for the preparation of tissue engineered scaffolds. Scaffolds produced by this technique have been used in a multitude of studies for bone and cartilage tissue engineering, with favourable results (Ochi et al., 2003). This method, first described by Mikos et al. in 1994, is based on dispersing mineral (e.g. sodium chloride, sodium tartrate and sodium citrate) or organic (e.g. saccharose) particles in a polymer solution. The dispersion process is then performed by casting or by freeze-drying in order to produce porous scaffolds. By modulation of the basic process, different researchers (Mikos et al,. 1994; Agraval et al., 2000; Yoon and Park, 2001; Murphy et al., 2002) aimed to improve the scaffold structure. They introduced variations of the basic processing principle to alter the polymer structure to that desired: i.e. to increase the porogen/polymer ratio, avoid crystal deposition, increase the pore interconnectivity, and obtain fully interconnected scaffolds with a high degree of porosity (Agraval et al., 2000; Murphy et al., 2002). Solvent casting/particulate leaching has been used, in particular, to fabricate poly(L-lactic acid) (PLLA) or poly(lactide-*co*-glycolide) (PLGA) scaffolds, but the method has also been applied to process other polymers (Gomes et al., 2002b). Despite the relative ease of fabricating scaffolds using this approach, the method has some inherent disadvantages such as the possible release of highly toxic solvents (Hutmacher, 2000; Yang et al., 2001; Gomes et al.,

2002a), the limitation of producing only thin scaffolds (Yang et al., 2001; Gomes et al., 2002b), and impaired mechanical properties (Gomes et al., 2002a).

Phase inversion/particulate leaching is a closely related technique to solvent casting. The difference from the previously described method is that instead of allowing the solvent to evaporate, the solution film is placed in water. The subsequent phase inversion causes the polymer to precipitate (Holy et al., 2000). The main advantage for tissue engineering purposes when compared to the basic solvent casting method is that crystal deposition is avoided, and this enables the production of thicker scaffolds. It was shown technically that using phase inversion, scaffolds with improved interconnectivity and morphologies mimicking trabecular bone could be fabricated (Holy et al., 2000). Based on experimental biological studies, these scaffolds have, on a number of occasions, been shown to support the growth of osteoblast-like cells and facilitate consequent bone matrix formation (Holy et al., 2000; Karp et al., 2003).

Fibre bonding is based on the presence of fibre-like polymer structures. In fibre bonding, individual fibres are woven or knitted into three-dimensional scaffolds having variable pore size. By using fibres with different diameters and by connecting the fibres in different special configurations, a high degree of variability in the scaffold structure can be achieved. Although this technique enables one to create large surface areas thereby improving nutrient diffusion (Mikos et al., 1993; Kim and Mooney, 1998), it is technically difficult to obtain the desired porosity and pore size. Additionally, there is a possibility of solvent residues in the scaffold that may be harmful to cells or cells at the host site (Lu and Mikos, 1996; Hutmacher, 2000; Yang et al., 2001; Leong et al., 2003).

Melt-based technologies are often used when it is desired to fabricate porous scaffolds. Melt moulding/particulate leaching is, of all the melt-based techniques, the most commonly used. Using this technique a polymer is mixed with a porogen prior loading into a mould (Thomson et al., 1995). The mould, shaped in the form of the desired defect geometry, is then heated above the glass transition temperature of the polymer used. After reaching the glass transition temperature, the composite material is immersed in a solvent for selective dissolution of the porogen (Thomson et al., 1995). As this technique enables one to fabricate porous scaffolds of defined shapes by creating a defined (external) mould geometry (Thomson et al., 1995; Lu and Mikos, 1996; Leong et al., 2003), this method has become popular in clinical tissue engineering strategies (Schiller et al., 2004; Meyer et al., 2005b). Furthermore, this method also offers independent control of the pore size and porosity, by varying the amount and size of the porogen crystals (Thomson et al., 1995; Lu and Mikos, 1996; Leong et al., 2003). Extrusion and injection moulding are other melt-based techniques used for the processing of scaffolds (Gomes et al., 2001; 2002a; 2002b). As with particulate leaching, generation of a scaffold (Gomes et al., 2002a) with a high degree of porosity and interconnectivity is possible. By resembling the porous structure of trabecular bone, the mechanical properties of such scaffolds can be adjusted in order to mimic the compressive modulus and compressive strength of trabecular bone. As the control of pore distribution is impaired using this method, nutritional demands of cells are difficult to meet.

Gas foaming under high pressure as another processing technique is based on the CO_2 saturation of polymer discs, through their exposure to high-pressure CO_2 (Mooney et al., 1996). An advantage of this method is the possibility of obtaining scaffolds with a high degree of porosity and at the same time, producing pores with a pore size in the range of 100 μm (Mooney et al., 1996). Scaffolds produced by this technique have the disadvantages of low mechanical strength and poorly defined pore structure, which limits widespread use of this technique (Shea et al., 2000).

A further method is based on thermally induced phase separation (freeze-drying), which occurs when the temperature of a homogeneous polymer solution, previously poured into a mould, is decreased. After the phase-separated system is stabilised, the solvent-rich phase is removed by vacuum sublimation leaving behind the polymeric foam. This technique allows the production of scaffolds consisting of natural and synthetic polymers (Malafaya and Reis, 2003; Mao et al., 2003). As the processing conditions are technically challenging and the scaffolds obtained have low mechanical competence accompanied by reduced pore size, application of this technique is rare (Hutmacher, 2000; Yang et al., 2001).

The varying success rates of scaffold fabrication by the above mentioned methods is, to some extent, technique-inherent. Additional limitations of conventional techniques are the need for manual intervention and the inconsistent and inflexible processing procedures. As an ideal scaffold material for bone and cartilage tissue engineering is unknown, it is speculative to comment on the feasibility of each processing technique. Much experimental work has to be performed to gain a more detailed insight into the success of the various conventionally fabricated scaffolds in terms of the biological and clinical outcome in bone and certilage tissue engineering strategies.

New processing technologies have been developed in recent decades, and have been applied in tissue engineering for scaffold fabrication to overcome the limitations of conventional processing techniques. Rapid prototyping (RP) (Hutmacher, 2000), a synonym for solid free-form fabrication (SFF) (Leong et al., 2003), is the most popular technique. Rapid prototyping is a computer-based design and fabrication techniques that enables one to produce ordered external and internal scaffold structures. The main advantages of the SFF techniques over conventional techniques are: the possibility of defined external and internal scaffold structure fabrication, computer-controlled fabrication processes, improved processing accuracy, and, eventually, the coating of scaffolds with cells. As with other computer-based techniques, automation and standardisation of processing protocols can be more easily achieved. The data sets used to design and fabricate scaffolds can be based on virtual data sets or computer-based medical imaging technologies (e.g. CT scans), and other technologies (Hutmacher, 2000; Leong et al., 2003). Rapid prototyping is a method that can not only individualise the external and internal defect geometry but can be envisioned in the future to produce controlled anisotrophic scaffold nanostructures. The solid free-form technique can be considered as a method of layered manufacturing. In the case of scaffold fabrication, the three-dimensional geometry is created layer-by-layer via defined processing techniques. Through the possibility of implementing macroscopic, microscopic and likely in the future, nanoscopic structural features in different areas of the scaffold, tissue-like structures may be obtained. A complex scaffold micro- and nanostructure, closely related to the desired biological defeet tissue, can be assumed to be advantageous when cell/scaffold constructs with multiple cell types (e.g. bone and endothelial cells), arranged in hierarchical orders, are desirable (Quarto et al., 2001; Vacanti et al., 2001). Solid free-form fabrication techniques currently used for tissue engineering purposes include: fused deposition modelling (FDM) (Hutmacher et al., 2001a; 2001b; Zein et al., 2002); three-dimensional printing (Cima et al., 1991; Park et al., 1998; Shen et al., 2000; Lam et al., 2002; Sherwood et al., 2002); three-dimensional plotting (Landers and Mühlhaupt, 2000; Ang et al., 2002; Landers et al., 2002) and a variety of other approaches (Fedchenko, 1996; Chu et al., 2001; Taboas et al., 2003). Whereas extensive research has been done at a material-based or cell biologically based level, only a small number of SFF techniques have been exploited for the clinical use of extracorporally grown tissues. As the advantages of these techniques are impressive and the logistic and technical problems seem capable of solution in the near future, it can be assumed that these techniques will become standard measures to create scaffolds.

Using fused deposition modelling, scaffolds with a highly ordered microstructure can be fabricated. The avoidance of organic solvents is the main advantage of this technique from a technical point of view. In contrast, incorporation of growth factors is difficult, because elevated temperatures during processing destroy the structure and activity of such growth factors (Leong et al., 2003). Fused deposition modelling was shown to generate scaffolds with adequate porosity supporting the ingrowth and survival of cells and tissues (Hutmacher et al., 2001a; Zein et al., 2002). It was demonstrated by Schantz et al. (2002) that osteoid formation could be obtained when these scaffolds, coated with periostal cells under osteogenic conditions in vitro, were implanted in vivo in a subcutaneous animal model. As the processing techniques leads to elevated material temperature, cells can be coated with the material only after the scaffold is produced.

From the viewpoint of tissue engineering, three-dimensional printing is a promising prototyping technique (Cima et al., 1991; Shen et al., 2000). The main advantage of three-dimensional printing is the fact that scaffolds can be created at room temperature. This method thus allows the seeding of cells or the incorporation of growth factors during the fabrication process (Hutmacher, 2000). The technique, based on the printing of a liquid binder onto thin layers of powder, enables one to coat cells with the polymer material during layered manufacturing and therefore locate cells in deeper structures of the scaffold (Park et al., 1998; Hutmacher, 2000; Leong et al., 2003). By stacking multiple cells containing material layers in a scaffold with a defined tunnel structure, the viability of cells in central parts of the scaffold can be envisioned. This promising technique has been successfully exploited in bone tissue engineering (Park et al., 1998; Hutmacher, 2000; Leong et al., 2003). In addition to the cell biological advantages of processing at room temperature, the deposition of cells in central areas of the scaffold and improved tube and pore geometry provide the further advantage of the possibility of fabricating complex scaffolds containing different materials with different substructures (Cima et al., 1991; Park et al., 1998; Lam et al., 2002; Sherwood et al., 2002). A main disadvantage of the three-dimensional printing technique is the fact that the microstructure of the scaffolds is dependent on the powder size of the stock material. An additional technical problem is the technique-related closure of the pores by the underlying material.

Three-dimensional plotting is a commonly used method of SFF fabrication for processing hydrogels (Landers and Mülhaupt, 2000; Ang et al., 2002; Landers et al., 2002). A hydrogel-based scaffold formation of special relevance in cartilage tissue engineering is achieved by chemical reactions of co-reactive components that are placed in two component dispensers, or one component can be plotted in a liquid medium containing a coreactive component (Landers et al., 2002). This technique has, like three-dimensional printing, the advantage of operating under physiological conditions (e.g. physiological temperature). Scaffolds can also be enriched homogenously throughout the scaffold volume with cells or growth factors during the fabrication process.

9.3 Scaffold-free Micromass Units

The in vitro formation of bone- or cartilage-like tissue for subsequent implantation (Lindenhayn et al., 1999; Hutmacher, 2000; Anderer and Libera, 2002) is, as described, commonly performed by using scaffolds. Recently, there has been controversy concerning the use of artificial scaffolds compared to the use of a natural matrix (van der Kraan et al., 2002). Skeletal defect regeneration by extracorporally created tissues commonly exploits a three-dimensional cell-containing artificial scaffold. As indicated earlier, a number of in vitro studies have been performed to evaluate the cell behaviour in various three-dimensional artificial scaffold materials. Whereas most of these materials were generally shown to allow spacing of skeletal cells in a three-dimensional space, not all materials promote the ingrowth of cells within the scaffolds (Freed et al., 1998). Rather, supporting cellular function depends, as described, on multiple parameters such as the chosen cell line, the underlying material, the surface properties and the scaffold structure. Some in vitro studies indicate that a material itself may impair the outcome of ex vivo tissue formation, when compared to a natural tissue-containing matrix. Additionally, in the in vivo situation defect regeneration can be critically impaired by the immunogenity of the material, the unpredictable degradation time and by side effects caused by degradation products (van der Kraan et al., 2002) (see Chap. 10). Based on these considerations, some researchers regard matrices close to the natural extracellular matrix as most promising for skeletal tissue engineering. A recently elaborated approach in extracorporal tissue engineering is therefore the avoidance of non-degradable scaffolds. These are resorbed at a different rate to skeletal tissue regeneration, which proceeds by itself. Therefore, new approaches have been invented to overcome these problems by renouncing scaffolds.

It is well known that tissue explants can be dissociated into dispersed cells and then reaggregated in vitro to regenerate complete organisms (Kelm and Fussenegger, 2004). Basic research has indicated that regeneration of simple animals, and of whole vertebrate tissues, can be achieved by reaggregation approaches using micromass technique. Investigations on skeletal development gave first insight into this micromass biology. The micromass technology relies to a great extent on the presence of the proteinacious extracellular matrix. As described earlier, the ECM may exert both direct and indirect influences on cells and consequently modulate their behaviour. At the same time, these cells alter the composition of the ECM. This may be accomplished in a variety of fashions, including differential expression of particular ECM components and/or proteases such as metalloproteinases by cells in the local microenvironment. A large body of evidence has confirmed that a minimal cell number is required in three-dimensional tissue-like constructs to induce the differentiation of mesenchymal precursors along the chondrogenic and osteogenic pathways (reviewed in Hall and Miyake, 1992). In contrast, mesenchymal precursors seeded in low-density micromasses adopt features of a fibroblastic phenotype and abolish cell differentiation, when mimicking a low-density condensation (Hattori and Ide, 1984; Cottrill et al., 1987; Hurle et al., 1989). These findings indicate that a critical cell mass is necessary to proceed with a specific ECM formation. A threshold amount of precursor cells is necessary to form a three-dimensional ECM structure around these cell masses promoting their differentiation. The ECM in the microenvironment then interacts with cells to further develop towards a specific tissue. The absence of the requisite ECM components would lead to decreased recruitment of precursors to the condensations, causing a subsequent deficiency in chondrocyte or osteoblast differentiation. In vitro studies with chondrocytes confirmed these findings, showing that the ability of mesenchymal precursors to initiate chondrogenic differentiation is dependent upon cell configuration within a condensation process, which varies with the density of the condensation (Archer et al., 1985).

In the context of tissue engineering, ex vivo tissue generation may be optimised by the use of cell reaggregation technology. The reaggregate approach is a method to generate, in an attempt to mimic the in vivo situation, a tissue-like construct from dispersed cells, under special culture conditions (Fig. 9.5). Therefore, the self-renewal (cell amplification), spatial sorting and self-organisation of multipotent stem cells in combination with the self-assembly of determined cells are the basis for such an engineering design option. Technically, cells are dissociated as indicated in the cell cultivation section, and the dispersed cells are then reaggregated into cellular spheres. In order to technically refine scaffold-free spheres, cells are kept either in regular culture dishes (as gravitory cultures), in spinner flasks, or in more sophisticated bioreactors. In contrast to conventional monolayer cell cultures, in which cells grow in only two dimensions on the flat surface of a plastic dish, suspension cultures allow tissue growth in all three dimensions. It has been observed that cells in spheres have higher proliferation rates than cells in monolayer cultures, and their differentiation more closely resembles that seen in situ. These findings may be based on the spatial configuration in a three-dimensional matrix network.

Different culture parameters (sizes of the culture plate, movement in a bioreactor, coating of culture walls) are all crucial to the process. Roller tube culture systems have been shown to be suitable for cultivation of tissue explants in suspension. The cultivated and fabricated tissues may be used to study the primary mixing of cells and the patterns of cell differentiation and growth within growing spheres in order to improve the outcome of microsphere cultivation. In addition, some culture conditions could aid the development of high-throughput systems and allow manipulation of individual spheres. It seems worthwhile elaborating new bioreactor technologies and culture techniques to improve the ex vivo growth of scaffold-free tissues. Technically, short-term reaggregation experiments, which last from minutes to a few hours, can be distinguished from long-term studies. Short-term reaggregation has been used widely to evaluate basic principles of cell–cell interactions and cell–matrix interactions, whereas long-term cultivation (days to several weeks) is suitable in ex vivo tissue engineering strategies. Recent studies of the reaggregation approach aim to solve two aspects: to fabricate scaffold-free, three-dimensional tissue formation and at the same time to investigate basic principles of cellular self-assembly. As in monolayer cultures, which facilitate the study of cell–material interactions, suspension cultures allow the evaluation of cell reactions towards a three-dimensional space. The reaggregate approach enables one to follow tissue formation from single cell sources to organised spheres in a controlled environment (Fig. 9.6). Thus, the inherent fundamentals of tissue engineering are better revealed. Additionally, as the

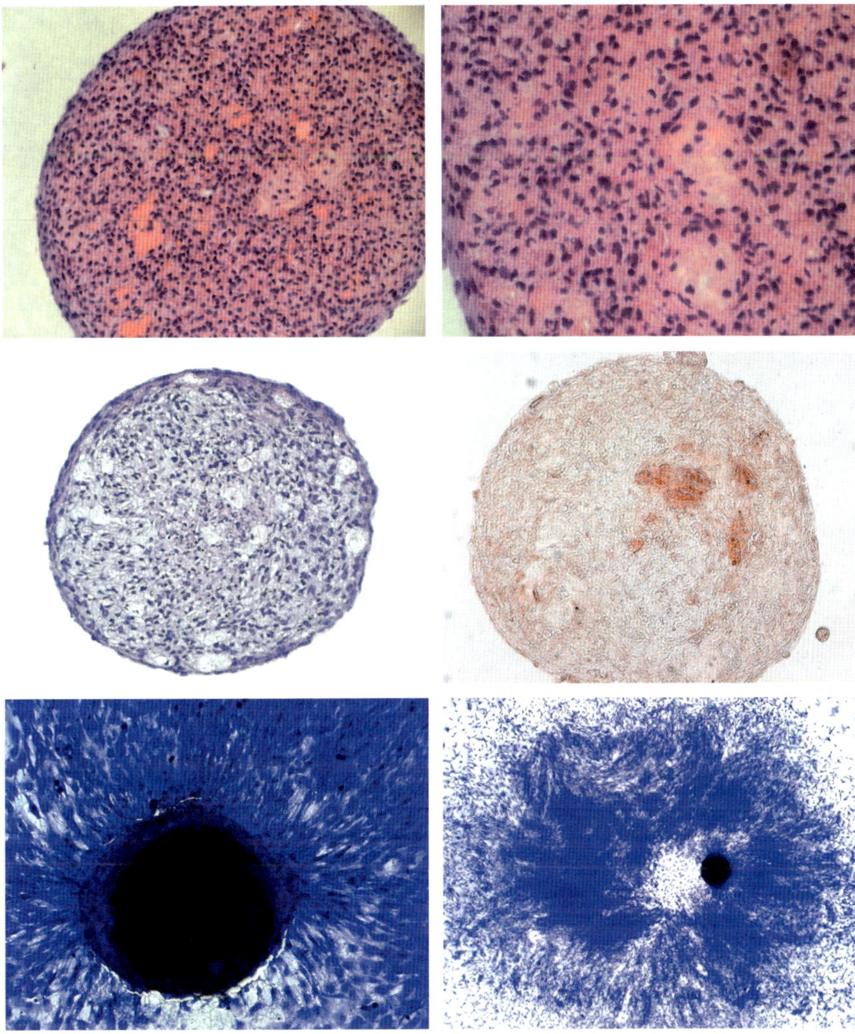

Fig. 9.5. Micromass culture of chondrocytes (*top*) (toluidine blue O staining) and osteoblasts (*middle*) (left: Richardson staining, right: Ostecalein expression). Cell outgrowth of osteoblasts from spheres to Petri dish (bottom) (Richardson son staining). Cultures are 100–300 μm in diameter

newly formed tissue is devoid of any artificial material, it more closely resembles the in vivo situation.

Skeletal cells were found to be a suitable cell source for such ex vivo reaggregate approaches. Anderer and Libera (2002) developed an autologous spheroid system to culture chondrocytes and osteoblasts without adding xenogenous serum, growth factors, or scaffolds, in consideration of the fact that several growth factors and scaffolds are not permitted for use in clinical applications. It was demonstrated that by such an approach autologous chondrocytes and osteoblasts cultered in the presence of autologous serum form a three-dimensional micro-tissue that had generated its

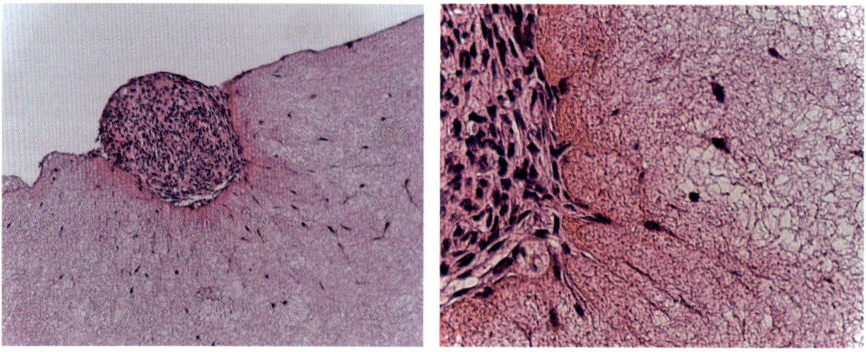

Fig. 9.6. Cell migration of micromass cultures of osteoblasts in a fibrin membrane

own extracellular matrix. Chondrocyte-based micro-tissues have a characteristic extracellular space that was similar to the natural matrix of hyaline cartilage. Osteoblasts were also able to build up a micro-tissue similar to that of bone repair tissue without collagen-associated mineral formation. The fabrication of a self-assembled skeletal tissue seems not to be limited to certain species, as results from bovine and porcine chondrocyte and osteoblast cultivation led to the formation of species-related cartilage-like or bone-like tissue.

It was recently observed that even complex cellular systems can be generated ex vivo without the use of scaffolds. Co-cultures of osteoblasts and endothelial cells, for example, resulted in the formation of a bi-cellular micromass tissue renouncing any other materials. Other organotypic cultures, used to develop engineered tissues other than of skeletal origin, confirm that it is feasible to create tissue substitutes based on reaggregated spheres technology. Examples of these strategies include liver reconstruction, synthesis of an artificial pancreas, restoration of heart valve tissue and cardiac organogenesis in vitro.

Several investigations have suggested that after in vivo transfer of such reaggregates, tissue healing is improved in the sense that the repair tissue mimics the features of the original skeletal tissue (Anderer and Libera, 2002; Meyer et al., 2005c). Preclinical and clinical cartilage repair studies, in particular, have demonstrated that tissue formation resembled more closely the natural situation. The transplantation of reassembled chondrogenic micro-tissues is able to impair the formation of fibrocartilage by suppression of type I collagen expression, while promoting the formation of proteoglycan accompanied by a distinct expression of type II collagen. It can be assumed that the volume of the observed repair tissue was formed by the implanted chondrospheres itself as well as by host cells located in the superficial cartilage defect. The mechanisms by which chondrospheres promote defect healing are complex and not completely understood. Van der Kraan et al. (2002) reviewed the role of the extracellular matrix in the regulation of chondrocyte function in the defect site and the relevance for cartilage tissue engineering. Numerous other studies have confirmed that extracellular matrix of articular cartilage can be maintained by a distinct number of chondrocytes and that the extracellular matrix plays an important role in the regulation of chondrocyte function. In in vitro generated cartilage-like tissue a time-dependent increase in the expression of collagen type II, S-100, and cartilage-specific proteoglycans paralleled by a reduced cell–matrix ratio was observed in the microspheres (Meyer et al., 2005c). The transplanted cell/matrix complex was attributed to be responsible for the observed chondrocyte proliferation, differentiation and hyaline cartilage-like matrix maturation in vivo.

The inductive properties of the implantation site may also be beneficial when a stem cell-based micro-tissue strategy is chosen. Stem cell tissue engineering using fetal or adult stem cells in combination with sphere technologies leads to implantable stem cell driven tissues. Typically, stem cells must be amplified to large quantities in suspension cultures and have access to appropriate growth factors to establish specially organised histotypical spheres. These spheres can then be implanted into the lesioned skeletal site. Although adult stem cells of various origins can transdifferentiate into distinct cell types, the transformation of these cell types into functioning tissues and their successful implantation by reaggregation technology needs further elaboration.

over other techniques relies greatly on the experimental model selected (Einhorn, 1999). Extracorporal bone tissue engineering is aimed at restoring large segments of the skeletal bone lost for various reasons, improving the healing of complicated fractures, and hopefully in the near future, fully regenerating complex skeletal defects (Puelacher et al., 1996; Bruder et al., 1998a; 1998b). Animal models should effectively mimic the clinical situation in human bone healing. However, it is often desired that bone defects in animal models should fail to heal unless they are treated with a cell-based tissue engineering strategy. Clinicians should be aware that bone tissue engineering approaches have unique features, as they differ in different fields of surgery. For example, bony regeneration is often observed after a sinus lift procedure in the maxillary sinus region, even in the absence of implanted biomaterial. In this case, elevation of the sinus mucosa seems to be the crucial procedure that induces bone growth. Bone regeneration in the maxillofacial area appears to take place in part by mechanisms distinct from those in the orthopaedic field. In particular, the response to scaffold materials may be different depending on the nature of the surrounding intact bone and soft tissue. As an initial approach to determine the osteogenic potential of tissue-engineered bone constructs in vivo, heterotopic animal models are of special interest. They allow the evaluation of the biological performance of the hybrid material commonly implanted in ectopic sites. Implantation is performed for example in muscle pouches, fascial pouches or subcutaneously. The investigation can be performed in immunocompetent as well as in immunocompromised animals. The next step of preclinical evaluation is the in vivo defect model. Schmitz and Hollinger (1986) were the first to postulate a rationale for testing bone tissue engineering by using critical size defects in a hierarchy of animal models. It is known that the rate of bone repair varies inversely with order along the phylogenetic scale (Enneking and Morris, 1972; Prolo et al., 1982). Moreover, bone regenerative capacities differ significantly among animals of the same species (Harris et al., 1968; Enneking et al., 1975) and among loaded and non-loaded skeletal sites (Figs 10.1 and 10.2). Bone defects regenerate more actively in immature animals of a given species than in older ones. Therefore, from a clinical point of view it is advisable to test cellular hybrid materials for their ability to repair an osseous defect in a mature, adult animal (Harris et al., 1968) (Figs 10.3–10.5). Mature dogs, goats, pigs and

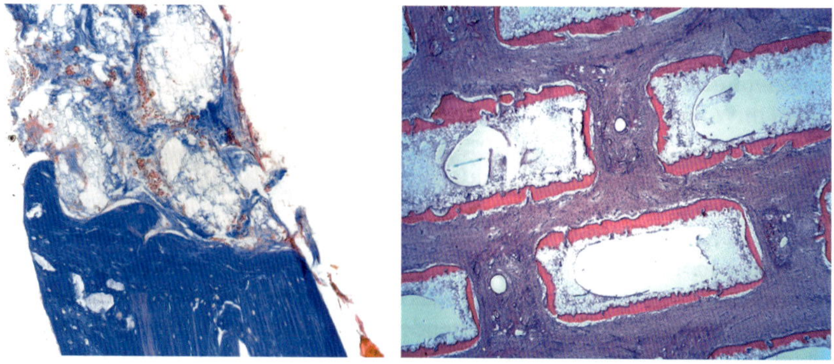

Fig. 10.1. Bone containing tricalcium phosphate-based bone substitutes after 4–6 months in rat calvaria (*left*) and sheep long bone (*right*)

non-human primates have been successfully used to examine the regeneration of mandibular discontinuity defects (Fennis et al., 2002). These animal models allow us to follow the fate of the implanted material in a functional environment which is comparable to the human situation. This is particularly important in preparation for future Food and Drug Administration trials (Slavkin, 2000). Furthermore, transgenic knock-in or knock-out animals may be attractive candidates for studying the functional role of a protein of interest in bone (or certilage) healing.

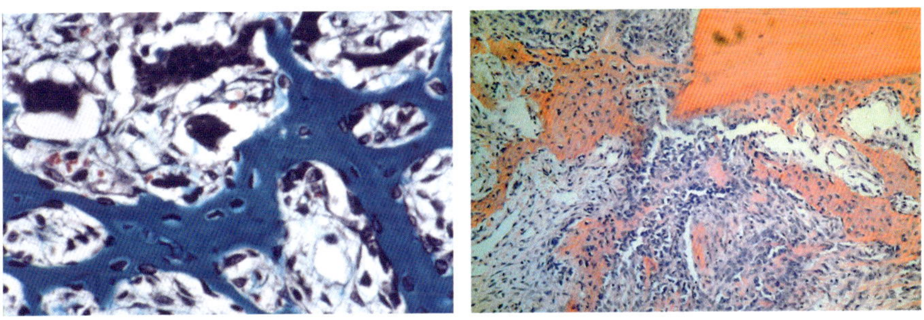

Fig. 10.2. New bone formation after extracorporal shock wave therapy

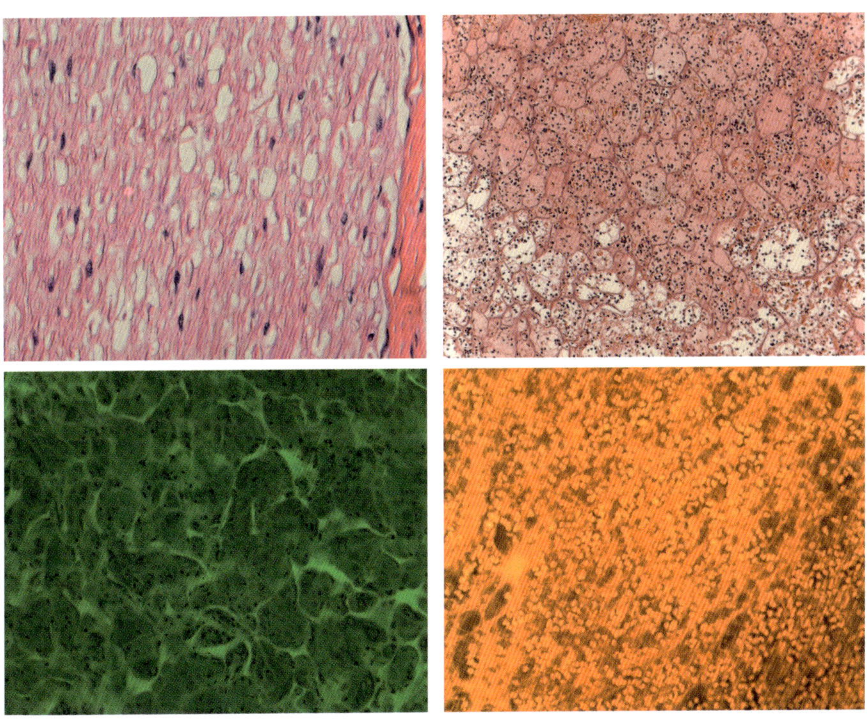

Fig. 10.3. Different matrices of biodegradable implants

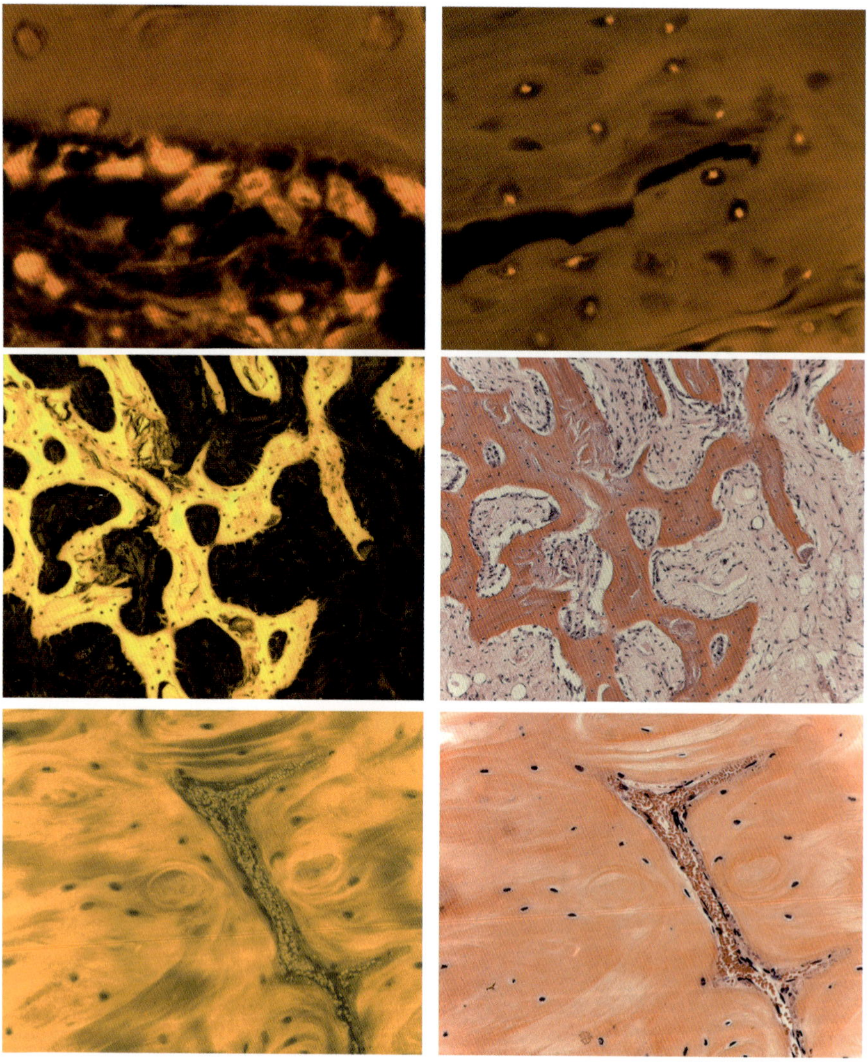

Fig. 10.4. Fluorescence and standard histology of bone healing at the scaffold/bone interface. *Top*: Autologous osteoblasts were fluorescence marked by a fluorescence dye in vitro and settled down on scaffolds. After cell/scaffold transplantation in minipigs, fluorescent cells indicate their ancestry from the ex vivo generated tissue-like construct. The technique enables not only to distinguish between resident and transplanted cells, but also to investigate the survival of cells after transplantation. In vivo, the marked cells are obvious during early bone formation (after 2 weeks) at the mineralization front (*left*) and in the newly formed bone (*right*). Midline: Auto fluorescence of hydroxyapatite (*left*) and alizarin red S staining in standard histology (*right*) can indicate the newly formed bone. Bottom: Newly formed blood vesicles can make out by auto fluorescence of erythrocytes (*left*) and in standard histology (*right*)

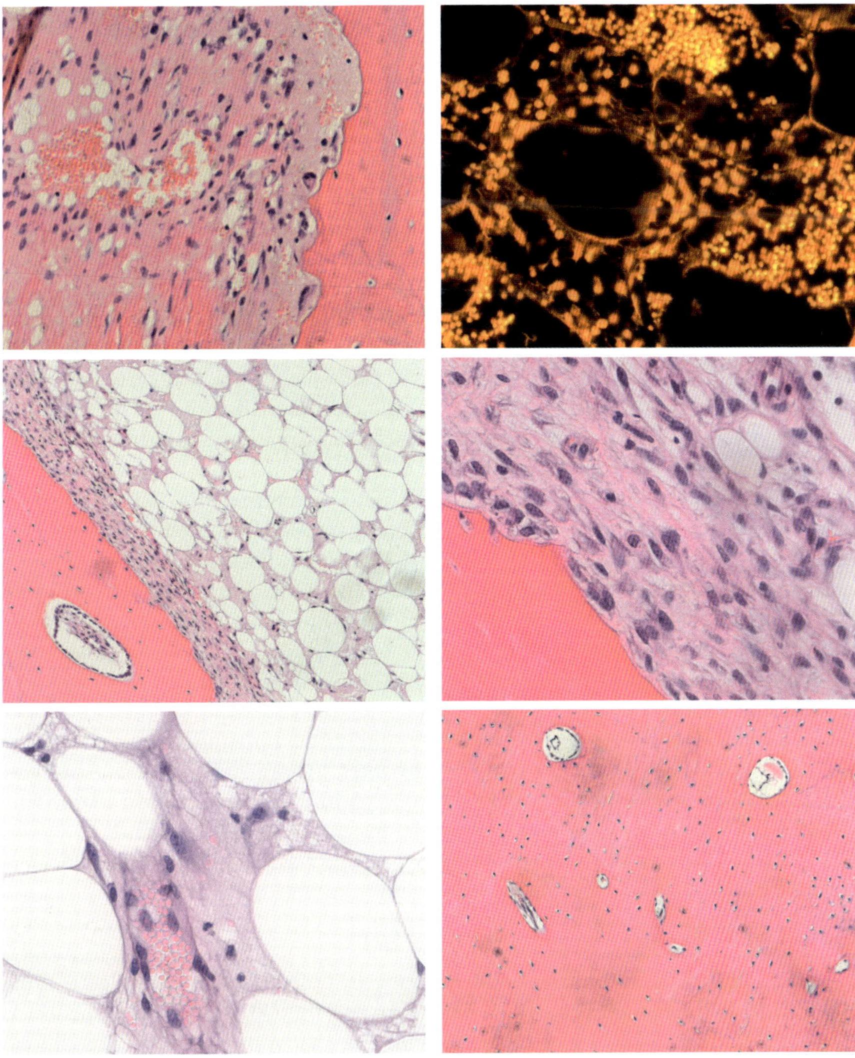

Fig. 10.5. Histological images of bone regeneration after cell/scaffold implantation. The bone repair tissue at early stages of bone regeneration (one week after transplantation) differs between various areas of the defect site (central scaffold area, superficial scaffold area). After 30 days bone regeneration is partly finished (*bottom, right*)

10.2 Animal Models used for Cartilage Tissue Engineering

As for bone tissue engineering, as a first step in determining the chondrogenic potential of tissue-engineered constructs in vivo, investigators have used small animal species in orthotopic sites or heterotopic animal models (Lipman et al., 1983; Nakahara et al., 1990b; Vacanti et al., 1991; Freed et al., 1993; Puelacher et al., 1994; Paige et al., 1996; Madry et al., 2002). Tissue-engineered cartilage constructs have, for example, been implanted in dorsal subcutaneous pouches of immunocompromised nude mice, since Vacanti and colleages were able to grow an ear on the back of a mouse. While heterotopic models may provide the first evidence of the nature of the tissue-engineered cartilage under in vivo conditions, different results may be observed when the construct is implanted into a cartilage defect or tested in immunocompetent animals. Therefore, further in vivo studies using articular cartilage defect models in a hierarchy of animal species should be conducted. However, heterotopic chondrogenesis models may provide some useful information concerning the basic biological phenomena of histogenesis. Due to the physiological and anatomical differences between the clinical situation of patients and those of experimental animals, there is no animal defect model that directly mimics the human situation. Additionally, many other variables are relevant when considering these experiments, such as age, gender, size and depth of the defect, age of the defect (i.e. intra-articular environment), post-operative treatment, etc. (An and Friedman, 1999; Hunziker, 1999; 2002). Whereas animals of a high phylogenetical scale like dogs, goats, pigs and horses more closely resemble the human situation compared to smaller animal models, it is usually not possible to conduct extended experimental series in larger animals. Therefore, the choice of a small-animal model for fundamental investigations (O´Driscoll, 2001) is well accepted. However, the preclinical assessment of an articular cartilage tissue engineering technique requires confirmation in a large animal model (Figs 10.6 and 10.7). The potential for cartilage repair depends to a great extent on the age of the animal. As is true for bone regeneration, cartilage defects can be repaired more successfully in immature animals than in skeletally mature animals. The capacity of articular cartilage repair potential is dependent on the state of the tissue (cartilage extracellular matrix, cell content), the inflammation at the defect site, and cartilage biomechanics (Stockwell, 1965; Stockwell and Scott, 1965; Meachim, 1969; Bonner et al., 1975; Roughley, 2001a; 2001b). In this respect it is of special concern in cartilage tissue engineering that most basic and preclinical results published originate from an optimally controlled laboratory environment or animal experimental work with healthy joint tissue where a surgically induced cartilage defect was treated using tissue engineering (Figs 10.7 and 10.8). In the clinical situation, the majority of patients have a chronic defect situation with a diseased peri-defect tissue before they are treated for their joint damage. This altered tissue environment is concomitant with an altered joint physiology. The impaired regenerative capacity of inflamed joint tissue, especially in cases of osteoarthritis, often associated with a disturbed biomechanical situation at the defect site, could provide an explanation for the confounding data concerning basic scientific results and the variable clinical results reported in the current literature (for a review see Salter, 1994). As mechanical factors influence chondrogenesis and articular cartilage healing in the in vivo situation, it is important to consider the post-operative treatment used after defect repair in designing experiments using animal defect models. Since

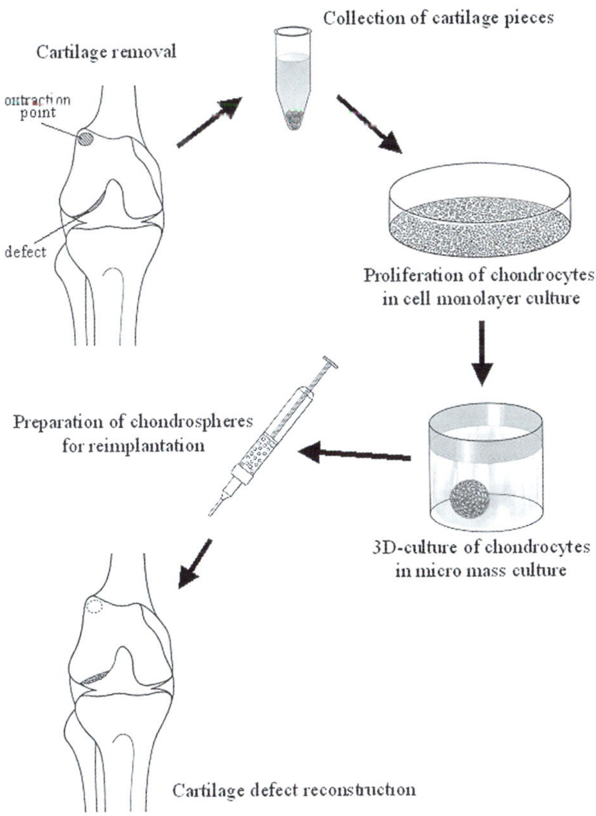

Fig. 10.6. Principle of cartilage tissue engineering

the use of continuous passive motion has been experimentally demonstrated to enhance the healing of articular cartilage in rabbits (Salter et al., 1980; O´Driscoll et al., 1983a; 1983b; O´Driscoll, 1984; O´Driscoll and Salter, 1984; 1986; Salter et al., 1984; Dhert et al., 1988; O´Driscoll et al., 1988; Salter, 1989; Kim et al., 1991; Moran et al., 1992) and in contrast, joint immobilisation has shown to decrease articular cartilage thickness, adjustment of the mechanical loading during the post-operation phase is a matter of relevance.

10.3 Clinical Applications

Tissue engineering demands that clinicians participate actively in the design, development, clinical introduction and informed use of this treatment option. The active participation requires that clinicians have a solid understanding of the biological and material-based principles of ex vivo tissue generation. To assess the efficacy and safety of tissue engineering, clinical studies must include a number of defined outcome measures. In contrast to animal studies in which the sacrificed animals are subjected to a variety of different investigations ranging from macroscopic to molecular level, clinical studies in humans use restricted outcome parameters (Figs 10.9 to 10.13).

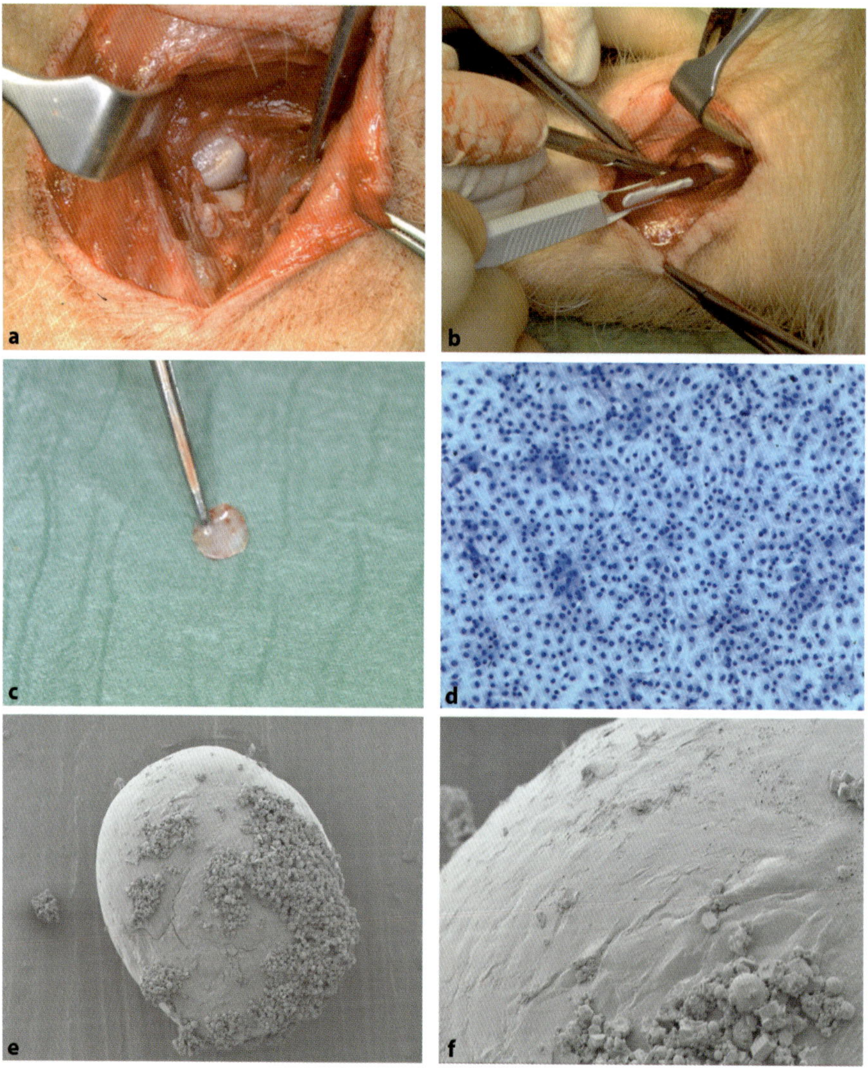

Fig. 10.7. Animal experiment using micromass culture for cartilage reconstruction in the knee; part I. **a** Exposure of joint prior to tissue harvesting. **b** Surgical removal of cartilage. **c** Explanted cartilage piece. **d** Cell growth in monolayer. **e** Gross and **f** detailed appearance of chondrospeheres, generated by micromass culture (**e**, **f** SEM micrographs)

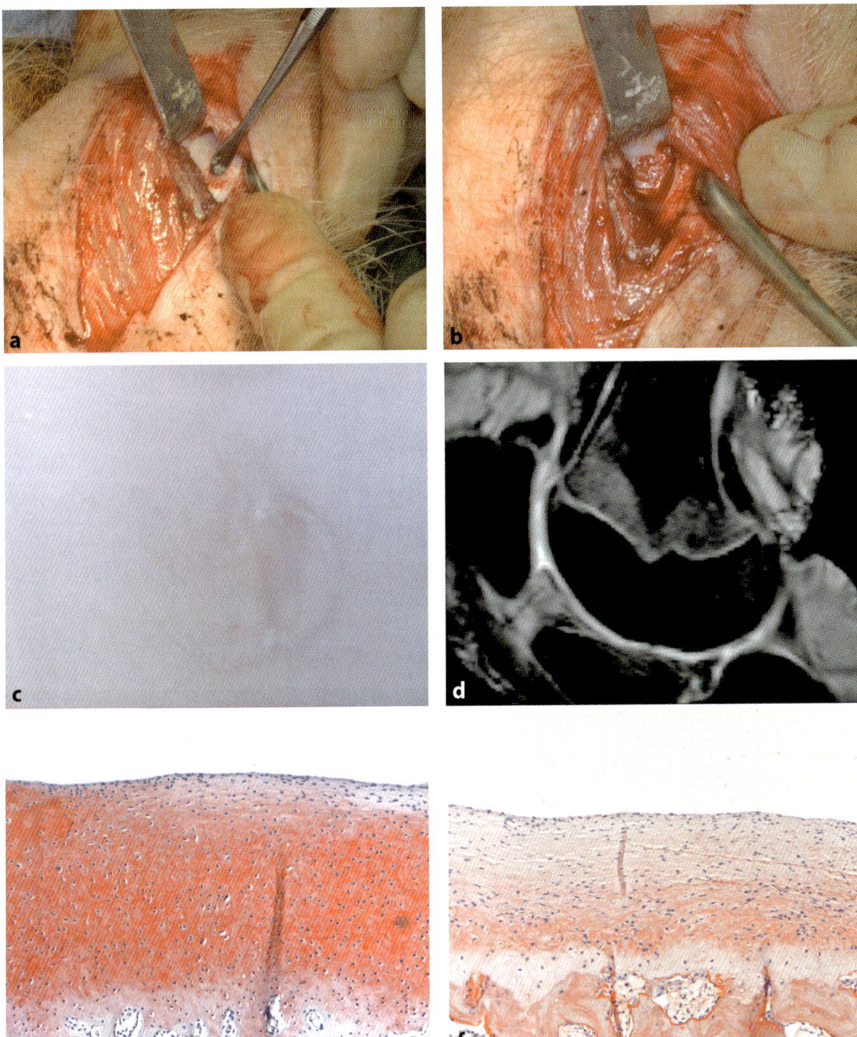

Fig. 10.8. Animal experiment using micromass culture for cartilage reconstruction in the knee; part II. **a** Overview. **b** Detail of the clinical replantation procedure. 20–25 chondrospheres are attached to the defect site. **c** Clinical and **d** NMR picture of the regenerate site. **e** Immunhistology revealed an enhanced expression of type II collagen, with **f** minor amounts of type I collagen, indicative of hyaline cartilage regeneration

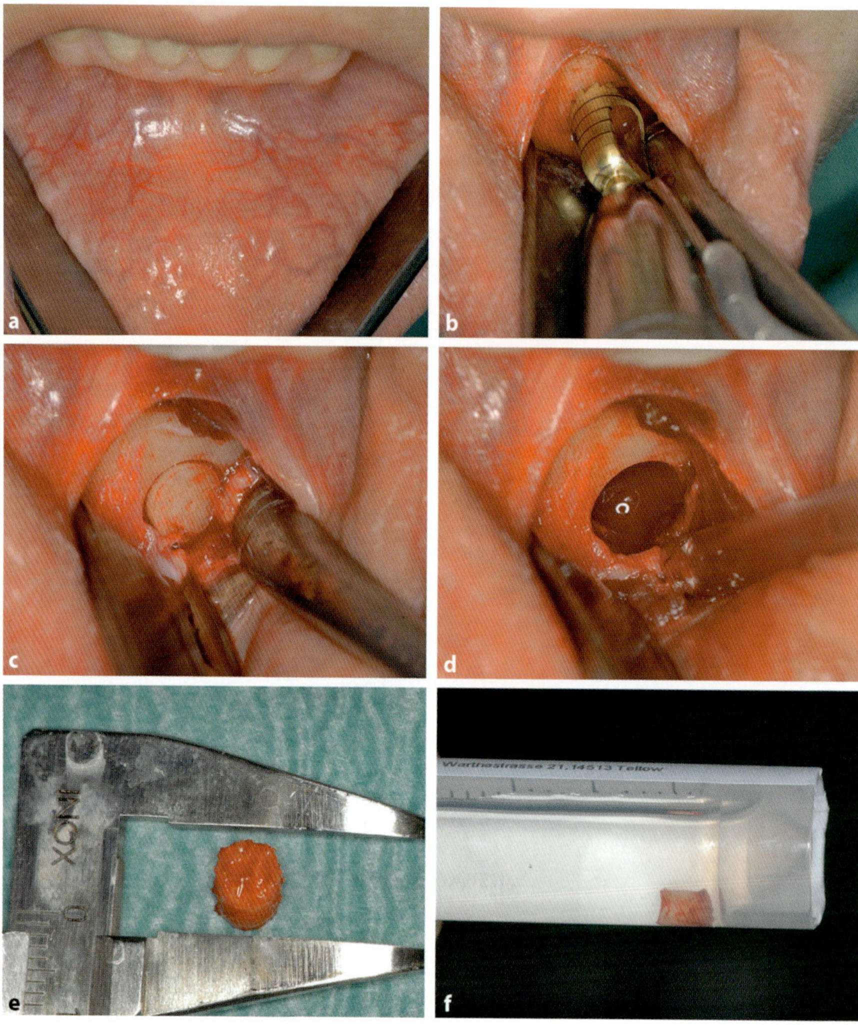

Fig. 10.9. Clinical bone tissue engineering procedure for bone reconstruction; part I. **a** View of the mucosa. **b**, **c**, **d** Different steps of bone harvesting by a trephane burr. **e** Size of the explanted bone piece. **f** Bone piece located in transport medium

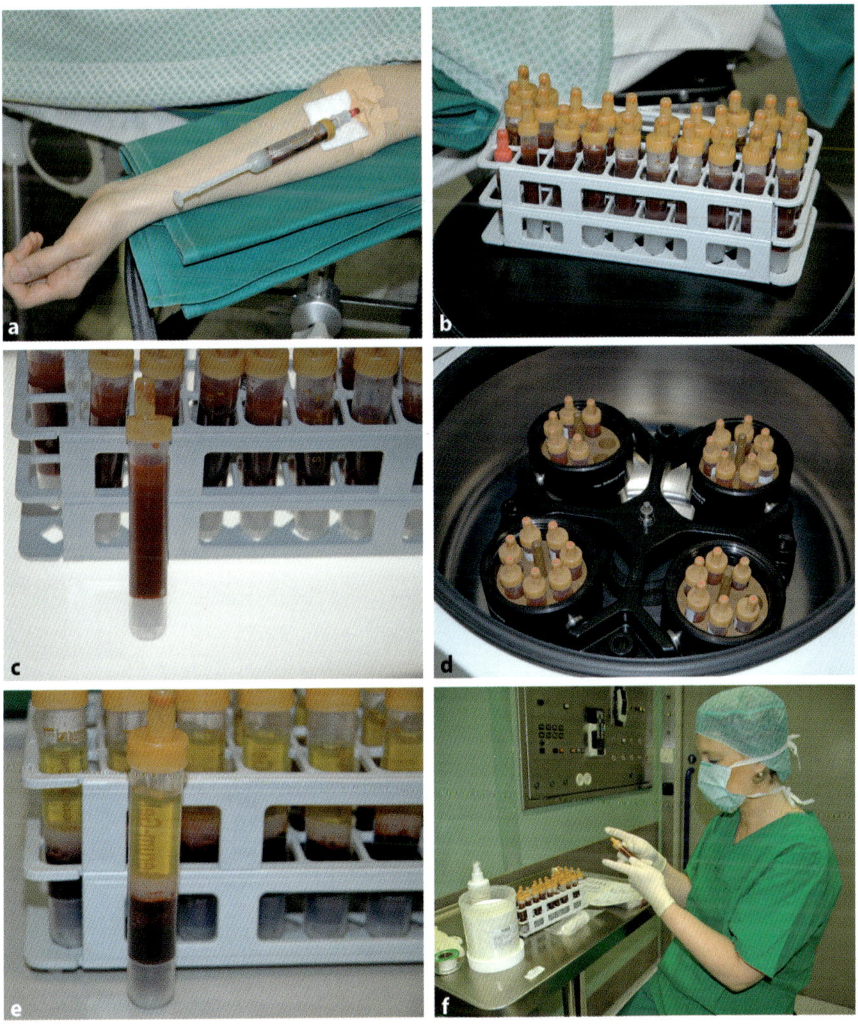

Fig. 10.10. Clinical bone tissue engineering procedure for bone reconstruction; part II. Different steps of autologous serum sample preparation

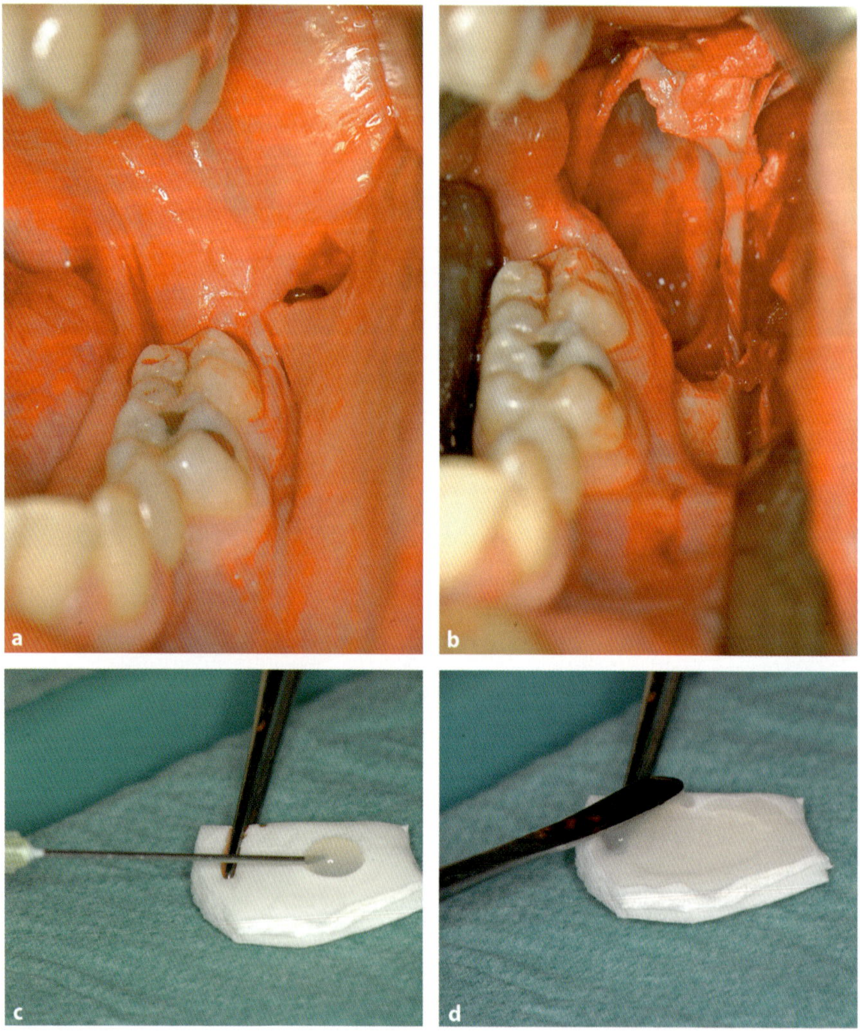

Fig. 10.11. Clinical bone tissue engineering procedure for bone reconstruction; part III. **a** Intraoral incision of the vestibular mucosa. **b** Critical size defect at the mandibular angle. **c** Attachment of the bone cell suspension to a collagen scaffold. **d** Coating the complete scaffold surface with cells

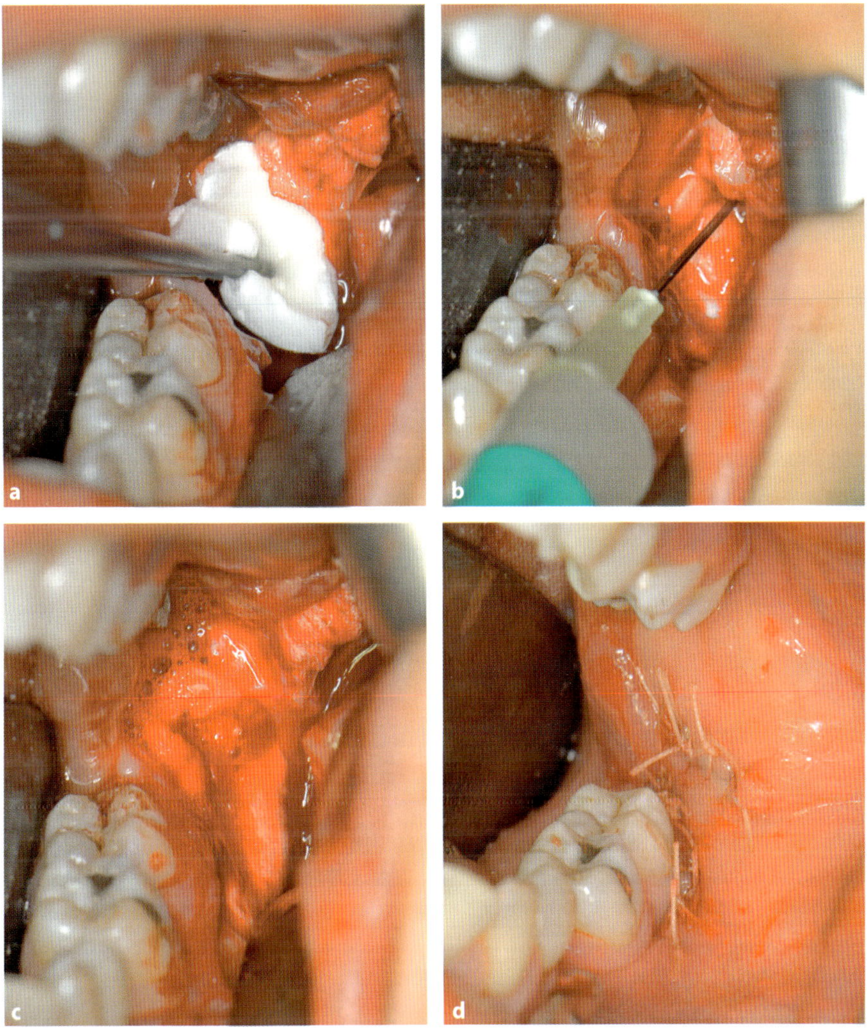

Fig. 10.12. Clinical bone tissue engineering procedure for bone reconstruction; part IV. **a** Defect filling by the cell/scaffold complex. **b** Injection of cells between defect border and scaffold. Clinical view after (**c**) defect filling and (**d**) wound closure

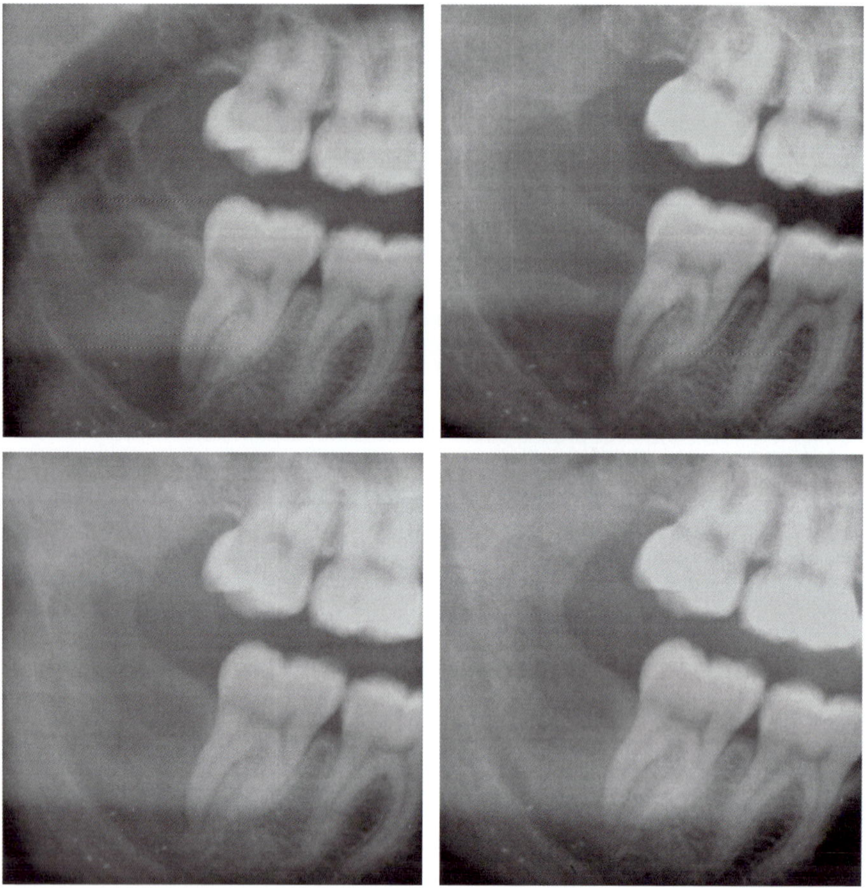

Fig. 10.13. Radiological control of bone regeneration. Time-dependent regeneration of bone. Pictures demonstrate successive mineralisation of a critical size defect from day of implatation to 3 months after

Animal studies should therefore include in addition to outcome measures similar to those that are anticipated in clinical studies also histological and biomechanical evaluations (Tables 10.3 and 10.4). When incorporating a cellular bone substitute in reconstructive surgery, radiographs and computed tomography should be routinely performed in order to link high resolution data with clinical findings. The repair response to a cellular bone construct varies substantially according to the mechanical stability of the defect site. In vivo remodelling either reinforces, maintains, or degrades the tissue formed during implant healing. Both the initial and long-term biological responses to tissue-engineered constructs are strongly influenced by mechanical interactions at the implant interface. The load transduction at the interface critically determines the fate of the implanted tissue substitute (Meyer et al., 1999b). In a changing strain environment these mechanical factors represent a key challenge in the surgical treatment of bone and cartilage defects.

Table 10.3. Biomechanical evaluation methods

Method
– Young`s modulus – Compressive strength – Bending strength – Shear stress – Hardness – Deformation – Dislocation

Table 10.4. Evaluation of in vivo models

Clinically
– Form – Function
Radiographically
– X-rays – Ultrasound – Computed tomography – Magnetic resonance tomography – Positron emission tomography – Szintigraphy
Structurally
– Histology – Immunohistochemistry – Ultrastructure
Mechanically
– E-modulus – Compression resistance

The integration of the extracorporally generated hybrid material into the surrounding tissue depends clinically, mainly on sufficient fixation of the transplanted construct, and biologically, mainly on the subsequent remodelling phase. Rigid fixation of bone constructs can be performed by plating, suturing or by a fit-in-fit system, covering the cell-containing hybrid material with membranes or soft tissues (e.g. periosteal flaps). In contrast, extracorporally grown cartilage tissue is mainly fixed by soft tissue flaps or artificial membranes. Loosening or loss of the transplanted construct should be considered as a currently unsolved aspect of tissue engineering. Additionally, whereas bone has a higher capacity for regeneration than cartilage tissue, both tissues retain their inherent biochemical property of forming new tissue in the presence of externally applied forces and strains. Implant integration into the host site depends on the strain and stress environment acting on the scaffold construct as well as on the surrounding implantation bed. Hyperphysiological loading may result in the destruction of scaffold integrity and also may induce cellular dedifferentiation, ultimately leading to fibrous tissue formation (Meyer et al., 2004b). Repeated disruption of vascular invasion at the construct interface resulting in impaired tissue formation is a clinically relevant problem mainly observed in bone tissue engineering. In the complete absence of adequate mechanical stimuli, however, implant integration may fail due to impaired bone or cartilage stimulation. Thus, mechanical factors can elicit both positive and negative effects on the biological response to implanted cell/scaffold constructs.

Guldberg (2002) was the first to study in vivo the influence of the mechanical environment on the formation and retention of bone within tissue-engineered constructs implanted into hydraulic bone chambers. He tested the hypothesis that tissue-engineered constructs under dynamic loading would promote bone repair in vivo. And indeed, it was found that, relative to the baseline bone formation, mechanical loading significantly increased the amount of mineralised matrix components. In contrast, the amount of mineralised matrix synthesised in the non-load control chambers was decreased. For load-bearing maxillofacial or orthopaedic defects, the implanted construct must provide adequate mechanical stability at the defect site, even under normal load when compressive strains have to be transferred to the newly formed tissue (Davy, 1999; Kon et al., 2000). Constructs possessing insufficient mechanical stability and fatigue resistance are at risk of plastic deformation or brittle fracture under functional loads, ultimately resulting in the collapse of the scaffold template. Only a very few in vivo applications in skeletal tissue engineering are non-load bearing. Calvarial critical sized defects for bone repair and non-load bearing sinus lift procedures for bone augmentation are two examples (Shang et al., 2001; Bidic et al., 2003). Although the impact of the local mechanical environment on bone remodelling has been appreciated (Meyer et al., 1999a), in the context of tissue-engineered constructs mechanical factors have not been systematically studied (Perka et al., 2000). Based on various clinical and experimental investigations it has been postulated that mechanical effects may overrule material-specific effects when biomaterials are tested in vivo (Handschel et al., 2002). Thus, mechanical effects should be anticipated when substitution with extracorporal bone or cartilage tissue is planned (Guldberg, 2002). An understanding of how mechanical signals affect the integration of the tissue construct may provide clinically relevant microstructural information for improved three-dimensional scaffold architecture. Models that take these three-dimensional, load-bearing functional requirements of skeletal tissues into account may be more predictive for human clinical trails.

10.4 Immunological Aspects

Despite the remarkable progress towards the generation of tissue-engineered bone or cartilage substitutes for therapeutical use, immunological problems associated with the recipient's response to the bioengineered tissue will have to be overcome. Although little has been published on the immune reaction toward bioengineered bone or cartilage tissue, it is known that the cell/scaffold complex will most likely induce a host reaction (Harlan et al., 2002). Both inflammatory and immune reactions can be anticipated, even with autologous tissue (Table 10.5). Clinical trials with allografts and xenografts have demonstrated that innate and adaptive immu-

Table 10.5. Inflammatory/immune responses

Aspect	Components
– Non-specific (innate)	– Cellular (granulocytes, macrophages, lymphocytes) – Non-cellular (complement system, lysozyme)
– Specific (acquired) – Naturally acquired – Artificially acquired	– Humoral (B-cells, immunoglobulins) – Cell-mediated (T-cells)

nity are serious barriers. Inflammation likewise influences cell/scaffold engraftment, and may also be pivotal for proper tissue remodelling. Therefore, it should not be assumed that an extracorporally bioengineered tissue will be inert. Rather, the host immune system will have a profound impact on the implanted bioengineered construct, and vice versa.

The two main components of an extracorporal tissue-engineered hybrid construct are the transplanted cells and the scaffold material. The implantation of a bone-like or cartilage-like polymer/cell construct combines concepts of both biomaterials and cell transplantation. Immune rejection is a common host response towards the cellular component of tissue-engineered devices containing allogeneic, xenogeneic or ex vivo manipulated immunogenic cells (Mikos et al., 1998).

The implantation of preformed scaffold materials without cells can initiate a sequence of events related to a foreign body reaction. Clinically, it may present as an acute inflammatory response and in other situations as a chronic inflammatory rejection (Anderson, 1993). The duration and intensity of the clinical response is dependent on patient-associated parameters (extent of tissue injury, age, immunological status) and scaffold parameters (chemical composition, porosity, roughness, implant size and shape) (Anderson, 1988). It has been shown that the intensity of the response is modulated by the biodegradation process itself (Lam et al., 1993; Nakaoka et al., 1996), determining to a great extent the clinical fate of the hybrid material (den Dunnen et al., 1997; Winet and Bao, 1997; Peter et al., 1998b). The immune response to common scaffold materials implanted into a defect region may result in a fibrous capsule containing macrophages and foreign body giant cells with needle-like, crystalline particles (Rozema et al., 1994). Some in vivo studies have suggested that particles released from a degrading implant may affect tissue regeneration or repair by direct interaction with cells (Lam et al., 1995; Winet and Bao, 1997). Indirect interactions through inflammatory cytokines released by macrophages upon particle phagocytosis will have to be examined in more detail.

Immunologic reactions against the transplanted cells and the host´s response towards the hybrid material are critical after transplantation of the extracorporally fabricated construct (Mikos et al., 1998). Implant rejection can be avoided or at least diminished in clinical practice by using autologous or isogeneic cells as the principal cell source. Obviously, cells derived from an autologous source can be rendered immunogenic if they are genetically modified (Verna and Somia, 1997) or extensively cultured in vitro (Sato, 1997) prior to their transplantation. If allogeneic or xenogeneic cells are incorporated into the device, the prevention of immune rejection by immune suppressive treatment, the induction of tolerance in the host

Table 10.6. Factors contributing to immunity

Non-specific	Specific
- Mechanical barriers (ext. surface) - Chemical barriers (pH) - Physiological factors (temperature) - Phagocytosis - Complement - Beta lysin	- T-cells - B-cells - Immunoglobulins - Interferons - Cytoriner - Chemotactic factors

or immuno-modulation of the graft become important clinical issues (Meiser and Reichart, 1994).

Immune rejection is the most important host response to the cellular component of tissue-engineered constructs containing non-autologous cells (Table 10.6). Xenografts were rejected hyperacutely by preformed natural antibodies and complement activation (Platt, 1992) or more slowly by cellular immunity (Dorling et al., 1996), when preventive measures were not taken. It should be emphasised that the immune response to a cellular bone or cartilage construct is critical for clinical success. Thus, the immunogenic nature of the biomaterial and the cellular components must be considered in the selection of both the scaffold material and the cell source. Future animal studies or clinical trials should evaluate thoroughly the immunological host response in order to improve clinical outcomes.

The use of allogeneic or xenogeneic cells has the clinical advantage of avoiding cell harvesting from the patient. Additionally, a time delay between the initial cell explantation and the final implantation does not occur when allogeneic or xenogeneic cells are employed. Methods for the use of these cells in extracorporal tissue engineering have been developed. Microencapsulation is a clinically applied method to prevent immune reaction against allogeneic or xenogeneic cells (Sefton et al., 2000). It places cells within a core such that the cells are sequestered by a material from direct contact with host cells and huge macromolecules. The wall thus formed, typically consisting of a polymer, is thought to provide immunoisolation by preventing contact between the encapsulated cells and the host immune system to allow for the transplantation of allogeneic or xenogeneic cells without extensive immunosuppressive therapy. Cartilage repair by xenogeneic chondrocytes placed in a polymer core is a recently established method in joint reconstruction. Similar approaches may also be successful in cellular bone tissue engineering despite the different cellular requirements between osteoblasts and chondrocytes.

Clinical Handling and Control 11

In order to provide safe cell/scaffold products of reliable quality, the principles of good manufacturing practice (GMP) must be followed in the selection of donors, retrieval of cells, testing of cells (e.g. after subculture), processing of cell/scaffold constructs, storage and delivery of finished tissues (for a review, see Hellman, 1997). To date, regulations governing these matters have been set up by individual countries. In Germany, for example, manufacturing is regulated by the German drug law and by the German operation ordinance for pharmaceutical entrepreneurs, if autologous cells are used.

Additionally, some institutions have set regulatory frameworks to guide the use of cell-containing products, initially implemented for tissue bank products. Codes of Practice (COP) for tissue banks specify the requirements for the activities of tissue banks that store and/or process human tissues for therapeutic use. The scope of these codes includes, in most instances, all human tissues used for therapeutic purposes including those tested in clinical trials. Musculoskeletal tissues (e.g. bone, cartilage, osteochondral tissues) or haemopoietic progenitor cells (e.g. bone marrow, peripheral blood, cord/placental blood) are typical examples of related items. Professional institutions and specialist societies have, in many instances, prepared standards and guidelines for specific procedures in order to introduce a framework for developing and supporting pre-existing standards and guidelines. An area where there is currently no specific guidance is that of tissue engineering, but where therapeutic products (including cells of human origin as is the case for tissue engineering applications) are processed by commercial or non-commercial organisations, this code applies. In addition the following principles apply.

- If autologous cells are cultured in vitro prior to implantation, the procedures must be validated or monitored, e.g. to ensure vitality of cells and sterility as well as identification of samples. In addition, lack of malignant transformation, and maintenance of relevant biological properties are desired properties of autologous cells that should ideally be documented by proper test systems.
- If allogeneic cells are used in tissue engineering applications (a strategy that has not yet been introduced into clinical bone or cartilage procedures), donors should be thoroughly evaluated to reduce the risk of transmitting diseases and immune rejections. Allogenic stem cells are commonly regulated by laws and regulations set up for tissue banks.

The intention to establish a code is based on Quality Management Systems (in Germany for example ISO 9000 series: ISO 9001–2000) This system refers to cell-based therapeuticals. The principles of good manufacturing practice concerning tissue banks differ in detail between countries (for example in Rules and Guidance for

Pharmaceutical Manufacturers and Distributors, Department of Health, 1997). The complexity of the ex vivo generation of artificial tissues and organs emphasises the need for compliance with an integrated quality assurance programme. As is the case for tissue banks, commercial or non-commercial organisations working in the cell-based tissue engineering field must adhere to the principles set out in other documents (e.g. Guidance on the Microbiological Safety of Human Organs, Tissues and Cells used in Transplantation; Department of Health, 2000). All stages of the selection and testing of donors, retrieval (harvesting) of cells or tissues, culturing, coating with materials, processing, storage and delivery of cell/scaffold constructs should meet the specified criteria. It is important to note that all institutions working in this field have a general duty and responsibility to comply with other statutory legislation of the countries that are involved in the performance and processing of tissue engineered products. Physicians and involved personnel must ensure that proper consent has been obtained for the retrieval of cells or tissue, as addressed by the UK Human Tissue Act 1961, the Human Fertilisation and Embryology Act 1990, the Human Fertilisation and Embryology (disclosure of information) Act 1992 and other professional guidelines.

The processes that are relevant for the clinical use of extracorporal fabricated bone and cartilage tissue constructs should be monitored by a quality system. Today, autologous cells are the sole cell source used in clinical bone and cartilage tissue engineering strategies. Quality management should include all aspects of tissue engineering: formal issues of tissue banks, managerial responsibilities, donor selection and testing, written agreements or contracts with third parties, specified testing of tissues, standards for the processing and storage of tissue, documentation and record keeping and transport of tissues. Formal issues of cell-based tissue engineering facilities include: buildings and premises, environmental controls, processing areas, personnel, ancillary materials, contamination from tissues of donors and equipment. A variety of donor criteria should be documented if allogenic or autologous cells are used, for example medical and behavioural history, pathology, microbiological testing, exclusion factors and consent. The above mentioned parameters are also relevant for donors donating tissue for autologous and/or directed allogeneic use. Ideally, the following parameters should be included in the whole process of clinical bone and cartilage tissue engineering, with respect to transplantation of an ex vivo grown cell/scaffold complex:

Manufacture

- Product consistency
- Product stability (functional, genetic)

Preclinical Safety

- Material sourcing
- Adventitious agents (testing process validation)
- Toxicity testing
- Sterility
- Sterilisation byproducts

Preclinical Activity

- Material characterisation (structural/functional)
- Biomaterial compatibility testing
- In vitro animal models (efficacy measures)

Clinical

- Indications
- Efficacy endpoints
- Safety monitoring
- Population exposure
- Post-market reporting

It is important to note that it is difficult to meet all of these criteria, since many of them are either ill or not defined in sufficient detail. Future developments will stress the need to monitor and eventually to refine such quality systems.

11.1 Regulatory Issues

Bone and cartilage tissue-engineered products act primarily in a functional way, thus resembling medical devices. As they act as pharmaceuticals (e.g. bone with its metabolic functions) they are regulated in some countries by drug-related laws (e.g. Germany: German Drug Law). As tissue-engineered products are a relatively new entity, existing regulatory frameworks are being reviewed and modified to ensure that these new procedures are covered.

Knowledge of the legal situation is important for all scientists and physicians working in all aspects of this new life science discipline. Currently, there is no common or specific regulation for human tissue-engineered products. The responsibilities as well as the regulations differ between countries. The regulatory framework in the USA and the European Community differs in various aspects, and this framework differs also between the various EU members. The Scientific Committee on Medicinal Products and Medical Devices (SCMPMD) of the European Commission stated that none of the existing European regulatory frameworks in their current form encompass tissue-engineered products appropriately (European Commission, 2001, http://europa.eu.int/). The special characteristics and the inherent risks concerning the cellular hybrid materials involved, the new kind of production process and the mode of action are only partially covered by existing regulations. Therefore, initiatives for a complementary regulatory framework have been commenced in the EU. The European Commission released in June 2002 (European Commission, 2002) a proposal for a directive on tissue banking, aimed at assuring quality and safety of human tissues and cells for medical purposes. The Directive is currently being discussed by the responsible institutions in order to implement common standards concerning the marketing of human tissue-engineered products, to safeguard consumers and to protect users (http://lifesciences.jrc.es). The Directive itself is supposed to cover only the donation, procurement, and testing of tissue in the context of tissue engineering, whereas processing, preservation, storage, and distribution are covered by other Community legislation. The current regulatory frameworks in some countries and the imposed problems of legal assessment of this new biotechnology can be gleaned from relevant society recommendations.

Ethical Considerations in Bone and Cartilage Tissue Engineering

12

T. Meyer

The rapid development of tissue engineering and in particular the introduction of gene therapy have elicited much interest among scientists, physicians, and the public in general. The implantation of artificially constructed bone-like tissue for research and therapeutical purposes raises major ethical and legal concerns, which must be considered by the medical profession as well as society. The recent acceleration of knowledge about tissue engineering, which stands currently at the threshold for routine clinical application, assures that the ethical problems presented will be significant and important (Longley and Lowford, 2001; Jenkins et al., 2003). However, it should be noted that from the standpoint of bioethics, scientific research on tissue engineering raises no completely novel ethical questions that have not been debated previously in the context of related advancements. This chapter deals with the stratification of risks and benefits in the development of artificial bone and cartilage tissue and focuses on appropriate and ethically acceptable ways of utilising the recent advances of stem cell derived therapies. Arguments are provided in support of the concept that bone and cartilage tissue engineering can be beneficial only when these ethical and moral issues are adequately addressed prior to its future clinical application. It is argued here that all research projects aimed at improving the outcome of bone and cartilage tissue engineering should be guided by ethical principles that respect and consider the patient´s interest and honour the moral, cultural, and religious values of society.

At the centre of all medical treatments, not limited to new or experimental therapies, stands the doctrine of informed consent, which is defined as the fundamental process of communication between a patient and physician that results in the patient´s authorisation or agreement to undergo a specific medical intervention (Churchill et al., 1998). Like all surgical procedures, this process begins long before the patient undergoes a surgical operation such as, for example, the implantation of extracorporally engineered bone and cartilage tissue. Moreover, the responsible physician has to assure the patient´s informed consent in all stages of the therapy starting from surgical planning to post-operative treatment. Informed consent in this respect means the interactive process by which a fully informed patient has the choice between newly developed techniques of tissue engineering and conventional methods of reconstructive bone surgery such as, for example, osteosynthesis of fractures. The treating physician has to comment on all relevant risks, benefits,

Author address: Thomas Meyer, Prof. Dr. Dr. Dr.
Forschungsinsitut für Molekulare Pharmakologie, Campus Berlin-Buch
Robert-Rössle-Str. 10, 13125 Berlin

and uncertainties related to each treatment strategy and must ensure that the patient is thereafter competent to decide which individual therapy should be favoured. To become a fully and emancipated participant, the patient must know about reasonable alternatives to the proposed treatment, since he holds the last decision on the nature of the intervention. Given that all possible and practicable alternatives are extensively discussed, the physician is not generally prohibited from providing a recommendation, but should share his/her reasoning process with the patient. Informed consent in this respect is regarded as an invitation to the patient to participate in his/her health care decisions. Provided that all relevant information are given and that comprehension is achieved, the patient has been offered the opportunity to either accept, refuse or modify the proposed intervention according to his/her own planning. This implies that the patient makes all therapeutical decisions on a rational and voluntary basis with the aid of professional medical advice. Given that the intervention is properly executed without negligence according to the prevailing standard of surgical care, the procedure of informed consent guarantees that the doctor is protected from financial liability.

Bone and cartilage tissue engineering holds great promise to ameliorate the regeneration of skeletal defects and has the potential to compensate for the loss of bone structures in cases when bone reconstruction is required to prevent a non-union defect. Currently, several groups worldwide are searching for the appropriate carriers and the right set of cells that, once retransplanted into the site of bone lesions, will ensure bony reunion (Lucarelli et al., 2004). Although a huge amount of knowledge has been gained so far, we are only at the beginning of our understanding, and the direction the field will take in the near future is not fully known. Nevertheless, it is inevitable that numerous ethical problems will have to be solved on the way. Generally, these ethical issues fall into three different categories: (1) conflicts arising from the allocation of donor cells and the general access to this surgical treatment; (2) problems concerning the use of stem cell technology, including foetal stem cells for ex vivo engineered bone and cartilage tissue; and (3) boundaries set by the genetic manipulation of transplanted cells.

In the first set of ethical issues we concentrate on bone cell allocation for use in reconstructive medicine and on general obligations associated with bone surgery. Two distinct treatment strategies are possible when attempting to engineer bone tissue substitutes for use in surgery. One approach involves the removal of osteoblasts from unaffected bones and their reimplantation in the patient´s body after they had been successfully seeded on bone-mimicking scaffolds (Lucarelli et al., 2004). The other approach is based on the allocation of bone-derived cells explanted from a donor and the reimplantation into a recipient after three-dimensional cultivation on devices (Strom et al., 2002). While the use of autologous cells is facilitated by less stringent ethical concerns, the transplantation of bone cells from a donor to a genetically different recipient gives rise to more serious ethical considerations (Lucarelli et al., 2004). In the former case there is no need for an immunosuppressive treatment, but the use of heterologous somatic or stem cells implies the long-term maintenance of an immunosuppressive state. The latter approach with heterologous cells carries the risk of graft rejection and graft failure depending on the histocompatibility match between the graft and the recipient. Grafting of engineered tissues derived from a genetically different donor requires the daily application of immunosuppressive drugs, which may compromise the patient´s resistance to infectious agents or result in otherwise serious side effects (Strom et al., 2002). These adverse reactions must be taken into account when deliberating on the use of grafting heterologous cells or tissues. Since reliance upon daily immunosuppressive medication is unacceptable for many clinical applications, it is important to develop new methods for the induction of immune tolerance. Moreover, the surgical explantation of bone cells from a living donor may cause harm by itself and is therefore only justified in severe cases where the surgical risk for the donor is acceptably low and when all other opportunities for bone reconstruction are either impracticable or have been exhausted. In addition to the usual iatrogenic risks attached to surgical procedures in general, such as local or systemic infections and damage to healthy tissues, certain potential health risks are specifically associated with the new approaches in regenerative medicine. Immune reactions against components of the device or against surface structures of the implanted allogeneic cell layer may cause graft rejection and finally result in an adverse outcome even under immunosuppressive treatment. Toxic effects or induction of auto-immune diseases may be other potentially harmful risks, which should be considered when cellular therapies using allogeneic cells are taken into account. Animal experimentation as an integrated part of tissue engineering helps to assess these risks (Nordgren, 2004).

The paucity of donor cells is another serious problem limiting the widespread application of such cell-based replacement therapies. This sourcing problem demands fair and transparent criteria for cell distribution and standardised procedures that assure equitable access to transplantation resources (Carter, 1999). It is advisable to fully exclude economic aspects of donor cell acquisition in order to prevent commercialism in handling and distribution of donor cells. However, there is some hope that the ability to establish stem cell lines in vitro will allow the production of large batches of terminally differentiated allogenic cells, which can be administered to patients for therapeutic grafting. When there is no need for a direct transplantation of freshly isolated cell preparations, the clinical utility of such cell lines is believed to ameliorate allocation problems and facilitate quality controls for minimalising the risk of disease transmission. Nevertheless, extensive controls of the cell-seeded devices are absolutely necessary to check that the applied donor cells are pathogen-free and unable to induce malignancies due to genetic transformation.

In this respect elaborated protocols for the handling, procurement, and delivery of cell-reconstituted devices would be helpful in order to avoid adverse side effects (Longley and Lawford, 2001). These protocols should follow strictly the guidelines for good manufacturing practice. It is important that for all stages of cellular replacement therapy, detailed protocols are established. Implementing guidelines for cell-derived replacement therapy will allow clinicians to pursue therapeutical advances in tissue engineering while maintaining the highest ethical and medical standards (Winter and Roger, 1995; Longley and Lawford, 2001). Provided all requirements for these new therapies fulfil the principles of good clinical practice and standardised quality control programmes exist, cell-based therapies may become acceptable and potentially important applications that in certain cases may be beneficial over conventional surgery. Furthermore, intervention-associated morbidity and mortality should be carefully documented, preferentially in central registries. Multicentre studies that are accompanied by a long-term scientific evaluation allow one to access the benefit of new therapies in a more reasonable timescale and are thus preferred over studies carried out at only one centre.

It is generally believed that human primary fetal bone cells could be of great interest for bone research, due to their fast growth rate and their ability to differentiate into mature osteoblasts (Cogle et al., 2003; Gilbert, 2004). A barrier, which hampers the progress in cell-derived replacement treatment, lies in the opposition to the use of embryonic stem cells because of moral and religious concerns over osteoblasts (Cogle et al., 2003; Gilbert, 2004). Objections are mainly raised because experimentation with embryonic stem cells derived from human blastocysts requires the destruction of human embryos. The current debate on the ethical status of the human embryo is focused on the fragility and defenceless of the human embryo, and the question as to what respect a human embryo should deserve in light of recent medical progress. It is generally accepted that the blastocyst contains a complete set of genetic instructions and the capacity for the epigenetic determinations needed to develop into a human being. However, there is a dispute on the ethical and legal implications of using human primordial stem cells for tissue engineering, which includes controversy over whether the absolute respect for individual human life begins already at conception osteoblasts (Cogle et al., 2003; Gilbert, 2004).

As it is evident that adult stem cells have the unexpected ability to differentiate into many specific cell types including those of skeletal origin, research with multipotent adult stem cells has become a promising alternative to embryonic stem cells for use in vivo (Colman and Burley, 2001; Gao et al, 2001; Im et al., 2001; Cogle et al., 2003; Tsuchida et al., 2003). Not all limitations on the use of adult stem cells have been solved so far, such as, for example, a comparably lower capacity to expand indefinitely without losing their differentiation potential. Furthermore, the initial number of adult stem cells obtained is lower than with stem cells of embryonic origin and it is apparently more difficult to genetically manipulate adult stem cells. Clearly, the ethical consequences of adult stem cell research are not so serious, making the use of stem cells obtained from adult tissue much less controversial.

The recent progress made in establishing stem cell lines in vitro implies that standardised therapeutical grafting of ex vivo generated bone substitutes will be applicable in the near future. In the context of the new cell-based therapies, genetic modification of stem cells used to cover implant carriers is a promising approach, which is expected to fulfil the requirements for better biocompatibility and immune tolerance (Jenkins et al., 2003). Up to now, experimental studies utilising somatic gene therapy have been restricted to treating serious, life-threatening or debilitating disorders and it is indeed questionable if clinical situations for which tissue-engineered implants are desired fall into this category. Nevertheless, despite the recent setbacks in the administration of gene constructs, there is some hope that future improvements in the efficacy and safety of somatic gene therapy will ultimately be integrated into the fast moving field of tissue engineering. Provided the problems with the design of the appropriate gene vectors are satisfactorily solved, it is assumed that future advances in somatic gene therapy will continue to shape the ethical debate and may influence the patient´s attitudes towards this therapeutical approach (Motulsky, 1983; Walters, 1991; Winter and Roger, 1995; Spink and Geddes, 2004). Genetic manipulation of cultured cells on carriers generated to be implanted into the body may be less harmful, compared to standard protocols for somatic gene therapy (Smith, 2003). This appears to be particularly true for the risk that the desired gene is unintentionally integrated into the germ line, however, this risk is commonly expected to be negligibly low.

Future Prospects 13

The most promising future areas in tissue engineering are in the fields of stem cell research, genetic engineering, customised tissue reconstructions and improvement of the nutritional features in the transplant.

13.1 Customised tissue reconstruction

A defined three-dimensional scaffold assembly of complex structure is needed for the development of unique bone or cartilage tissue substitutes. Present day computer-aided technologies, medical imaging, and modern techniques offer elegant solutions and create new possibilities in the design and application of bone tissue substitutes. Non-invasive computed tomography (CT) and magnetic resonance imaging (MRI) generate accurate anatomical information for scaffold design, and computer-aided design/computer-aided manufacturing (CAD/CAM) and rapid prototyping (RP) technology allow the production and insertion of individualised scaffolds (Coward et al., 1999; Zonneveld, 2000; Runte et al., 2002) (Table 13.1). Implant prostheses, custom-made according to the size and shape of an individual defect site, can thus be produced (Fig. 13.1). The utilisation of these technologies has evolved into a new emerging field of computer-aided tissue engineering (CATE) (Sun and Lal, 2002). Driven by computer imaging and modern manufacturing technology, regenerative surgery may in future be directed towards individualised fabrication of bone and cartilage substitutes (Meyer et al., 2003). The principle steps of computer aided tissue engineering are given in Fig. 13.2.

Table 13.1. Aspects of computer aided tissue engineering

Modelling	Tissue classification	Implantation
- Anatomical modelling - Physical modelling - Physiological modelling - CAD-based modelling - Prototype modelling	- Defect identification - 3D quantification - Tissue measurement - Tissue structure analysis	- Surgical planning - Surgical guidance - Robotics

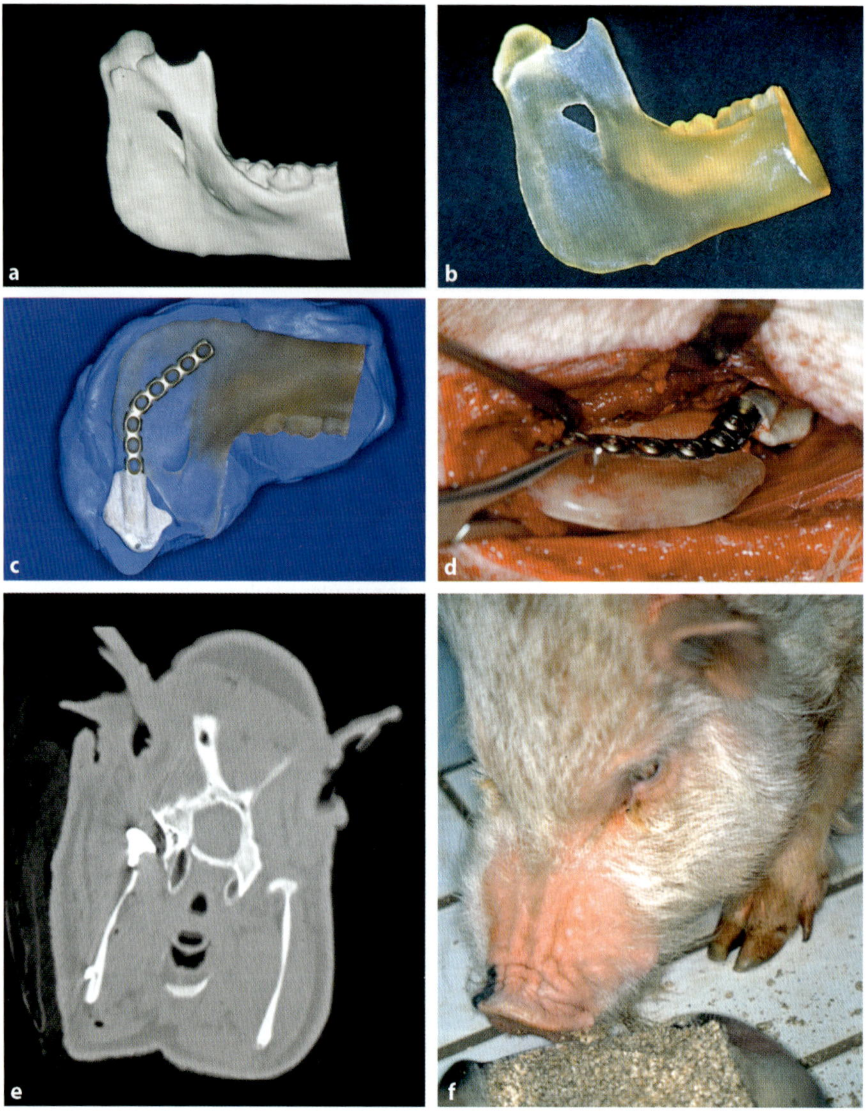

Fig. 13.1. Individual computer-aided reconstruction of temporomandibular joint. **a** STL model of the mandible. **b** stereolithography model. **c** Fabrication of a PLA/PGA condyle attached to a reconstruction plate. **d** Template-driven insertion of the artificial TMJ. **e** CT scan one month after insertion. **f** Clinical view of masticating animal

13.2 Vascularisation

One future development in clinically applied bone tissue engineering will have to focus on the vascularisation of the regenerate tissue. Angiogenesis is crucial for the survival of tissue-engineered constructs. The need for a prompt restart of blood sup-

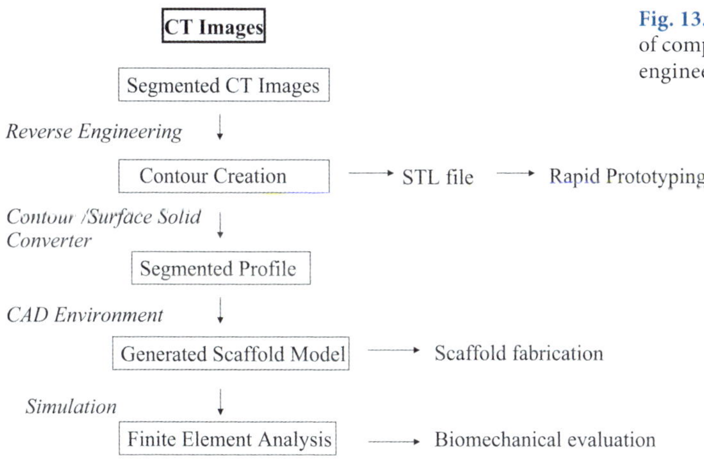

Fig. 13.2. Principal steps of computer-aided tissue engineering

ply is underlined by the observation that a delayed and inadequate neovascularisation of the graft implant is likely to account for implant failure. However, it appears unlikely that the final vascular structure can be predetermined in the micro-fabrication of the tissue construct in the near future, despite the improvements in vascular-like structure function ex vivo. Rather, the natural adaptive power of resident cells will be needed to achieve a vasculature that is sufficient for large, complex tissues. Recent advances indicate that the goal of providing a tissue-engineered vascular graft that will remain patent in vivo for substantial periods of time is achievable. It was shown by Ratcliffe that a non-degradable polyurethane scaffold cultured with smooth muscle cells generated a construct with mechanical properties similar to native vessels (Ratcliffe, 2000). These results show that tissue engineering of vascular grafts has true potential for application in the clinical situation. Adding growth factors such as vascular endothelial growth factor (VEGF) to the scaffold material is another promising approach to support vascular assembly (Nomi et al., 2002).

13.3 Genetic Engineering

The prospect of gene therapy in the context of tissue engineering is offered by recent advances in gene delivery techniques. Gene therapy itself can be defined as the introduction of nucleic acid into cells in order to alter their genetic constitution. Application of gene therapy to control cellular behaviour has a number of advantages above conventional, protein-based therapies (for a review, see Klamut et al., 2004). Genetic modification of cells has some advantages over protein delivery approaches to the ex vivo generation of a bone- or cartilage-like tissue. The advantages associated with genetic modification of cells are:

- Expression of the desired transgene is prolonged compared to the effects of added proteins
- Proteins often require hyperphysiological doses to execute specific effects
- Expression of protein restricted to forget cell

- Transgenes do not have to be produced in large amounts with recombinant expression technology
- Transgene production can be regulated by the use of controllable or tissue-specific promoters.

Various genetic engineering strategies can be used for gene transfer to tissues of bone and cartilage (Evans and Robbins, 1995; Robbins and Ghivizzani, 1998; Hannallah et al., 2002) (Fig. 13.3) The strategies include, beneath local or systemic delivery approaches in vivo, the transfection of cells ex vivo (for a review, see Baltzer and Lieberman, 2004; Partridge and Oreffo, 2004). Systemic delivery, performed by administration of the vector into the bloodstream, allows gene application and dissemination into all organs of the body. This method has advantages in bone or cartilage tissue engineering (as referred to in the extended definition of tissue engineering) only under some circumstances. It is a favourable approach when the target tissue is located in different regions of the body or when it cannot be reached directly.

Major limitations of systemic delivery include:

- The low specificity of gene expression
- The high vector concentration required to attain therapeutic effects
- The lack of blood supply in cartilage tissue
- The non-specific dissemination of the vectors to all areas of the body
- Immuno-reactions against components of the delivery systems (vectors).

In contrast to systemic delivery, local gene therapy in bone and cartilage healing has been investigated in a number of studies (Evans and Robbins, 1995; Robbins and Ghivizzani, 1998; Hannallah et al., 2002). Two approaches can be distinguished: first, vectors can be applied directly into the host tissue (in vivo) (Alden et al., 1999; Musgrave et al., 1999; Baltzer et al., 2000; Okubo et al., 2000), and secondly, cells harvested from the patient can be genetically modified by DNA transfection in vitro.

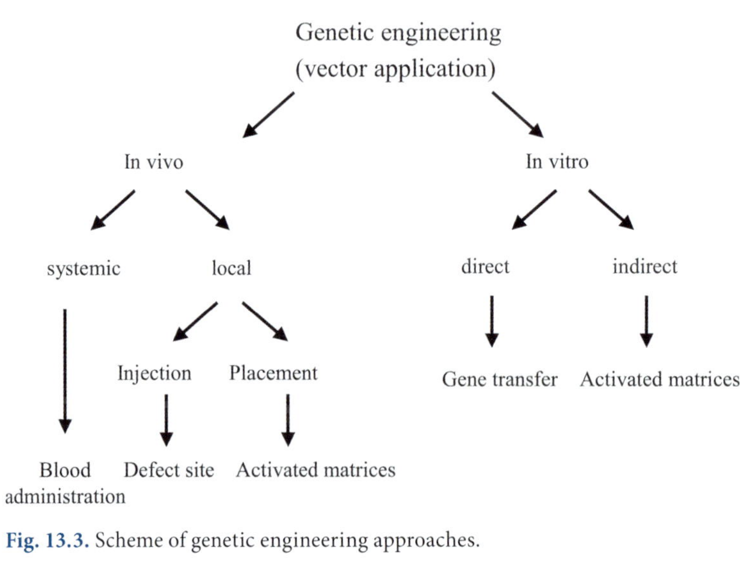

Fig. 13.3. Scheme of genetic engineering approaches.

For the ex vivo tissue engineering approach, genetically altered cells are then coated with a scaffold in order to extracorporally fabricate bone or cartilage tissue. Ex vivo gene delivery can be considered as a more defined method of genetic engineering. In addition to the gene transfer under controlled in vitro conditions, this technique is safer since the gene manipulation takes place under controlled conditions outside the body. An additional advantage of this method is that nearly all cells can be transfected which is very hard to achieve in vivo. Successful gene therapy involves four key steps: effective transfection followed by transcription, translation, and sustained expression of the reccombinant target gene. The uptake of new genetic material and the expression of the introduced foreign gene have to be facilitated by advanced transfection protocols (Fig. 13.4.). Generally, virus-based vectors (adenovirus, adeno-associated virus, lentivirus and Herpes simplex virus) are more efficient than non-viral vector systems (e.g. liposomes). A variety of cDNAs have been cloned aimed to improve tissue healing by (1) inducing mitosis or the synthesis and deposition of tissue-specific extracellular matrix components by autochthonous cells, (2) induction of cell differentiation by mesenchymal progenitor cells, or (3) inhibiting cellular responses to inflammatory stimuli. (Fig. 13.4)

Experimental studies have shown that gene therapy is effective for both bone and cartilage tissue engineering. The effectiveness of gene therapy has been demonstrated by in vitro and in vivo studies. Several investigators have, for example,

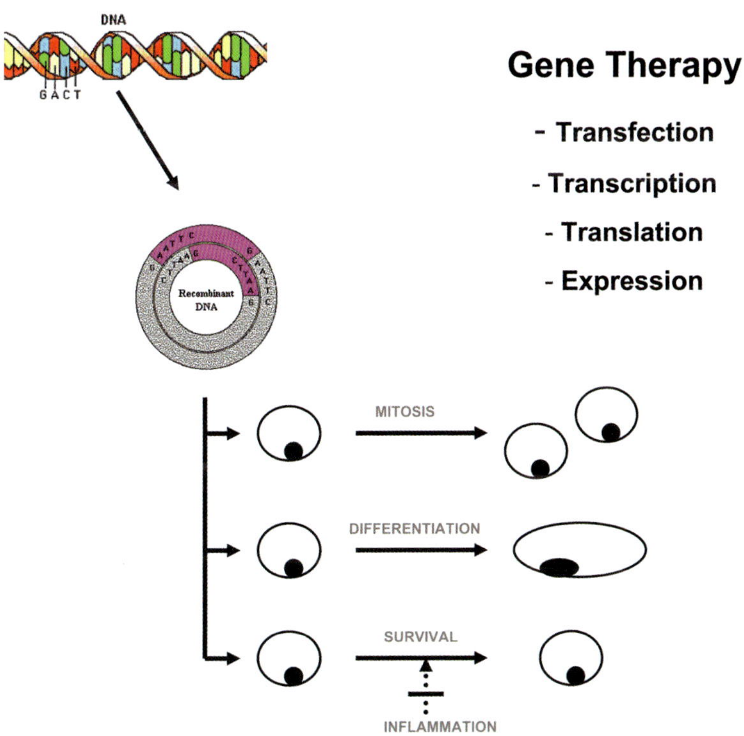

Fig. 13.4. Scheme of gene transfer and cellular actions.

demonstrated that viral vectors can be used to deliver genes to chondrocytes in vitro (Arai et al., 1997; Wehling et al., 1997; Doherty et al., 1998; Smith et al., 2000). The genetically altered chondrocytes have been cultured ex vivo in a three-dimensional space without loss of cell viability or differentiation characteristics (Doherty et al., 1998; Ikeda et al., 2000). Cells were commonly transduced with genes that are involved in chondrocyte development. It was demonstrated that the in vitro delivery of these genes (encoding for BMP-2, IGF-1, and TGF-β) to articular chondrocytes leads to an increase in proteoglycan synthesis by the cells in culture (Arai et al., 1997; Smith et al., 2000). In addition to chondrocyte-based studies, Lieberman and collegues. (1999) were able to successfully present an ex vivo gene therapy approach to enhance the osteogenic potential of bone marrow cells. In general, cells from various mesenchymal cell lines were able to induce bone- or cartilage-like cell differentiation by incorporating cell differentiation genes.

The local gene therapy approach was also applied to experimental animal studies as revealed by investigations on in vitro cartilage or bone healing (Baragi et al., 1997; Kang et al., 1997; Mason et al., 1998; Goomer et al., 2000; 2001). Mason et al., for example, demonstrated improved healing of articular defects by using a retroviral vector to transduce mesenchymal stem cells with a gene for BMP-7 in a rabbit model (Mason et al., 1998). Gene delivery methods have also been successful in the promotion of bone healing in various animal experimental settings (Beresford, 1989; Fang et al., 1996; Bruder et al., 1998a; b; Bonadio et al., 1999). In this respect, gene therapy and the use of gene activated matrices offers great promise in the field of tissue engineering.

Importantly, gene therapy has not only advantages but also risks. The integration of viral vectors into the genome of cells bears the risk of mutagenesis and oncogenesis (Crystal, 1995). Abnormal regulation of cell growth, toxicity due to chronic overexpression of the gene product, dysregulated development and induction of malignant tumours are currently unsolved problems associated with gene therapy. Despite their promising expectations all gene therapy protocols should be regarded with extreme caution and should be conducted only in specialised centres with long-standing expertise in recombinant DNA technologies. The effect of genetic tissue engineering has therefore to be tested at different experimental levels. Basic evaluation can be performed in in vitro systems and in small animals in order to prove basic concepts of genetic engineering (such as the regulation of gene expression). Large animal models are the next step to study the effectiveness as well as to evaluate possible adverse effects of gene therapy at an in vivo level, before clinical trials can be started. A special model system that can be used as a proof of the system concept system is the immunodeficient mouse model, since this model allows one to study the effect of transgene expression on tissue formation without having additional interactions by immune mechanisms.

References

Aarden, E. M., E. H. Burger and P. J. Nijweide (1994) Function of osteocytes in bone. J Cell Biochem **55**(3): 287–99.

Abdel-Aleem, S., J. D. St Louis, G. C. Hughes and J. E. Lowe (1999) Metabolic changes in the normal and hypoxic neonatal myocardium. Ann NY Acad Sci **874**: 254–61.

Abott, N. L., J. P. Folkers and G. M. Whitesides (1992) Manipulation of the wettability of surfaces on the 0.1–1-micrometer scale through micromachining and molecular self-assembly. Science **257**: 1380–2.

Aegerter, E. and J. A. Kirkpatrick (1973) Orthopedic Diseases; Physiology, Pathology, Radiology. W. B. Saunders, Philadelphia.

Agrawal, C. M., J. S. Mckinney, D. Huang and K. A. Athanasiou (2000) Synthetic Bioabsorbable Polymers for Implants, 1st edn. ASTM, Philadelphia.

Agrawal, C. M. and R. B. Ray (2001) Biodegradable polymeric scaffolds for musculoskeletal tissue engineering. J Biomed Mater Res **55**(2): 141–50.

Ahmad, R., J. F. Bates and T. T. Lewis (1982) Measurement of strain rate behaviour in complete mandibular dentures. Biomaterials **3**(2): 87–92.

Ahmad, M., M. B. McCarthy and G. Gronowicz (1999) An in vitro model for mineralization of human osteoblast-like cells on implant materials. Biomaterials **20**(3): 211–20.

Akagawa, K. S., N. Takasuka, Y. Nozaki, I. Komuro, M. Azuma, M. Ueda, M. Naito and K. Takahashi (1996) Generation of CD1+RelB+ dendritic cells and tartrate-resistant acid phosphatase-positive osteoclast-like multinucleated giant cells from human monocytes. Blood **88**(10): 4029–39.

Akita, J., M. Takahashi, M. Hojo, A. Nishida, M. Haruta and Y. Honda (2002) Neuronal differentiation of adult rat hippocampus-derived neural stem cells transplanted into embryonic rat explanted retinas with retinoic acid pretreatment. Brain Res **954**(2): 286–93.

Alam, M. I., I. Asahina, I. Seto, M. Oda and S. Enomoto (2003) Prefabrication of vascularized bone flap induced by recombinant human bone morphogenetic protein 2 (rhBMP-2). Int J Oral Maxillofac Surg **32**(5): 508–14.

Alden, T. D., D. D. Pittman, G. R. Hankins, E. J. Beres, J. A. Engh, S. Das, S. B. Hudson, K. M. Kerns, D. F. Kallmes and G. A. Helm (1999) In vivo endochondral bone formation using a bone morphogenetic protein 2 adenoviral vector. Hum Gene Ther **10**(13): 2245–53.

Alini, M., Y. Matsui, G. R. Dodge and A. R. Poole (1992) The extracellular matrix of cartilage in the growth plate before and during calcification: changes in composition and degradation of type II collagen. Calcif Tissue Int **50**(4): 327–35.

Alison, M. R., R. Poulsom, S. Forbes and N. A. Wright (2002) An introduction to stem cells. J Pathol **197**(4): 419–23.

Al-Khadi, A., N. Eliopoulos, K. Lachapelle and J. Galipeau (2001) EGF-dependent angiogenic response induced by in situ cultured marrow stromal cells. Anaheim, Calif: American Heart Association Scientific Session, November: 11–14.

Alsberg, E., E. E. Hill and D. J. Mooney (2001) Craniofacial tissue engineering. Crit Rev Oral Biol Med **12**(1): 64–75.

An, Y. H. and R. J. Friedman (1999) Animal models of articular cartilage defect. Animal models in orthopaedic research. Boca Raton, FL: CRC Press LLC.

Anderer, U. and J. Libera (2002) In vitro engineering of human autogenous cartilage. J Bone Miner Res **17**(8): 1420–9.

Anderson, H. C. (1967) Electron microscopic studies of induced cartilage development and calcification. J Cell Biol **35**(1): 81–101.

Anderson, J. M. (1988) Inflammatory response to implants. ASAIO Trans **34**(2): 101–7.

Anderson, J. M. (1993) Mechanisms of inflammation and infection with implanted devices. Cardiovasc Pathol **2**: 33–41.

Anderson, H. C. (1995) Molecular biology of matrix vesicles. Clin Orthop Relat Res (314): 266–80.

Ando, J., T. Komatsuda and A. Kamiya (1988) Cytoplasmic calcium response to fluid shear stress in cultured vascular endothelial cells. In Vitro Cell Dev Biol **24**(9): 871–7.

Andrade, J. D. (1973) Interfacial phenomena and biomaterials. Med Instrum **7**(2): 110–9.

Ang, T. H., F. S. A. Sultana, D. W. Hutmacher, Y. S. Wong, J. Y. H. Fuh, X. M. Mo, H. T. Loh, E. Burdet and S. H. Teoh (2002) Fabrication of 3D chitosan-hydroxyapatite scaffolds using a robotic dispensing system. Mater Sci Eng C **20**(1–2): 35–42.

Anselme, K. (2000) Osteoblast adhesion on biomaterials. Biomaterials **21**(7): 667–81.

Arai, Y., T. Kubo, K. Kobayashi, K. Takeshita, K. Takahashi, T. Ikeda, J. Imanishi, M. Takigawa and Y. Hirasawa (1997) Adenovirus vector-mediated gene transduction to chondrocytes: in vitro evaluation of therapeutic efficacy of transforming growth factor-beta 1 and heat shock protein 70 gene transduction. J Rheumatol **24**(9): 1787–95.

Archer, C. W., P. Rooney and C. P. Cottrill (1985) Cartilage morphogenesis in vitro. J Embryol Exp Morphol **90**: 33–48.

Arendts, F. J. and C. Sigolotto (1989) [Standard measurements, elasticity values and tensile strength behavior of the human mandible, a contribution to the biomechanics of the mandible--I]. Biomed Tech (Berlin) **34**(10): 248–55.

Arendts, F. J. and C. Sigolotto (1990) [Mechanical characteristics of the human mandible and study of in vivo behavior of compact bone tissue, a contribution to the description of biomechanics of the mandible--II]. Biomed Tech (Berlin) **35**(6): 123–30.

Aronson, J. (1992) Mechanical factors generated during distraction osteogenesis. The International Society for Fracture Repair, Ottrot, France, April, 1992.

Asahara, T., T. Murohara, A. Sullivan, M. Silver, R. van der Zee, T. Li, B. Witzenbichler, G. Schatteman and J. M. Isner (1997) Isolation of putative progenitor endothelial cells for angiogenesis. Science **275**(5302): 964–7.

Asahara, T., H. Masuda, T. Takahashi, C. Kalka, C. Pastore, M. Silver, M. Kearne, M. Magner and J. M. Isner (1999) Bone marrow origin of endothelial progenitor cells responsible for postnatal vasculogenesis in physiological and pathological neovascularization. Circ Res **85**(3): 221–8.

Ashton, B. A., T. D. Allen, C. R. Howlett, C. C. Eaglesom, A. Hattori and M. Owen (1980) Formation of bone and cartilage by marrow stromal cells in diffusion chambers in vivo. Clin Orthop Relat Res (151): 294–307.

Askew, M. J. and V. C. Mow (1978) The biomechanical function of the collagen fibril ultrastructure of articular cartilage. J Biomech Eng **100**: 105–15.

Ateshian, G. A. and H. Wang (1995) A theoretical solution for the frictionless rolling contact of cylindrical biphasic articular cartilage layers. J Biomech **28**(11): 1341–55.

Athanasiou, K. A., A. R. Shah, R. J. Hernandez and R. G. LeBaron (2001) Basic science of articular cartilage repair. Clin Sports Med **20**(2): 223–47.

Aubin, J. E. and F. Liu (1996) The osteoblast lineage. In Bilezikian, J. P., Raisz, L. G. and Rodan, G. A. (eds) Principles of Bone Biology. Academic Press, San Diego, CA. 51–67.

Aubin, J. E. (1998a) Bone stem cells. J Cell Biochem Suppl **30–31**: 73–82.

Aubin, J. E. (1998b) Advances in the osteoblast lineage. Biochem Cell Biol **76**(6): 899–910.

Aubin, J. E. (2001) Regulation of osteoblast formation and function. Rev Endocr Metab Disord **2**(1): 81–94.

Ayad, S., A. P. Kwan and M. E. Grant (1987) Partial characterization of type X collagen from bovine growth-plate cartilage. Evidence that type X collagen is processed in vivo. FEBS Lett **220**(1): 181–6.

Bagi, C. and E. H. Burger (1989) Mechanical stimulation by intermittent compression stimulates sulfate incorporation and matrix mineralization in fetal mouse long-bone rudiments under serum-free conditions. Calcif Tissue Int **45**(6): 342–7.

Bahrami, S., U. Stratmann, H. P. Wiesmann, K. Mokrys, P. Bruckner and T. Szuwart (2000) Periosteally derived osteoblast-like cells differentiate into chondrocytes in suspension culture in agarose. Anat Rec **259**(2): 124–30.

Baier, R. E., A. E. Meyer, J. R. Natiella, R. R. Natiella and J. M. Carter (1984) Surface properties determine bioadhesive outcomes: methods and results. J Biomed Mater Res **18**(4): 327–55.

Baker, S. R. (1989) Microsurgical Reconstruction of the Head and Neck, Churchill Livingstone, New York, 159.

Baksh, D., J. E. Davies and S. Kim (1998) Three-dimensional matrices of calcium polyphosphates support bone growth in vitro and in vivo. J Mater Sci Mater Med **9**(12): 743–8.

Balaban, N. Q., U. S. Schwarz, D. Riveline, P. Goichberg, G. Tzur, I. Sabanay, D. Mahalu, S. Safran, A. Bershadsky, L. Addadi and B. Geiger (2001) Force and focal adhesion assembly: a close relationship studied using elastic micropatterned substrates. Nat Cell Biol **3**(5): 466–72.

Baltzer, A. W., C. Lattermann, J. D. Whalen, P. Wooley, K. Weiss, M. Grimm, S. C. Ghivizzani, P. D. Robbins and C. H. Evans (2000) Genetic enhancement of fracture repair: healing of an experimental segmental defect by adenoviral transfer of the BMP-2 gene. Gene Ther **7**(9): 734–9.

Baltzer, A. W. and J. R. Lieberman (2004) Regional gene therapy to enhance bone repair. Gene Ther **11**(4): 344–50.

Baragi, V. M., R. R. Renkiewicz, L. Qiu, D. Brammer, J. M. Riley, R. E. Sigler, S. R. Frenkel, A. Amin, S. B. Abramson and B. J. Roessler (1997) Transplantation of adenovirally transduced allogeneic chondrocytes into articular cartilage defects in vivo. Osteoarthritis Cartilage **5**(4): 275–82.

Barnes, G. L., P. J. Kostenuik, L. C. Gerstenfeld and T. A. Einhorn (1999) Growth factor regulation of fracture repair. J Bone Miner Res **14**(11): 1805–15.

Barthlott, W. and C. Neinhuis (1997) Purity of the sacred lotus, or escape from contamination in biological surfaces. Planta **202**(1): 1–8.

Beaupre, G. S., S. S. Stevens and D. R. Carter (2000) Mechanobiology in the development, maintenance, and degeneration of articular cartilage. J Rehabil Res Dev **37**(2): 145–51.

Behonick, D. J. and Z. Werb (2003) A bit of give and take: the relationship between the extracellular matrix and the developing chondrocyte. Mech Dev **120**(11): 1327–36.

Berger, J., M. Reist, J. M. Mayer, O. Felt, N. A. Peppas and R. Gurny (2004a) Structure and interactions in covalently and ionically cross-linked chitosan hydrogels for biomedical applications. Eur J Pharm Biopharm **57**(1): 19–34.

Berger, J., M. Reist, J. M. Mayer, O. Felt and R. Gurny (2004b) Structure and interactions in chitosan hydrogels formed by complexation or aggregation for biomedical applications. Eur J Pharm Biopharm **57**(1): 35–52.

Berglundh, T. and J. Lindhe (1997) Healing around implants placed in bone defects treated with Bio-Oss. An experimental study in the dog. Clin Oral Implants Res **8**(2): 117–24.

Bianco, P., M. Riminucci, S. Gronthos and P. G. Robey (2001) Bone marrow stromal stem cells: nature, biology, and potential applications. Stem Cells **19**(3): 180–92.

Bidic, S. M., J. W. Calvert, K. Marra, P. Kumta, P. Campbell, R. Mitchell, W. Wigginton, J. O. Hollinger, L. Weiss and M. P. Mooney (2003) Rabbit calvarial wound healing by means of seeded Caprotite scaffolds. J Dent Res **82**(2): 131–5.

Biebuyck, H. A. and G. M. Whitesides (1994) Self-organisation of organic liquids on patterned self-assembled monolayers of alkanthiols on gold. Langmuir **10**: 2790–3.

Biewener, A. A. (1993) Safety factors in bone strength. Calcif Tissue Int **53 Suppl 1**: 68–74.

Binderman, I., U. Zor, A. M. Kaye, Z. Shimshoni, A. Harell and D. Somjen (1988) The transduction of mechanical force into biochemical events in bone cells may involve activation of phospholipase A2. Calcif Tissue Int **42**(4): 261–6.

Binderman, I. and N. Fin (1990) Bone substitutes organic, inorganic, and polymeric: Cell material interactions. In: Yamamuro, T., Hench, L. and Wilson J. (eds) CRC Handbook of Bioactive Ceramics. CRC Press, Boca Raton, FL, 45–51.

Blair, H. C., S. L. Teitelbaum, R. Ghiselli and S. Gluck (1989) Osteoclastic bone resorption by a polarized vacuolar proton pump. Science **245**(4920): 855–7.

Blankevoort, L., J. H. Kuiper, R. Huiskes and H. J. Grootenboer (1991) Articular contact in a three-dimensional model of the knee. J Biomech **24**(11): 1019–31.

Boden, S. D., L. Titus, G. Hair, Y. Liu, M. Viggeswarapu, M. S. Nanes and C. Baranowski (1998) Lumbar spine fusion by local gene therapy with a cDNA encoding a novel osteoinductive protein (LMP-1) Spine **23**(23): 2486–92.

Böltau, M., S. Walheim, J. Mlynek, G. Krausch and U. Steiner (1998) Surface-induced structure formation of polymer blends on patterned substrates. Nature **391**(6670): 887–9.

Bonadio, J., E. Smiley, P. Patil and S. Goldstein (1999) Localized, direct plasmid gene delivery in vivo: prolonged therapy results in reproducible tissue regeneration. Nat Med **5**(7): 753–9.

Bonner, W. M., H. Jonsson, C. Malanos and M. Bryant (1975) Changes in the lipids of human articular cartilage with age. Arthritis Rheum **18**(5): 461–73.

Bonucci, E. (1967) Fine structure of early cartilage calcification. J Ultrastruct Res **20**(1): 33–50.

Bostrom, M. P., J. M. Lane, W. S. Berberian, A. A. Missri, E. Tomin, A. Weiland, S. B. Doty, D. Glaser and V. M. Rosen (1995) Immunolocalization and expression of bone morphogenetic proteins 2 and 4 in fracture healing. J Orthop Res **13**(3): 357–67.

Botchwey, E. A., S. R. Pollack, E. M. Levine and C. T. Laurencin (2001) Bone tissue engineering in a rotating bioreactor using a microcarrier matrix system. J Biomed Mater Res **55**(2): 242–53.

Bottlang, M., M. Simnacher, H. Schmitt, R. A. Brand and L. Claes (1997) A cell strain system for small homogeneous strain applications. Biomed Tech (Berlin) **42**(11): 305–9.

Bouletreau, P. J., S. M. Warren and M. T. Longaker (2002a) The molecular biology of distraction osteogenesis. J Craniomaxillofac Surg **30**(1): 1–11.

Bouletreau, P. J., S. M. Warren, J. A. Spector, Z. M. Peled, R. P. Gerrets, J. A. Greenwald and M. T. Longaker (2002b) Hypoxia and VEGF up-regulate BMP-2 mRNA and protein expression in microvascular endothelial cells: implications for fracture healing. Plast Reconstr Surg **109**(7): 2384–97.

Bowers, K. T., J. C. Keller, B. A. Randolph, D. G. Wick and C. M. Michaels (1992) Optimization of surface micromorphology for enhanced osteoblast responses in vitro. Int J Oral Maxillofac Implants **7**(3): 302–10.

Boyan, B. D., T. W. Hummert, D. D. Dean and Z. Schwartz (1996) Role of material surfaces in regulating bone and cartilage cell response. Biomaterials **17**(2): 137–46.

Boyce, B. F., D. E. Hughes, K. R. Wright, L. Xing and A. Dai (1999) Recent advances in bone biology provide insight into the pathogenesis of bone diseases. Lab Invest **79**(2): 83–94.

Brighton, C. T. (1998) Breakout session. 4: Biophysical enhancement. Clin Orthop Relat Res (355 Suppl): S357–8.

Brittberg, M., A. Lindahl, A. Nilsson, C. Ohlsson, O. Isaksson and L. Peterson (1994) Treatment of deep cartilage defects in the knee with autologous chondrocyte transplantation. N Engl J Med **331**(14): 889–95.

Brittberg, M. (1996) Cartilage repair: On cartilaginous tissue engineering with the emphasis on chondrocyte transplantation. PhD Thesis, Göteborg, Sweden, Göteborg University.

Brittberg, M. (1999) Autologous chondrocyte transplantation. Clin Orthop Relat Res (367 Suppl): S147–55.

Brown, T. D. and A. B. Ferguson, Jr. (1978) The development of a computational stress analysis of the femoral head. Mapping tensile, compressive, and shear stress for the varus and valgus positions. J Bone Joint Surg Am **60**(5): 619–29.

Brown, T. D. and D. T. Shaw (1983) In vitro contact stress distributions in the natural human hip. J Biomech **16**(6): 373–84.

Brown, T. D., D. F. Pope, J. E. Hale, J. A. Buckwalter and R. A. Brand (1991) Effects of osteochondral defect size on cartilage contact stress. J Orthop Res **9**(4): 559–67.

Brown, T. D. (2000) Techniques for mechanical stimulation of cells in vitro: a review. J Biomech **33**(1): 3–14.

Bruder, S. P., N. Jaiswal and S. E. Haynesworth (1997) Growth kinetics, self-renewal, and the osteogenic potential of purified human mesenchymal stem cells during extensive subcultivation and following cryopreservation. J Cell Biochem **64**(2): 278–94.

Bruder, S. P., K. H. Kraus, V. M. Goldberg and S. Kadiyala (1998a) The effect of implants loaded with autologous mesenchymal stem cells on the healing of canine segmental bone defects. J Bone Joint Surg Am **80**(7): 985–96.

Bruder, S. P., A. A. Kurth, M. Shea, W. C. Hayes, N. Jaiswal and S. Kadiyala (1998b) Bone regeneration by implantation of purified, culture-expanded human mesenchymal stem cells. J Orthop Res **16**(2): 155–62.

Büchter, A., J. Kleinheinz, H. P. Wiesmann, L. Seper, U. Joos and U. Meyer (2004) [Peri-implant bone formation around cylindrical and conical implant systems]. Mund Kiefer Gesichtschir **8**(5): 282–8.

Buckwalter, J. A., E. B. Hunziker, L. C. Rosenberg and e. al. (1988a) Articular Cartilage: Composition and Structure. In Woo, S. L. and Buckwalter, J. A. (eds) Injury and Repair of the Musculoskeletal Soft Tissues. American Academy of Orthopaedic Surgeons, Park Ridge, IL, 405–25.

Buckwalter, J. A., L. C. Rosenberg, R. Coutts and e. al. (1988b) Articular Cartilage: Injury and Repair. In Woo, S. L. and Buckwalter, J. A. (eds) Injury and Repair of the Musculoskeletal Soft Tissues. American Academy of Orthopaedic Surgeons, Park Ridge, IL, 465–82.

Buckwalter, J. A., L. A. Rosenberg and E. B. Hunziker (1990) Articular Cartilage: Composition, Structure, Response to Injury, and Methods of Facilitation Repair. In Ewing, J. W. (ed) Articular Cartilage and Knee Joint Function: Basic Science and Arthroscopy. Raven Press, New York, 19–56.

Buckwalter, J. A. and V. C. Mow (1991) Cartilage Repair in Osteoarthritis. In Moskowitz, R. W., Howell, D. S., Goldberg, V. M. and Mankin, H. J. (eds) Osteoarthritis: Diagnosis and Management. 2nd edn. W. B. Saunders, Philadelphia, 71–107.

Buckwalter, J. A. (1992) Mechanical Injuries of Articular Cartilage. In Finerman, G. (ed.) Biology and Biomechanics of the Traumatized Synovial Joint. American Academy of Orthopaedic Surgeons, Park Ridge, IL, 83–96.

Buckwalter, J. A. and H. J. Mankin (1997a) Articular cartilage: I. Tissue design and chondrocyte-matrix interactions. J Bone Joint Surg Am **79A**: 600–11.

Buckwalter, J. A. and H. J. Mankin (1997b) Articular cartilage: II. Degeneration and osteoarthrosis, repair, regeneration and transplantation. J Bone Joint Surg Am **79A**: 612–32.

Buckwalter, J. A., T. A. Einhorn and J. L. Marsh (2001) Bone and Joint Healing. In Rockwood, C. A., Green, D. P., Bucholz, R. W. and Heckman, J. D. (eds) Fractures. Lippincott, Philadelphia, 245–71.

Buckwalter, J. A., J. A. Martin, M. Olmstead, K. A. Athanasiou, M. P. Rosenwasser and V. C. Mow (2003) Osteochondral repair of primate knee femoral and patellar articular surfaces: implications for preventing post-traumatic osteoarthritis. Iowa Orthop J **23**: 66–74.

Buckwalter, J. A. and T. D. Brown (2004) Joint injury, repair, and remodeling: roles in post-traumatic osteoarthritis. Clin Orthop Relat Res (423): 7–16.

Burg, K. J., W. D. Holder, Jr., C. R. Culberson, R. J. Beiler, K. G. Greene, A. B. Loebsack, W. D. Roland, P. Eiselt, D. J. Mooney and C. R. Halberstadt (2000a) Comparative study of seeding methods for three-dimensional polymeric scaffolds. J Biomed Mater Res **51**(4): 642–9.

Burg, K. J., S. Porter and J. F. Kellam (2000b) Biomaterial developments for bone tissue engineering. Biomaterials **21**(23): 2347–59.

Burger, E. H. and J. P. Veldhuijzen (1993) Influence of mechanical factors on bone formation, resorption, and growth in vitro. In Hall, B. K. Bone, Vol. 7, CRC Press, Boca Raton, 37–56.

Burkart, A. C., P. B. Schoettle and A. B. Imhoff (2001) [Surgical therapeutic possibilities of cartilage damage]. Unfallchirurg **104**(9): 798–807.

Burr, D. B. (2004) Anatomy and physiology of the mineralized tissues: role in the pathogenesis of osteoarthrosis. Osteoarthritis Cartilage **12 Suppl A**: 20–30.

Burwell, R. G. (1964) Studies in the Transplantation of Bone. VII. The fresh composite homograft–autograft of cancellous bone; an analysis of factors leading to osteogenesis in marrow transplants and in marrow–containing bone grafts. J Bone Joint Surg Br **46**: 110–40.

Burwell, R. G. (1966) Studies in the transplantation of bone. 8. Treated composite homograft–autografts of cancellous bone: an analysis of inductive mechanisms in bone transplantation. J Bone Joint Surg Br **48**(3): 532–66.

Burwell, R. G. (1985) The function of bone marrow in the incorporation of a bone graft. Clin Orthop Relat Res (200): 125–41.

Buschmann, M. D., Y. A. Gluzband, A. J. Grodzinsky and E. B. Hunziker (1995) Mechanical compression modulates matrix biosynthesis in chondrocyte/agarose culture. J Cell Sci **108** (**Pt 4**): 1497–508.

Buser, D., K. Dula, H. P. Hirt and R. K. Schenk (1996) Lateral ridge augmentation using autografts and barrier membranes: a clinical study with 40 partially edentulous patients. J Oral Maxillofac Surg **54**(4): 420–32; discussion 432–3.

Butler, W. T. and H. Ritchie (1995) The nature and functional significance of dentin extracellular matrix proteins. Int J Dev Biol **39**(1): 169–79.

Butler, D. L., S. A. Goldstein and F. Guilak (2000) Functional tissue engineering: the role of biomechanics. J Biomech Eng **122**(6): 570–5.

Buttery, L. D., S. Bourne, J. D. Xynos, H. Wood, F. J. Hughes, S. P. Hughes, V. Episkopou and J. M. Polak (2001) Differentiation of osteoblasts and in vitro bone formation from murine embryonic stem cells. Tissue Eng **7**(1): 89–99.

Calvert, J. M. (1993) Lithographic patterning of self-assembled films. J Vac Sci Technol B **11**: 2155–63.

Calvert, J. W., L. E. Weiss and M. J. Sundine (2003) New frontiers in bone tissue engineering. Clin Plast Surg **30**(4): 641–8.

Campagnoli, C., I. A. Roberts, S. Kumar, P. R. Bennett, I. Bellantuono and N. M. Fisk (2001) Identification of mesenchymal stem/progenitor cells in human first-trimester fetal blood, liver, and bone marrow. Blood **98**(8): 2396–402.

Cao, Y., J. P. Vacanti, K. T. Paige, J. Upton and C. A. Vacanti (1997) Transplantation of chondrocytes utilizing a polymer–cell construct to produce tissue–engineered cartilage in the shape of a human ear. Plast Reconstr Surg **100**(2): 297–302; discussion 303–4.

Caplan, A. I. (1984) Cartilage. Sci Am **251**(4): 84–7, 90–4.

Caplan, A. L. (1985) Ethical issues raised by research involving xenografts. J Am Med Assoc **254**(23): 3339–43.

Caplan, A. I. (1991) Mesenchymal stem cells. J Orthop Res **9**(5): 641–50.

Caplan, A. I. (2000) Mesenchymal stem cells and gene therapy. Clin Orthop Relat Res (379 Suppl): S67–70.

Carter, D. R., T. E. Orr, D. P. Fyhrie and D. J. Schurman (1987) Influences of mechanical stress on prenatal and postnatal skeletal development. Clin Orthop Relat Res (219): 237–50.

Carter, D. R. and M. Wong (1990) Mechanical stresses in joint morphogenesis and maintenance. In Mow, V. C., Ratcliffe, A. and Woo, S. L. Y. (eds) Biomechanics of Diarthrodial Joints. Springer–Verlag, New York, 155–74.

Carter, D. R. and T. E. Orr (1992) Skeletal development and bone functional adaptation. J Bone Miner Res **7 Suppl 2**: S389–95.

Carter, G. (1999) Harvesting and implanting allograft bone. AORN J **70**(4): 660–70; quiz 672–6.

Casser-Bette, M., A. B. Murray, E. I. Closs, V. Erfle and J. Schmidt (1990) Bone formation by osteoblast-like cells in a three-dimensional cell culture. Calcif Tissue Int **46**(1): 46–56.

Catledge, S. A., M. D. Fries, Y. K. Vohra, W. R. Lacefield, J. E. Lemons, S. Woodard and R. Venugopalan (2002) Nanostructured ceramics for biomedical implants. J Nanosci Nanotechnol **2**(3–4): 293–312.

Chamay, A. (1970) Mechanical and morphological aspects of experimental overload and fatigue in bone. J Biomech **3**(3): 263–70.

Chambers, T. J. (2000) Regulation of the differentiation and function of osteoclasts. J Pathol **192**(1): 4–13.

Chao, E. Y. and N. Inoue (2003) Biophysical stimulation of bone fracture repair, regeneration and remodelling. Eur Cell Mater **6**: 72–84; discussion 84–5.

Chen, W. T. and S. J. Singer (1982) Immunoelectron microscopic studies of the sites of cell–substratum and cell–cell contacts in cultured fibroblasts. J Cell Biol **95**(1): 205–22.

Chen, N. T., J. Glowacki, L. P. Bucky, H. Z. Hong, W. K. Kim and M. J. Yaremchuk (1994) The roles of revascularization and resorption on endurance of craniofacial onlay bone grafts in the rabbit. Plast Reconstr Surg **93**(4): 714–22; discussion 723–4.

Chen, A. C., J. P. Nagrampa, R. M. Schinagl, L. M. Lottman and R. L. Sah (1997) Chondrocyte transplantation to articular cartilage explants in vitro. J Orthop Res **15**(6): 791–802.

Cheng, M. Z., G. Zaman, S. C. Rawlinson, R. F. Suswillo and L. E. Lanyon (1996) Mechanical loading and sex hormone interactions in organ cultures of rat ulna. J Bone Miner Res **11**(4): 502–11.

Cheng, G. C., W. H. Briggs, D. S. Gerson, P. Libby, A. J. Grodzinsky, M. L. Gray and R. T. Lee (1997) Mechanical strain tightly controls fibroblast growth factor-2 release from cultured human vascular smooth muscle cells. Circ Res **80**(1): 28–36.

Cho, T. J., L. C. Gerstenfeld and T. A. Einhorn (2002) Differential temporal expression of members of the transforming growth factor beta superfamily during murine fracture healing. J Bone Miner Res **17**(3): 513–20.

Choi, I. H., J. H. Ahn, C. Y. Chung and T. J. Cho (2000) Vascular proliferation and blood supply during distraction osteogenesis: a scanning electron microscopic observation. J Orthop Res **18**(5): 698–705.

Chu, C. R., R. D. Coutts, M. Yoshioka, F. L. Harwood, A. Z. Monosov and D. Amiel (1995) Articular cartilage repair using allogeneic perichondrocyte-seeded biodegradable porous polylactic acid (PLA): a tissue-engineering study. J Biomed Mater Res **29**(9): 1147–54.

Chu, T. M., J. W. Halloran, S. J. Hollister and S. E. Feinberg (2001) Hydroxyapatite implants with designed internal architecture. J Mater Sci Mater Med **12**(6): 471–8.

Chung, S., A. Hazen, J. P. Levine, G. Baux, W. A. Olivier, H. T. Yee, M. S. Margiotta, N. S. Karp and G. C. Gurtner (2003) Vascularized acellular dermal matrix island flaps for the repair of abdominal muscle defects. Plast Reconstr Surg **111**(1): 225–32.

Chuong, C. J. and Y. C. Fung (1983) Three-dimensional stress distribution in arteries. J Biomech Eng **105**(3): 268–74.

Churchill, L. R., M. L. Collins, N. M. King, S. G. Pemberton and K. A. Wailoo (1998) Genetic research as therapy: implications of gene therapy for informed consent. J Law Med Ethics **26**(1): 38–47, 3.

Cima, L. G., J. P. Vacanti, C. Vacanti, D. Ingber, D. Mooney and R. Langer (1991) Tissue engineering by cell transplantation using degradable polymer substrates. J Biomech Eng **113**(2): 143–51.

Coelho, M. J. and M. H. Fernandes (2000) Human bone cell cultures in biocompatibility testing. Part II: effect of ascorbic acid, beta-glycerophosphate and dexamethasone on osteoblastic differentiation. Biomaterials **21**(11): 1095–102.

Cogle, C. R., S. M. Guthrie, R. C. Sanders, W. L. Allen, E. W. Scott and B. E. Petersen (2003) An overview of stem cell research and regulatory issues. Mayo Clin Proc **78**(8): 993–1003.

Colman, A. and J. C. Burley (2001) A legal and ethical tightrope. Science, ethics and legislation of stem cell research. EMBO Rep **2**(1): 2–5.

Combe, E. C., B. A. Owen and J. S. Hodges (2004) A protocol for determining the surface free energy of dental materials. Dent Mater **20**(3): 262–8.

Conley, J. (1972) Use of composite flaps containing bone for major repairs in the head and neck. Plast Reconstr Surg **49**(5): 522–6.

Connolly, J. F. (1981) Repair of fractures. In: DePalma AF. DePalma's the management of fractures and dislocations: an atlas. 3rd edn. W. B. Saunders, Philadelphia. 17–8.

Connolly, J., R. Guse, L. Lippiello and R. Dehne (1989) Development of an osteogenic bone-marrow preparation. J Bone Joint Surg Am **71**(5): 684–91.

Cooper, L. F. (2000) A role for surface topography in creating and maintaining bone at titanium endosseous implants. J Prosthet Dent **84**(5): 522–34.
Cottrill, C. P., C. W. Archer and L. Wolpert (1987) Cell sorting and chondrogenic aggregate formation in micromass culture. Dev Biol **122**(2): 503–15.
Coutts, R. D., R. M. Healey, R. Ostrander, R. L. Sah, R. Goomer and D. Amiel (2001) Matrices for cartilage repair. Clin Orthop Relat Res (391 Suppl): s271–9.
Coward, T. J., R. M. Watson and I. C. Wilkinson (1999) Fabrication of a wax ear by rapid-process modeling using stereolithography. Int J Prosthodont **12**(1): 20–7.
Cram, D. J. (1988) The design of molecular hosts, guests, and their complexes. Science **240**: 760–7.
Crystal, R. G. (1995) Transfer of genes to humans: early lessons and obstacles to success. Science **270**(5235): 404–10.
Cuono, C. B. and S. Ariyan (1980) Immediate reconstruction of a composite mandibular defect with a regional osteomusculocutaneous flap. Plast Reconstr Surg **65**(4): 477–84.
Curey, J. D. (1962) Stress concentration in bone. Q J Microsc Sci **103**: 111–33.
Curtis, A. and C. Wilkinson (1997) Topographical control of cells. Biomaterials **18**(24): 1573–83.
Curtis, A. and C. Wilkinson (1999) New depths in cell behaviour: reactions of cells to nanotopography. Biochem Soc Symp **65**: 15–26.
Curtis, A. S., B. Casey, J. O. Gallagher, D. Pasqui, M. A. Wood and C. D. Wilkinson (2001) Substratum nanotopography and the adhesion of biological cells. Are symmetry or regularity of nanotopography important? Biophys Chem **94**(3): 275–83.
Curtis, A. and M. Riehle (2001) Tissue engineering: the biophysical background. Phys Med Biol **46**(4): R47–65.
Curtis, A. and C. Wilkinson (2001) Nanotechniques and approaches in biotechnology. Trends Biotechnol **19**(3): 97–101.
Cutler, S. M. and A. J. Garcia (2003) Engineering cell adhesive surfaces that direct integrin alpha5beta1 binding using a recombinant fragment of fibronectin. Biomaterials **24**(10): 1759–70.
Dahir, G. A., Q. Cui, P. Anderson, C. Simon, C. Joyner, J. T. Triffitt and G. Balian (2000) Pluripotential mesenchymal cells repopulate bone marrow and retain osteogenic properties. Clin Orthop Relat Res (379 Suppl): S134–45.
Dalby, M. J., L. Di Silvio, G. W. Davies and W. Bonfield (2000) Surface topography and HA filler volume effect on primary human osteoblasts in vitro. J Mater Sci Mater Med **11**(12): 805–10.
Dalby, M. J., M. O. Riehle, H. Johnstone, S. Affrossman and A. S. Curtis (2002) In vitro reaction of endothelial cells to polymer demixed nanotopography. Biomaterials **23**(14): 2945–54.
Damien, C. J. and J. R. Parsons (1991) Bone graft and bone graft substitutes: a review of current technology and applications. J Appl Biomater **2**(3): 187–208.
Damien, E., J. S. Price and L. E. Lanyon (1998) The estrogen receptor's involvement in osteoblasts' adaptive response to mechanical strain. J Bone Miner Res **13**(8): 1275–82.
Darling, E. M. and K. A. Athanasiou (2003) Articular cartilage bioreactors and bioprocesses. Tissue Eng **9**(1): 9–26.
Davies, J. E., B. Lowenberg and A. Shiga (1990) The bone-titanium interface in vitro. J Biomed Mater Res **24**(10): 1289–306.
Davisson, T., S. Kunig, A. Chen, R. Sah and A. Ratcliffe (2002) Static and dynamic compression modulate matrix metabolism in tissue engineered cartilage. J Orthop Res **20**(4): 842–8.
Davy, D. T. (1999) Biomechanical issues in bone transplantation. Orthop Clin North Am **30**(4): 553–63.
Dekker, A., K. Reitsma, T. Beugeling, A. Bantjes, J. Feijen and W. G. van Aken (1991) Adhesion of endothelial cells and adsorption of serum proteins on gas plasma-treated polytetrafluoroethylene. Biomaterials **12**(2): 130–8.
Delamarche, E., A. Bernard, H. Schmid, B. Michel and H. Biebuyck (1997) Patterned delivery of immunoglobulins to surfaces using microfluidic networks. Science **276**(5313): 779–81.

Delany, A. M., Y. Dong and E. Canalis (1994) Mechanisms of glucocorticoid action in bone cells. J Cell Biochem **56**(3): 295–302.

Demergasso, F. and M. V. Piazza (1979) Trapezius myocutaneous flap in reconstructive surgery for head and neck cancer: an original technique. Am J Surg **138**(4): 533–6.

Dempster, D. W., F. Cosman, M. Parisien, V. Shen and R. Lindsay (1993) Anabolic actions of parathyroid hormone on bone. Endocr Rev **14**(6): 690–709.

Dempster, D. W., F. Cosman, M. Parisien, V. Shen and R. Lindsay (1995) Anabolic actions of par athyroid hormone on bone: update 1995. In Bikle, D. D. and Negro-Vilar, A. (eds) Endocrine Reviews Monographs. 4. Hormonal Regulation of Bone Mineral Metabolism. The Endocrine Society, Bethesda, MD. 247–50.

den Dunnen, W. F., P. H. Robinson, R. van Wessel, A. J. Pennings, M. B. van Leeuwen and J. M. Schakenraad (1997) Long-term evaluation of degradation and foreign-body reaction of subcutaneously implanted poly(DL-lactide-epsilon-caprolactone). J Biomed Mater Res **36**(3): 337–46.

Deutsch, M., J. Meinhart, T. Fischlein, P. Preiss and P. Zilla (1999) Clinical autologous in vitro endothelialization of infrainguinal ePTFE grafts in 100 patients: a 9-year experience. Surgery **126**(5): 847–55.

Dhert, W. J., S. W. O'Driscoll, B. J. van Royen and R. B. Salter (1988) Effects of immobilization and continuous passive motion on postoperative muscle atrophy in mature rabbits. Can J Surg **31**(3): 185–8.

Di Silvio, L., M. J. Dalby and W. Bonfield (2002) Osteoblast behaviour on HA/PE composite surfaces with different HA volumes. Biomaterials **23**(1): 101–7.

Doherty, P. J., H. Zhang, L. Tremblay, V. Manolopoulos and K. W. Marshall (1998) Resurfacing of articular cartilage explants with genetically-modified human chondrocytes in vitro. Osteoarthritis Cartilage **6**(3): 153–9.

Domen, J., S. H. Cheshier and I. L. Weissman (2000) The role of apoptosis in the regulation of hematopoietic stem cells: Overexpression of Bcl-2 increases both their number and repopulation potential. J Exp Med **191**(2): 253–64.

Domke, J., S. Dannohl, W. J. Parak, O. Muller, W. K. Aicher and M. Radmacher (2000) Substrate dependent differences in morphology and elasticity of living osteoblasts investigated by atomic force microscopy. Colloids Surf B Biointerfaces **19**(4): 367–379.

Donzelli, P. S., R. L. Spilker, G. A. Ateshian and V. C. Mow (1999) Contact analysis of biphasic transversely isotropic cartilage layers and correlations with tissue failure. J Biomech **32**(10): 1037–47.

Dorling, A., K. Riesbeck and R. I. Lechler (1996) The T-cell response to xenografts: molecular interactions and graft-specific immunosuppression. Xeno **4**: 68–76.

dos Santos, L. F. (1984) The vascular anatomy and dissection of the free scapular flap. Plast Reconstr Surg **73**(4): 599–604.

Dowthwaite, G. P., J. C. Bishop, S. N. Redman, I. M. Khan, P. Rooney, D. J. Evans, L. Haughton, Z. Bayram, S. Boyer, B. Thomson, M. S. Wolfe and C. W. Archer (2004) The surface of articular cartilage contains a progenitor cell population. J Cell Sci **117**(Pt 6): 889–97.

Ducheyne, P. (1988) Titanium and calcium phosphate ceramic dental implants, surfaces, coatings and interfaces. J Oral Implantol **14**(3): 325–40.

Duncan, R. L. and C. H. Turner (1995) Mechanotransduction and the functional response of bone to mechanical strain. Calcif Tissue Int **57**(5): 344–58.

Ecarot-Charrier, B., F. H. Glorieux, M. van der Rest and G. Pereira (1983) Osteoblasts isolated from mouse calvaria initiate matrix mineralization in culture. J Cell Biol **96**(3): 639–43.

Egrise, D., D. Martin, A. Vienne, P. Neve and A. Schoutens (1992) The number of fibroblastic colonies formed from bone marrow is decreased and the in vitro proliferation rate of trabecular bone cells increased in aged rats. Bone **13**(5): 355–61.

Einhorn, T. A., R. J. Majeska, E. B. Rush, P. M. Levine and M. C. Horowitz (1995) The expression of cytokine activity by fracture callus. J Bone Miner Res **10**(8): 1272–81.

Einhorn, T. A. (1996) Biomechanics of bone. In Bilezikian, J., Raisz, L. and Rodan, G. (eds) Principles of Bone Biology. Academic Press, New York. 25–37.

Einhorn, T. A. (1999) Clinically applied models of bone regeneration in tissue engineering research. Clin Orthop Relat Res (367 Suppl): S59–67.

Einhorn, T. A. and C. A. Lee (2001) Bone regeneration: new findings and potential clinical applications. J Am Acad Orthop Surg **9**(3): 157–65.

Elema, H., J. H. de Groot, A. J. Nijenhuis, A. J. Pennings, R. P. Veth, J. Klompmaker and H. W. Jansen (1990) Use of biodegradable polymer implants in meniscus reconstruction. 2. Biological evaluation of porous biodegradable implants in menisci. Colloid Polym Sci **268**: 1082–8.

Elgendy, H. M., M. E. Norman, A. R. Keaton and C. T. Laurencin (1993) Osteoblast-like cell (MC3T3-E1) proliferation on bioerodible polymers: an approach towards the development of a bone-bioerodible polymer composite material. Biomaterials **14**(4): 263–9.

Elwing, H. (1998) Protein absorption and ellipsometry in biomaterial research. Biomaterials **19**(4–5): 397–406.

Enneking, W. F. and J. L. Morris (1972) Human autologous cortical bone transplants. Clin Orthop Relat Res **87**: 28–35.

Enneking, W. F., H. Burchardt, J. J. Puhl and G. Piotrowski (1975) Physical and biological aspects of repair in dog cortical-bone transplants. J Bone Joint Surg Am **57**(2): 237–52.

Erices, A., P. Conget and J. J. Minguell (2000) Mesenchymal progenitor cells in human umbilical cord blood. Br J Haematol **109**(1): 235–42.

Erikson, L. G. T., P. M. Cleasson, S. Ohnishi and M. Hato (1997) Stability of dimethyl-dioctadecylammonium bromide Langmuir–Blodgett films on mica in aqueous salt solutions – implications for surface force measurements. Thin Solid Films **300**: 240–55.

Esenwein, S. A., S. Esenwein, G. Herr, G. Muhr, W. Kusswetter and C. H. Hartwig (2003) [Histologic and histomorphometric follow–up observations of osseointegration of corundum–blasted BMP–3 coated titanium test implants (Ti6Al4V) at orthotopic site in the giant rabbit]. Biomed Tech (Berlin) **48**(7–8): 217–24.

Evans, S. D., T. M. Flynn and A. Ulman (1995) Self–assembled multilayer formation on predefined templates. Langmuir **11**: 3811–4.

Evans, C. H. and P. D. Robbins (1995) Possible orthopaedic applications of gene therapy. J Bone Joint Surg Am **77**(7): 1103–14.

Fang, J., Y. Y. Zhu, E. Smiley, J. Bonadio, J. P. Rouleau, S. A. Goldstein, L. K. McCauley, B. L. Davidson and B. J. Roessler (1996) Stimulation of new bone formation by direct transfer of osteogenic plasmid genes. Proc Natl Acad Sci USA **93**(12): 5753–8.

Fedchenko, F. (1996) Stereolithography and other RP&M Technologies, ASME Press, Dearborn. 2.

Fennis, J. P., P. J. Stoelinga and J. A. Jansen (2002) Mandibular reconstruction: a clinical and radiographic animal study on the use of autogenous scaffolds and platelet-rich plasma. Int J Oral Maxillofac Surg **31**(3): 281–6.

Ferguson, C., E. Alpern, T. Miclau and J. A. Helms (1999) Does adult fracture repair recapitulate embryonic skeletal formation? Mech Dev **87**(1–2): 57–66.

Ferrara, N. and T. Davis–Smyth (1997) The biology of vascular endothelial growth factor. Endocr Rev **18**(1): 4–25.

Ferre, J. C., R. Legoux, J. L. Helary, F. Albugues, C. Le Floc'h, J. Bouteyre, J. P. Lumineau, C. Chevalier, A. Y. Le Cloarec, E. Orio, et al. (1985) Study of the mandible under static constraints by holographic interferometry. New biomechanical deductions. Anat Clin **7**(3): 193–201.

Ferris, D. M., G. D. Moodie, P. M. Dimond, C. W. Gioranni, M. G. Ehrlich and R. F. Valentini (1999) RGD–coated titanium implants stimulate increased bone formation in vivo. Biomaterials **20**: 2323–31.

Findlay, M., J. Dolderer, J. Cooper-White, E. Thompson, A. Penington and W. A. Morrison (2003) Creating large amounts of tissue for reconstructive surgery – a porcine model. Aust N Z J Surg **73**: 240.

Fiorellini, J. P., S. P. Engebretson, K. Donath and H. P. Weber (1998) Guided bone regeneration utilizing expanded polytetrafluoroethylene membranes in combination with submerged and nonsubmerged dental implants in beagle dogs. J Periodontol **69**(5): 528–35.

Fisher, J. and M. B. Wood (1987) Experimental comparison of bone revascularization by musculocutaneous and cutaneous flaps. Plast Reconstr Surg **79**(1): 81–90.
Fodor, W. L. (2003) Tissue engineering and cell based therapies, from the bench to the clinic: the potential to replace, repair and regenerate. Reprod Biol Endocrinol **1**(1): 102.
Frank, E. H. and A. J. Grodzinsky (1987) Cartilage electromechanics – II. A continuum model of cartilage electrokinetics and correlation with experiments. J Biomech **20**(6): 629–39.
Freed, L. E., J. C. Marquis, A. Nohria, J. Emmanual, A. G. Mikos and R. Langer (1993) Neocartilage formation in vitro and in vivo using cells cultured on synthetic biodegradable polymers. J Biomed Mater Res **27**(1): 11–23.
Freed, L. E., D. A. Grande, Z. Lingbin, J. Emmanual, J. C. Marquis and R. Langer (1994) Joint resurfacing using allograft chondrocytes and synthetic biodegradable polymer scaffolds. J Biomed Mater Res **28**(8): 891–9.
Freed, L. E. and G. Vunjak-Novakovic (1997) Microgravity tissue engineering. In Vitro Cell Dev Biol Anim **33**(5): 381–5.
Freed, L. E., A. P. Hollander, I. Martin, J. R. Barry, R. Langer and G. Vunjak-Novakovic (1998) Chondrogenesis in a cell-polymer-bioreactor system. Exp Cell Res **240**(1): 58–65.
Frenz, D. A., W. Liu, J. D. Williams, V. Hatcher, V. Galinovic-Schwartz, K. C. Flanders and T. R. Van de Water (1994) Induction of chondrogenesis: requirement for synergistic interaction of basic fibroblast growth factor and transforming growth factor-beta. Development **120**(2): 415–24.
Friedenstein, A. J. (1976) Precursor cells of mechanocytes. Int Rev Cytol **47**: 327–59.
Friedman, C. D., P. D. Costantino, S. Takagi and L. C. Chow (1998) BoneSource hydroxyapatite cement: a novel biomaterial for craniofacial skeletal tissue engineering and reconstruction. J Biomed Mater Res **43**(4): 428–32.
Frodel, J. L., Jr., G. F. Funk, D. T. Capper, K. L. Fridrich, J. R. Blumer, J. R. Haller and H. T. Hoffman (1993) Osseointegrated implants: a comparative study of bone thickness in four vascularized bone flaps. Plast Reconstr Surg **92**(3): 449–55; discussion 456–8.
Frondoza, C. G., R. Z. LeGeros and D. S. Hungerford (1998) Effect of bovine bone derived materials on human osteoblast-like cells in vitro. In LeGeros, R. Z. and LeGeros, J. P. (eds) Bioceramics 11. World Scientific, Singapore, 289–91.
Frost, H. M. (1964a) Laws of Bone Structure. Charles C. Thomas, Springfield.
Frost, H. M. (1964b) Mathematical Elements of Lamellar Bone Remodeling. Charles C. Thomas, Springfield
Frost, H. M. (1983) The regional acceleratory phenomenon: a review. Henry Ford Hosp Med J **31**(1): 3–9.
Frost, H. M. (1986) Intermediary Organization of the Skeleton, Vols I and II. CRC Press, Boca Raton.
Frost, H. M. (1992) Perspectives: bone's mechanical usage windows. Bone Miner **19**(3): 257–71.
Frost, H. M. (1996) Perspectives: a proposed general model of the mechanostat (suggestions from a new skeletal-biologic paradigm) Anat Rec **244**(2): 139–47.
Frost, H. M. (2000a) The Utah paradigm of skeletal physiology: an overview of its insights for bone, cartilage and collagenous tissue organs. J Bone Miner Metab **18**(6): 305–16.
Frost, H. M. (2000b) Why the ISMNI and the Utah paradigm? Their role in skeletal and extraskeletal disorders. J Musculoskeletal Interactions **1**: 29–30.
Frost, H. M. and E. Schonau (2000) The muscle-bone unit in children and adolescents: a 2000 overview. J Pediatr Endocrinol Metab **13**(6): 571–90.
Frost, H. M., U. Meyer, U. Joos and O. T. Jensen (2002) Dental alveolar distraction and the Utah paradigm. In Jensen, O. T. (ed.) Alveolar distraction osteogenesis. Quintessence Publishing, Chicago.
Fukada, E. and I. Yasuda (1957) On the piezoelectric effect of bone. J Phys Soc **12**: 1158–62.
Fukuda, K. (2002) Molecular characterization of regenerated cardiomyocytes derived from adult mesenchymal stem cells. Congenit Anom (Kyoto) **42**(1): 1–9.
Fukumoto, T., J. W. Sperling, A. Sanyal, J. S. Fitzsimmons, G. G. Reinholz, C. A. Conover and S. W. O'Driscoll (2003) Combined effects of insulin-like growth factor-1 and transforming

growth factor-beta1 on periosteal mesenchymal cells during chondrogenesis in vitro. Osteoarthritis Cartilage **11**(1): 55–64.
Galletti, G., S. Gogolewski, G. Ussia and F. Farruggia (1989) Long-term patency of regenerated neoaortic wall following the implant of a fully biodegradable polyurethane prosthesis: experimental lipid diet model in pigs. Ann Vasc Surg **3**(3): 236–43.
Gao, J., J. E. Dennis, L. A. Solchaga, A. S. Awadallah, V. M. Goldberg and A. I. Caplan (2001) Tissue-engineered fabrication of an osteochondral composite graft using rat bone marrow-derived mesenchymal stem cells. Tissue Eng **7**(4): 363–71.
Garcia, A. J. and B. G. Keselowsky (2002) Biomimetic surfaces for control of cell adhesion to facilitate bone formation. Crit Rev Eukaryot Gene Expr **12**(2): 151–62.
Garfein, E. S., D. P. Orgill and J. J. Pribaz (2003) Clinical applications of tissue engineered constructs. Clin Plast Surg **30**(4): 485–98.
Gatti, A., R. Z. LeGeros, E. Monari and e. al. (1998) Preliminary in vivo evaluation of synthetic CaP materials. In LeGeros, R. Z. and LeGeros, J. P. (eds) Bioceramics 11. World Scientific, Singapore, 399–402.
Gau, H., S. Herminghaus, P. Lenz and R. Lipowsky (1999) Liquid morphologies on structured surfaces: from microchannels to microchips. Science **283**(5398): 46–9.
Geiger, B., K. T. Tokuyasu, A. H. Dutton and S. J. Singer (1980) Vinculin, an intracellular protein localized at specialized sites where microfilament bundles terminate at cell membranes. Proc Natl Acad Sci USA **77**(7): 4127–31.
Gelse, K., K. von der Mark and H. Schneider (2003) Cartilage regeneration by gene therapy. Curr Gene Ther **3**(4): 305–17.
Gerber, H. P. and N. Ferrara (2000) Angiogenesis and bone growth. Trends Cardiovasc Med **10**(5): 223–8.
Gerstenfeld, L. C., D. M. Cullinane, G. L. Barnes, D. T. Graves and T. A. Einhorn (2003a) Fracture healing as a post-natal developmental process: molecular, spatial, and temporal aspects of its regulation. J Cell Biochem **88**(5): 873–84.
Gerstenfeld, L. C., M. Thiede, K. Seibert, C. Mielke, D. Phippard, B. Svagr, D. Cullinane and T. A. Einhorn (2003b) Differential inhibition of fracture healing by non-selective and cyclooxygenase-2 selective non-steroidal anti-inflammatory drugs. J Orthop Res **21**(4): 670–5.
Giannoni, P., M. Siegrist, E. B. Hunziker and M. Wong (2003) The mechanosensitivity of cartilage oligomeric matrix protein (COMP) Biorheology **40**(1–3): 101–9.
Gilbert, D. M. (2004) The future of human embryonic stem cell research: addressing ethical conflict with responsible scientific research. Med Sci Monit **10**(5): RA99–103.
Girdler, N. M. and M. Hosseini (1992) Orbital floor reconstruction with autogenous bone harvested from the mandibular lingual cortex. Br J Oral Maxillofac Surg **30**(1): 36–8.
Gleiche, M., L. F. Chi and H. Fuchs (2000) Nanoscopic channel lattices with controlled anisotropic wetting. Nature **403**(6766): 173–5.
Globus, R. K., S. B. Doty, J. C. Lull, E. Holmuhamedov, M. J. Humphries and C. H. Damsky (1998) Fibronectin is a survival factor for differentiated osteoblasts. J Cell Sci **111 (Pt 10)**: 1385–93.
Glowacki, J. (1998) Angiogenesis in fracture repair. Clin Orthop Relat Res (355 Suppl): 82–9.
Gogolewski, S. and A. J. Pennings (1982) Biodegradable materials of polylactides. IV. Porous biomedical materials based on mixtures of polylactides and polyurethanes. Macromol Chem Rapid Commun **3**: 839–45.
Gogolewski, S. and A. J. Pennings (1983) An artificial skin based on biodegradable mixtures of polylactides and polyurethanes for full thickness wound covering. Macromol Chem Rapid Commun **4**: 675–80.
Gogolewski, S., A. J. Pennings, E. Lommen, P. Nieuwenhuis and C. R. H. Wildevuur (1983) Growth of a neo-artery induced by a biodegradable polymeric vascular prosthesis. Macromol Chem Rapid Commun **4**: 213–9.
Gogolewski, S. and G. Galletti (1986) Degradable vascular prosthesis from segmented polyurethanes. Colloid Polym Sci **264**: 854–8.

Gogolewski, S., G. Galletti and G. Ussia (1987a) Polyurethane vascular prosthesis in pigs. Colloid Polym Sci **265**: 774–8.

Gogolewski, S., B. Walpoth and P. Rheiner (1987b) Polyurethane microporous membranes as pericardial substitutes. Colloid Polym Sci **265**: 971–7.

Gogolewski, S., K. Gorna, B. Rahn and R. Wieling (2001) Biodegradable polyurethane cancellous bone graft substitute promotes bone regeneration in the iliac crest defects. Transactions 24, 573, 27th Annual Meeting, Society for Biomaterials, Saint Paul, MN, USA.

Gogolewski, S., K. Gorna and A. S. Turner (2002) Regeneration of bicortical defects in the iliac crest of estrogen deficient sheep using new biodegradable polyurethane cancellous bone graft substitutes. A pilot study. 48th Annual Meeting, Orthopaedic Research Society, Dallas, TX, USA.

Goldsborough, M. D., M. L. Tilkins, P. J. Price, J. Lobo-Alfonso, J. R. Morrison and M. E. Stevens (1998) Serum-free culture of murine embryonic stem (ES) cells. Focus **20**: 8–12.

Gomes, M. E., A. S. Ribeiro, P. B. Malafaya, R. L. Reis and A. M. Cunha (2001) A new approach based on injection moulding to produce biodegradable starch-based polymeric scaffolds: morphology, mechanical and degradation behaviour. Biomaterials **22**(9): 883–9.

Gomes, M. E., J. S. Godinho, D. Tchalamov, A. M. Cunha and R. L. Reis (2002a) Alternative tissue engineering scaffolds based on starch: processing methodologies, morphology, degradation and mechanical properties. Mater Sci Eng C **20**(1–2): 19–26.

Gomes, M. E., A. J. Salgado and R. L. Reis (2002b) Polymer Based Systems on Tissue Engineering, Replacement and Regeneration, 1st edn, Kluwer, Dordrecht, The Netherlands, 221.

Gomes, R. R., Jr., M. C. Farach-Carson and D. D. Carson (2004) Perlecan functions in chondrogenesis: insights from in vitro and in vivo models. Cells Tissues Organs **176**(1–3): 79–86.

Goomer, R. S., T. M. Maris, R. Gelberman, M. Boyer, M. Silva and D. Amiel (2000) Nonviral in vivo gene therapy for tissue engineering of articular cartilage and tendon repair. Clin Orthop Relat Res (379 Suppl): S189–200.

Goomer, R. S., L. J. Deftos, R. Terkeltaub, T. Maris, M. C. Lee, F. L. Harwood and D. Amiel (2001) High-efficiency non-viral transfection of primary chondrocytes and perichondrial cells for ex-vivo gene therapy to repair articular cartilage defects. Osteoarthritis Cartilage **9**(3): 248–56.

Gowen, M., D. D. Wood, E. J. Ihrie, M. K. McGuire and R. G. Russell (1983) An interleukin 1 like factor stimulates bone resorption in vitro. Nature **306**(5941): 378–80.

Grad, S., L. Zhou, S. Gogolewski and M. Alini (2003) Chondrocytes seeded onto poly (L/DL-lactide) 80%/20% porous scaffolds: a biochemical evaluation. J Biomed Mater Res A **66**(3): 571–9.

Grande, D. A., C. Halberstadt, G. Naughton, R. Schwartz and R. Manji (1997) Evaluation of matrix scaffolds for tissue engineering of articular cartilage grafts. J Biomed Mater Res **34**(2): 211–20.

Granet, C., N. Laroche, L. Vico, C. Alexandre and M. H. Lafage-Proust (1998) Rotating-wall vessels, promising bioreactors for osteoblastic cell culture: comparison with other 3D conditions. Med Biol Eng Comput **36**(4): 513–9.

Granick, M. S., S. S. Ramasastry, E. D. Newton, M. P. Solomon, D. C. Hanna and S. Kaltman (1990) Reconstruction of complex maxillectomy defects with the scapular-free flap. Head Neck **12**(5): 377–85.

Green, M. F., J. R. Gibson, J. R. Bryson and E. Thomson (1981) A one-stage correction of mandibular defects using a split sternum pectoralis major osteo-musculocutaneous transfer. Br J Plast Surg **34**(1): 11–6.

Griffith, L. G. and G. Naughton (2002) Tissue engineering – current challenges and expanding opportunities. Science **295**(5557): 1009–14.

Grigoriadis, A. E., J. N. Heersche and J. E. Aubin (1988) Differentiation of muscle, fat, cartilage, and bone from progenitor cells present in a bone-derived clonal cell population: effect of dexamethasone. J Cell Biol **106**(6): 2139–51.

Groessner-Schreiber, B. and R. S. Tuan (1992) Enhanced extracellular matrix production and mineralization by osteoblasts cultured on titanium surfaces in vitro. J Cell Sci **101 (Pt 1)**: 209–17.

Gross, D. and W. S. Williams (1982) Streaming potential and the electromechanical response of physiologically-moist bone. J Biomech **15**(4): 277–95.

Grundel, R. E., M. W. Chapman, T. Yee and D. C. Moore (1991) Autogeneic bone marrow and porous biphasic calcium phosphate ceramic for segmental bone defects in the canine ulna. Clin Orthop Relat Res (266): 244–58.

Guan, K., H. Chang, A. Rolletschek and A. M. Wobus (2001) Embryonic stem cell–derived neurogenesis. Retinoic acid induction and lineage selection of neuronal cells. Cell Tissue Res **305**(2): 171–6.

Gugala, Z. and S. Gogolewski (2000) In vitro growth and activity of primary chondrocytes on a resorbable polylactide three-dimensional scaffold. J Biomed Mater Res **49**(2): 183–91.

Guilak, F. (1995) Compression-induced changes in the shape and volume of the chondrocyte nucleus. J Biomech **28**(12): 1529–41.

Guilak, F., A. Ratcliffe and V. C. Mow (1995) Chondrocyte deformation and local tissue strain in articular cartilage: a confocal microscopy study. J Orthop Res **13**(3): 410–21.

Guilak, F., R. L. Sah and L. A. Setton (1997) Physical regulation of cartilage metabolism. In: Mow, V. C. and Hayes, W. C. (eds) Basic Orthopaedic Biomechanics. Lippincott–Raven, Philadelphia, 179–207.

Guilak, F., W. R. Jones, H. P. Ting–Beall and G. M. Lee (1999) The deformation behavior and mechanical properties of chondrocytes in articular cartilage. Osteoarthritis Cartilage **7**(1): 59–70.

Guilak, F. and V. C. Mow (2000) The mechanical environment of the chondrocyte: a biphasic finite element model of cell–matrix interactions in articular cartilage. J Biomech **33**(12): 1663–73.

Guilak, F., D. L. Butler and S. A. Goldstein (2001) Functional tissue engineering: the role of biomechanics in articular cartilage repair. Clin Orthop Relat Res (391 Suppl): S295–305.

Guilak, F., B. Fermor, F. J. Keefe, V. B. Kraus, S. A. Olson, D. S. Pisetsky, L. A. Setton and J. B. Weinberg (2004) The role of biomechanics and inflammation in cartilage injury and repair. Clin Orthop Relat Res (423): 17–26.

Guillamondegui, O. M. and D. L. Larson (1981) The lateral trapezius musculocutaneous flap: its use in head and neck reconstruction. Plast Reconstr Surg **67**(2): 143–50.

Guldberg, R. E. (2002) Consideration of mechanical factors. Ann NY Acad Sci **961**: 312–4.

Gundle, R., C. J. Joyner and J. T. Triffitt (1995) Human bone tissue formation in diffusion chamber culture in vivo by bone–derived cells and marrow stromal fibroblastic cells. Bone **16**(6): 597–601.

Gutierrez-Rodriguez, M., E. Reyes-Maldonado and H. Mayani (2000) Characterization of the adherent cells developed in Dexter-type long-term cultures from human umbilical cord blood. Stem Cells **18**(1): 46–52.

Gutowska, A., B. Jeong and M. Jasionowski (2001) Injectable gels for tissue engineering. Anat Rec **263**(4): 342–9.

Hall, B. K. and T. Miyake (1992) The membranous skeleton: the role of cell condensations in vertebrate skeletogenesis. Anat Embryol (Berlin) **186**(2): 107–24.

Hallgren, C., H. Reimers, J. Gold and A. Wennerberg (2001) The importance of surface texture for bone integration of screw shaped implants: an in vivo study of implants patterned by photolithography. J Biomed Mater Res **57**(4): 485–96.

Ham, A. W. (1969) Histology. J. B. Lippincott Co., Philadelphia, 247.

Hammerle, C. H., G. C. Chiantella, T. Karring and N. P. Lang (1998) The effect of a deproteinized bovine bone mineral on bone regeneration around titanium dental implants. Clin Oral Implants Res **9**(3): 151–62.

Han, H. C. and Y. C. Fung (1995) Longitudinal strain of canine and porcine aortas. J Biomech **28**(5): 637–41.

Handschel, J., H. P. Wiesmann, U. Stratmann, J. Kleinheinz, U. Meyer and U. Joos (2002) TCP is hardly resorbed and not osteoconductive in a non-loading calvarial model. Biomaterials **23**(7): 1689–95.

Hannallah, D., B. Peterson, J. R. Lieberman, F. H. Fu and J. Huard (2002) Gene therapy in orthopaedic surgery. J Bone Joint Surg Am **84**(6): 1046–1061.

Harlan, D. M., C. L. Karp, P. Matzinger, D. H. Munn, R. M. Ransohoff and D. W. Metzger (2002) Immunological concerns with bioengineering approaches. Ann NY Acad Sci **961**: 323–30.

Harris, W. H., E. A. Haywood, J. Lavorgna and D. L. Hamblen (1968) Spatial and temporal variation in cortical bone formation in dogs: a long term study. J Bone Joint Surg **50**: 1118–28.

Hart, R. T., V. V. Hennebel, N. Thongpreda, W. C. Van Buskirk and R. C. Anderson (1992) Modeling the biomechanics of the mandible: a three-dimensional finite element study. J Biomech **25**(3): 261–86.

Harter, L. V., K. A. Hruska and R. L. Duncan (1995) Human osteoblast-like cells respond to mechanical strain with increased bone matrix protein production independent of hormonal regulation. Endocrinology **136**(2): 528–35.

Hartgerink, J. D., E. Beniash and S. I. Stupp (2001) Self-assembly and mineralization of peptide-amphiphile nanofibers. Science **294**(5547): 1684–8.

Hartig, M., U. Joos and H. P. Wiesmann (2000) Capacitively coupled electric fields accelerate proliferation of osteoblast-like primary cells and increase bone extracellular matrix formation in vitro. Eur Biophys J **29**(7): 499–506.

Hartwig, C. H., S. A. Esenwein, A. Pfund, W. K. Dagger and G. Herr (2003) [Improved osseointegration of titanium implants of different surface characteristics by the use of bone morphogenetic protein (BMP–3): an animal study performed at the metaphyseal bone bed in dogs]. Z Orthop Ihre Grenzgeb **141**(6): 705–11.

Hastings, G. W. and F. A. Mahmud (1988) Electrical effects in bone. J Biomed Eng **10**(6): 515–21.

Hattori, T. and H. Ide (1984) Limb bud chondrogenesis in cell culture, with particular reference to serum concentration in the culture medium. Exp Cell Res **150**(2): 338–46.

Hauselmann, H. J., T. Flura, C. Marti, N. Hauser and E. Hedbom (1998) [From chondrocyte culture to joint cartilage replacement. Development of de novo cartilage in vitro]. Schweiz Med Wochenschr **128**(21): 824–32.

Hayashi, S., T. Yamane, A. Miyamoto, H. Hemmi, H. Tagaya, Y. Tanio, H. Kanda, H. Yamazaki and T. Kunisada (1998) Commitment and differentiation of stem cells to the osteoclast lineage. Biochem Cell Biol **76**(6): 911–22.

Hayes, D. W., Jr. and R. K. Averett (2001) Articular cartilage transplantation. Current and future limitations and solutions. Clin Podiatr Med Surg **18**(1): 161–76.

Haynesworth, S. E., J. Goshima, V. M. Goldberg and A. I. Caplan (1992) Characterization of cells with osteogenic potential from human marrow. Bone **13**(1): 81–8.

Hellman, K. B. (1997) Bioartificial organs as outcomes of tissue engineering. Scientific and regulatory issues. Ann NY Acad Sci **831**: 1–9.

Hidalgo, D. A. (1989) Fibula free flap: a new method of mandible reconstruction. Plast Reconstr Surg **84**(1): 71–9.

Higginson, G. R. and J. Snaith (1979) The mechanical stiffness of articular cartilage in confined oscillating compression. Eng Med **8**: 11–4.

Hillsley, M. V. and J. A. Frangos (1994) Bone tissue engineering: the role of interstitial fluid flow. Biotechnol Bioeng **43**(7): 573–81.

Hiltunen, A., H. T. Aro and E. Vuorio (1993) Regulation of extracellular matrix genes during fracture healing in mice. Clin Orthop Relat Res (297): 23–7.

Hing, K. A. (2004) Bone repair in the twenty–first century: biology, chemistry or engineering? Philos Trans A Math Phys Eng Sci **362**(1825): 2821–50.

Hirschi, K. K., T. C. Skalak, S. M. Peirce and C. D. Little (2002) Vascular assembly in natural and engineered tissues. Ann NY Acad Sci **961**: 223–42.

Hodge, W. A., K. L. Carlson, R. S. Fijan, R. G. Burgess, P. O. Riley, W. H. Harris and R. W. Mann (1989) Contact pressures from an instrumented hip endoprosthesis. J Bone Joint Surg Am **71**(9): 1378–86.

Hogan, B. L. (1996) Bone morphogenetic proteins: multifunctional regulators of vertebrate development. Genes Dev **10**(13): 1580–94.

Höhling, H. J., R. H. Barckhaus, E. R. Krefting, J. Althoff and P. Quint (1990) Collagen mineralization: aspects of the structural relationships between collagen and the apatitic crystallites. In Bonucci, E. and Motte, P. M. (eds) Ultrastructure of Skeletal Tissues. Academic Press, 41–62.

Höhling, H. J., S. Arnold, R. H. Barckhaus, U. Plate and H. P. Wiesmann (1995) Structural relationship between the primary crystal formations and the matrix macromolecules in different hard tissues. Discussion of a general principle. Connect Tissue Res **33**(1–3): 171–8.

Holmes, R. E. (1979) Bone regeneration within a coralline hydroxyapatite implant. Plast Reconstr Surg **63**(5): 626–33.

Holmvall, K., L. Camper, S. Johansson, J. H. Kimura and E. Lundgren-Akerlund (1995) Chondrocyte and chondrosarcoma cell integrins with affinity for collagen type II and their response to mechanical stress. Exp Cell Res **221**(2): 496–503.

Holy, C. E., M. S. Shoichet and J. E. Davies (2000) Engineering three-dimensional bone tissue in vitro using biodegradable scaffolds: investigating initial cell-seeding density and culture period. J Biomed Mater Res **51**(3): 376–82.

Horton, W. A. (1993) Morphology of connective tissue: cartilage. In Royce, R. N. and Steinmann, B. (eds.) Connective Tissue and its Heritable Disorders. Molecular Genetic, and Medical Aspects. Wiley-Liss, New York, 73–84.

Hsu, H., D. L. Lacey, C. R. Dunstan, I. Solovyev, A. Colombero, E. Timms, H. L. Tan, G. Elliott, M. J. Kelley, I. Sarosi, L. Wang, X. Z. Xia, R. Elliott, L. Chiu, T. Black, S. Scully, C. Capparelli, S. Morony, G. Shimamoto, M. B. Bass and W. J. Boyle (1999) Tumor necrosis factor receptor family member RANK mediates osteoclast differentiation and activation induced by osteoprotegerin ligand. Proc Natl Acad Sci USA **96**(7): 3540–5.

Huang, H., Y. Zhao, Z. Liu, Y. Zhang, H. Zhang, T. Fu and X. Ma (2003) Enhanced osteoblast functions on RGD immobilized surface. J Oral Implantol **29**(2): 73–9.

Hubbell, J. A. (2003) Materials as morphogenetic guides in tissue engineering. Curr Opin Biotechnol **14**(5): 551–8.

Hung, C. T., R. L. Mauck, C. C. Wang, E. G. Lima and G. A. Ateshian (2004) A paradigm for functional tissue engineering of articular cartilage via applied physiologic deformational loading. Ann Biomed Eng **32**(1): 35–49.

Hunt, T. R., J. R. Schwappach and H. C. Anderson (1996) Healing of a segmental defect in the rat femur with use of an extract from a cultured human osteosarcoma cell-line (Saos-2). A preliminary report. J Bone Joint Surg Am **78**(1): 41–8.

Hunziker, E. B. (1992) Articular cartilage structure in humans and experimental animals. In Kuettner, K. E., Schleyerbach, R., Peyron, J. G., Hascall and V. C. (eds) Articular Cartilage and Osteoarthritis. Raven Press, Raven Press, 183–99.

Hunziker, E. B. (1994) Mechanism of longitudinal bone growth and its regulation by growth plate chondrocytes. Microsc Res Tech **28**(6): 505–19.

Hunziker, E. B. (1999) Biologic repair of articular cartilage. Defect models in experimental animals and matrix requirements. Clin Orthop Relat Res (367 Suppl): S135–46.

Hunziker, E. B. (2002) Articular cartilage repair: basic science and clinical progress. A review of the current status and prospects. Osteoarthritis Cartilage **10**(6): 432–63.

Hurle, J. M., Y. Ganan and D. Macias (1989) Experimental analysis of the in vivo chondrogenic potential of the interdigital mesenchyme of the chick leg bud subjected to local ectodermal removal. Dev Biol **132**(2): 368–74.

Hutmacher, D. W. (2000) Scaffolds in tissue engineering bone and cartilage. Biomaterials **21**(24): 2529–43.

Hutmacher, D. W. (2001) Scaffold design and fabrication technologies for engineering tissues–state of the art and future perspectives. J Biomater Sci Polym Ed **12**(1): 107–24.

Hutmacher, D. W., J. C. Goh and S. H. Teoh (2001a) An introduction to biodegradable materials for tissue engineering applications. Ann Acad Med Singapore **30**(2): 183–91.

Hutmacher, D. W., T. Schantz, I. Zein, K. W. Ng, S. H. Teoh and K. C. Tan (2001b) Mechanical properties and cell cultural response of polycaprolactone scaffolds designed and fabricated via fused deposition modeling. J Biomed Mater Res **55**(2): 203–16.

Hutmacher, D. W. and M. Sittinger (2003) Periosteal cells in bone tissue engineering. Tissue Eng **9 Suppl 1**: S45–64.

Ikeda, T., T. Kubo, T. Nakanishi, Y. Arai, K. Kobayashi, O. Mazda, S. Ohashi, K. Takahashi, J. Imanishi, M. Takigawa and Y. Hirasawa (2000) Ex vivo gene delivery using an adenovirus vector in treatment for cartilage defects. J Rheumatol **27**(4): 990–6.

Ilizarov, G. A. (1992) The Transosseous Osteosynthesis. Theoretical and Clinical Aspects of the Regeneration and Growth of Tissue. Springer, New York.

Im, G. I., D. Y. Kim, J. H. Shin, C. W. Hyun and W. H. Cho (2001) Repair of cartilage defect in the rabbit with cultured mesenchymal stem cells from bone marrow. J Bone Joint Surg Br **83**(2): 289–94.

Ishida, Y. and J. N. Heersche (1998) Glucocorticoid-induced osteoporosis: both in vivo and in vitro concentrations of glucocorticoids higher than physiological levels attenuate osteoblast differentiation. J Bone Miner Res **13**(12): 1822–6.

Ivanovic, Z., B. Bartolozzi, P. A. Bernabei, M. G. Cipolleschi, E. Rovida, P. Milenkovic, V. Praloran and P. Dello Sbarba (2000) Incubation of murine bone marrow cells in hypoxia ensures the maintenance of marrow-repopulating ability together with the expansion of committed progenitors. Br J Haematol **108**(2): 424–9.

Jackson, I. T., L. R. Scheker, J. G. Vandervord and J. G. McLennan (1981) Bone marrow grafting in the secondary closure of alveolar-palatal defects in children. Br J Plast Surg **34**(4): 422–5.

Jaiswal, N., S. E. Haynesworth, A. I. Caplan and S. P. Bruder (1997) Osteogenic differentiation of purified, culture-expanded human mesenchymal stem cells in vitro. J Cell Biochem **64**(2): 295–312.

Jaquiery, C., D. Rohner, C. Kunz, P. Bucher, F. Peters, R. K. Schenk and B. Hammer (2004) Reconstruction of maxillary and mandibular defects using prefabricated microvascular fibular grafts and osseointegrated dental implants – a prospective study. Clin Oral Implants Res **15**(5): 598–606.

Jargiello, D. M. and A. I. Caplan (1983) The establishment of vascular-derived microenvironments in the developing chick wing. Dev Biol **97**(2): 364–74.

Jarrell, B. E., S. K. Williams, G. Stokes, F. A. Hubbard, R. A. Carabasi, E. Koolpe, D. Greener, K. Pratt, M. J. Moritz, J. Radomski, et al. (1986) Use of freshly isolated capillary endothelial cells for the immediate establishment of a monolayer on a vascular graft at surgery. Surgery **100**(2): 392–9.

Jayaraman, M., U. Meyer, M. Buhner, U. Joos and H. P. Wiesmann (2004) Influence of titanium surfaces on attachment of osteoblast-like cells in vitro. Biomaterials **25**(4): 625–31.

Jeansonne, B. G., F. F. Feagin, R. W. McMinn, R. L. Shoemaker and W. S. Rehm (1979) Cell-to-cell communication of osteoblasts. J Dent Res **58**(4): 1415–23.

Jee, W. S. S. (1999) The interactions of muscles and skeletal tissue. In Lyritis, G. P. (ed.) Musculoskeletal Interactions, Vol. II. Hylonome, Athens, 35–46.

Jenkins, D. D., G. P. Yang, H. P. Lorenz, M. T. Longaker and K. G. Sylvester (2003) Tissue engineering and regenerative medicine. Clin Plast Surg **30**(4): 581–8.

Johnstone, B., T. M. Hering, A. I. Caplan, V. M. Goldberg and J. U. Yoo (1998) In vitro chondrogenesis of bone marrow-derived mesenchymal progenitor cells. Exp Cell Res **238**(1): 265–72.

Jones, D. B., H. Nolte, J. G. Scholubbers, E. Turner and D. Veltel (1991) Biochemical signal transduction of mechanical strain in osteoblast-like cells. Biomaterials **12**(2): 101–10.

Jones, D., G. Leivseth and J. Tenbosch (1995) Mechano-reception in osteoblast-like cells. Biochem Cell Biol **73**(7–8): 525–34.

Jones, D. B., E. Broeckmann, T. Pohl and E. L. Smith (2003) Development of a mechanical testing and loading system for trabecular bone studies for long term culture. Eur Cell Mater **5**: 48–59; discussion 59–60.

Joyce, M. E., S. Jingushi and M. E. Bolander (1990) Transforming growth factor-beta in the regulation of fracture repair. Orthop Clin North Am **21**(1): 199–209.

Joyner, C. J., A. Bennett and J. T. Triffitt (1997) Identification and enrichment of human osteoprogenitor cells by using differentiation stage-specific monoclonal antibodies. Bone **21**(1): 1–6.

Jung, D. R., R. Kapur, T. Adams, K. A. Giuliano, M. Mrksich, H. G. Craighead and D. L. Taylor (2001) Topographical and physicochemical modification of material surface to enable patterning of living cells. Crit Rev Biotechnol **21**(2): 111–54.

Juppner, H. (2000) Role of parathyroid hormone-related peptide and Indian hedgehog in skeletal development. Pediatr Nephrol **14**(7): 606–11.

Kale, S. and M. W. Long (2000) Osteopoiesis: the early development of bone cells. Crit Rev Eukaryot Gene Expr **10**(3–4): 259–71.

Kamakura, S., Y. Sasano, H. Homma, O. Suzuki, M. Kagayama and K. Motegi (1999) Implantation of octacalcium phosphate (OCP) in rat skull defects enhances bone repair. J Dent Res **78**(11): 1682–7.

Kandziora, F., G. Schmidmaier, G. Schollmeier, H. Bail, R. Pflugmacher, T. Gorke, M. Wagner, M. Raschke, T. Mittlmeier and N. P. Haas (2002) IGF–I and TGF–beta1 application by a poly-(D,L-lactide)-coated cage promotes intervertebral bone matrix formation in the sheep cervical spine. Spine **27**(16): 1710–23.

Kang, R., T. Marui, S. C. Ghivizzani, I. M. Nita, H. I. Georgescu, J. K. Suh, P. D. Robbins and C. H. Evans (1997) Ex vivo gene transfer to chondrocytes in full-thickness articular cartilage defects: a feasibility study. Osteoarthritis Cartilage **5**(2): 139–43.

Karp, J. M., M. S. Shoichet and J. E. Davies (2003) Bone formation on two-dimensional poly(DL-lactide-co-glycolide) (PLGA) films and three-dimensional PLGA tissue engineering scaffolds in vitro. J Biomed Mater Res A **64**(2): 388–96.

Karsenty, G. and E. F. Wagner (2002) Reaching a genetic and molecular understanding of skeletal development. Dev Cell **2**(4): 389–406.

Katagiri, T. and N. Takahashi (2002) Regulatory mechanisms of osteoblast and osteoclast differentiation. Oral Dis **8**(3): 147–59.

Kaufman, M. R. and G. W. Tobias (2003) Engineering cartilage growth and development. Clin Plast Surg **30**(4): 539–46.

Kaushal, S., G. E. Amiel, K. J. Guleserian, O. M. Shapira, T. Perry, F. W. Sutherland, E. Rabkin, A. M. Moran, F. J. Schoen, A. Atala, S. Soker, J. Bischoff and J. E. Mayer, Jr. (2001) Functional small-diameter neovessels created using endothelial progenitor cells expanded ex vivo. Nat Med **7**(9): 1035–40.

Kawamura, H., A. Ito, S. Miyakawa, P. Layrolle, K. Ojima, N. Ichinose and T. Tateishi (2000) Stimulatory effect of zinc-releasing calcium phosphate implant on bone formation in rabbit femora. J Biomed Mater Res **50**(2): 184–90.

Kawashima, K., R. Shibata, Y. Negishi and H. Endo (1998) Stimulative effect of high-level hypergravity on differentiated functions of osteoblast-like cells. Cell Struct Funct **23**(4): 221–9.

Kay, S., A. Thapa, K. M. Haberstroh and T. J. Webster (2002) Nanostructured polymer/nanophase ceramic composites enhance osteoblast and chondrocyte adhesion. Tissue Eng **8**(5): 753–61.

Kazimiroff, J., S. R. Frankel and R. Z. LeGeros (1996) Bone/biomaterial interface: autoradiographic assessment. In Kokubo, T., Nakamura, T. and Mijaji, F. (eds) Bioceramics 9. Elsevier, London, 169–72.

Kelm, J. M. and M. Fussenegger (2004) Microscale tissue engineering using gravity-enforced cell assembly. Trends Biotechnol **22**(4): 195–202.

Keser, A., M. Bozkurt, O. F. Taner, M. Akan and O. Sensoz (2004) Prefabrication of bone by vascular induction: an experimental study in rabbits. Scand J Plast Reconstr Surg Hand Surg **38**(5): 257–60.

Kim, H. K., M. E. Moran and R. B. Salter (1991) The potential for regeneration of articular cartilage in defects created by chondral shaving and subchondral abrasion. An experimental investigation in rabbits. J Bone Joint Surg Am **73**(9): 1301–15.

Kim, W. S., J. P. Vacanti, L. Cima, D. Mooney, J. Upton, W. C. Puelacher and C. A. Vacanti (1994) Cartilage engineered in predetermined shapes employing cell transplantation on synthetic biodegradable polymers. Plast Reconstr Surg **94**(2): 233–7; discussion 238–40.

Kim, E., Y. Xia and G. M. Whitesides (1995) Polymer microstructures formed by moulding in capillaries. Nature **376**: 581–4.

Kim, B. S. and D. J. Mooney (1998) Engineering smooth muscle tissue with a predefined structure. J Biomed Mater Res **41**(2): 322–32.

Kim, B. J., J. H. Seo, J. K. Bubien and Y. S. Oh (2002) Differentiation of adult bone marrow stem cells into neuroprogenitor cells in vitro. Neuroreport **13**(9): 1185–8.

Kimble, R. B., J. L. Vannice, D. C. Bloedow, R. C. Thompson, W. Hopfer, V. T. Kung, C. Brownfield and R. Pacifici (1994) Interleukin-1 receptor antagonist decreases bone loss and bone resorption in ovariectomized rats. J Clin Invest **93**(5): 1959–67.

Kimble, R. B., S. Bain and R. Pacifici (1997) The functional block of TNF but not of IL-6 prevents bone loss in ovariectomized mice. J Bone Miner Res **12**(6): 935–41.

Kirsch, T., G. Harrison, K. P. Worch and E. E. Golub (2000) Regulatory roles of zinc in matrix vesicle-mediated mineralization of growth plate cartilage. J Bone Miner Res **15**(2): 261–70.

Klamut, H. J., S. T. Chen, K. H. Lau and D. J. Baylink (2004) Progress toward skeletal gene therapy. Crit Rev Eukaryot Gene Expr **14**(1–2): 89–136.

Klompmaker, J., H. W. Jansen, R. P. Veth, J. H. de Groot, A. J. Nijenhuis and A. J. Pennings (1991) Porous polymer implant for repair of meniscal lesions: a preliminary study in dogs. Biomaterials **12**(9): 810–16.

Knott, L. and A. J. Bailey (1998) Collagen cross-links in mineralizing tissues: a review of their chemistry, function, and clinical relevance. Bone **22**(3): 181–7.

Knudson, W., D. J. Aguiar, Q. Hua and C. B. Knudson (1996) CD44-anchored hyaluronan-rich pericellular matrices: an ultrastructural and biochemical analysis. Exp Cell Res **228**(2): 216–28.

Kon, E., A. Muraglia, A. Corsi, P. Bianco, M. Marcacci, I. Martin, A. Boyde, I. Ruspantini, P. Chistolini, M. Rocca, R. Giardino, R. Cancedda and R. Quarto (2000) Autologous bone marrow stromal cells loaded onto porous hydroxyapatite ceramic accelerate bone repair in critical-size defects of sheep long bones. J Biomed Mater Res **49**(3): 328–37.

Kong, Y. Y., H. Yoshida, I. Sarosi, H. L. Tan, E. Timms, C. Capparelli, S. Morony, A. J. Oliveira-dos-Santos, G. Van, A. Itie, W. Khoo, A. Wakeham, C. R. Dunstan, D. L. Lacey, T. W. Mak, W. J. Boyle and J. M. Penninger (1999) OPGL is a key regulator of osteoclastogenesis, lymphocyte development and lymph-node organogenesis. Nature **397**(6717): 315–23.

Korioth, T. W. and A. Versluis (1997) Modeling the mechanical behavior of the jaws and their related structures by finite element (FE) analysis. Crit Rev Oral Biol Med **8**(1): 90–104.

Korvick, D. L., J. F. Cummings, E. S. Grood, J. P. Holden, S. M. Feder and D. L. Butler (1996) The use of an implantable force transducer to measure patellar tendon forces in goats. J Biomech **29**(4): 557–61.

Krause, A., E. A. Cowles and G. Gronowicz (2000) Integrin-mediated signaling in osteoblasts on titanium implant materials. J Biomed Mater Res **52**(4): 738–47.

Krishnan, L., J. A. Weiss, M. D. Wessman and J. B. Hoying (2004) Design and application of a test system for viscoelastic characterization of collagen gels. Tissue Eng **10**(1–2): 241–52.

Kucich, U., J. C. Rosenbloom, D. J. Herrick, W. R. Abrams, A. D. Hamilton, S. M. Sebti and J. Rosenbloom (2001) Signaling events required for transforming growth factor-beta stimulation of connective tissue growth factor expression by cultured human lung fibroblasts. Arch Biochem Biophys **395**(1): 103–12.

Kudawara, I., N. Araki, A. Myoui, Y. Kato, A. Uchida and H. Yoshikawa (2004) New cell lines with chondrocytic phenotypes from human chondrosarcoma. Virchows Arch **444**(6): 577–86.

Kumar, A., H. A. Biebuyk and G. M. Whitesides (1994) Patterning self-assembled monolayers: applications in materials science. Langmuir **10**: 1498–511.

Lacey, D. L., E. Timms, H. L. Tan, M. J. Kelley, C. R. Dunstan, T. Burgess, R. Elliott, A. Colombero, G. Elliott, S. Scully, H. Hsu, J. Sullivan, N. Hawkins, E. Davy, C. Capparelli, A. Eli, Y. X. Qian, S. Kaufman, I. Sarosi, V. Shalhoub, G. Senaldi, J. Guo, J. Delaney and W. J. Boyle (1998) Osteoprotegerin ligand is a cytokine that regulates osteoclast differentiation and activation. Cell **93**(2): 165–76.

Lai, W. M., J. S. Hou and V. C. Mow (1991) A triphasic theory for the swelling and deformation behaviors of articular cartilage. J Biomech Eng **113**(3): 245–58.

Lam, K. H., W. I. Wei and K. F. Siu (1984) The pectoralis major costomyocutaneous flap for mandibular reconstruction. Plast Reconstr Surg **73**(6): 904–10.

Lam, K. H., J. M. Schakenraad, H. Esselbrugge, J. Feijen and P. Nieuwenhuis (1993) The effect of phagocytosis of poly(L-lactic acid) fragments on cellular morphology and viability. J Biomed Mater Res **27**(12): 1569–77.

Lam, K. H., J. M. Schakenraad, H. Groen, H. Esselbrugge, P. J. Dijkstra, J. Feijen and P. Nieuwenhuis (1995) The influence of surface morphology and wettability on the inflammatory response against poly(L-lactic acid): a semi-quantitative study with monoclonal antibodies. J Biomed Mater Res **29**(8): 929–42.

Lam, C. X. F., X. M. Mo, S. H. Teoh and D. W. Hutmacher (2002) Scaffold development using 3D printing with a starch-based polymer. Mater Sci Eng C **20**(1–2): 49–56.

Landers, R. and R. Mulhaupt (2000) Desktop manufacturing of complex objects, prototypes and biomedical scaffolds by means of computer-assisted design combined with computer-guided 3D plotting of polymers and reactive oligomers. Macromol Mater Eng **282**: 17–21.

Landers, R., U. Hubner, R. Schmelzeisen and R. Mulhaupt (2002) Rapid prototyping of scaffolds derived from thermoreversible hydrogels and tailored for applications in tissue engineering. Biomaterials **23**(23): 4437–47.

Lane, J. M., M. Suda, K. von der Mark and R. Timpl (1986) Immunofluorescent localization of structural collagen types in endochondral fracture repair. J Orthop Res **4**(3): 318–29.

Lang, N. P., C. H. Hammerle, U. Bragger, B. Lehmann and S. R. Nyman (1994) Guided tissue regeneration in jawbone defects prior to implant placement. Clin Oral Implants Res **5**(2): 92–7.

Lange, R., F. Luthen, U. Beck, J. Rychly, A. Baumann and B. Nebe (2002) Cell-extracellular matrix interaction and physico-chemical characteristics of titanium surfaces depend on the roughness of the material. Biomol Eng **19**(2–6): 255–61.

Langer, R. and J. P. Vacanti (1993) Tissue engineering. Science **260**(5110): 920–6.

Lanyon, L. E., W. G. Hampson, A. E. Goodship and J. S. Shah (1975) Bone deformation recorded in vivo from strain gauges attached to the human tibial shaft. Acta Orthop Scand **46**(2): 256–68.

Lavik, E. and R. Langer (2004) Tissue engineering: current state and perspectives. Appl Microbiol Biotechnol **65**(1): 1–8.

Leach, J. K. and D. J. Mooney (2004) Bone engineering by controlled delivery of osteoinductive molecules and cells. Expert Opin Biol Ther **4**(7): 1015–27.

Lee, A. A., T. Delhaas, L. K. Waldman, D. A. MacKenna, F. J. Villarreal and A. D. McCulloch (1996) An equibiaxial strain system for cultured cells. Am J Physiol **271**(4 Pt 1): C1400–8.

Lee, D. A., T. Noguchi, S. P. Frean, P. Lees and D. L. Bader (2000) The influence of mechanical loading on isolated chondrocytes seeded in agarose constructs. Biorheology **37**(1–2): 149–61.

LeGeros, R. Z., O. R. Trautz, J. P. LeGeros, et al. (1967) Apatite crystallites: effect of carbonate on morphology. Science **155**(1409–11)

LeGeros, R. Z., J. P. LeGeros, O. R. Trautz, et al. (1971) Conversion of monetite, CaHPO4, to apatites: Effect of carbonate on the crystallinity and the morphology of the apatite crystallites. Adv Xray Anal **14**: 57–66.

LeGeros, R. Z. (1981) Apatites in biological systems. Prog Cryst Growth Charact **4**: 1–45.

LeGeros, R. Z. and M. S. Tung (1983) Chemical stability of carbonate- and fluoride-containing apatites. Caries Res **17**(5): 419–29.

LeGeros, R. Z. (1988) Calcium phosphate materials in restorative dentistry: a review. Adv Dent Res **2**(1): 164–80.

LeGeros, R. Z., I. Orly and M. Gregoire (1988) Comparative properties and in vitro transformation of HA ceramics in serum. J Dent Res **67**: 177.

LeGeros, R. Z., G. Daculsi and R. Kijkowska (1989) The effect of magnesium on the formation of apatites and whitlockites. In Itokawa, Y. and Durlach, J. (eds) Magnesium in Health and Disease. J Libbey & Co., New York, 11–19.

LeGeros, R. Z. (1991) Calcium phosphates in oral biology and medicine. Monogr Oral Sci **15**: 1–201.

LeGeros, R. Z., G. Daculsi, I. Orly, et al. (1991) Substrate surface dissolution and interfacial biological mineralization. In Davies, J. E. D. (ed.) The Bone Biomaterial Interface. University of Toronto Press, Toronto, 76–88.

LeGeros, R. Z. (1992) Materials for bone repair, augmentation and implant coatings. In Niwa, S. (ed.) Proceedings of the International Seminar of Orthopedic Research, Nagoya, 1990. Springer–Verlag, Tokyo, 147–74.

LeGeros, R. Z., C. Bautista and J. P. LeGeros (1995a) Comparative properties of bioactive bone graft materials. In Hench, L. and Wilson-Hench, J. (eds) Bioceramics 8. Pergamon Press, New York, 81–7.

LeGeros, R. Z., R. Kijkowska, C. Bautista and J. P. LeGeros (1995b) Synergistic effects of magnesium and carbonate on properties of biological and synthetic apatites. Connect Tissue Res **33**(1–3): 203–9.

LeGeros, R. Z., J. P. LeGeros, G. Daculsi and et. al. (1995c) CaP biomaterials: preparation, properties and biodegradation. In Wise, D. L., Trantolo, D. J. and Altobelli, D. E. (eds) Encyclopedic Handbook of Biomaterials and Bioengineering Part 1. Marcel Dekker, New York, 1429–63.

LeGeros, R. Z., T. Sakae, C. Bautista, M. Retino and J. P. LeGeros (1996) Magnesium and carbonate in enamel and synthetic apatites. Adv Dent Res **10**(2): 225–31.

LeGeros, R. Z., C. B. Bleiwas, M. Retino, R. Rohanizadeh and J. P. LeGeros (1999) Zinc effect on the in vitro formation of calcium phosphates: relevance to clinical inhibition of calculus formation. Am J Dent **12**(2): 65–71.

LeGeros, R. Z. (2002) Properties of osteoconductive biomaterials: calcium phosphates. Clin Orthop Relat Res (395): 81–98.

Lenhert, S., M. B. Meier, U. Meyer, L. Chi and H. P. Wiesmann (2005) Osteoblast alignment, elongation and migration on grooved polystyrene surfaces patterned by Langmuir–Blodgett lithography. Biomaterials **26**(5): 563–70.

Lennon, D. P., J. M. Edmison and A. I. Caplan (2001) Cultivation of rat marrow-derived mesenchymal stem cells in reduced oxygen tension: effects on in vitro and in vivo osteochondrogenesis. J Cell Physiol **187**(3): 345–55.

Leong, K. F., C. M. Cheah and C. K. Chua (2003) Solid freeform fabrication of three-dimensional scaffolds for engineering replacement tissues and organs. Biomaterials **24**(13): 2363–78.

L'Heureux, N., S. Paquet, R. Labbe, L. Germain and F. A. Auger (1998) A completely biological tissue-engineered human blood vessel. FASEB J **12**(1): 47–56.

Lian, J. B., G. S. Stein, J. L. Stein and A. J. van Wijnen (1999) Regulated expression of the bone-specific osteocalcin gene by vitamins and hormones. Vitam Horm **55**: 443–509.

Liao, H., A. S. Andersson, D. Sutherland, S. Petronis, B. Kasemo and P. Thomsen (2003) Response of rat osteoblast-like cells to microstructured model surfaces in vitro. Biomaterials **24**(4): 649–54.

Lieberman, J. R., L. Q. Le, L. Wu, G. A. Finerman, A. Berk, O. N. Witte and S. Stevenson (1998) Regional gene therapy with a BMP-2-producing murine stromal cell line induces heterotopic and orthotopic bone formation in rodents. J Orthop Res **16**(3): 330–9.

Lieberman, J. R., A. Daluiski, S. Stevenson, L. Wu, P. McAllister, Y. P. Lee, J. M. Kabo, G. A. Finerman, A. J. Berk and O. N. Witte (1999) The effect of regional gene therapy with bone morphogenetic protein-2-producing bone-marrow cells on the repair of segmental femoral defects in rats. J Bone Joint Surg Am **81**(7): 905–17.

Lieberman, J. R., A. Daluiski and T. A. Einhorn (2002) The role of growth factors in the repair of bone. Biology and clinical applications. J Bone Joint Surg Am **84–A**(6): 1032–44.

Liebschner, M. A. (2004) Biomechanical considerations of animal models used in tissue engineering of bone. Biomaterials **25**(9): 1697–714.

Lindenhayn, K., C. Perka, R. Spitzer, H. Heilmann, K. Pommerening, J. Mennicke and M. Sittinger (1999) Retention of hyaluronic acid in alginate beads: aspects for in vitro cartilage engineering. J Biomed Mater Res **44**(2): 149–55.

Linhart, W., F. Peters, W. Lehmann, K. Schwarz, A. F. Schilling, M. Amling, J. M. Rueger and M. Epple (2001) Biologically and chemically optimized composites of carbonated apatite and polyglycolide as bone substitution materials. J Biomed Mater Res **54**(2): 162–71.

Lipman, J. M., C. A. McDevitt and L. Sokoloff (1983) Xenografts of articular chondrocytes in the nude mouse. Calcif Tissue Int **35**(6): 767–72.

Liu, F., L. Malaval and J. E. Aubin (1997) The mature osteoblast phenotype is characterized by extensive plasticity. Exp Cell Res **232**(1): 97–105.

Liu, S., Y. Qu, T. J. Stewart, M. J. Howard, S. Chakrabortty, T. F. Holekamp and J. W. McDonald (2000) Embryonic stem cells differentiate into oligodendrocytes and myelinate in culture and after spinal cord transplantation. Proc Natl Acad Sci USA **97**(11): 6126–31.

Liu, J., Q. Zhang, E. E. Remsen and K. L. Wooley (2001) Nanostructured materials designed for cell binding and transduction. Biomacromolecules **2**(2): 362–8.

Liu, X. and P. X. Ma (2004) Polymeric scaffolds for bone tissue engineering. Ann Biomed Eng **32**(3): 477–86.

Liu, Y., E. B. Hunziker, P. Layrolle, J. D. De Bruijn and K. De Groot (2004) Bone morphogenetic protein 2 incorporated into biomimetic coatings retains its biological activity. Tissue Eng **10**(1–2): 101–8.

Loeser, R. F. (2000) Chondrocyte integrin expression and function. Biorheology **37**(1–2): 109–16.

Lohmander, L. S. (2003) Tissue engineering of cartilage: do we need it, can we do it, is it good and can we prove it? Novartis Found Symp **249**: 2–10; discussion 10–6, 170–4, 239–41.

Longley, D. and P. Lawford (2001) Engineering human tissue and regulation: confronting biology and law to bridge the gaps. Med Law Int **5**(2): 101–15.

Losos, J. B. (2001) Evolution: a lizard's tale. Sci Am **284**(3): 64–9.

Loty, C., J. M. Sautier, H. Boulekbache, T. Kokubo, H. M. Kim and N. Forest (2000) In vitro bone formation on a bone-like apatite layer prepared by a biomimetic process on a bioactive glass-ceramic. J Biomed Mater Res **49**(4): 423–34.

Lu, L. and A. G. Mikos (1996) The importance of new processing techniques in tissue engineering. MRS Bull **21**(11): 28–32.

Lu, L., X. Zhu, R. G. Valenzuela, B. L. Currier and M. J. Yaszemski (2001) Biodegradable polymer scaffolds for cartilage tissue engineering. Clin Orthop Relat Res (391 Suppl): S251–70.

Lucarelli, E., D. Donati, A. Cenacchi and P. M. Fornasari (2004) Bone reconstruction of large defects using bone-marrow derived autologous stem cells. Transfus Apheresis Sci **30**(2): 169–74.

Lysaght, M. J. and J. Reyes (2001) The growth of tissue engineering. Tissue Eng **7**(5): 485–93.

Macdonald, W., P. Campbell, J. Fisher and A. Wennerberg (2004) Variation in surface texture measurements. J Biomed Mater Res **70B**(2): 262–9.

Macirowski, T., S. Tepic and R. W. Mann (1994) Cartilage stresses in the human hip joint. J Biomech Eng **116**(1): 10–8.

Madry, H., R. Padera, J. Seidel, R. Langer, L. E. Freed, S. B. Trippel and G. Vunjak-Novakovic (2002) Gene transfer of a human insulin-like growth factor I cDNA enhances tissue engineering of cartilage. Hum Gene Ther **13**(13): 1621–30.

Malafaya, P. B. and R. L. Reis (2003) Key Engineering Materials. Trans Tech Pub, Zurich **240–2**: 39.

Malaviya, P., D. L. Butler, D. L. Korvick and F. S. Proch (1998) In vivo tendon forces correlate with activity level and remain bounded: evidence in a rabbit flexor tendon model. J Biomech **31**(11): 1043–9.

Malda, J., D. E. Martens, J. Tramper, C. A. van Blitterswijk and J. Riesle (2003) Cartilage tissue engineering: controversy in the effect of oxygen. Crit Rev Biotechnol **23**(3): 175–94.

Mandelbaum, B. R., J. E. Browne, F. Fu, L. Micheli, J. B. Mosely, Jr., C. Erggelet, T. Minas and L. Peterson (1998) Articular cartilage lesions of the knee. Am J Sports Med **26**(6): 853–61.

Manso, M., S. Ogueta, J. Perez-Rigueiro, J. P. Garcia and J. M. Martinez-Duart (2002) Testing biomaterials by the in-situ evaluation of cell response. Biomol Eng **19**(2–6): 239–42.

Mao, J. S., L. G. Zhao, Y. J. Yin and K. D. Yao (2003) Structure and properties of bilayer chitosan–gelatin scaffolds. Biomaterials **24**(6): 1067–74.

Mareschi, K., E. Biasin, W. Piacibello, M. Aglietta, E. Madon and F. Fagioli (2001) Isolation of human mesenchymal stem cells: bone marrow versus umbilical cord blood. Haematologica **86**(10): 1099–100.

Marino, A. A., B. D. Gross and R. D. Specian (1986) Electrical stimulation of mandibular osteotomies in rabbits. Oral Surg Oral Med Oral Pathol **62**(1): 20–4.

Maroudas, A. and P. Bullough (1968) Permeability of articular cartilage. Nature **219**(160): 1260–1.

Maroudas, A. (1979) Physicochemical properties of articular cartilage. In Freeman, M. (ed.) Adult Articular Cartilage. Pitman Medical, Tunbridge Wells, 215–90.

Martin, G. R. (1981) Isolation of a pluripotent cell line from early mouse embryos cultured in medium conditioned by teratocarcinoma stem cells. Proc Natl Acad Sci USA **78**(12): 7634–8.

Martin, J. Y., Z. Schwartz, T. W. Hummert, D. M. Schraub, J. Simpson, J. Lankford, Jr., D. D. Dean, D. L. Cochran and B. D. Boyan (1995) Effect of titanium surface roughness on proliferation, differentiation, and protein synthesis of human osteoblast-like cells (MG63) J Biomed Mater Res **29**(3): 389–401.

Martin, R. B., D. B. Burr and N. A. Sharkey (1998) Skeletal Tissue Mechanics. Springer, New York.

Martin, J. A. and J. A. Buckwalter (2000) The role of chondrocyte-matrix interactions in maintaining and repairing articular cartilage. Biorheology **37**(1–2): 129–40.

Martin, I., B. Obradovic, S. Treppo, A. J. Grodzinsky, R. Langer, L. E. Freed and G. Vunjak-Novakovic (2000) Modulation of the mechanical properties of tissue engineered cartilage. Biorheology **37**(1–2): 141–7.

Martin, I., M. Jakob, D. Schafer, W. Dick, G. Spagnoli and M. Heberer (2001) Quantitative analysis of gene expression in human articular cartilage from normal and osteoarthritic joints. Osteoarthritis Cartilage **9**(2): 112–18.

Martin, J. A., B. A. Miller, M. B. Scherb, L. A. Lembke and J. A. Buckwalter (2002) Co-localization of insulin-like growth factor binding protein 3 and fibronectin in human articular cartilage. Osteoarthritis Cartilage **10**(7): 556–63.

Martin, I., D. Wendt and M. Heberer (2004) The role of bioreactors in tissue engineering. Trends Biotechnol **22**(2): 80–6.

Martines, E., K. McGhee, C. Wilkinson and A. Curtis (2004) A parallel-plate flow chamber to study initial cell adhesion on a nanofeatured surface. IEEE Trans Nanobiosci **3**(2): 90–5.

Maruyama, Y., Y. Urita and K. Ohnishi (1985) Rib-latissimus dorsi osteomyocutaneous flap in reconstruction of a mandibular defect. Br J Plast Surg **38**(2): 234–7.

Marx, R. E., R. I. Miller, W. J. Ehler, G. Hubbard and T. I. Malinin (1984) A comparison of particulate allogeneic and particulate autogenous bone grafts into maxillary alveolar clefts in dogs. J Oral Maxillofac Surg **42**(1): 3–9.

Marx, G. (2003) Evolution of fibrin glue applicators. Transfus Med Rev **17**(4): 287–98.

Masi, L., A. Franchi, M. Santucci, D. Danielli, L. Arganini, V. Giannone, L. Formigli, S. Benvenuti, A. Tanini, F. Beghe, et al. (1992) Adhesion, growth, and matrix production by osteoblasts on collagen substrata. Calcif Tissue Int **51**(3): 202–12.

Mason, J. M., D. A. Grande, M. Barcia, R. Grant, R. G. Pergolizzi and A. S. Breitbart (1998) Expression of human bone morphogenic protein 7 in primary rabbit periosteal cells: potential utility in gene therapy for osteochondral repair. Gene Ther **5**(8): 1098–104.

Matsuda, N., N. Morita, K. Matsuda and M. Watanabe (1998) Proliferation and differentiation of human osteoblastic cells associated with differential activation of MAP kinases in response to epidermal growth factor, hypoxia, and mechanical stress in vitro. Biochem Biophys Res Commun **249**(2): 350–4.

Matsuoka, H., H. Akiyama, Y. Okada, H. Ito, C. Shigeno, J. Konishi, T. Kokubo and T. Nakamura (1999) In vitro analysis of the stimulation of bone formation by highly bioactive apatite- and wollastonite-containing glass–ceramic: released calcium ions promote osteogenic differentiation in osteoblastic ROS17/2.8 cells. J Biomed Mater Res **47**(2): 176–88.

Matsuzaka, K., F. Walboomers, A. de Ruijter and J. A. Jansen (2000) Effect of microgrooved poly-l-lactic (PLA) surfaces on proliferation, cytoskeletal organization, and mineralized matrix formation of rat bone marrow cells. Clin Oral Implants Res **11**(4): 325–33.

Mauck, R. L., M. A. Soltz, C. C. Wang, D. D. Wong, P. H. Chao, W. B. Valhmu, C. T. Hung and G. A. Ateshian (2000) Functional tissue engineering of articular cartilage through dynamic loading of chondrocyte-seeded agarose gels. J Biomech Eng **122**(3): 252–60.

Mayne, R. and R. G. Brewton (1993) New members of the collagen superfamily. Curr Opin Cell Biol **5**(5): 883–90.

McCarthy, J. G. and B. M. Zide (1984) The spectrum of calvarial bone grafting: introduction of the vascularized calvarial bone flap. Plast Reconstr Surg **74**(1): 10–8.

McCarthy, J. G., C. B. Cutting and W. W. Shaw (1987) Vascularized calvarial flaps. Clin Plast Surg **14**(1): 37–47.

McCutchen, C. W. (1959) Mechanisms of animal joints: sponge-hydrostatic and weeping bearings. Nature **184**: 1284–5.

McCutchen, C. W. (1962) The frictional properties of animal joints. Wear **1**: 1–7.

Meachim, G. (1969) Age changes in articular cartilage. Clin Orthop Relat Res **64**: 33–44.

Meazzini, M. C., C. D. Toma, J. L. Schaffer, M. L. Gray and L. C. Gerstenfeld (1998) Osteoblast cytoskeletal modulation in response to mechanical strain in vitro. J Orthop Res **16**(2): 170–80.

Meiser, B. M. and B. Reichart (1994) New trends in clinical immunosuppression. Transplant Proc **26**(6): 3181–3.

Mendler, M., S. G. Eich-Bender, L. Vaughan, K. H. Winterhalter and P. Bruckner (1989) Cartilage contains mixed fibrils of collagen types II, IX, and XI. J Cell Biol **108**(1): 191–7.

Meyer, U., D. H. Szulczewski, R. H. Barckhaus, M. Atkinson and D. B. Jones (1993a) Biological evaluation of an ionomeric bone cement by osteoblast cell culture methods. Biomaterials **14**(12): 917–24.

Meyer, U., H. D. Szulczewski, K. Möller, H. Heide and D. B. Jones (1993b) Attachment kinetics and differentiation of osteoblasts on different biomaterials. Cells Mater **3**: 129–40.

Meyer, U., J. Kleinheinz, D. H. Szulczewski, D. B. Jones and U. Joos (1997a) Strain application for evaluation of mechano-transduction in osteoblasts. In Diner, P. A. and Vasquez, M. P. (eds) International Congress on Craniofacial and Facial Bone Distraction Processes, Paris, France. Monduzzi Editore, Bologna, Italy.

Meyer, U., T. Meyer and D. B. Jones (1997b) No mechanical role for vinculin in strain transduction in primary bovine osteoblasts. Biochem Cell Biol **75**(1): 81–7.

Meyer, U., T. Meyer and D. B. Jones (1998) Attachment kinetics, proliferation rates and vinculin assembly of bovine osteoblasts cultured on different pre-coated artificial substrates. J Mater Sci Mater Med **9**(6): 301–7.

Meyer, U., T. Meyer, J. Vosshans and U. Joos (1999a) Decreased expression of osteocalcin and osteonectin in relation to high strains and decreased mineralization in mandibular distraction osteogenesis. J Craniomaxillofac Surg **27**(4): 222–7.

Meyer, U., H. P. Wiesmann, B. Kruse-Losler, J. Handschel, U. Stratmann and U. Joos (1999b) Strain-related bone remodeling in distraction osteogenesis of the mandible. Plast Reconstr Surg **103**(3): 800–7.

Meyer, U., D. Vollmer, C. Homann, R. Schuon, S. Benthaus, A. Vegh, E. Felszegi, U. Joos and J. Piffko (2000) [Experimental and finite-element models for the assessment of mandibular deformation under mechanical loading]. Mund Kiefer Gesichtschir **4**(1): 14–20.
Meyer, U., U. Joos, T. Szuwart and H. P. Wiesmann (2001a) Mineralized 3D bone tissue engineered by osteoblasts cultured in a collagen gel. Tissue Eng **7**: 671.
Meyer, U., T. Meyer, W. Schlegel, H. Scholz and U. Joos (2001b) Tissue differentiation and cytokine synthesis during strain-related bone formation in distraction osteogenesis. Br J Oral Maxillofac Surg **39**(1): 22–9.
Meyer, U., M. Terodde, U. Joos and H. P. Wiesmann (2001c) [Mechanical stimulation of osteoblasts in cell culture]. Mund Kiefer Gesichtschir **5**(3): 166–72.
Meyer, U., C. Runte, D. Dirksen, T. Stamm, T. Fillies, U. Joos and H. P. Wiesmann (2003) Image-based biomimetric approach to design and fabrication of tissue engineered bone. Comp Assist Radiol Surg **1256**: 726–32.
Meyer, U., U. Joos, J. Mythili, T. Stamm, A. Hohoff, T. Fillies, U. Stratmann and H. P. Wiesmann (2004a) Ultrastructural characterization of the implant/bone interface of immediately loaded dental implants. Biomaterials **25**(10): 1959–67.
Meyer, U., U. Joos and H. P. Wiesmann (2004b) Biological and biophysical principles in extracorporal bone tissue engineering. Part I. Int J Oral Maxillofac Surg **33**(4): 325–32.
Meyer, U., U. Joos and H. P. Wiesmann (2004c) Biological and biophysical principles in extracorporal bone tissue engineering. Part III. Int J Oral Maxillofac Surg **33**(7): 635–41.
Meyer, U., J. Kleinheinz and U. Joos (2004d) Biomechanical and clinical implications of distraction osteogenesis in craniofacial surgery. J Craniomaxillofac Surg **32**(3): 140–9.
Meyer, U., N. Nazer and H. P. Wiesmann (2005a) Design and performance of a bioreactor to mechanically promote bone and cartilage tissue formation. Br J Oral Maxillofac Surg, 15
Meyer, U., T. Szuwart, C. Runte, D. Dierksen, A. Büchter and H. P. Wiesmann (2005b) Computer-aided bone tissue engineering. Int J Oral Maxillofac Implants **20:** 855–863.
Meyer, U., H. P. Wiesmann, A. Büchter and J. Libera (2005c) Cartilage defect regeneration by ex-vivo engineered autologous micro-tissue. Osteoarthritis Cartilage: submitted.
Michel, D. and M. F. Harmand (1990) Fibrin seal in wound healing: effect of thrombin and [Ca2+] on human skin fibroblast growth and collagen production. J Dermatol Sci **1**(5): 325–33.
Midy, V., M. Dard and E. Hollande (2001) Evaluation of the effect of three calcium phosphate powders on osteoblast cells. J Mater Sci Mater Med **12**(3): 259–65.
Mikos, A. G., Y. Bao, L. G. Cima, D. E. Ingber, J. P. Vacanti and R. Langer (1993) Preparation of poly(glycolic acid) bonded fiber structures for cell attachment and transplantation. J Biomed Mater Res **27**(2): 183–9.
Mikos, A. G., A. J. Thorsen, L. A. Czerwonka, Y. Bao, R. Langer, D. N. Winslow and J. P. Vacanti (1994) Preparation and characterization of poly(L-lactic acid) foams. Polymer **35**: 1068.
Mikos, A. G., L. V. McIntire, J. M. Anderson and J. E. Babensee (1998) Host response to tissue engineered devices. Adv Drug Deliv Rev **33**(1–2): 111–39.
Milgrom, C., A. Finestone, A. Simkin, I. Ekenman, S. Mendelson, M. Millgram, M. Nyska, E. Larsson and D. Burr (2000) In-vivo strain measurements to evaluate the strengthening potential of exercises on the tibial bone. J Bone Joint Surg Br **82**(4): 591–4.
Minas, T. (2001) Autologous chondrocyte implantation for focal chondral defects of the knee. Clin Orthop Relat Res (391 Suppl): S349–61.
Minguell, J. J., A. Erices and P. Conget (2001) Mesenchymal stem cells. Exp Biol Med (Maywood) **226**(6): 507–20.
Mitchell, N. and N. Shepard (1980) Healing of articular cartilage in intra-articular fractures in rabbits. J Bone Joint Surg Am **62**(4): 628–34.
Möller, K., U. Meyer, D. H. Szulczewski, H. Heide, B. Priessnitz and D. B. Jones (1994) The influence of zeta potential and interfacial tension on osteoblast-like cells. Cell Mater **4**: 263–74.
Mogi, M., K. Fukuo, J. Yang, T. Suhara and T. Ogihara (2001) Hypoxia stimulates release of the soluble form of fas ligand that inhibits endothelial cell apoptosis. Lab Invest **81**(2): 177–84.
Monroe, E. A., W. Votava, D. B. Bass and J. McMullen (1971) New calcium phosphate ceramic material for bone and tooth implants. J Dent Res **50**(4): 860–1.

Mooney, D. J., D. F. Baldwin, N. P. Suh, J. P. Vacanti and R. Langer (1996) Novel approach to fabricate porous sponges of poly(D,L-lactic-co-glycolic acid) without the use of organic solvents. Biomaterials **17**(14): 1417–22.

Moran, M. E., H. K. Kim and R. B. Salter (1992) Biological resurfacing of full-thickness defects in patellar articular cartilage of the rabbit. Investigation of autogenous periosteal grafts subjected to continuous passive motion. J Bone Joint Surg Br **74**(5): 659–67.

Moreno, E. C., M. Kresak and R. T. Zahradnik (1977) Physicochemical aspects of fluoride–apatite systems relevant to the study of dental caries. Caries Res **11 Suppl 1**: 142–71.

Morrison, S. J., M. Csete, A. K. Groves, W. Melega, B. Wold and D. J. Anderson (2000) Culture in reduced levels of oxygen promotes clonogenic sympathoadrenal differentiation by isolated neural crest stem cells. J Neurosci **20**(19): 7370–6.

Mosbach, K. and O. Ramstrom (1996) The emerging technique of molecular imprinting and its future impact on biotechnology. Biotechnology **14**: 163–70.

Mosley, J. R., B. M. March, J. Lynch and L. E. Lanyon (1997) Strain magnitude related changes in whole bone architecture in growing rats. Bone **20**(3): 191–8.

Motulsky, A. G. (1983) Impact of genetic manipulation on society and medicine. Science **219**(4581): 135–40.

Moursi, A. M., R. K. Globus and C. H. Damsky (1997) Interactions between integrin receptors and fibronectin are required for calvarial osteoblast differentiation in vitro. J Cell Sci **110 (Pt 18)**: 2187–96.

Mow, V. C., A. Ratcliffe and A. R. Poole (1992) Cartilage and diarthrodial joints as paradigms for hierarchical materials and structures. Biomaterials **13**(2): 67–97.

Mow, V. C., N. Bachrach, L. A. Setton and e. al. (1994) Stress, strain, pressure, and flow fields in articular cartilage. In Mow, V. C., Guilak, F., Tran-Son-Tay, R. and Hochmuth, R. M. (eds) Cell Mechanics and Cellular Engineering. Springer Verlag, New York, 345–79.

Mow, V. C. and G. A. Ateshian (1997) Lubrication and wear of diarthrodial joints. In Mow, V. C. and Hayes, W. C. (eds) Basic Orthopaedic Biomechanics. Lippencott-Raven. Philadelphia, 275–315.

Muraglia, A., R. Cancedda and R. Quarto (2000) Clonal mesenchymal progenitors from human bone marrow differentiate in vitro according to a hierarchical model. J Cell Sci **113 (Pt 7)**: 1161–6.

Murayama, T., O. M. Tepper, M. Silver, H. Ma, D. W. Losordo, J. M. Isner, T. Asahara and C. Kalka (2002) Determination of bone marrow-derived endothelial progenitor cell significance in angiogenic growth factor-induced neovascularization in vivo. Exp Hematol **30**(8): 967–72.

Murphy, W. L., R. G. Dennis, J. L. Kileny and D. J. Mooney (2002) Salt fusion: an approach to improve pore interconnectivity within tissue engineering scaffolds. Tissue Eng **8**(1): 43–52.

Muschler, G. F., H. Nitto, Y. Matsukura, C. Boehm, A. Valdevit, H. Kambic, W. Davros, K. Powell and K. Easley (2003) Spine fusion using cell matrix composites enriched in bone marrow–derived cells. Clin Orthop Relat Res (407): 102–18.

Muschler, G. F., C. Nakamoto and L. G. Griffith (2004) Engineering principles of clinical cell–based tissue engineering. J Bone Joint Surg Am **86–A**(7): 1541–58.

Musgrave, D. S., P. Bosch, S. Ghivizzani, P. D. Robbins, C. H. Evans and J. Huard (1999) Adenovirus-mediated direct gene therapy with bone morphogenetic protein-2 produces bone. Bone **24**(6): 541–7.

Nagai, M., T. Hayakawa, A. Fukatsu, M. Yamamoto, M. Fukumoto, F. Nagahama, H. Mishima, M. Yoshinari, K. Nemoto and T. Kato (2002) In vitro study of collagen coating of titanium implants for initial cell attachment. Dent Mater J **21**(3): 250–60.

Nakahara, H., S. P. Bruder, V. M. Goldberg and A. I. Caplan (1990a) In vivo osteochondrogenic potential of cultured cells derived from the periosteum. Clin Orthop Relat Res (259): 223–32.

Nakahara, H., S. P. Bruder, S. E. Haynesworth, J. J. Holecek, M. A. Baber, V. M. Goldberg and A. I. Caplan (1990b) Bone and cartilage formation in diffusion chambers by subcultured cells derived from the periosteum. Bone **11**(3): 181–8.

Nakahara, H., J. E. Dennis, S. P. Bruder, S. E. Haynesworth, D. P. Lennon and A. I. Caplan (1991) In vitro differentiation of bone and hypertrophic cartilage from periosteal-derived cells. Exp Cell Res **195**(2): 492–503.

Nakahara, H., V. M. Goldberg and A. I. Caplan (1992) Culture-expanded periosteal-derived cells exhibit osteochondrogenic potential in porous calcium phosphate ceramics in vivo. Clin Orthop Relat Res (276): 291–8.

Nakaoka, R., Y. Tabata and Y. Ikada (1996) Production of interleukin 1 from macrophages incubated with poly (DL-lactic acid) granules containing ovalbumin. Biomaterials **17**(23): 2253–8.

Nathanson, M. A. (1985) Bone matrix-directed chondrogenesis of muscle in vitro. Clin Orthop Relat Res (200): 142–58.

Nesbitt, S. A. and M. A. Horton (1997) Trafficking of matrix collagens through bone-resorbing osteoclasts. Science **276**(5310): 266–9.

Nielsen, H. M., T. T. Andreassen, T. Ledet and H. Oxlund (1994) Local injection of TGF-beta increases the strength of tibial fractures in the rat. Acta Orthop Scand **65**(1): 37–41.

Nishimura, K., L. A. Solchaga, A. I. Caplan, J. U. Yoo, V. M. Goldberg and B. Johnstone (1999) Chondroprogenitor cells of synovial tissue. Arthritis Rheum **42**(12): 2631–7.

Nishimura, I., R. L. Garrell, M. Hedrick, K. Iida, S. Osher and B. Wu (2003) Precursor tissue analogs as a tissue-engineering strategy. Tissue Eng **9 Suppl 1**: S77–89.

Nishio, K., M. Neo, H. Akiyama, S. Nishiguchi, H. M. Kim, T. Kokubo and T. Nakamura (2000) The effect of alkali- and heat-treated titanium and apatite-formed titanium on osteoblastic differentiation of bone marrow cells. J Biomed Mater Res **52**(4): 652–61.

Nomi, M., A. Atala, P. D. Coppi and S. Soker (2002) Principals of neovascularization for tissue engineering. Mol Aspects Med **23**(6): 463–83.

Nomura, S., A. J. Wills, D. R. Edwards, J. K. Heath and B. L. Hogan (1989) Expression of genes for non–collagenous proteins during embryonic bone formation. Connect Tissue Res **21**(1–4): 31–5; discussion 36–9.

Nordgren, A. (2004) Moral imagination in tissue engineering research on animal models. Biomaterials **25**(9): 1723–34.

Nutt, S. L., B. Heavey, A. G. Rolink and M. Busslinger (1999) Commitment to the B-lymphoid lineage depends on the transcription factor Pax5. Nature **401**(6753): 556–62

Nuttall, M. E., A. J. Patton, D. L. Olivera, D. P. Nadeau and M. Gowen (1998) Human trabecular bone cells are able to express both osteoblastic and adipocytic phenotype: implications for osteopenic disorders. J Bone Miner Res **13**(3): 371–82.

Oakes, D. A. and J. R. Lieberman (2000) Osteoinductive applications of regional gene therapy: ex vivo gene transfer. Clin Orthop Relat Res (379 Suppl): S101–12.

Ochi, K., G. Chen, T. Ushida, S. Gojo, K. Segawa, H. Tai, K. Ueno, H. Ohkawa, T. Mori, A. Yamaguchi, Y. Toyama, J. Hata and A. Umezawa (2003) Use of isolated mature osteoblasts in abundance acts as desired-shaped bone regeneration in combination with a modified poly-DL-lactic-co-glycolic acid (PLGA)-collagen sponge. J Cell Physiol **194**(1): 45–53.

O'Driscoll, S. W., A. Kumar and R. B. Salter (1983a) The effect of continuous passive motion on the clearance of a hemarthrosis from a synovial joint. An experimental investigation in the rabbit. Clin Orthop Relat Res (176): 305–11.

O'Driscoll, S. W., A. Kumar and R. B. Salter (1983b) The effect of the volume of effusion, joint position and continuous passive motion on intraarticular pressure in the rabbit knee. J Rheumatol **10**(3): 360–3.

O'Driscoll, S. W. (1984) The chondrogenic potential of free periosteal grafts for biological resurfacing of joints under the influence of continuous passive motion. PhD thesis, University of Toronto.

O'Driscoll, S. W. and R. B. Salter (1984) The induction of neochondrogenesis in free intra–articular periosteal autografts under the influence of continuous passive motion. An experimental investigation in the rabbit. J Bone Joint Surg Am **66**(8): 1248–57.

O'Driscoll, S. W. and R. B. Salter (1986) The repair of major osteochondral defects in joint surfaces by neochondrogenesis with autogenous osteoperiosteal grafts stimulated by continuous passive motion. An experimental investigation in the rabbit. Clin Orthop Relat Res (208): 131–40.

O'Driscoll, S. W., F. W. Keeley and R. B. Salter (1988) Durability of regenerated articular cartilage produced by free autogenous periosteal grafts in major full-thickness defects in joint surfaces under the influence of continuous passive motion. A follow-up report at one year. J Bone Joint Surg Am **70**(4): 595–606.

O'Driscoll, S. W. (2001) Preclinical cartilage repair: current status and future perspectives. Clin Orthop Relat Res (391 Suppl): S397–401.

Ogata, T. (2000) Fluid flow-induced tyrosine phosphorylation and participation of growth factor signaling pathway in osteoblast-like cells. J Cell Biochem **76**(4): 529–38.

Ohgushi, H., V. M. Goldberg and A. I. Caplan (1989a) Repair of bone defects with marrow cells and porous ceramic. Experiments in rats. Acta Orthop Scand **60**(3): 334–9.

Ohgushi, H., V. M. Goldberg and A. I. Caplan (1989b) Heterotopic osteogenesis in porous ceramics induced by marrow cells. J Orthop Res **7**(4): 568–78.

Ohgushi, H. and A. I. Caplan (1999) Stem cell technology and bioceramics: from cell to gene engineering. J Biomed Mater Res **48**(6): 913–27.

Ohgushi, H., J. Miyake and T. Tateishi (2003) Mesenchymal stem cells and bioceramics: strategies to regenerate the skeleton. Novartis Found Symp **249**: 118–27; discussion 127–32, 170–4, 239–41.

Ohma, N., Y. Takagi and Y. Takano (2000) Distribution of non-collagenous dentin matrix proteins and proteoglycans, and their relation to calcium accumulation in bisphosphonate-affected rat incisors. Eur J Oral Sci **108**(3): 222–32.

Okazaki, M. and R. Z. LeGeros (1992) Crystallographic and chemical properties of Mg-containing apatites before and after suspension in solutions. Magnesium Res **5**(2): 103–8.

Okazaki, M., T. Matsumoto, M. Taira and e. al. (1998) CO3apatite preparations with solubility gradient: potential degradable biomaterials. In LeGeros, R. Z. and LeGeros, J. P. (eds) Bioceramics 11. World Scientific, Singapore, 85–8.

Okubo, Y., K. Bessho, K. Fujimura, T. Iizuka and S. I. Miyatake (2000) Osteoinduction by bone morphogenetic protein-2 via adenoviral vector under transient immunosuppression. Biochem Biophys Res Commun **267**(1): 382–7.

Oloyede, A. and N. Broom (1993) Stress-sharing between the fluid and solid components of articular cartilage under varying rates of compression. Connect Tissue Res **30**(2): 127–41.

Orban, J. M., K. G. Marra and J. O. Hollinger (2002) Composition options for tissue-engineered bone. Tissue Eng **8**(4): 529–39.

Oreffo, R. O. and J. T. Triffitt (1999) Future potentials for using osteogenic stem cells and biomaterials in orthopedics. Bone **25**(2 Suppl): 5S–9S.

Ortega, N., D. Behonick, D. Stickens and Z. Werb (2003) How proteases regulate bone morphogenesis. Ann NY Acad Sci **995**: 109–16.

O'Toole, G. C., E. Salih, C. Gallagher, D. Fitzatrick, N. O'Higgins and S. K. O'Rourke (2004) Bone sialoprotein-coated femoral implants are osteoinductive but mechanically compromised. J Orthop Res **22**(3): 641–6.

Otto, W. R. and J. Rao (2004) Tomorrow's skeleton staff: mesenchymal stem cells and the repair of bone and cartilage. Cell Prolif **37**(1): 97–110.

Owan, I., D. B. Burr, C. H. Turner, J. Qiu, Y. Tu, J. E. Onyia and R. L. Duncan (1997) Mechanotransduction in bone: osteoblasts are more responsive to fluid forces than mechanical strain. Am J Physiol **273**(3 Pt 1): 810–5.

Owen, M. (1988) Marrow stromal stem cells. J Cell Sci Suppl **10**: 63–76.

Owen, M. and A. J. Friedenstein (1988) Stromal stem cells: marrow-derived osteogenic precursors. Ciba Found Symp **136**: 42–60.

Owen, T. A., M. Aronow, V. Shalhoub, L. M. Barone, L. Wilming, M. S. Tassinari, M. B. Kennedy, S. Pockwinse, J. B. Lian and G. S. Stein (1990) Progressive development of the rat osteoblast phenotype in vitro: reciprocal relationships in expression of genes associated with osteoblast proliferation and differentiation during formation of the bone extracellular matrix. J Cell Physiol **143**(3): 420–30.

Ozawa, H., K. Imamura, E. Abe, N. Takahashi, T. Hiraide, Y. Shibasaki, T. Fukuhara and T. Suda (1990) Effect of a continuously applied compressive pressure on mouse osteoblast-like cells (MC3T3-E1) in vitro. J Cell Physiol **142**(1): 177–85.
Ozkaynak, E., D. C. Rueger, E. A. Drier, C. Corbett, R. J. Ridge, T. K. Sampath and H. Oppermann (1990) OP 1 cDNA encodes an osteogenic protein in the TGF-beta family. Embo J **9**(7): 2085–93.
Paige, K. T., L. G. Cima, M. J. Yaremchuk, B. L. Schloo, J. P. Vacanti and C. A. Vacanti (1996) De novo cartilage generation using calcium alginate–chondrocyte constructs. Plast Reconstr Surg **97**(1): 168–78; discussion 179–80.
Pan, T. C., R. Z. Zhang, M. G. Mattei, R. Timpl and M. L. Chu (1992) Cloning and chromosomal location of human alpha 1(XVI) collagen. Proc Natl Acad Sci USA **89**(14): 6565–9.
Panje, W. and C. Cutting (1980) Trapezius osteomyocutaneous island flap for reconstruction of the anterior floor of the mouth and the mandible. Head Neck Surg **3**(1): 66–71.
Parfitt, A. M. (1977) The cellular basis of bone turnover and bone loss: a rebuttal of the osteocytic resorption–bone flow theory. Clin Orthop Relat Res (127): 236–47.
Parikh, S. N. (2002) Bone graft substitutes: past, present, future. J Postgrad Med **48**(2): 142–8.
Park, A., B. Wu and L. G. Griffith (1998) Integration of surface modification and 3D fabrication techniques to prepare patterned poly(L–lactide) substrates allowing regionally selective cell adhesion. J Biomater Sci Polym Ed **9**(2): 89–110.
Park, S. R., R. O. Oreffo and J. T. Triffitt (1999) Interconversion potential of cloned human marrow adipocytes in vitro. Bone **24**(6): 549–54.
Partridge, K. A. and R. O. Oreffo (2004) Gene delivery in bone tissue engineering: progress and prospects using viral and nonviral strategies. Tissue Eng **10**(1–2): 295–307.
Pavalko, F. M., N. X. Chen, C. H. Turner, D. B. Burr, S. Atkinson, Y. F. Hsieh, J. Qiu and R. L. Duncan (1998) Fluid shear-induced mechanical signaling in MC3T3-E1 osteoblasts requires cytoskeleton–integrin interactions. Am J Physiol **275**(6 Pt 1): C1591–601.
Pavesio, A., G. Abatangelo, A. Borrione, D. Brocchetta, A. P. Hollander, E. Kon, F. Torasso, S. Zanasi and M. Marcacci (2003) Hyaluronan-based scaffolds (Hyalograft C) in the treatment of knee cartilage defects: preliminary clinical findings. Novartis Found Symp **249**: 203–17; discussion 229–33, 234 8, 239–41.
Perka, C., O. Schultz, R. S. Spitzer, K. Lindenhayn, G. R. Burmester and M. Sittinger (2000) Segmental bone repair by tissue-engineered periosteal cell transplants with bioresorbable fleece and fibrin scaffolds in rabbits. Biomaterials **21**(11): 1145–53.
Peter, S. J., M. J. Miller, A. W. Yasko, M. J. Yaszemski and A. G. Mikos (1998a) Polymer concepts in tissue engineering. J Biomed Mater Res **43**(4): 422–7.
Peter, S. J., S. T. Miller, G. Zhu, A. W. Yasko and A. G. Mikos (1998b) In vivo degradation of a poly(propylene fumarate)/beta–tricalcium phosphate injectable composite scaffold. J Biomed Mater Res **41**(1): 1–7.
Peterson, L., T. Minas, M. Brittberg, A. Nilsson, E. Sjogren–Jansson and A. Lindahl (2000) Two– to 9–year outcome after autologous chondrocyte transplantation of the knee. Clin Orthop Relat Res (374): 212–34.
Phillips, B. W., C. Vernochet and C. Dani (2003) Differentiation of embryonic stem cells for pharmacological studies on adipose cells. Pharmacol Res **47**(4): 263–8.
Piekarski, K. and M. Munro (1977) Transport mechanism operating between blood supply and osteocytes in long bones. Nature **269**(5623): 80–2.
Pienkowski, D. and S. R. Pollack (1983) The origin of stress-generated potentials in fluid-saturated bone. J Orthop Res **1**(1): 30–41.
Pittenger, M. F., A. M. Mackay, S. C. Beck, R. K. Jaiswal, R. Douglas, J. D. Mosca, M. A. Moorman, D. W. Simonetti, S. Craig and D. R. Marshak (1999) Multilineage potential of adult human mesenchymal stem cells. Science **284**(5411): 143–7.
Plate, U., S. Arnold, U. Stratmann, H. P. Wiesmann and H. J. Höhling (1998) General principle of ordered apatitic crystal formation in enamel and collagen rich hard tissues. Connect Tissue Res **38**(1–4): 149–57; discussion 201–5.

Platt, J. L. (1992) Mechanisms of tissue injury in hyperacute xenograft rejection. Asaio J **38**(1): 8–16.

Pockwinse, S. M., L. G. Wilming, D. M. Conlon, G. S. Stein and J. B. Lian (1992) Expression of cell growth and bone specific genes at single cell resolution during development of bone tissue-like organization in primary osteoblast cultures. J Cell Biochem **49**(3): 310–23.

Poole, A. R., I. Pidoux, A. Reiner and L. Rosenberg (1982) An immunoelectron microscope study of the organization of proteoglycan monomer, link protein, and collagen in the matrix of articular cartilage. J Cell Biol **93**(3): 921–37.

Poole, A. R. (1991) The growth plate: cellular physiology, cartilage assembly and mineralization. In Hall, B. K. and Newman, S.A. (eds), Cartilage: Molecular Aspects, CRC Press, Boca Raton, 179–221.

Poole, A. R., T. Kojima, T. Yasuda, F. Mwale, M. Kobayashi and S. Laverty (2001) Composition and structure of articular cartilage: a template for tissue repair. Clin Orthop Relat Res (391 Suppl): S26–33.

Price, R. L., K. M. Haberstroh and T. J. Webster (2003a) Enhanced functions of osteoblasts on nanostructured surfaces of carbon and alumina. Med Biol Eng Comput **41**(3): 372–5.

Price, R. L., M. C. Waid, K. M. Haberstroh and T. J. Webster (2003b) Selective bone cell adhesion on formulations containing carbon nanofibers. Biomaterials **24**(11): 1877–87.

Prolo, D. J., P. W. Pedrotti, K. P. Burres and S. Oklund (1982) Superior osteogenesis in transplanted allogeneic canine skull following chemical sterilization. Clin Orthop Relat Res(168): 230–42.

Puelacher, W. C., D. Mooney, R. Langer, J. Upton, J. P. Vacanti and C. A. Vacanti (1994) Design of nasoseptal cartilage replacements synthesized from biodegradable polymers and chondrocytes. Biomaterials **15**(10): 774–8.

Puelacher, W. C., J. P. Vacanti, N. F. Ferraro, B. Schloo and C. A. Vacanti (1996) Femoral shaft reconstruction using tissue-engineered growth of bone. Int J Oral Maxillofac Surg **25**(3): 223–8.

Quarto, R., D. Thomas and C. T. Liang (1995) Bone progenitor cell deficits and the age-associated decline in bone repair capacity. Calcif Tissue Int **56**(2): 123–9.

Quarto, R., M. Mastrogiacomo, R. Cancedda, S. M. Kutepov, V. Mukhachev, A. Lavroukov, E. Kon and M. Marcacci (2001) Repair of large bone defects with the use of autologous bone marrow stromal cells. N Engl J Med **344**(5): 385–6.

Ragan, P. M., V. I. Chin, H. H. Hung, K. Masuda, E. J. Thonar, E. C. Arner, A. J. Grodzinsky and J. D. Sandy (2000) Chondrocyte extracellular matrix synthesis and turnover are influenced by static compression in a new alginate disk culture system. Arch Biochem Biophys **383**(2): 256–64.

Ramirez-Bergeron, D. L. and M. C. Simon (2001) Hypoxia-inducible factor and the development of stem cells of the cardiovascular system. Stem Cells **19**(4): 279–86.

Rammelt, S., E. Schulze, R. Bernhardt, U. Hanisch, D. Scharnweber, H. Worch, H. Zwipp and A. Biewener (2004) Coating of titanium implants with type-I collagen. J Orthop Res **22**(5): 1025–34.

Rangappa, S., J. W. Entwistle, A. S. Wechsler and J. Y. Kresh (2003) Cardiomyocyte-mediated contact programs human mesenchymal stem cells to express cardiogenic phenotype. J Thorac Cardiovasc Surg **126**(1): 124–32.

Ratcliffe, A. (2000) Tissue engineering of vascular grafts. Matrix Biol **19**(4): 353–7.

Ratcliffe, A. and L. E. Niklason (2002) Bioreactors and bioprocessing for tissue engineering. Ann NY Acad Sci **961**: 210–5.

Reddi, A. H., R. Gay, S. Gay and E. J. Miller (1977) Transitions in collagen types during matrix-induced cartilage, bone, and bone marrow formation. Proc Natl Acad Sci USA **74**(12): 5589–92.

Reddi, A. H. (1994) Symbiosis of biotechnology and biomaterials: applications in tissue engineering of bone and cartilage. J Cell Biochem **56**(2): 192–5.

Reddi, A. H. (2000) Morphogenesis and tissue engineering of bone and cartilage: inductive signals, stem cells, and biomimetic biomaterials. Tissue Eng **6**(4): 351–9.

Redman, S. N., S. F. Oldfield and C. W. Archer (2005) Current strategies for articular cartilage repair. Eur Cell Mater **9**: 23–32; discussion 23–32.
Rehn, M. and T. Pihlajaniemi (1994) Alpha 1(XVIII), a collagen chain with frequent interruptions in the collagenous sequence, a distinct tissue distribution, and homology with type XV collagen. Proc Natl Acad Sci USA **91**(10). 4234–8
Reid, D. L., M. B. Aydelotte and J. Mollenhauer (2000) Cell attachment, collagen binding, and receptor analysis on bovine articular chondrocytes. J Orthop Res **18**(3): 364–73.
Reinholz, G. G., L. Lu, D. B. Saris, M. J. Yaszemski and S. W. O'Driscoll (2004) Animal models for cartilage reconstruction. Biomaterials **25**(9): 1511–21.
Reyes, M., T. Lund, T. Lenvik, D. Aguiar, L. Koodie and C. M. Verfaillie (2001) Purification and ex vivo expansion of postnatal human marrow mesodermal progenitor cells. Blood **98**(9): 2615–25.
Rezania, A. and K. E. Healy (2000) The effect of peptide surface density on mineralization of a matrix deposited by osteogenic cells. J Biomed Mater Res **52**(4): 595–600.
Rice, J. M., J. A. Hunt, J. A. Gallagher, P. Hanarp, D. S. Sutherland and J. Gold (2003) Quantitative assessment of the response of primary derived human osteoblasts and macrophages to a range of nanotopography surfaces in a single culture model in vitro. Biomaterials **24**(26): 4799–818.
Richards, M., C. Y. Fong, W. K. Chan, P. C. Wong and A. Bongso (2002) Human feeders support prolonged undifferentiated growth of human inner cell masses and embryonic stem cells. Nat Biotechnol **20**(9): 933–6.
Richardson, J. B., B. Caterson, E. H. Evans, B. A. Ashton and S. Roberts (1999) Repair of human articular cartilage after implantation of autologous chondrocytes. J Bone Joint Surg Br **81**(6): 1064–8.
Ripamonti, U. and J. R. Tasker (2000) Advances in biotechnology for tissue engineering of bone. Curr Pharm Biotechnol **1**(1): 47–55.
Risbud, M. V. and M. Sittinger (2002) Tissue engineering: advances in in vitro cartilage generation. Trends Biotechnol **20**(8): 351–6.
Robbins, P. D. and S. C. Ghivizzani (1998) Viral vectors for gene therapy. Pharmacol Ther **80**(1): 35–47.
Robey, P. G., P. Bianco and J. D. Termine (1992) The cell biology and molecular biochemistry of bone formation. In Favus, M. J. and Coe, F. L. (eds) Disorders of Mineral Metabolism. Raven Press, New York, 241–63.
Robey, P. G. (1996) Vertebrate mineralized matrix proteins: structure and function. Connect Tissue Res **35**(1–4): 131–6.
Robey, P. G. and A. L. Boskey (1996) The biochemistry of bone.In Macus, R., Feldman, D. and Kelsey, J. (eds) Osteoporosis, Academic Press, New York.
Rogers, J. J., H. E. Young, L. R. Adkison, P. A. Lucas and A. C. Black, Jr. (1995) Differentiation factors induce expression of muscle, fat, cartilage, and bone in a clone of mouse pluripotent mesenchymal stem cells. Am Surg **61**(3): 231–6.
Rolink, A. G., S. L. Nutt, F. Melchers and M. Busslinger (1999) Long-term in vivo reconstitution of T-cell development by Pax5-deficient B-cell progenitors. Nature **401**(6753): 603–6.
Ronsky, J. L., W. Herzog, T. D. Brown, D. R. Pedersen, E. S. Grood and D. L. Butler (1995) In vivo quantification of the cat patellofemoral joint contact stresses and areas. J Biomech **28**(8): 977–83.
Rosado, E., Z. Schwartz, V. L. Sylvia, D. D. Dean and B. D. Boyan (2002) Transforming growth factor–beta1 regulation of growth zone chondrocytes is mediated by multiple interacting pathways. Biochim Biophys Acta **1590**(1–3): 1–15.
Rose, E. H. and M. S. Norris (1990) The versatile temporoparietal fascial flap: adaptability to a variety of composite defects. Plast Reconstr Surg **85**(2): 224–32.
Rose, F. R. and R. O. Oreffo (2002) Bone tissue engineering: hope vs hype. Biochem Biophys Res Commun **292**(1): 1–7.
Rose, F. R., Q. Hou and R. O. Oreffo (2004) Delivery systems for bone growth factors – the new players in skeletal regeneration. J Pharm Pharmacol **56**(4): 415–27.

Rosier, R. N., R. J. O'Keefe and D. G. Hicks (1998) The potential role of transforming growth factor beta in fracture healing. Clin Orthop Relat Res (355 Suppl): 294–300.

Roughley, P. J. (2001a) Articular cartilage and changes in arthritis: noncollagenous proteins and proteoglycans in the extracellular matrix of cartilage. Arthritis Res **3**(6): 342–7.

Roughley, P. J. (2001b) Age-associated changes in cartilage matrix: implications for tissue repair. Clin Orthop Relat Res (391 Suppl): S153–60.

Rowe, N. M., B. J. Mehrara, J. S. Luchs, M. E. Dudziak, D. S. Steinbrech, P. B. Illei, G. J. Fernandez, G. K. Gittes and M. T. Longaker (1999) Angiogenesis during mandibular distraction osteogenesis. Ann Plast Surg **42**(5): 470–5.

Rozema, F. R., J. E. Bergsma, R. R. M. Bos, G. Boering, A. J. Nijenhuis, A. J. Pennings and W. C. De Bruijn (1994) Late tissue response to bone-plates and screws of poly(L-lactide) used for fixation of zygomatic fractures. J Mater Sci Mater Med **5**(575–81)

Rubin, C. T. and L. E. Lanyon (1987) Kappa Delta Award paper. Osteoregulatory nature of mechanical stimuli: function as a determinant for adaptive remodeling in bone. J Orthop Res **5**(2): 300–10.

Ruiz-Hitzky, E. (2003) Functionalizing inorganic solids: towards organic–inorganic nanostructured materials for intelligent and bioinspired systems. Chem Rec **3**(2): 88–100.

Runte, C., D. Dirksen, H. Delere, C. Thomas, B. Runte, U. Meyer, G. von Bally and F. Bollmann (2002) Optical data acquisition for computer-assisted design of facial prostheses. Int J Prosthodont **15**(2): 129–32.

Saad, B., P. Neuenschwander, G. K. Uhlschmid and U. W. Suter (1999) New versatile, elastomeric, degradable polymeric materials for medicine. Int J Biol Macromol **25**(1–3): 293–301.

Sachlos, E. and J. T. Czernuszka (2003) Making tissue engineering scaffolds work. Review: the application of solid freeform fabrication technology to the production of tissue engineering scaffolds. Eur Cell Mater **5**: 29–39; discussion 39–40.

Salgado, A. J., O. P. Coutinho and R. L. Reis (2004) Bone tissue engineering: state of the art and future trends. Macromol Biosci **4**(8): 743–65.

Salo, J., P. Lehenkari, M. Mulari, K. Metsikko and H. K. Väänänen (1997) Removal of osteoclast bone resorption products by transcytosis. Science **276**(5310): 270–3.

Salter, R. B., D. F. Simmonds, B. W. Malcolm, E. J. Rumble, D. MacMichael and N. D. Clements (1980) The biological effect of continuous passive motion on the healing of full-thickness defects in articular cartilage. An experimental investigation in the rabbit. J Bone Joint Surg Am **62**(8): 1232–51.

Salter, R. B., H. W. Hamilton, J. H. Wedge, M. Tile, I. P. Torode, S. W. O'Driscoll, J. J. Murnaghan and J. H. Saringer (1984) Clinical application of basic research on continuous passive motion for disorders and injuries of synovial joints: a preliminary report of a feasibility study. J Orthop Res **1**(3): 325–42.

Salter, R. B. (1989) The biologic concept of continuous passive motion of synovial joints. The first 18 years of basic research and its clinical application. Clin Orthop Relat Res (242): 12–25.

Salter, R. B. (1994) The physiologic basis of continuous passive motion for articular cartilage healing and regeneration. Hand Clin **10**(2): 211–9.

Sanchez, C., H. Arribart and M. M. Guille (2005) Biomimetism and bioinspiration as tools for the design of innovative materials and systems. Nat Mater **4**(4): 277–88.

Sarikaya, M., C. Tamerler, A. K. Jen, K. Schulten and F. Baneyx (2003) Molecular biomimetics: nanotechnology through biology. Nat Mater **2**(9): 577–85.

Sato, G. H. (1997) Animal cell culture. In Lanza, R., Langer, R. and Chick, W. (eds) Principles of Tissue Engineering. R.G. Landes Company, Austin, TX, 101–9.

Sato, M., T. Ochi, T. Nakase, S. Hirota, Y. Kitamura, S. Nomura and N. Yasui (1999) Mechanical tension-stress induces expression of bone morphogenetic protein (BMP)-2 and BMP-4, but not BMP-6, BMP-7, and GDF-5 mRNA, during distraction osteogenesis. J Bone Miner Res **14**(7): 1084–95.

Schaefer, J. F., M. L. Millham, B. de Crombrugghe and L. Buckbinder (2003) FGF signaling antagonizes cytokine-mediated repression of Sox9 in SW1353 chondrosarcoma cells. Osteoarthritis Cartilage **11**(4): 233–41.

minimize the possibility that we may miss a correct segment by using only one method.

The third strategy is to incorporate active learning [24] into the bootstrapping framework to ensure that the framework is scalable to larger problems. This is because mistakes will be made during co-training and the degradation in quality of the "automatically labeled sample set" might be too large for the bootstrapping process to proceed effectively. Thus, in addition to selecting those unlabeled training samples that the co-training approach is most confident of, active learning selects those that the co-training approach is least confident with and repeatedly asks the human users to label and includes them into the "expanded" labeled sample set.

We test our bootstrapping framework using a mid-sized image collection (comprising about 6,000 images from photoCD, CorelCD and Web) and demonstrate that our co-training approach without active learning could improve the performance of annotation by about 4% in terms of F_1 measure as compared to the best traditional supervised learning approach. Of course, the co-training approach has the added benefit of requiring much fewer labeled samples during training. To address the concern that the co-training framework is not scalable, we evaluate the accuracy of the resulting labeled set and found that it is only 78%. This suggests that further bootstrapping using this erroneous labeled set might be a problem since a reasonably accurate labeled set is assumed in most learning scenario. By applying active learning that requires users to label a small set of additional samples, we found that the accuracy of the resulting labeled set is improved dramatically to over 85%. Moreover, it leads to significant improvement in performance of annotation with an F_1 measure of over 58%. The results confirm that co-training with active learning is effective and is scalable to large image collections.

The main contribution of this research is two-fold. First, we devise a co-training and active learning framework to bootstrap the process of annotating large image collections starting from a small number of labeled samples. Second, we demonstrate that the framework is effective and scalable.

The rest of the chapter is organized as follows: Section 2 reviews related research, and Section 3 presents our bootstrapping framework. Section 4 presents the initial experimental results and discussion. Section 5 concludes the chapter with discussion for future work.

2 Related Work

Our work is related to research in three areas: auto image annotation, co-training and active learning. Several recent works deal with the automated or semi-automated attachment of keywords [2, 7, 13] to image databases. Mori et al. [13] were among the earliest to perform "image-to-word" transformation. They divided the images into fixed-size blocks and trained the clusters of blocks to predict keywords for new images. Barnard and Forsyth [2] segmented the images into regions using Blobworld segmentation [6] and associated keywords to regions in the training set. Chang et al. [7] employed image level content analysis and associated keywords with each image through the application of BPM (Bayes Point Machine). Wang and Li [23] performed image analysis on a fixed size blocks using a 2-D multi-resolution HMM to capture the cross blocks and cross resolution dependencies between blocks for the entire image collection. Jeon et al. [11] also used Blobworld to segment images into regions, and learned the joint distribution of blob regions and concepts.

The above approaches are based on the traditional supervised learning scheme. The training sample set is fixed and much manual effort is needed to come up with a reasonable sized labeled training set. To overcome this problem, Blum and Mitchell [4] proposed a co-training algorithm based on the conditional (view) independence assumption. The algorithm repeatedly trains two classifiers from the labeled data, labels some unlabeled data with the two classifiers, and exchanges the newly labeled data between the two classifiers. In this algorithm, one classifier always asks the other classifier to label the most certain data for the collaborator. Since the assumption of view independence cannot always be met in practice, Collins and Singer [8] proposed a co-training algorithm based on "agreement" between the classifiers. Muslea et al. [14] introduced the idea of co-testing which is designed for problems with redundant views or with multiple disjoint sets of features that can be used to learn the target concepts. Nigam and Ghani [15] empirically demonstrated that even bootstrapping (co-training) that violates the view independent assumption can still work better than the traditional learning approach. Cao et al. [5] proposed the use of uncertainty reduction in co-training, in which one classifier selects the most uncertain unlabeled data and asks the other classifier to label. They showed that the natural split of features in co-training algorithm produces the best results. Finally Pierce and Cardie [16] proposed a moderately supervised variant of co-training in which human corrects mistakes made during automatic labeling.

The main issue in active learning is how to choose the most critical instances for users to label manually. The use of uncertainty measurement is one of the popular strategies. Lewis and Gale [12] performed uncertainty sampling to compute an uncertain score to each sample and chose the next sample that the classifier has the least confidence. Zhang and Chen [24] proposed an active learning framework that selects samples automatically based on the criterion that annotating these samples will lead to an overall decrease in the uncertainty of the system.

3 The Co-Training Framework for Image Annotation

Given a scenario that we have a (small) set of labeled regions $\underline{R}_L$ and a (large) set of unlabeled regions $\underline{R}_U$, we discuss our proposed framework based on co-training and active learning to annotate large image collections. To accomplish this, we break the task of annotating images into three sub-stages of: (a) segmenting images into meaningful units, (b) extracting appropriate features for the units, and (c) associating the units in images with concepts. Thus, the problem of auto image annotation can be expressed as:

$$S^p(I_i) \approx \sum R^p_{ij} \approx \sum F^q(R^p_{ij}) \quad (1)$$

$$G^a(I_i) \approx G^a(S^p(I_i)) \approx \sum G^a(F^q(R^p_{ij})) \rightarrow \underline{L}_c \quad (2)$$

In (1), function $S^p(I_i)$ performs the transformation of the contents of image I_i. An example of such transformation is the segmentation of the image by converting its contents into meaningful units (or regions/ blocks), i.e. $S^p(I_i) \rightarrow \sum R^p_{ij}$. The function $F^q(R_{ij})$ selects a set of features to model each unit/region, R_{ij}. In (2), function $G^a(I_i)$ performs the auto-annotation that maps an image to a set of concepts in $\underline{L}_c$. Here $\underline{L}_c$ is the set of lexicon or concepts used to annotate the images. As expressed in (2), if we adopt an approach to segment the image contents into sub-units R_{ij}, then $G^a(I_i)$ can be approximated by an equivalent function to annotate each sub-unit separately and integrating the results of annotations for the overall image.

Equations (1-2) allow us to substitute different models to accomplish each stage of the annotation process independently. For example, we may choose to perform $S^p(I_i)$ by either segmenting the image I_i into regions [6, 9] or dividing it equally into fixed blocks [13] in Stage (a). We may use different function $F^q(R_{ij})$ to map the content of each sub-unit R_{ij} into different set of features in Stage (b). Finally, we may choose different machine learning methods, including the bootstrapping technique, to perform the auto-annotation of image I_i in Stage (c).

Here, we detail our bootstrapping cum active learning approach to perform auto image annotation using three strategies. The first strategy performs bootstrapping [1] at the region level by using two different classifiers derived using two orthogonal sets of content features. The second strategy employs a contextual model at the image level to disambiguate the set of concepts learned at the image level using the overlapping set of regions generated from two separate image segmentation methods. The third strategy incorporates active learning [24] into the bootstrapping framework to ensure that the framework is scalable to larger problems.

3.1 Region Classifiers for Bootstrapping Process

Given a set of regions for each image, we first discuss how to employ the co-training framework to derive the concepts for each region independently. To initiate the co-training process, we need to develop two (weakly) view independent classifiers. To this end, we adopt different function $F^q(R_{ij})$, $q \in [1, 2]$, in Stage (b), to select different set of features to represent the contents of each unit R_{ij} in the image. Here, we simply split the feature set into two disjoint sets as: (a) Set 1: color histogram, and, (b) Set 2: texture and shape features. We denote the feature sets as $F^1(R^p_{ij})$ and $F^2(R^p_{ij})$.

Next we employ a learning function $G^a(R_{ij})$ to perform the annotation by associating the contents of sub-unit R_{ij} with a set of concepts in $\underline{L}_c$. Here we adopt the probabilistic SVM method to train $G^a(R_{ij})$. For different feature sets $F^1(R^p_{ij})$ and $F^2(R^p_{ij})$, we develop two independent classifiers, H^{p1} and H^{p2}, using SVM to map a region into a confident vector of concepts as:

$$H^{p1}:\ G^a\,(S^p(F^1(R^p_{ij}))\rightarrow \underline{\Phi}^{p1} \qquad (3)$$

$$H^{p2}:\ G^a\,(S^p(F^2(R^p_{ij}))\rightarrow \underline{\Phi}^{p2}$$

where $\underline{\Phi}^{pq} = \{\ v^{pq}_1, v^{pq}_2, .., v^{pq}_N\}$ with $q\in[1,2]$. v^{pq}_j is the confident value for concept $c_j\in\underline{L}_c$, and N is the total number of concepts in $\underline{L}_c$. By combining the outputs from H^{p1} and H^{p2}, we derive the final confidence vector for region R^p_{ij} as:

$$\underline{\Phi}^P_{ij} = \frac{\sum_{k=1}^{n} v_k^{p1} * v_k^{p2}}{\underline{\Phi}_{ij}^{p1} \bullet \underline{\Phi}_{ij}^{p2}} \qquad (4)$$

The final confidence vector $\underline{\Phi}^p_{ij}$ can be used to control the assignment of concepts to region. Due to the unreliability of region segmentation method, a single concept may be insufficient to describe the region's contents. We therefore adopt two strategies to assign concepts from $\underline{\Phi}^p_{ij}$ to region R^p_{ij} as: (a) Strategy 1: select only one concept per region; and (b) Strategy 2: select the top *k* concepts.

We now outline the details of the co-training framework for annotating each region as follows.

- Inputs:

  $\underline{R}_L$: an initial collection of (small) labeled regions;

  $\underline{R}_U$: a large set of unlabeled regions;

  c_z: the concept label of the current classifiers;

  β: the number of unlabeled regions to be considered in each iteration of co-training;

  M: maximum number of iterations of the co-training process;

  m: the iteration number (m=0 initially);

  θ: the predefined threshold for selecting the most confident class label;

  τ_1, τ_2: the thresholds for selecting one classifier to label over the other.

  ε: the tolerance for the least uncertainty regions.

- LOOP:

  While there exist regions without concept labels and $m \le M$:

  - Train classifiers H^{p1} and H^{p2} from the current labeled training set $\underline{R}_L$.
  - Randomly select next set of β unlabeled regions $\underline{R}_\beta$ from $\underline{R}_U$:
    - For each $r_i \in \underline{R}_\beta$, compute the confidence values for all concepts in r_i using classifiers H^{p1} and H^{p2} based on (3).

- The following conditions are used to determine the assignment of concepts c_z to region r_i:
  - Condition 1 (when both Classifiers have high confidence in c_z): When the confidence value for c_z is larger than θ for both H^{p1} and H^{p2}, simply label r_i with concept c_z and add it to the labeled set $\underline{R}_L$.
  - Condition 2 (when only one Classifier has high confidence in c_z): If condition 1 is not satisfied, but the confidence value of concept c_z for one classifier is larger than τ_1, while that of the other classifier is less than τ_2, then use the classifier that gives higher confidence value to label the region and add it to the labeled set $\underline{R}_L$.
  - Condition 3 (when both Classifiers are uncertain) – to perform the optional active learning step: If the above two conditions are not met, but the confidence values of two classifiers for the class label c_z are around $0.5\pm\varepsilon$, then choose k such instances with the lowest entropy values and optionally asks the user/expert to label the region and add it to the labeled set $\underline{R}_L$.
- Outputs: Two updated Classifiers H^{p1} and H^{p2} and an expanded labeled set $\underline{R}_L$.

The above procedure for co-training the classifiers is performed for each segmentation method $S^p(I_i)$ separately. Optionally, it also incorporates strategy 3 by employing active learning to improve the quality of the automatically annotated sample set.

3.2 Concept Disambiguation at the Image Level

Because of the unreliability and uncertainty in image segmentation, the use of only one segmentation method runs the risk of missing or wrongly segmenting important regions, thus resulting in the missing of key concepts. In this research, we explore the use of different function $S^p(I_i)$ to segment the image into regions at the same time. In other words, we employ two different segmentation methods based on Blobworld [6] and JSEG [9]. They are denoted as $S^B(I_i)$ and $S^U(I_i)$ respectively. The idea here is to use these two different segmentation methods to segment the image into two separate sets of possibly overlapping regions. We then employ the function $G^a()$ of (3) to map each region independently into concepts, and develop a contextual model that uses the correlations between the overlapping regions and conflicting concepts to disambiguate the learnt concepts to arrive at the final annotation for each region. We call this process *concept disambiguation*.

A naïve approach to generate the overall annotation for the entire image is simply to aggregate the annotations of all regions. This, however, will not work well because although the concepts for regions are generated independently, there are dependencies between concepts or against concepts and/or regions. For example, certain concepts should not co-occur in adjacent regions or in the same image. To derive such knowledge, we need to make use of the context between regions and concepts to perform concept disambiguation. The contextual relationships between regions can be modeled by computing the overlaps between regions generated from different methods as:

$$Mc_{jk} = U_{R^b_{ij}, R^u_{ik}} = \frac{R^b_{ij} \cap R^u_{ik}}{|\text{Image } I_i|} \tag{5}$$

where Mc_{jk} contains the overlap between region R^b_{ij} and region R^u_{ik}, normalized by the size of image I_i. The Mc_{jk} values are stored in the overlapping matrix that encodes the overlaps between all regions in the same image.

As we expect the regions generated by different methods to be correlated, we expect the regions R^b_{ij} and R^u_{ik} to have some overlaps (i.e. $Mc_{jk} \neq 0$ for some j and k) and that they share common concepts (i.e. $\underline{\Phi}(R^b_{ij}) \cap \underline{\Phi}(R^u_{ik}) \neq 0$ for some j and k). The disambiguation process will make use of a decision model based on SEE5 to identify the best set of concepts for each region based on this contextual information. The inputs to the decision tree are the region id, its concept vector $\underline{\Phi}^M$, and the list of overlapping regions and their corresponding concept vector $\underline{\Phi}^S$'s. The output of the decision tree is a confidence vector for the main region, $\underline{\Phi}^M$, where the elements of $\underline{\Phi}^M$ are as defined in (3). From $\underline{\Phi}^M$, it is easy to choose the concept(s) for the region. We again employ the same strategies as in Section 3.1 to select one or more concepts to annotate the region. The unions of all resulting concepts are used as the final annotation of the image.

The overall process of our concept disambiguation process is given in Fig. 1.

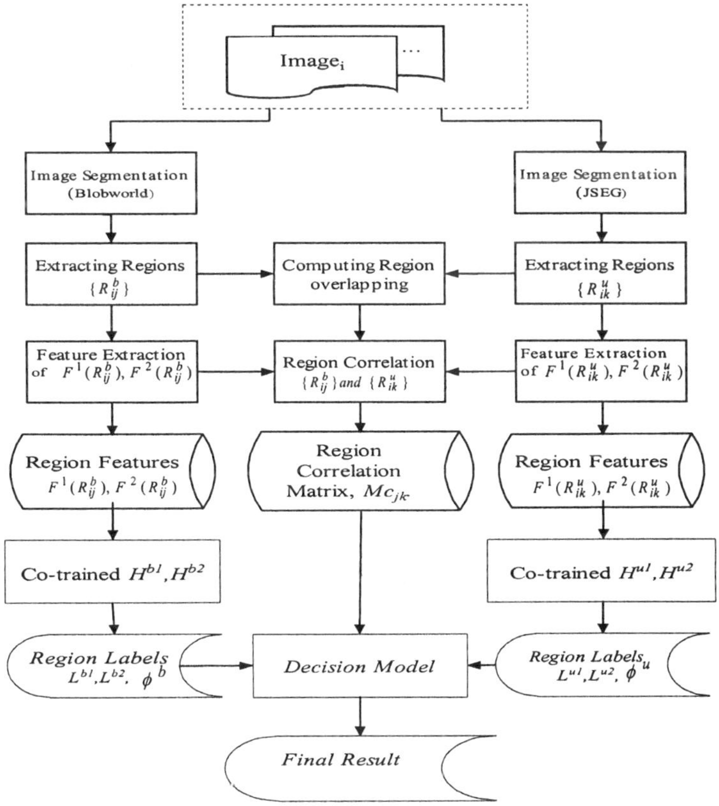

Fig. 1. The concept disambiguation framework at the image level

4 Experimental Results and Discussions

4.1 Test Data and Methods

To test the effectiveness of our approach, we use an image collection comprising about 6,000 images. The images come from PhotoCD, Web and parts from CorelCD. We randomly selected as sub-set of about 780 images for training, and the rest for testing. We test the annotation of images using 20 concepts derived from Corel CD. Some concepts are general while others are more specific. Examples of general concepts are: animals, computer, food, industry, transport, indoor, etc. Examples of more specific concepts include: people, plant, sports, rock, water, vegetation, snow, sky, beach, road, table, field, aircraft, sunset, etc.

For the co-training framework described earlier, we need to select different models at different stages of the process. The models we use are summarized as follows:

a) Feature selection function $F^q(R^p_{ij})$. For each region R^p_{ij}, we use the standard color histogram, texture and shape as the features. For the co-training experiments, we divide the feature set as: F^1 contains the color histogram, and F^2 includes only the texture and shape features.

b) Segmentation methods $S^p(I_i)$. We employ two segmentation methods based on Blobworld [6] ($S^B(I_i)$) and JSEG [9] ($S^U(I_i)$).

c) Image annotation function $G^a(I_i)$. Here we use SVM to train the classifiers, and Decision Tree in the contextual model to disambiguate the concepts learned from different classifiers based on different segmentation methods. Here we experiment with using two types of SVM -- the hard SVM that returns only a single binary decision and the probabilistic SVM (or pSVM) that returns multiple decisions with confidence values. We select SVM with radial basis function (RBF) kernel [22], and use logistic regression to compute the probability of pSVM [17].

In order to test the effectiveness of our co-training method with and without active learning against the traditional machine learning methods, we carry out experiments using the following methods:

a) Traditional machine learning approaches based on probabilistic-SVM. Our earlier work [10] showed that probabilistic-SVM is superior to hard-SVM for this task, thus we consider only the use of probabilistic-pSVM in the experiments here. We combine the feature sets F^1 and F^2 into one set, and choose 400 labeled regions for each concept label to train the classifiers. We experiment with two variants of method as follows:

   pSVM-single: Employ both the Blobworld and JSEG segmentation methods separately and use Decision Tree to perform concept disambiguation. It uses strategy 1 to select only one concept for each region.

   pSVM-multiple: Same as pSVM-single except that it selects multiple concepts for each region.

b) Co-training framework: For the co-training experiment, we choose only 20 labeled seed regions for each concept label to kick-start the co-training process. We again experiment with two variants of co-training methods -- one without active learning and the other with. The resulting methods are denoted as **co-Train(M)** and **co-Train-Active(M)** respectively, where M denotes the maximum of iterations to be performed during co-training.

4.2 Co-Training Experiment

We first test the feasibility of our co-training framework in annotating images. Here we consider only co-training without active learning. Table 1 summarizes our initial results, in which we present the results of **co-Train** with M =50 and 100. The results are presented in terms of recall, precision and F_1 measures [18]. In addition, we also differentiate between two kinds of results. The first set, which we termed ACR ("Automatically Checked Result"), compares the learned concepts for each image against the "original annotation" come with the image collection. It does not consider whether the additional concepts learned by the system that are not present in the original annotation are correct. In general, we observe that most images are only assigned with one or few keywords, and they often miss some details of images that are found by the automated methods. As a result, ACR tends to report lower precision for automated methods, as we tend to find more concepts that are correct. In order to fairly evaluate the automated techniques, we present another set of results, which we termed MCR ("Manually Checked Result"). In MCR, we manually check the learned concepts against the image contents. We consider the learned keywords as correct if it is present in the original annotation or in the image contents. MCR allows us to add more meaningful keywords into the original annotation. For example, the image with only the keywords plane often has sky, cloud, etc. The cloud and sky are likely to be learned in the automated approach, which should be considered as correct.

Table 1. Comparison between Co-training (without active learning) and traditional methods (Note: ACR: Automatically Checked Results; and MCR: Manually Checked Results)

Method	ACR			MCR		
	Re.	**Pr.**	F_1	**Re.**	**Pr.**	F_1
pSVM-single	45.0	26.5	33.4	50.5	39.0	44.0
pSVM-multiple	47.6	28.5	**35.4**	51.1	44.2	**47.4**
co-Train (50)	48.3	34.3	40.9	51.8	41.0	45.8
co-Train (100)	34.4	57.1	**42.8**	43.1	57.7	**49.3**

From Table 1, we found that the traditional method **pSVM-multiple** performs better than **pSVM-single**, indicating that the strategy of annotating "one region" with "one or more concepts" is more effective. The **pSVM-multiple** could attain an F_1 measure of 35.4% for ACR and 47.4% for MCR.

Table 1 also indicates that by using **co-Train (100)**, we could achieve a superior performance of over 42.8% for ACR and 49.3% for MCR cases. This is about 4% better than the best of the traditional method for the MCR case. The results indicate that co-training without active learning is more effective, while requiring much fewer training samples (20 times less than the traditional method) as compared to the traditional supervised learning approach.

Table 1 also shows that by performing more iterations, the performance of **co-Train(M)** improves steadily from M=50 to M=100. This indicates that our method is consistent.

4.3 Scalability Experiment

One major concern with using the co-training framework is that it might not scale up to larger problems. This is because the mistakes made during the co-training process will degrade the quality of the resulting "automatically labeled set". Thus we investigate the incorporation of active learning in the co-training process and evaluate the quality of labeled training set as compared to co-training without active learning. Table 2 lists the accuracy of the resulting labeled sets for both **co-Train(100)** and **co-Train-Active(100)**. We found that the accuracy of resulting labeled set for **co-Train (100)** is about 78.5%, whereas with **co-Train-Active(100)**, the accuracy of the labeled set improves dramatically to 85.7%. As part of the underlying assumption of co-training is that the labeled set should be sufficiently accurate, higher accuracy in the resulting labeled set suggests that further co-training is feasible and that the process is scalable. The active learning process requires users to annotate about 150 additional samples for each class. This is a relatively small amount of efforts for users to achieve superior performance.

Table 3 shows that the incorporation of active learning leads to significant improvement in the performance of annotation with an F_1 measure of over 58.4%.

Table 2: Accuracy of resulting labeled set after training (Note for pSVM, no new labeled sets are added, and hence the error rate is 0)

Method	# of initial labeled set	# of labeled samples at the end of Co-Training	Accuracy of expanded labeled set
pSVM	25 * 400	10,000	100%
co-Train(100)	25 * 20	4,595	78.5%
co-Train-Active(100)	25 * 20	4,652	85.7%

Table 3: Results of co-training with active learning (Note: ACR: Automatically Checked Results; and MCR: Manually Checked Results)

Method	ACR			MCR		
	Re.	**Pr.**	**F_1**	**Re.**	**Pr.**	**F_1**
co-Train-Active (50)	36.9	27.2	31.3	58.6	47.5	52.5
co-Train-Active (100)	34.4	57.1	**42.9**	57.3	59.6	**58.4**

4.4 Examples of Image Annotation

Fig. 2 shows some examples of images annotated using our approach. Column 2 of Fig. 2 gives both the original annotation provided by the authors, as well as the annotation learned by our system. The results show that our annotation scheme could give reasonably accurate and complete annotation. Note that as we support only "animal" as the general concept for all types of animals, specific animals such as "dog", "tiger", etc. are tagged as "animals", which are considered to be correct.

(1) Image	(2) Keywords
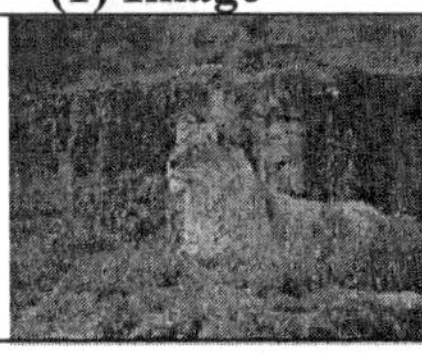	Original: tiger, grass, rock Learned: animals, grass
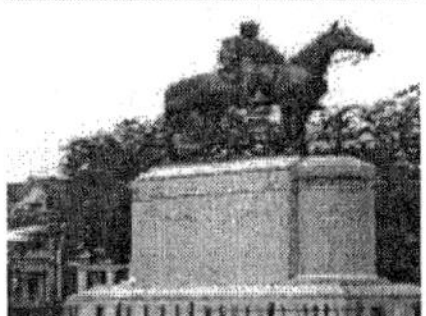	Original: travel Learned: plant, rock
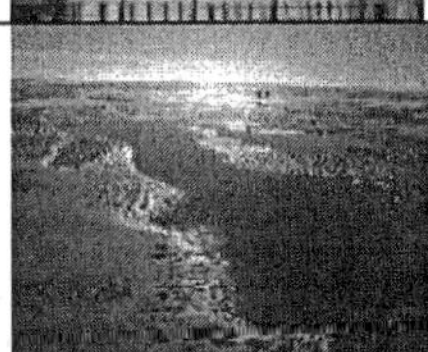	Original: water, beach Learned: water, beach, sunset, sky
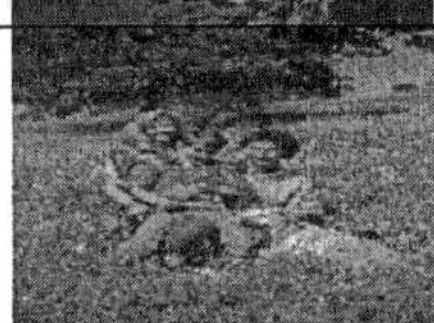	Original: people, plant, travel, animals Learned: people, grass, sky
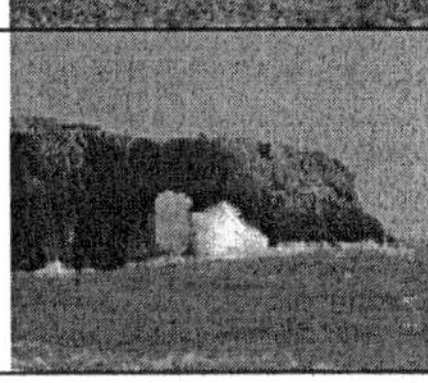	Original: water Learned: rock, water

Fig. 2. Examples of image annotation using our approach

5 Summary

Because of the ambiguity in content-based retrieval techniques, most users prefer to access images using keywords. This brings in a major practical problem of how to (semi-) automatically annotate large image/video archives with text annotations. This research explores the use of bootstrapping approach to perform auto image annotation that requires a small number of labeled training samples to kick start the training process. We carried out experiments using a mid-sized image collection (comprising about 6,000 images). We demonstrated that our co-training framework is able to improve the accuracy of annotation by over 4% in F_1 measure as compared to the traditional supervised learning approach, while requiring only 5% of the labeled samples to kick start the training process. Further we addressed the concern of scalability with co-training by incorporating active learning into the framework. We demonstrated that the use of active learning could further improve the performance of annotation significantly by over 18%, and that the accuracy of the resulting labeled set remains high (>85%), thus ensuring that the co-training framework is scalable.

In evaluating the effectiveness of the bootstrapping techniques, one should also consider the enormous benefits of requiring much fewer training samples (20 times less) as compared to the traditional supervised learning approach to kick start the learning process. This provides a practical approach to deploy the system to handle dynamic environment.

Our results demonstrated that the collaborative bootstrapping approach, initially developed for text processing, could be effectively employed to tackle the challenging problems of multimedia information retrieval. We will carry out further research in the following areas. First, we will further investigate the consistency and scalability of co-training approach by carrying out both theoretical study and large-scale empirical experiments. Second, we will explore the use of better content features to model images' contents. Finally, we will research into web image mining based on the images obtained from the web and their surrounding context.

Acknowledgment

The first author would like to thank the National University of Singapore (NUS) for the provision of a scholarship, under which this research is carried out.

References

1. Abney, S. (2002) Bootstrapping, Association for Computational Linguistics (ACL'02).
2. Barnard, K., Forsyth, D. A. (2001) Learning the semantics of words and pictures, IEEE International Conference on Computer Vision II, 408-415
3. Barnard, K., Duygulu, P., Forsyth, D. (2001) Clustering Art, IEEE Computer Vision and Pattern Recognition, 434-441
4. Blum, A., Mitchell, T. (1998) Combined labeled data and unlabelled data with co-training, Proceeding of the 11th Annual Conference on Computational Learning Theory.
5. Cao, Y., Li, H., Lian, L. (2003) Uncertainty reduction in collaborative bootstrapping: measure and algorithm, Association for computational Linguistics (ACL'03).
6. Carson, C., Thomas, M., Hellerstein, J. M., Malik, J. (1999) BlobWorld: A system for region-based image indexing and retrieval, International Conf Visual Info Sys.
7. Chang, E., Goh, K., Sychay, G., Wu, G. (2003) CBSA: content-based soft annotation for multimodal image retrieval using Bayes Point Machines, IEEE Transactions on Circuits and Systems for Video Technology, Special Issue on Conceptual and Dynamical Aspects of Multimedia Content Description **13**, 26-38
8. Collins, M., Singer, Y. (1999) Unsupervised models for name entity classification, Proceedings of the Joint SIGDAT Conference on Empirical Methods in Natural language Processing and Very Large Corpora.
9. Deng, Y., Manjunath, B. S. (2001) Unsupervised segmentation of color-texture regions in images and video, IEEE Trans on Pattern Analysis and Machine Intelligence, **23**, 800-810
10. Feng, H., Chua, T.-S., (2003) A bootstrapping approach to annotating large image collection, Workshop on Multimedia Information Retrieval, organized in part of ACM Multimedia 2003, 55-62
11. Jeon, J., Lavrenko, V., Manmatha, R. (2003) Automatic image annotation and retrieval using cross-media relevance models, ACM AIGIR, 119-126
12. Lewis, D. D., Gale, W. A. (1994) A sequential algorithm for training text classifiers, in proceeding of ACM SIGIR, 3-12
13. Mori, Y., Takahashi, H., Oka, R. (1999) Image-to-word transformation based on dividing and vector quantizing images with words, First International Workshop on multimedia Intelligent Storage and Retrieval Management.
14. Muslea, I., Minton, S., Knoblock, C. A. (2000) Selective sampling with co-testing, CRM Workshop on Combining and Selecting Multiple Models with Machine Learning.

15. Nigam, K., Ghani, R. (2000) Analyzing the effectiveness and applicability of co-training, Proceedings of the 9th International Conference on Information and Knowledge management.
16. Pierce, D., Cardie, C. (2001) Limitations of co-training for natural language learning from large datasets, Proceeding of the Conference on Empirical Methods in Natural Language Processing.
17. Platt, J. C. (1999) Probabilistic outputs for support vector machines and comparisons to regularized likelihood methods, in 'Advances in Large Margin Classifiers', Smola, A. J., Bartlett, P., Scholkopf, B., Schuurmans, D. (Eds). MIT Press.
18. Salton, G., McGill, M. J. (1983) Introduction to modern information retrieval, McGraw Hill.
19. Smith, J. R., Chang, S.-F. (1996) VisualSeek: A fully automated content-based query system, ACM Multimedia, 87-92
20. Smith, J. R., Naphade, M., Natsev, A. (2003) Multimedia semantic indexing using model vectors. ICME '03.
21. Shi, R., Feng, H., Chua, T.-S., Lee, C.-H. (2004) An adaptive image content representation and segmentation approach to automatic image annotation, Conference on Image and Video Retrieval (CIVR'04).
22. Vapnik, Vladimir. (1995) The nature of statistical learning theory, Springer, New York.
23. Wang, J. Z., Li, J. (2002) Learning-based linguistic indexing of pictures with 2-D MHHMs, ACM Multimedia '2002, 436-445
24. Zhang C., Chen, T. (2002) An active learning framework for content-based information retrieval, IEEE transactions on multimedia, **4**, 260-268

Moderate Vocabulary Visual Concept Detection for the TRECVID 2002

Milind R. Naphade and John R. Smith

IBM Thomas J. Watson Research Center
19 Skyline Drive
Hawthorne, NY 10532
http://www.research.ibm.com/people/m/milind
{naphade,jsmith}@us.ibm.com

Abstract. The explosion in multimodal content availability underlines the necessity for content management at a semantic level. We have cast the problem of detecting semantics in multimedia content as a pattern classification problem and the problem of building models of multimodal semantics as a learning problem. Recent trends show increasing use of statistical machine learning providing a computational framework for mapping low level media features to high level semantic concepts. In this chapter we expose the challenges that these techniques face. We show that if a lexicon of visual concepts is identified a priori, a statistical framework can be used to build visual feature models for the concepts in the lexicon. Using support vector machine (SVM) classification we build models for 34 semantic concepts for the TREC 2002 benchmark corpus. We study the effect of number of examples available for training with respect to their impact on detection. We also examine low level feature fusion as well as parameter sensitivity with SVM classifiers.

Keywords: TRECVID, support vector machines, mean average precision, visual concept detection

1 Introduction

The age of multimedia content explosion is upon us thanks to the recent advances in technology and reductions in costs of capture, storage and transmission of content. This starkly exposes the limitation of processing and management of the content using low-level features and underlines the need for intelligent analysis that exposes the semantics of the content. Analyzing the semantics of multimedia content is essential and for popular utilization of multimedia repositories. Various multimedia applications such as storage and retrieval, transmission, editing, mining, commerce, etc. increasingly require the availability of semantic metadata along with the content. The MPEG-7

[1] standard provides a mechanism for describing this metadata. But the challenge is to encode MPEG-7 descriptions automatically or semi-automatically. This is possible if computational multimedia features can be mapped to high-level semantic concepts represented by the media. Semantic analysis of multimedia content is necessary to support search and retrieval of content based on the presence (or absence) of semantic concepts such as *Explosion* [2], sunset [3], Outdoors, Rocket-launch [4], Cityscape [5], genre [6], sports video classification [7], meeting video analysis [8], broadcast news analysis [9], commercials [10], hunt videos [11], etc. There is a shift in focus from query by example techniques [12, 13] and relevance feedback [14] to model based fixed-lexicon concept detection. This has to do as much with the difficulty in phrasing a query in terms of very few exemplars as it has to do with the difference in complexity of semantic concepts for which models can be built as against that of the run-time semantic concepts that the selected examples in relevance feedback are supposed to abstract. Obviously the former task is less formidable than the latter. By confining the lexicon to a set of mid-level semantic concepts and coupling this with greater supervision in terms of number of positive exemplars, model-based concept detection is able to perform multimedia analysis and retrieval. The concept modeling framework can also assist the query by example paradigm by complementing low-level feature based similarity with mid-level semantic concept-based similarity [15] as well as context modeling and enforcement [16]. The assumption is that a limited set of concept detectors can help expand richly semantic user queries [17].

The National Institute for Standards and Technology (NIST) established a TREC Video benchmark [17] to evaluate progress in multimedia retrieval for semantic queries. One task was to use 24 hours of video data for concept modeling and detect ten benchmark semantic concepts on a different 5 hours test collection. This explicit concept detection task galvanized research in many groups worldwide resulting in participation of 10 groups in the task for TRECVID 2002 [17, 18, 19, 20, 21, 22, 23, 24, 25]. In this chapter we discuss a generic trainable framework using support vector machine classifiers to build models for the 6 visual concepts from among the 10 benchmark concepts. The same framework has also been applied to model 34 visual semantic concepts (either sites or objects). Specifically we will discuss issues such as early fusion of multiple visual features. We will also discuss simple methods of overcoming performance sensitivity to various model parameters.

The chapter is organized as follows. In Section 2 we present our framework for modeling a moderate sized lexicon of visual semantic concepts. In Section 3 we discuss the experimental setup used in this chapter. In Section 4 we report the results using the TREC Video corpus. Conclusions and directions for future research are presented in Section 5.

2 Modeling Visual Semantic Concepts

The generic framework for modeling semantic concepts from multimedia features [2] includes an annotation interface, a learning framework for building models and a detection module for ranking unseen content based on detection confidence for the models (which can be interpreted as keywords). Suitable learning models include generative models [4] as well as discriminant techniques. Positive examples for interesting semantic concepts are usually rare.

2.1 Support Vector Machines

The approach used in the IBM TRECVID 2001 concept modeling system [26] required modeling of conditional densities that describe the distribution of a semantic concept in a given feature space under the two possible hypotheses. On the other hand the approach described in this chapter uses the discriminant approach that is focussed only on those characteristics of a given feature set that can discriminate between the two hypotheses of interest. Vapnik [27] proposed the idea of constructing learning algorithms based on the structural risk minimization inductive principle. Vapnik introduced *Support vector machine* (SVM) classifiers that implement the idea of mapping a feature vector into a high dimensional space through some nonlinear mapping and then constructing an optimal separating hyperplane in this space.

Consider a set of patterns $\{\mathbf{x_1}, \ldots, \mathbf{x_n}\}$ with a corresponding set of labels $\{y_1, \ldots, y_n\}$ where $y \in \{-1, 1\}$. The idea is to use a nonlinear transformation $\Phi(x)$ and a kernel $K(\mathbf{x}_i, \mathbf{x}_j)$, such that this kernel K can be used in place of an inner product defined on the transformed non-linear feature vectors $< \Phi(\mathbf{x}_i), \Phi(\mathbf{x}_j) >$. The optimal hyperplane for classification in the nonlinear transformed space is then computed by converting this constrained optimization problem into its dual problem, using Lagrange multipliers and then solving the dual problem.

Introducing slack in terms of soft margins and using a 2-norm soft margin, this is then equivalent to solving the constrained optimization problem stated in Eq. (1)

$$\min_{W,b,\xi} \quad 0.5 < W, W > +c \sum_{i=1}^{i=n} \xi_i^2 \tag{1}$$

subject to the constraints in Eq. (2)

$$y_i(< W, x_i > +b) \geq 1 - \xi_i \quad \xi_i \geq 0 \tag{2}$$

Here ξ is the slack or soft margin and W and b are the parameters of the separating hyperplane. It turns out that using Lagrange multipliers and the saddle point theorem [28], the primal problem of minimization can be converted to a dual problem of maximization of the expression in Eq. (3)

$$\max_{\alpha \in \Lambda} \tilde{L}(\alpha) = \sum_{i=1}^{n} \alpha_i - 0.5 \sum_{i=1}^{n} \sum_{i=1}^{n} \alpha_i \alpha_j y_i y_j < \Phi(\mathbf{x}_i), \Phi(\mathbf{x}_j) > \quad (3)$$

subject to the constraints

$$\sum_{i=1}^{n} \alpha_i y_i = 0 \;\; \alpha_i \geq 0 \quad (4)$$

where α_i are the Lagrange multipliers introduced to solve the constrained optimization problems under inequality constraints. If the non-linear transformation $\Phi()$ is chosen carefully, such that the Kernel can be used to replace inner product in the transformed space Eq. (3) reduces to

$$\max_{\alpha \in \Lambda} \tilde{L}(\alpha) = \sum_{i=1}^{n} \alpha_i - 0.5 \sum_{i=1}^{n} \sum_{i=1}^{n} \alpha_i \alpha_j y_i y_j K(\mathbf{x}_i, \mathbf{x}_j) \quad (5)$$

where the operations are now performed using the kernel in the original feature space. The problem then reduces to finding the right kernel.

For the experiments in this chapter we have reported results using the radial basis kernel function defined in Eq. (6)

$$K(x_i, x_j) = e^{\frac{-||x_i - x_j||^2}{2\sigma^2}} \quad (6)$$

We compared the SVM classifier with the GMM (Gaussian Mixture Model) classifier on TRECVID 2001 data, and observed that the SVM classifiers perform better with fewer training samples. They also perform better in the range of 100 to 500 training samples [29].

For annotating video content so as to train models, a lexicon is needed. An annotation tool that allows the user to associate the object-labels with an individual region in a key-frame image or with the entire image was used[1] to create a labeled training set. For experiments reported here the models were built using features extracted from key-frames. Fig. 1 shows the feature and parameter selection process incorporated in the learning framework for optimal model selection and is described below.

2.2 Early Feature Fusion

Assuming that we extract features for color, texture, shape, structure, etc. It is important to fuse information from across these feature types. One way is to build models for each feature type including color, structure, texture and shape and combine their confidence scores post-detection [4]. We also experiment with early feature fusion by combining multiple feature types at an early stage to construct a single model across different features. This approach is

[1] Available at http://www.alphaworks.ibm.com/tech/videoannex

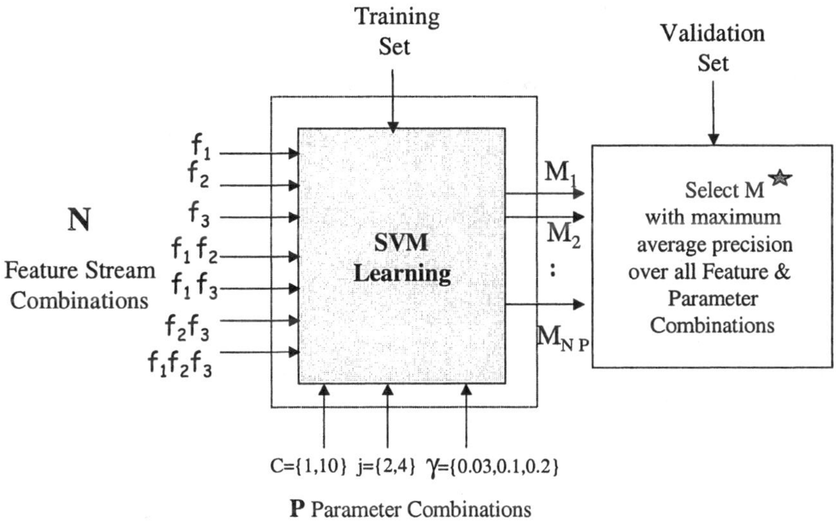

Fig. 1. SVM learning: optimizing over multiple possible feature combinations and model parameters.

suitable for concepts that have sufficiently large number of training set exemplars and feature types, which are believed to be correlated and dependent. We can simply concatenate one or more of these feature types (appropriately normalized). Different combinations can then be used to construct models and the validation set is used to choose the optimal combination. This is feature selection at the coarse level of feature types. Results of this feature type combination selection and early fusion are presented in Section 4.

2.3 Minimizing Sensitivity to Kernel Parameters

Performance of SVM classifiers can vary significantly with variation in parameters of the models. Choice of the kernels and their parameters is therefore crucial. To minimize sensitivity to these design choices, we experiment with different kernels and for each kernel we build models for several combinations of the parameters. Radial basis function kernels usually perform better than other kernels. In our experiments we built models for different values of the RBF parameter γ (variance), relative significance of positive vs. negative examples j (necessitated also by the imbalance in the number of positive vs. negative training samples) and trade-off between training error and margin c. While a coarse to fine search is ideal, we tried 3 values of γ, 2 values of j and 2 of c. Using the validation set we then performed a grid search for the combination that resulted in highest average precision.

3 Experimental Setup

3.1 TREC Video 2002 Corpus: Training & Validation

NIST provided the following data sets for the TRECVID 2002 Video Benchmark:

- Training Set: 24 hours
- Feature (Concept) Detection Test Set: 5 hours
- Search Test Set: 40 hours

The above sets were obtained by random selection from the master set of 69 hours of video content. We further partitioned the NIST training set into a 19 hour IBM training set and left out the remaining 5 hours as a validation set. The idea is to annotate the training set to construct the models and then annotate the validation set and measure the performance of the constructed models using the validation set. This is essential for parameter selection and to avoid over-fitting on the training set. Only a validation set that was drawn randomly from the original NIST training set was used to tune the performance of all the models. An ideal approach would have been to dynamically partition the 24 hour NIST training set into several pairs of complementary training and validation sets and construct an ensemble of models. Given the limited time for the experiments we however persisted with a single fixed partition that was decided before starting the modeling experiments. NIST defined non-interpolated average precision over 1000 retrieved shots as a measure of retrieval effectiveness. Let R be the number of true relevant documents in a set of size S; L the ranked list of documents returned. At any given index j let R_j be the number of relevant documents in the top j documents. Let $I_j = 1$ if the jth document is relevant and 0 otherwise. Assuming $R < S$, the non-interpolated average precision **(AP)** is then defined in Eq. (7)

$$\frac{1}{R}\sum_{j=1}^{S}\frac{R_j}{j} * I_j \tag{7}$$

3.2 Lexicon

We created a lexicon with more than hundred semantic concepts for describing events, sites, and objects [2]. However only 34 concepts had support of more than 20 shots in the training set and were modeled:

- Scenes: Outdoors, Indoors, Landscape, Cityscape, Sky, Greenery, Waterbody, Beach, Mountain, Land, Farm Setting, Farm Field, Household Setting, Factory Setting, Office Setting.
- Objects: Face, Person, People, Road, Building, Transportation Vehicle, Car, Train, Tractor, Airplane, Boat, Tree, Flowers, Fire/smoke, Animal, Text Overlay, Chicken, Cloud, Household Appliances.

3.3 Feature Extraction

After performing shot boundary detection and key-frame extraction [30], each keyframe was analyzed to detect the 5 largest regions described by their bounding boxes. The system then extracts the following low level visual features at the frame-level or global level as well as the region level for the entire frame as well as each of the regions in the keyframes.

- Color Histogram (72): 72-bin YCbCr color space ($8 \times 3 \times 3$).
- Color Correlogram (72): Single-banded auto-correlogram coefficients extracted for 8 radii depths in a 72-bin YCbCr color space [31].
- Edge Orientation Histogram (32): Using a Sobel filtered image and quantized to 8 angles and 4 magnitudes.
- Co-occurrence Texture (48): Based on entropy, energy, contrast, and homogeneity features extracted from gray-level co-occurrence matrices at 24 orientations (c.f. [32]),
- Moment Invariants (6): Based on Dudani's moment invariants [33] for shape description modified to take into the account the gray-level intensities instead of binary intensities.
- Normalized Bounding Box Shape (2): The width and the height of the bounding box normalized by that of the image.

4 Results

4.1 Validation Set Performance

Fig. 2 shows the precision recall curve as well as the average precision curve for the concept *Outdoors* based on early feature fusion. The average precision as defined in Eq. (7) is plotted against the number of documents retrieved and is a non-decreasing function in terms of the number of documents.

Fig. 3 demonstrates the importance of parameter selection of the SVM models. Exhaustive modeling for different parameter combinations and use of validation set for selection helps significantly in minimizing sensitivity of the model performance as seen from the range of average precision (AP) from 0.15 to 0.53 in this case.

Fig. 3 in particular shows the precision recall curves for 12 parameter combinations of γ, j and c of the RBF kernel for the cooccurrence feature type. In this case it is clear that $j = 4$ is a bad choice irrespective of the other parameters. In Table 1 we list the average precision computed over a fixed number of total documents retrieved. Fig. 4 displays bar plots for all 34 semantic concepts. We compare average precision for each concept with the ratio of positive training samples to the total number of training samples for that concept. The number of positive training samples vary from 20 (Beach with AP 0.17) to 2809 (Outdoors with AP 0.59).

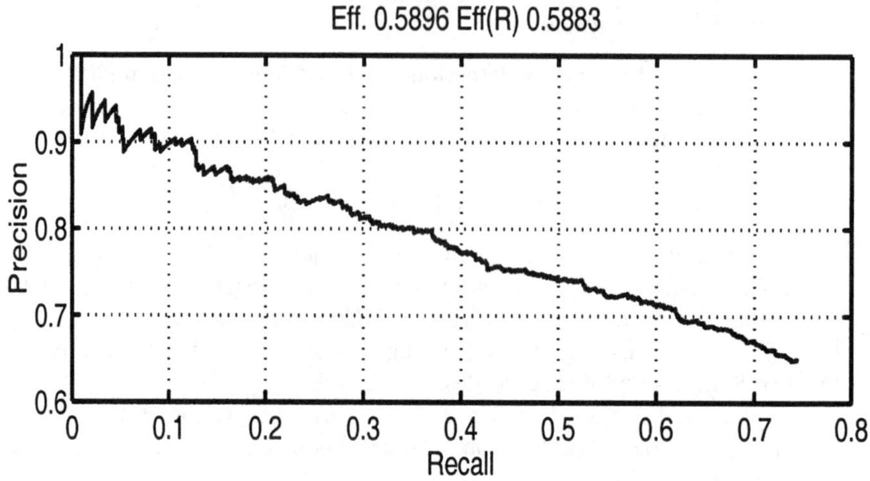

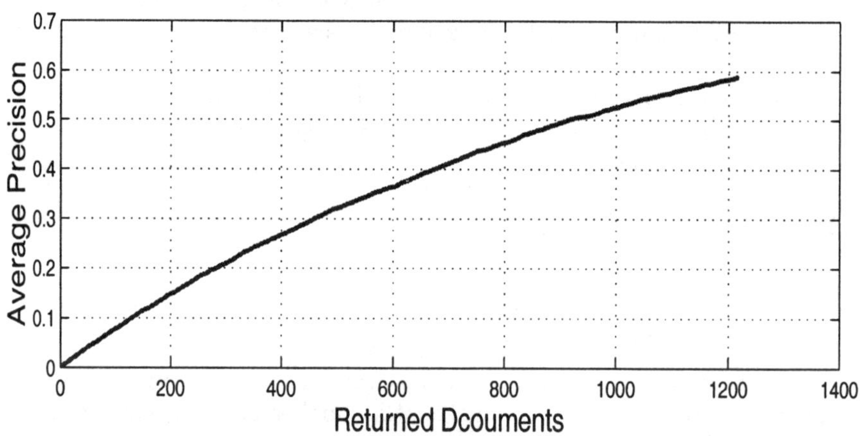

Fig. 2. Comparing Validation Set Detection performance for concept *Outdoors* with the precision recall curve and the average precision curve.

Fig. 5 plots average precision as a function of number of training samples. In Fig. 5 each point is a different concept, so the plot does not track the progress of a single concept as the number of samples in the training set are increased. Each point is a snapshot (which can also be seen in Table 1) using the maximum number of positive training samples available in the training set. This is one way to analyze the complexity of concepts. In general as the number of training samples increases the average precision improves significantly in the beginning and then the growth rate decreases. The exceptions to the general nature of the curve also indicate the complexity of the concept. Concepts like *Beach* perform better than other concepts which have more

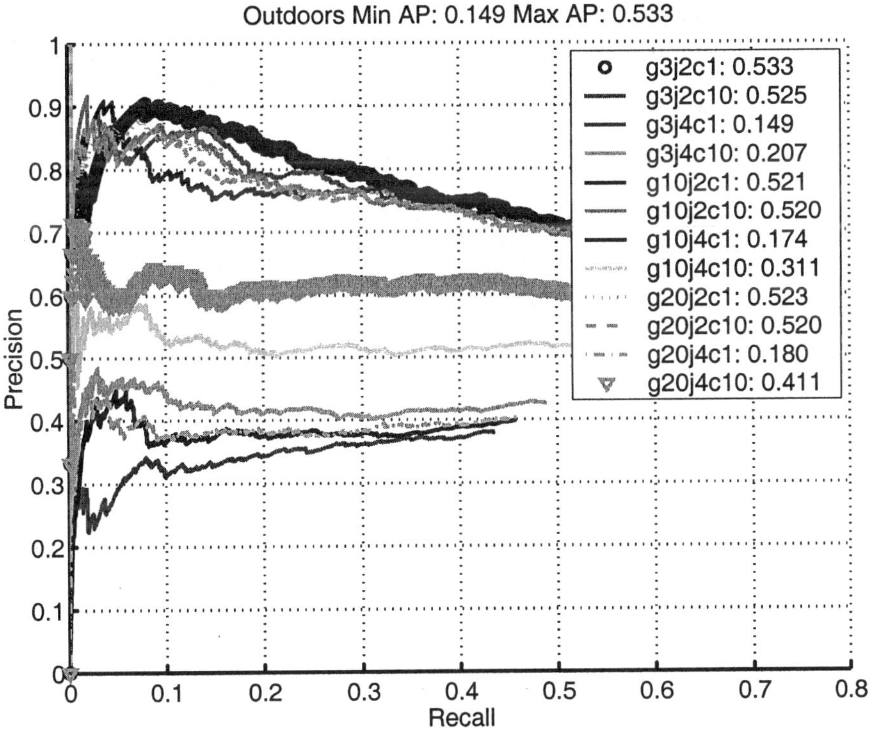

Fig. 3. Comparing Validation Set Detection performance for concept *Outdoors* across color, texture and structure features and a combination of all three types. Legend lists average precision in each case.

samples. Conversely a concept like *Water-body* performs worse than other concepts which have roughly the same number of training samples.

4.2 Test Set Performance

Seven of the ten TRECVID benchmark concepts are visual: Outdoors, Indoors, Face, People, Landscape, Cityscape, Text Overlay. Table 2 lists the test set concept detection performance for 6 of the 7 concepts where models were based on generic SVM classification. The validation set performance carries over to the test set.

Early feature fusion described in Section 2 demonstrates improvement in performance over any single feature for all six concepts (Table 2). Figs. 6 and 7 show precision recall curves comparing the early fusion performance for color, texture and structure features for *Outdoors* and *Indoors* respectively.

Semantic concepts are interlinked. Naphade et al. [16] have explicitly modeled and utilized this interaction. Here we see how effectively simple dependencies may be used. Fig. 8 shows the precision recall curve for ranking all

Table 1. Concept Detection Performance Measure listed in the decreasing order of number of positive examples in a training set of 9603 keyframes.

Semantic Concept	# Training Examples	Average Precision
Outdoors	2809	0.59
Person	2238	0.53
People	1710	0.4
Sky	1441	0.43
Indoors	1392	0.39
Face	1059	0.26
Building	881	0.174
Greenery	755	0.173
Transportation	713	0.2947
Text Overlay	444	0.12
Tree	431	0.146
Road	332	0.27
Water-body	327	0.133
Landscape	292	0.217
HouseSetting	238	0.09
Car	220	0.227
Cloud	217	0.07
OfficeSetting	213	0.024
FactorySetting	191	0.033
Animal	142	0.067
Land	139	0.059
Train	126	0.06
Flower	125	0.132
Mountain	120	0.02
Farm	103	0.017
Airplane	96	0.1
Household Appliance	84	0.009
Farmfield	83	0.016
Boat	68	0.07
Cityscape	66	0.067
Tractor	51	0.012
Fire/Smoke	37	0.1386
Beach	20	0.173

Outdoor shots based on the detection of *Sky* in them. The high average precision is not surprising. Fig. 9 illustrates a similar correlation between *Building* and *Cityscape*.

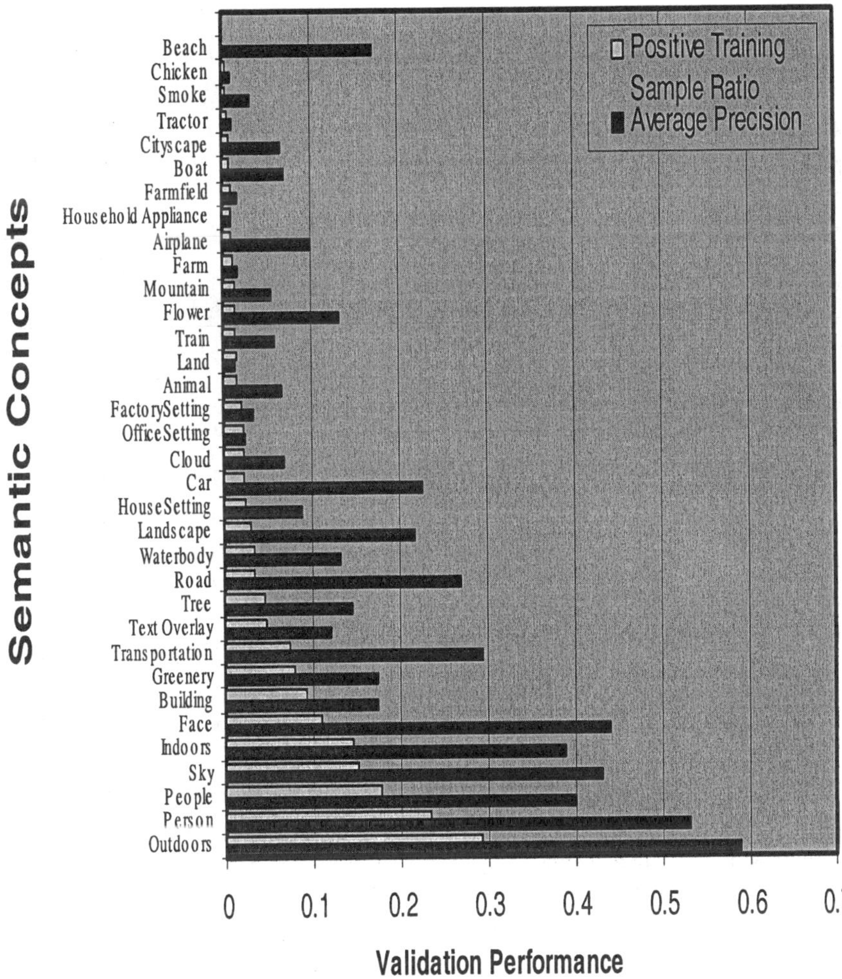

Fig. 4. Validation Set Average Precision and the Training Set Positive Example Ratio for the 34 concept models. Training set consists of 9603 shots.

5 Conclusion and Future Directions

We present a framework for modeling visual concepts using low-level features and support vector machine learning. Using the TRECVID Video corpus we develop a novel and comprehensive vocabulary of 34 visual semantic concepts. With reasonable number of training examples, this results in satisfactory detection performance. If the number of positive training examples is reasonable, early feature fusion with SVM classification improves detection over any sin-

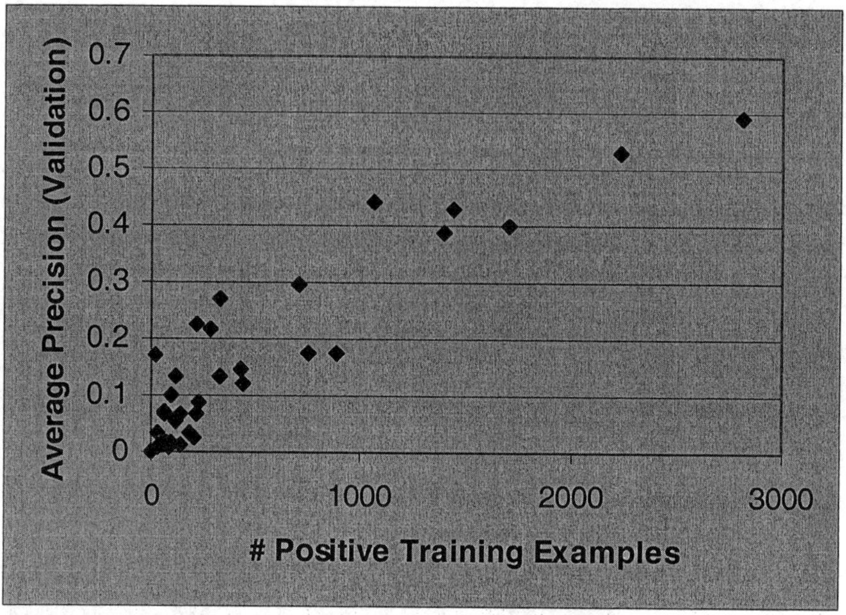

Fig. 5. Validation Set Average Precision and the Training Set Positive Example Ratio for the 34 concept models. Training set consists of 9603 shots.

Table 2. Test Set Detection Performance of 6 visual Benchmark concepts. Ground Truth provided by NIST. Concepts marked by ⋆ were used in 4 of the 7 IBM detectors that resulted in highest average precision among all participants.

Semantic Concept	Average Precision
Outdoors⋆	0.55
People⋆	0.244
Indoors⋆	0.281
Face	0.231
Landscape	0.178
Cityscape⋆	0.315

gle feature type. We examine how sensitivity to parameters can be minimized. Future research aims at improving detection especially for rare classes using context and multimodality. Future research also aims at increasing the size of the lexicon so as to improve the coverage of the lexicon and its effective utilization for semantic search.

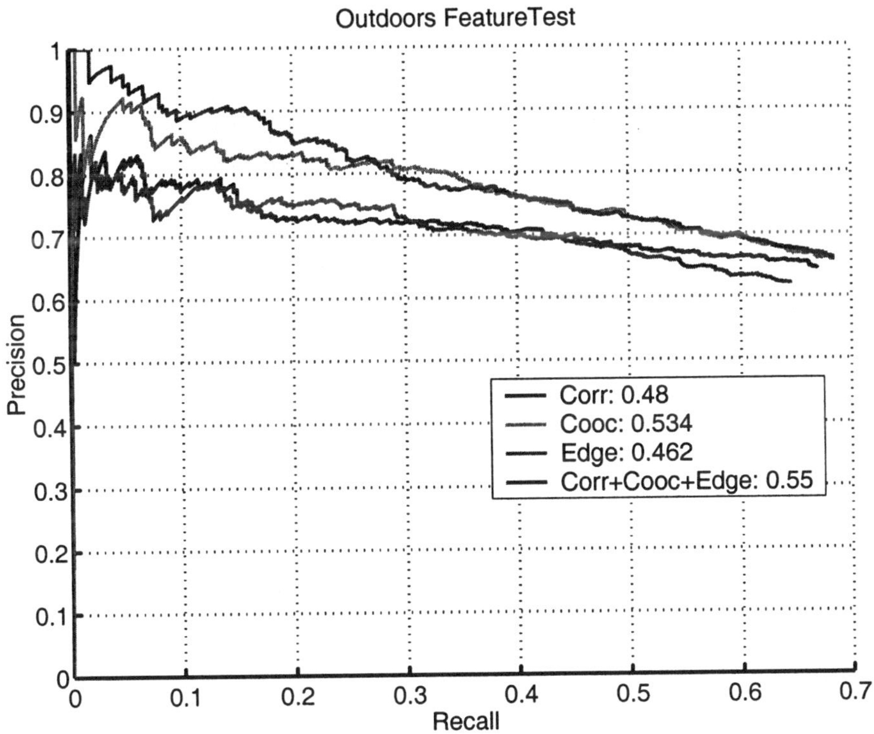

Fig. 6. Test Set Detection Comparison for *Outdoors* across feature types. Legend lists AP in each case.

6 Acknowledgements

The IBM TREC team (annotation, shot detection). NIST (performance evaluation). In particular, the authors would like to thank C. Lin for the bounding boxes in keyframes from which regional features were extracted, A. Natsev for help with feature extraction, and A. Amir for the CueVideo shot boundary detection.

References

1. ISO/IEC JTC 1/SC 29/WG 11/N3966 (2001) *Text of 15938-5 FCD Information Technology - Multimedia Content Description Interface - Part 5 Multimedia Description Schemes*, Final Committee Draft (FCD) edition.
2. Naphade, M., Kristjansson, T., Frey, B., Huang, T. S. (1998) Probabilistic multimedia objects (multijects): A novel approach to indexing and retrieval in multimedia systems, IEEE International Conference on Image Processing, vol. 3, pp. 536–540.

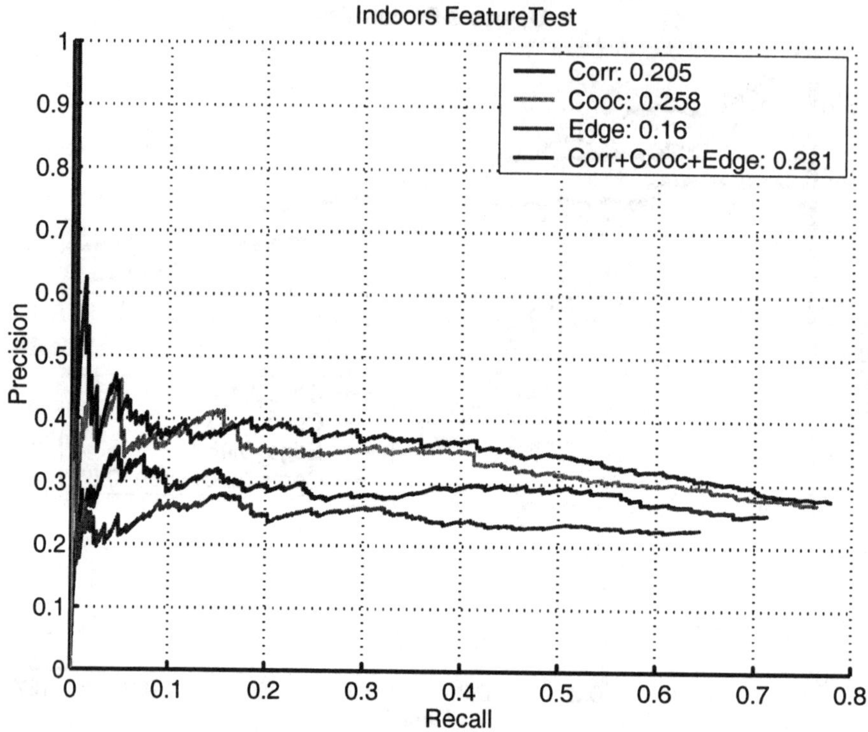

Fig. 7. Test Set Detection Comparison for *Indoors* across feature types. Legend lists AP in each case.

3. Chang, S. F., Chen, W., Sundaram, H. (1998) Semantic visual templates - linking features to semantics, IEEE International Conference on Image Processing, vol. 3, pp. 531–535.
4. Naphade, M., Basu, S., Smith, J., Lin, C., Tseng, B. (2002) Modeling semnatic concepts to support query by keywords in video, International Confernce on Image Processing.
5. Vailaya, A., Jain, A., Zhang, H. (1998) On image classification: City images vs. landscapes, Pattern Recognition, vol. 31, pp. 1921–1936.
6. Iyengar, G., Lippman, A. (1998) Models for automatic classification of video sequences, SPIE Conference on Storage and Retrieval for Still Image and Video Databases, pp. 216–227.
7. Saur, D. D., Tan, Y.-P., Kulkarni, S. R., Ramadge, P. J. (1997) Automated analysis and annotation of basketball video, SPIE Symposium, vol. 3022, pp. 176–187.
8. Foote, J., Boreczky, J., Wilcox, L. (1999) Finding presentations in recorded meetings using audio and video features, IEEE International Conference on Speech Accoustics and Signal Processing, pp. 3029–3032.
9. Brown, M. G., Foote, J. T., Jones, G., Jones, K., Young, S. (1995) Automatic content-based retrieval of broadcast news, ACM International Conference on Multimedia, pp. 35–43.

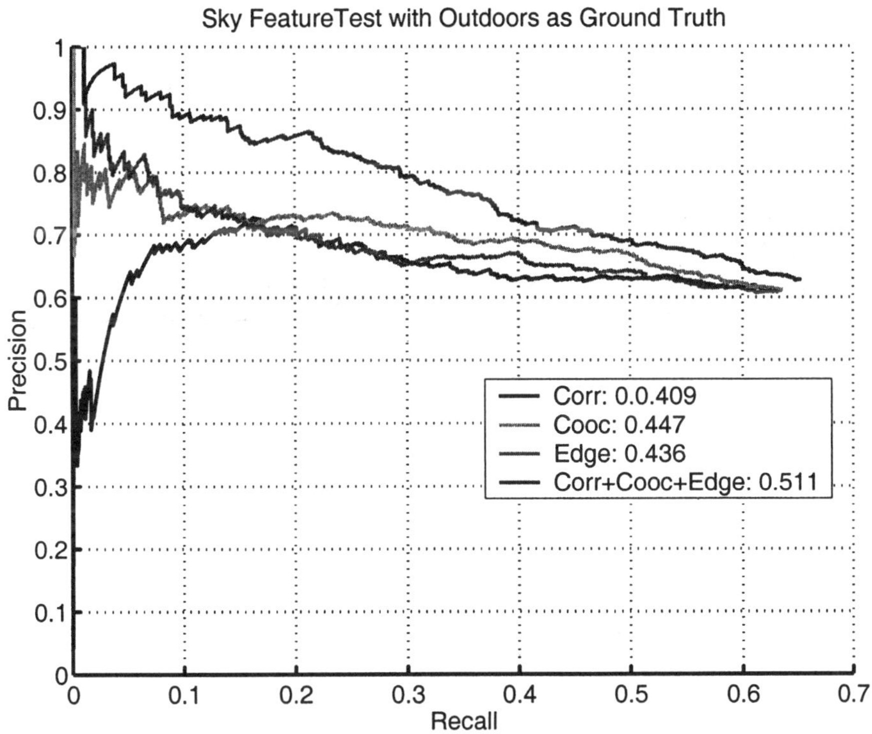

Fig. 8. Using *Sky* detection to predict *Outdoors.*

10. DelBimbo, A., Pala, P., Tanganelli, L. (2000) Retrieval by contents of commercials based on dynamics of color flows, IEEE International Confernece on Multimedia and Expo, vol. 1, pp. 479–482.
11. Qian, R., Hearing, N., Sezan, I. (1999) A computational approach to semantic event detection, Computer Vision and Pattern Recognition, vol. 1, pp. 200–206.
12. Smith, J. R., Chang, S. F. (1996) Visualseek: A fully automated content-based image query system, ACM Multimedia.
13. Flickner, M., Sawhney, H., Niblack, W., Ashley, J., Huang, Q., Dom, B., Gorkani, M., Hafner, J., Lee, D., Petkovic, D., Steele, D., Yanker, P. (1995) Query by image and video content: The QBIC system, IEEE Computer, vol. 28, no. 9, pp. 23–32.
14. Rui, Y., Huang, T. S. Ortega, M., Mehrotra, S. (1998) Relevance feedback: A power tool in interactive content-based image retrieval, IEEE Transactions on Circuits and Systems for Video Technology, Special issue on Segmentation, Description, and Retrieval of Video Content, vol. 8, no. 5, pp. 644–655.
15. Smith, J., Naphade, M., Natsev, A. (2003) Multimedia semantic indexing using model vectors, IEEE International Conference on Multimedia and Expo.
16. Naphade, M., Smith, J. R. (2003) A hybrid framework for detecting the semantics of concepts and context, Lecture Notes in Computer Science: Image and Video Retrieval, Lew, M., Sebe, N., Eakins, J., Eds. Springer.

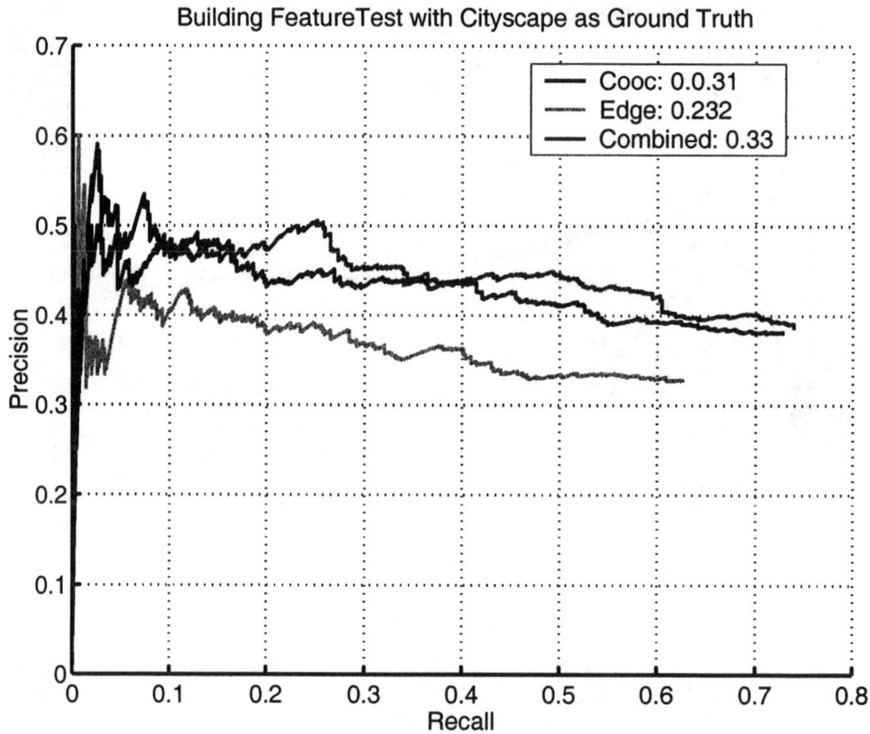

Fig. 9. Using *Building* detection to predict *Cityscape*.

17. Adams, W. H., Amir, A., Dorai, C., Ghoshal, S., Iyengar, G., Jaimes, A., Lang, C., Lin, C. Y., Naphade, M. R., Natsev, A., Neti, C., Nock, H. J., Permutter, H., Singh, R., Srinivasan, S., Smith, J. R. Tseng, B. L. Varadaraju, A. T. Zhang, D. (2002) IBM research TREC-2002 video retrieval system, Text Retrieval Conference (TREC), pp. 289–298.
18. Hauptmann, A., Yan, R., Qi, Y., Jin, R., Christel, M., Derthick, M., Chen, M., Baron, R., Lin, W., Ng, T. (2002) Video classification and retrieval with the informedia digital video library system, The Eleventh Text Retrieval Conference, TREC 2002, pp. 119–127.
19. Vendrig, J., Hartog, J., Leeuwen, D., Patras, I., Raaijmakers, S., Best, J., Snoek, C., Worring, M. (2002) TREC feature extraction by active learning, The Eleventh Text Retrieval Conference, TREC 2002, pp. 429–438.
20. Rautiainen, M., Pebttila, J., Peterila, P., Vorobiev, D., Noponen, K., Hosio, M., Matinmikko, E., Makela, S., Peltola, J., Ojala, T., Seppanen, T. (2002) TRECVID 2002 experiments at mediateam oulu and VTT, The Eleventh Text Retrieval Conference, TREC 2002, pp. 417–428.
21. Wu, L., Huang, X., Niu, J., Xia, Y., Feng, Z., Zhou, Y. (2002) FDU at TREC 2002: Filtering, q&a and video tasks, The Eleventh Text Retrieval Conference, TREC 2002, pp. 232–247.

22. Souvannavong, F., Merialdo, B., Huet, B. (2002) Semantic feature extraction using mpeg macro-block classification, The Eleventh Text Retrieval Conference, TREC 2002, pp. 227–231.
23. Westerveld, T., deVries, A., Ballegooij, A. (2002) Cwi at trec 2002 video track, The Eleventh Text Retrieval Conference, TREC 2002, pp. 207–216.
24. Quenot, G., Moraru, D., Besacier, L., Muthem, P. (2002) Clips at trec 11: Experiments in video retrieval, The Eleventh Text Retrieval Conference, TREC 2002, pp. 181–187.
25. Browne, P., Czirjek, C., Gurrin, C., Jarina, R., Lee, H., Markow, S., McDonald, K., Murphy, N., O'Connor, N., Smeaton, A., Ye, J. (2002) Dublin city university video track experiments for TREC 2002, The Eleventh Text Retrieval Conference, TREC 2002, pp. 217–226.
26. Basu, S., Naphade, M., Smith, J. (2002) A statistical modeling approach to content-based video retrieval, IEEE International Conference on Acoustics Signal and Speech Processing.
27. Vapnik, V. (1995) The Nature of Statistical Learning Theory, Springer, New York.
28. Bertsekas, D. (1995) Nonlinear Programming, Athena Scientific, Belmont, MA.
29. Naphade, M., Smith, J. (2003) The role of classifiers in multimedia content management, in SPIE Storage and Retrieval for Media Databases, vol. 5021.
30. Srinivasan, S., Ponceleon, D., Amir, A., Petkovic, D. (2000) What is that video anyway? In search of better browsing, IEEE International Conference on Multimedia and Expo, pp. 388–392.
31. Huang, J., Kumar, S., Mitra, M., Zhu, W., Zabih, R. (1999) Spatial color indexing and applications, International Journal of Computer Vision, vol. 35, no. 3, pp. 245–268.
32. Jain, R., Kasturi, R., Schunck, B. (1995) Machine Vision, MIT Press and McGraw-Hill, New York.
33. Dudani, S., Breeding, K., McGhee, R. (1977) Aircraft identification by moment invariants, IEEE Transactions on Computers, vol. C-26, no. 1, pp. 39–45.

Automatic Visual Concept Training Using Imperfect Cross-Modality Information

Xiaodan Song[1], Ching-Yung Lin[2], and Ming-Ting Sun[1]

[1]Department of Electrical Engineering, University of Washington, Seattle, WA 98195, USA

[2]IBM T. J. Watson Research Center, 19 Skyline Dr., Hawthorne, NY 10532, USA

Abstract. In this chapter, we show an autonomous learning scheme to automatically build visual semantic concept models from video sequences or the searched data of Internet search engines without any manual labeling work. First of all, system users specify some specific concept models to be learned automatically. Example videos or images can be obtained from the large video databases based on the result of keyword search on the automatic speech recognition transcripts. Another alternative method is to gather them by using the Internet search engines. Then, we propose to model the searched results as a term of "Quasi-Positive Bags" in the Multiple-Instance Learning (MIL). We call this as the generalized MIL (GMIL). In some of the scenarios, there is also no "Negative Bags" in the GMIL. We propose an algorithm called "Bag K-Means" to find out the maximum Diverse Density (DD) without the existence of negative bags. A cost function is found as K-Means with special "Bag Distance". We also show a solution called "Uncertain Labeling Density" (ULD) which describes the target density distribution of instances in the case of quasi-positive bags. A "Bag Fuzzy K-Means" is presented to get the maximum of ULD. Utilizing this generalized MIL with ULD framework, the model for a particular concept can then be learned through general supervised learning methods. Experiments show that our algorithm get correct models for the concepts we are interested in.

Keywords: autonomous learning, imperfect learning, cross-modality training, image retrieval, semantic concept training

1 Introduction

As the amount of image data increases, content-based image indexing and retrieval is becoming increasingly important. Semantic model-based indexing has been proposed as an efficient method, which matches human experience in search. Supervised learning has been used as a successful method to build generic semantic models [11]. This approach performed the best in the NIST TRECVID concept detection benchmarking in 2002 and 2003 [17][11]. However, in this approach, tedious manual labeling is needed to build tens or hundreds of models for various visual concepts. For example, in 2003, 111 researchers from 23 institutes spent 220+ hours to annotate 63 hours of TREC 2003 development corpus [16]. This manual annotating process is usually time- and cost-consuming, and, thus, makes the system hard to scale. Even with this enormous labeling effort, any new instances not previously labeled would not be able to be dealt with. It is desirable to have an automatic learning algorithm, which totally does not need the costly manual labeling process.

In [1], we proposed a solution by making use of the correlation between audio and visual data in video sequences. We proposed that visual models can be built based on imperfect labeling process from other detectors, either from another modality or other pre-established models. These weak associations of some labels on the unlabeled training data can be used to build models. In [18], we proposed another solution by using the search results from Internet search engines to build visual models. The correlation between the textual and the visual modalities for the huge amount of image data available on the web would be another possibility for our autonomous learning scheme to build models for concepts for content-based retrieval.

Multiple Instance Learning (MIL) was proposed to solve the ambiguity in the manual labeling process by making weaker assumptions about the labeling information [2][3][4]. In this learning scheme, instead of giving the learner labels for individual examples, the trainer only labels collections of examples, which are called bags. A bag is labeled negative if all the examples in it are negative. It is labeled positive if there is at least one positive example in it. The key challenge in MIL is to cope with the ambiguity of not knowing which instances in a positive bag are actually positive and which are not. Based on that, the learner attempts to find the desired concept.

MIL helps to deal with the ambiguity in the manual labeling process. However, users still have to label the bags in the MIL framework. To prevent the tedious manual labeling work, we need to generate the positive bags and negative bags automatically. In practical applications, it is very difficult if not impossible to generate the positive bags reliably. Also, negative bags are often not available. In this chapter, we propose a generalized MIL (GMIL) concept by introducing "Quasi-Positive bags" to remove the strong requirement of using strictly positive bags in the MIL framework. In the GMIL framework, we also avoid the strong dependency on the appearance of negative bags. Maron et al. proposed a Diverse Density algorithm as a efficient solution for MIL [2]. In this chapter, we first propose an efficient algorithm called "Bag K-Means" to find the maximum Diverse Density (DD) with the absence of negative bags and the existence of positive bags. We develop a cost function, which uses K-Means with special "Bag Distance". We also propose a term of "Uncertain Labeling Density" (ULD) to describe the "quasi-positive bags" issues in the generalized MIL problem. Comparing with DD, ULD pays more attention to the structure of the "Quasi-Positive bags" instead of depending on the distribution of the negative instances like many traditional MIL algorithms do. A "Bag Fuzzy K-Means" is proposed to efficiently obtain the maximum of ULD. Comparing with what we proposed in [1], a more general formulation for ULD and theoretical analysis are given in this chapter. Based on our proposed GMIL and ULD approach, we propose an automatic learning scheme to generate models for various concepts from cross-textual and visual information.

The overall process of the cross-modality automatic learning scheme on the Internet search results is shown in Fig. 1. The framework of using such technique on videos is shown in [1]. In this Internet search scenario, first of all, images are gathered by image crawling from the Google search results. Then, using the GMIL solved by ULD, the most informative examples are learned and the model of the named concept is built. This learned model can be used for concept indexing in other test sets. One of the applications is to use it as a "quasi-relevance feedback" mechanism which can be used to improve the accuracy of the original retrieved image dataset. For instance, a revised relevance score rank list can be generated by the distance from the model and the retrieved image dataset. Thus, this can also be used to improve retrieval accuracy.

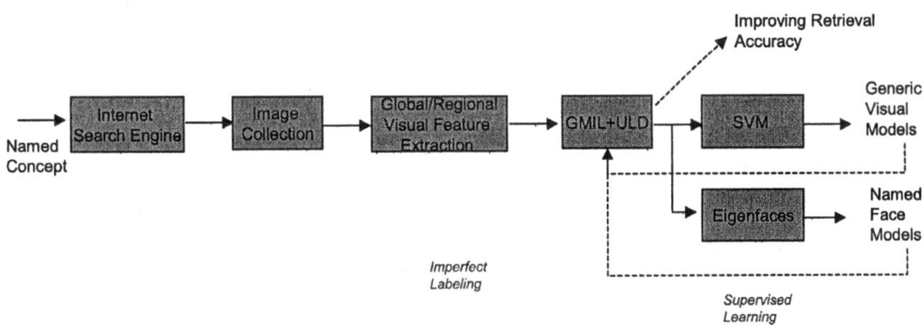

Fig. 1. A framework for autonomous concept learning based on image crawling through Internet

The rest of this chapter is organized as follows. In Section 2, we briefly review MIL and generalize it by introducing "Quasi-Positive bags" so that the learning process can be done based on the cross-modality correlation without any manual labeling work. In Section 3, DD for solving the MIL problem is introduced. The MIL is then generalized to allow false-positive bags, and ULD is proposed to solve the generalized MIL problem. Both theoretical and experimental analyses will be given for ULD. The details of our autonomous learning algorithm are described in Section 4. Finally, experimental results and conclusions are given in Sections 5 and 6, respectively.

2 Generalized Multiple-Instance Learning

In this section, we present a brief introduction to Multiple-Instance Learning, and generalize it for autonomous learning by introducing the concept of "Quasi-Positive Bags".

2.1 Multiple-Instance Learning

Given a set of instances $x_1, x_2 ..., x_N$, the task in a typical machine learning problem is to learn a function

$$y = f(x_1, x_2, \cdots, x_N) \tag{1}$$

so that the function can be used to classify the data. In traditional supervised learning, some training data are given in terms of (y_i, x_i). Based on those training data, the function is learned and used to classify the data outside the training set. In MIL, the training data are grouped into bags $X_1, X_2, \cdots, X_M$, with $X_j = \{\mathbf{x}_i : i \in I_j\}$ and $I_j \subseteq \{1, \cdots K\}$. Instead of giving the labels y_i for each instance, we have the label Y_i for each bag. A bag is labeled negative ($Y_j = -1$), if all the instances in it are negative. A bag is positive ($Y_j = 1$), if at least one instance in it is positive.

The MIL model was first formalized by Dietterich et al. [5] to deal with the drug activity prediction problem. Following that, an algorithm called Diverse Density (DD) was developed in [3] to provide a solution to MIL, which performs well on a variety of problems such as drug activity prediction, stock selection, and image retrieval [4]. Later, the method is extended in [6] to deal with the real-valued instead of binary labels. Many other algorithms, such as k-*NN* algorithms [7], Support Vector Machine (SVM) [8], and EM combined with DD [15] are proposed to solve MIL. However, most of the algorithms are sensitive to the distribution of the instances in the positive bags, and cannot work without negative bags.

In the MIL framework, users still have to label the bags. To prevent the tedious manual labeling work, we need to generate the positive bags and negative bags automatically. However, in practical applications, it is very difficult if not impossible to generate the positive and negative bags reliably. Without reliable positive and negative bags, DD may not give reliable solutions. To solve the problem, we generalize the concept of "Positive bags" to "Quasi-Positive bags", and propose "Uncertain Labeling Density" (ULD) to solve this GMIL problem.

2.2 Quasi-Positive Bag

In our scenario, although there is a relatively high probability that the concept of interest (e.g. a person's face) will appear in the crawled images, there are many cases that no such association exists (e.g. Fig. 4 in Section 4). If these images are used as the positive bags, we may have false-positive bags that do not contain the concept of interest. To overcome this problem, we extend the concept of "Positive bags" to "Quasi-Positive bags". A "Quasi-Positive bag" has a high probability to contain a positive instance, but may not be guaranteed to contain one. The introduction of "Quasi-Positive bags" removes a major limitation of applying MIL to many practical problems.

Definition: Generalized Multiple Instance Learning (GMIL)

In the generalized MIL, a bag is labeled negative ($Y_j = -1$), if all the instances in it are negative. A bag is Quasi-Positive ($Y_j = 1$), if in a high probability, at least one instance in it is positive.

3. Diversity Density and Uncertain Labeling Density

In this section, we first have a brief overview of Diverse Density proposed by Moron et al. [2]. We show that it has a similar cost function as the K-Means algorithm but with a different definition of distance, which we call "bag distance". Then, an efficient Bag K-Means algorithm is presented to efficiently find the maximum of DD instead of using the time-consuming gradient descent algorithm. We also prove the convergence property of this Bag K-Means algorithm. This algorithm can be used to find the maximum DD solutions in MIL with the existence of positive bags but without the negative bags. Then, for the GMIL, we introduce a concept called Uncertain Labeling Density (ULD) to solve the problem of quasi-positive bags. A Bag Fuzzy K-Means algorithm is presented to find the maximum of ULD.

3.1 Diverse Density

One way to solve MIL problems is to examine the distribution of the instance vectors, and look for a feature vector that is close to the instances in different positive bags and far from all the instances in the negative bags. Such a vector represents the concept we are trying to learn. This is the basic idea of the Diverse Density algorithm [2].

Diverse Density is a measure of the intersection of the positive bags minus the union of the negative bags. By maximizing Diverse Density, we can find the point of intersection (the desired concept). Here a simple probabilistic measure of Diverse Density is explained. We use the same notation as in [2]. We denote the *i*th positive bag as B_i^+, the *j*th instance in that bag as B_{ij}^+, and the *i*th instance from a negative bag as B_i^-. Assume the intersection of all positive bags minus the union of all negative bags is a single point *t*, we can find this point by

$$\arg\max_t \prod_i \Pr\left(t \mid B_i^+\right) \prod_i \left(1 - \Pr\left(t \mid B_i^-\right)\right). \tag{2}$$

This is the formal definition of Diverse Density. $\Pr\left(t \mid B_i^-\right)$ is estimated by the most-likely-cause estimator, in which only the instance in the bag which is most likely to be in the concept c_t is considered:

$$\Pr(t \mid B_i) = \max_j \{\Pr(t \mid B_{ij})\}. \tag{3}$$

The distribution is estimated as a Gaussian-like distribution of

$$\Pr(t \mid B_{ij}) = \exp\left(-\|B_{ij} - t\|^2\right), \tag{4}$$

where $\|B_{ij} - t\|^2 = \sum_k (B_{ijk} - t_k)^2$. For the convenience of discussion, we define "Bag Distance" as:

$$d_i^t \triangleq \min_j \|B_{ij} - t\|^2 \tag{5}$$

3.2 The Bag K-Means Algorithm for Diverse Density with the Absence of Negative Bags

In our special application, where negative bags are not provided, (2) can be simplified as:

$$\arg\max_t \prod_i \Pr(t \mid B_i^+) = \arg\min_t \sum_i d_i^t \triangleq J, \tag{6}$$

which has the same form of the cost function J as K-Means' with the different definition of d in (5). We call it Bag K-Means in this chapter. Basically, when there is no negative bag, the DD algorithm is trying to find the centroid of the cluster by K-Means with $K = 1$. With this, we propose an efficient algorithm to find the maximum DD by the Bag K-Means algorithm as follows:

(1) Choose an initial seed t
(2) Choose a convergence threshold ε
(3) For each bag i, choose one example s_i which is closest to the seed t, and calculate the distance d_i^t
(4) Calculate $t_{new} = \sum_i s_i / N$, where N is the total number of bags.
(5) If $\|t - t_{new}\| \le \varepsilon$, stop, otherwise, update $t = t_{new}$, and repeat (3) to (5).

Theorem: The Bag K-Means algorithm converges.
Proof: Assume t_i is the centroid we found in the iteration i, and s_{ij} is the sample obtained in step (3) for bag j. By step (4), we get a new centroid t_{i+1}. We have:

$$\sum_j \|s_{ij} - t_{i+1}\|^2 \le \sum_j \|s_{ij} - t_i\|^2 \tag{7}$$

because of the property of the traditional K-Means algorithm.

Because of the criterion of choosing new s_{i+1j}, we have:

$$\sum_j \left\| s_{i+1j} - t_{i+1} \right\|^2 \le \sum_j \left\| s_{ij} - t_{i+1} \right\|^2 \tag{8}$$

Thus, combine (7) and (8), we will get

$$\sum_j \left\| s_{i+1j} - t_{i+1} \right\|^2 \le \sum_j \left\| s_{ij} - t_i \right\|^2 \tag{9}$$

which means the algorithm decreases the cost function J in (6) each time. Therefore, this process will converge.

3.3 Uncertain Labeling Density

In our generalized MIL, what we have are Quasi-Positive bags, i.e., some false-positive bags do not include positive instances at all. In a false-positive bag, by the original DD definition, $\Pr\left(t \mid B_i^+\right)$ will be very small or even zero. These outliers will influence the DD significantly due to the multiplication of the probabilities. The outlier problem is also a challenge to the traditional K-Means algorithm [9][10]. Many algorithms have been proposed to handle this problem. Among them, fuzzy K-Means algorithm is the most well known [9][10]. The intuition of the algorithm is to give different measurements (weights) on the relationship of each example belonging to any cluster. The weights indicate the possibility that a given example belongs to any cluster. By assigning low weight values to outliers, the effect of noisy data on the clustering process is reduced. In this chapter, based on the similar idea from fuzzy K-Means, we propose an Uncertain Labeling Density (ULD) algorithm to handle the Quasi-Positive bag problem for MIL.

Definition: Uncertain Labeling Density (ULD)

$$\begin{aligned} ULD(t) &= \prod_i \left(\Pr\left(t \middle| B_i^+\right)^{\left(\mu_i^t\right)^b} \right) \\ \sum_i \mu_i^t &= N, \end{aligned} \tag{10}$$

where μ_i^t represents the weight of bag i belonging to concept t, and $b > 1$ is the fuzzy exponent. It determines the degree of fuzziness of the final solution. Usually $b = 2$.

Similarly, we conclude that the maximum of ULD can be obtained by Fuzzy K-Means with the definition of "Bag Distance" (5), with the cost function as:

$$\arg\max_t \prod_i \Pr\left(t \mid B_i^+\right)^{\left(\mu_i^t\right)^b} = \arg\min_t \sum_i \left(\mu_i^t\right)^b d_i^t \tag{11}$$

3.4 The Bag Fuzzy K-Mean Algorithm for Uncertain Labeling Density

The Bag Fuzzy K-Means algorithm is proposed as follows:

(1) Choose an initial seed t

(2) Choose a convergence threshold ε

(3) For each bag i, choose one example s_i which is closest to seed t, and calculate the Bag Distance d_i^t

(4) Calculate

$$t_{new} = \frac{\sum_{i=1}^{N} (\mu_i^t)^b s_i}{\sum_{i=1}^{N} (\mu_i^t)^b}$$
$$\mu_i^t = \frac{N(1/d_i^t)^{1/(b-1)}}{\sum_{j=1}^{N} (1/d_j^t)^{1/(b-1)}} \tag{12}$$

where N is the total number of bags.[1]

(5) If $\|t - t_{new}\| \le \varepsilon$, stop; otherwise, update $t = t_{new}$, and repeat (3) to (5).

The basic idea is to update the weight according to the distance to the centroid, and use the weighted mean as the new centroid.

Fig. 2 shows an example with Quasi-Positive bags and without negative bags. Different symbols represent various Quasi-Positive bags. There are two false-positive bags, which are illustrated by the inverse-triangles and circles, in this example. The true intersection point is the instance with the value (9, 9) with intersections from four different positive bags. Just by finding the maximum of the original Diverse Density, the algorithm will converge to (5, 5) (labeled with a "+" symbol) because of the influence of the false-positive bags. Fig. 2(b) illustrates the corresponding Diverse Density values. By using the ULD method, it is easy to obtain the correct intersection point with the ULD as shown in Fig. 2(c).

---

[1] In practice, we add a small number ε' to d_i^t to avoid the situation of division by 0.

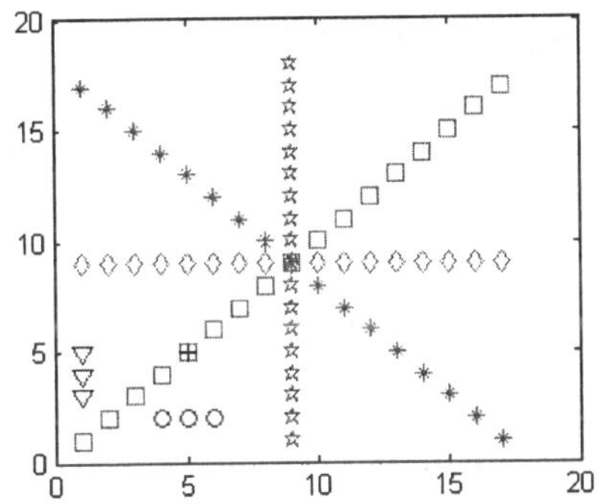

(a) An example with Quasi-Positive bags

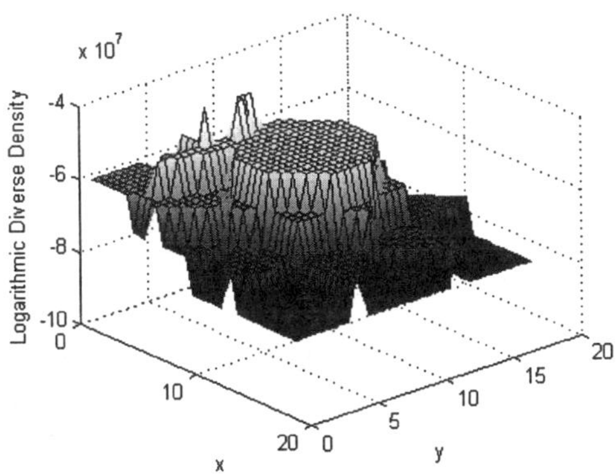

(b) The corresponding Diverse Density

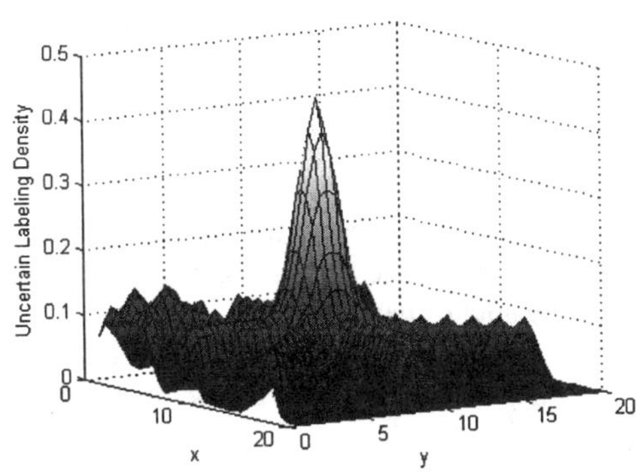

(c) Using Uncertain Labeling Density

Fig. 2 Comparison of MIL using Diversity Density and Uncertain Labeling Density Algorithms in the case of quasi-positive bags

4. Cross-Modality Automatic Training

In this section, we describe two scenarios that we have used to build models: the news videos and the image searches from Internet Engines.

4.1 Automatic Training from Videos

We first describe how to find the quasi-positive bags and the negative bags for learning the model based on MIL in news videos. First, we describe how to generate the quasi-positive bags, and a method is introduced to exclude the anchor persons; then, we describe how to get the visual rank list from the ASR analysis results by using the MIL-ULD algorithm, and how to build regression models of generic visual concepts from the rank list.

4.1.1 Quasi-positive bag generation

The quasi-positive bags are those frames which are associated with the names mentioned in the audio data.

When an anchor person tells a story about someone, usually that person will appear in the following scenes. Therefore, our algorithm automatically selects candidate frames, which are believed to be with high probability to have the face of that person, according to the association between the speech and the images. Here, we choose the keyframes of four shots after the frame in which the name or specific concept is mentioned from the Automatic Speech Recognition (ASR) or Closed Captions (CC) data as the candidate frames because those four frames have this face with a relatively high probability based on our observation.

4.1.2 Negative bag generation

Our objective is to find a common point from all the quasi-positive bags. The useful negative instances are those confusing negative examples in the quasi-positive bags, such as the anchor persons.

1) Anchor person detection: We propose to detect the anchor persons based on a model based clustering method. In model based clustering, each cluster is represented as a Gaussian model:

$$\phi_k(\mathbf{x} \mid \mu_k, \Sigma_k) = (2\pi)^{-\frac{p}{2}} |\Sigma_k|^{-\frac{1}{2}} \exp\left\{-\frac{1}{2}(\mathbf{x}_i - \mu_k)^T \Sigma_k^{-1} (\mathbf{x}_i - \mu_k)\right\} \tag{13}$$

with mean μ_k and covariance Σ_k, where $\mathbf{x}$ represents the data and k is an integer subscript specifying a particular cluster.

We set the covariance matrix Σ_k as a diagonal matrix. We use Bayesian Information Criterion (BIC) to determine the size of clusters. BIC is a value of the maximized log-likelihood with a penalty for the number of parameters in the model. It allows comparisons of models with different parameterizations and numbers of clusters. In general, the larger the value of the BIC, the stronger the evidence for the model and the number of clusters.

Since the anchor is the host of the program, the anchor cluster is in a relatively large size with high density. Therefore, after we get the clusters by the model based clustering, we choose the cluster with both large size and high density as the anchor person cluster. Here we define a new concept "Relative Sparsity" to recognize the anchor person from the cluster obtained above:

$$RSpars = \frac{Cov(i,i)}{N_i} \tag{14}$$

where $Cov(i,i)$ represents the variance, and N_i is the size of cluster i respectively. Heuristically, the larger the variance for a cluster, the lower density it is in, and so, we will get larger *RSpars*. Also, the larger the cluster, the smaller the *RSpars*. Therefore, the smaller *RSpars* is, the more possible the cluster belongs to an anchor person.

4.1.3 Generating rank list

Based on the ASR unimodal analysis results, each shot will be associated with a confidence score in the range of $[0,1]$, showing how likely this shot belongs to this concept from the view point of audio features. Based on these scores, we choose the shots with nonzero confidence scores as the Quasi-Positive bags. Generally, we do not use negative bags when calculating the ULD values because ASR based analysis is not so accurate to tell which examples are definitely unrelated, except in some special cases we have prior information, which can help us to find the negative bags; for example, when a particular person is the concept we are interested in, anchor persons are set as the negative bags.

Considering the reliability of each positive bag, $\Pr(t \mid B_i^+)$ can be calculated as:

$$\Pr(t \mid B_i^+) = 1 - \prod_j \left[\left(1 - \Pr(t \mid B_{ij}^+)\right) \cdot CS(i) \right], \tag{15}$$

where $CS(i)$ represents the confidence score for the ith shot. The more reliable the positive bag, the more contribution to the whole density it provides.

Based on those Quasi-Positive bags and the MIL-ULD algorithm, the point with the highest ULD value is chosen as the visual model for the concept we are trying to learn, denoted as x_E.

Then, the visual rank list is generated by considering both the distances between the instances and the learned most informative example, and the ULD values:

$$CS_v(i) = ULD(i) \cdot Dist(x_i, x_E) \tag{16}$$

where

$$Dist(x_i, x_E) = \exp\left(\frac{\left\| x_i - x_E \right\|^2}{Z_E}\right) \tag{17}$$

where Z_E is a normalization constant, and both *ULD* values and the *Dist* are normalized in the range of $[0,1]$. Based on the rank list generated above, Support Vector Regression (SVR) is used to build models for general visual concepts.

Fig. 3 shows an illustration of the process described in this section.

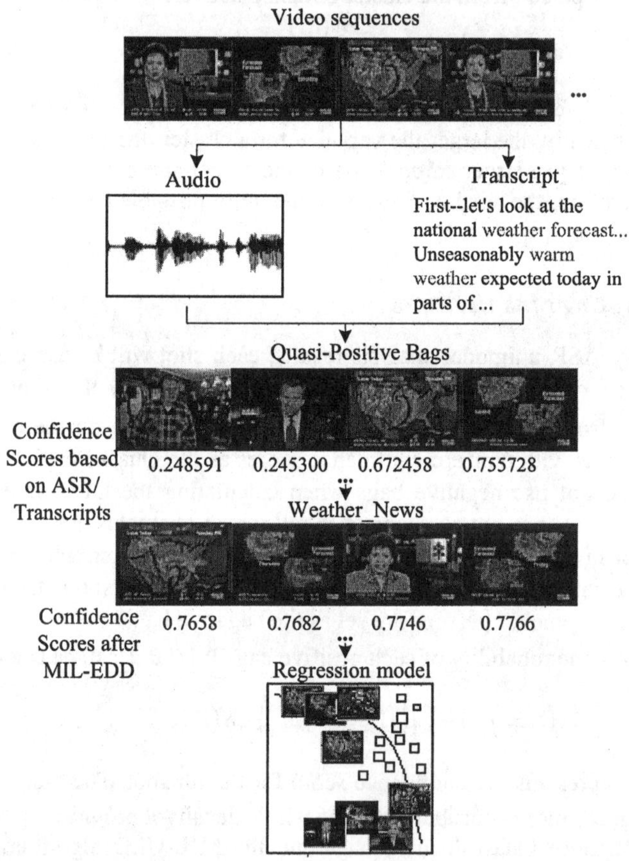

Fig. 3. An example of building weather model from news video

4.2 Automatic Visual Model Training from Crawled Image through Internet Search Engines

In this chapter, we only show detailed procedure of the cross-modality training on building face models based on Internet search engines. For generic visual models, the system can use a region segmentation, feature extraction and supervised learning framework as in [17].

4.2.1 Feature generation

We focus on the frontal face model. We first extract frontal faces from the images obtained from the search engine, use skin detection to exclude some false alarm detections, and then obtain the projection coefficients based on eigenfaces for the face recognition.

Face detection

The face detection algorithm we used is based on the approach proposed in [12], which extends Viola et al.'s rapid object detection scheme [13]. It is based on a boosted cascade of simple features by enriching the basic set of simple Haar-like features and incorporating a post optimization procedure. This algorithm reduces the false alarm rate significantly with a relative high hit-rate and fast speed. However, there are still some false detections since it is based on gray value features only. We propose to reduce those false alarms by skin color detection. Our skin detection algorithm is based on a skin pixel classifier, which is derived using the standard likelihood ratio approach in [14]. After getting skin pixel candidates, we post-process the candidates to determine the skin regions, using techniques including Gaussian blurring, thresholding, and mathematical morphological operations such as closing and opening.

Eigenface generation

The eigenfaces we use in this chapter are the same as what we obtained in [1]. The frontal faces, which are in a relatively large scale (larger than 48×48) and include certain skin regions (face regions which cover more than a quarter of the whole image), are detected from the crawled images. After normalized to a size of 64×64 and a median value 128 of gray level, they are used to get the top 22 eigenfaces with 85% energy for recognition. The features used throughout this chapter are the projection coefficients based on these eigenfaces.

4.2.2 Quasi-positive bag generation

The quasi-positive bags are just those images with the extracted frontal faces as the instances. An illustration of the quasi-positive bags is shown in the bottom part of Fig. 4.

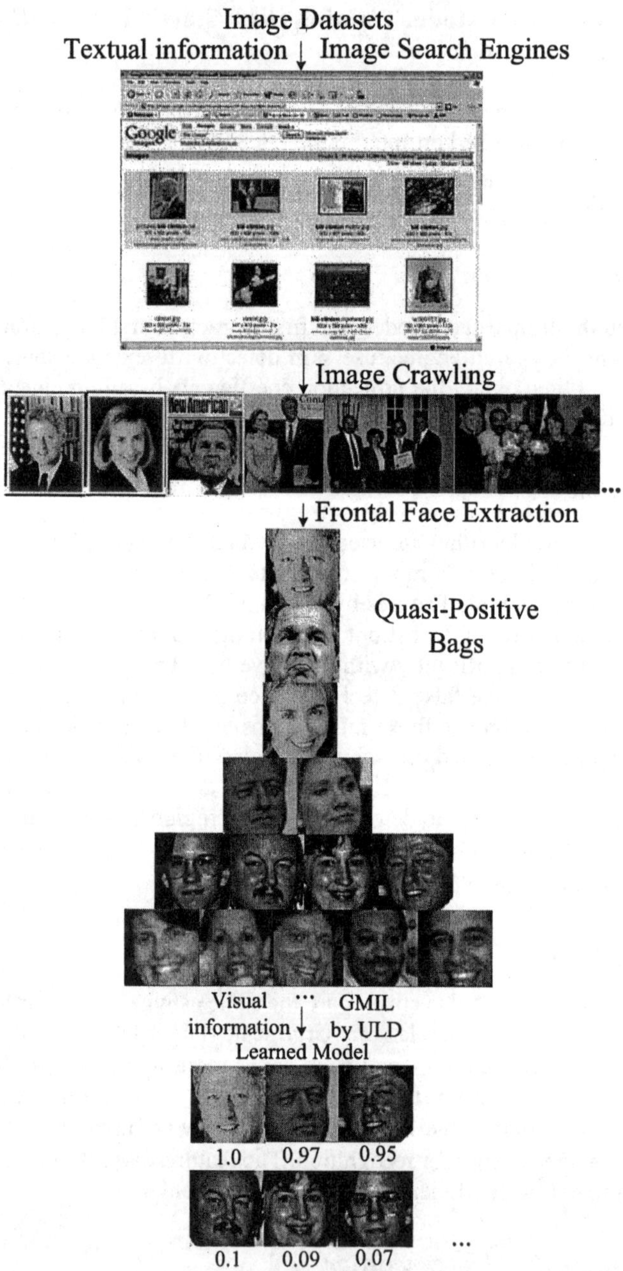

Fig. 4. An example of building the face model of "Bill Clinton" from results of Internet search engine

5. Experimental Results

We now demonstrate the performance of our algorithm using the NIST Video TRECVID 2003 corpus. The whole video dataset is divided into five parts: ConceptTraining, ConceptFusion1, ConceptFusion2, ConceptValidate, and ConceptTesting [11]. In the first experiment, we set ConceptValidate, a dataset of small size which includes 13 video sequences with 4420 shots/key frames, as the training set in our experiment. We try the MIL-ULD+SVR algorithm to train models for the concept "Weather_News", and "Airplane".

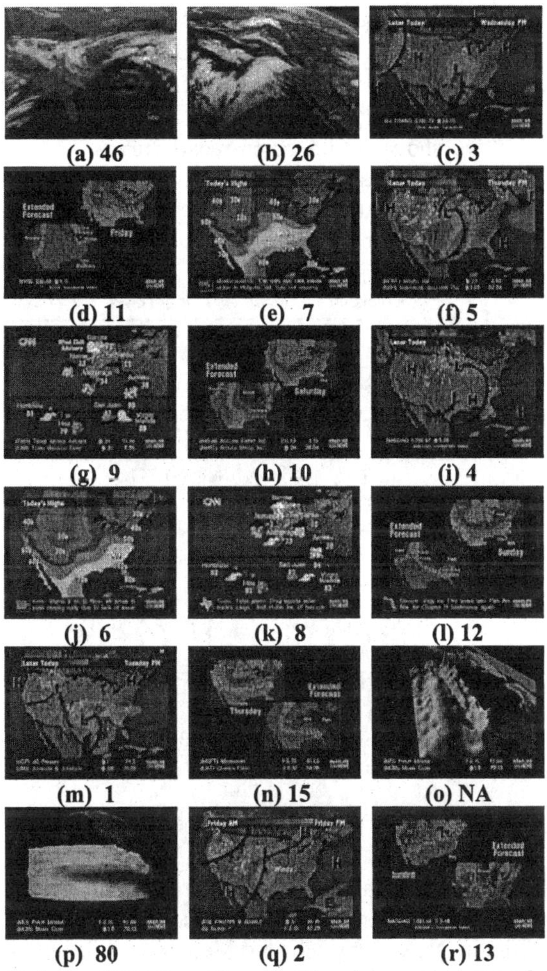

Fig. 5. Training Data for "Weather_News" with relevance score ranks based on MIL-ULD (Note: The number below the picture shows the rank based on the relevance score. NA means it cannot be obtained by the ASR unimodal analysis)

There are 1696 Quasi-Positive bags for "Weather_News", based on the ASR unimodal analysis. Using a 512-bin color histogram as the feature, the MIL-ULD algorithm provides relevance scores for each key frame. The ranks are shown in Fig. 5. We can see that the most informative visual model for the concept "Weather_News" is close to (m). In Fig. 5, (p) is not so frequently shown for this concept, thus its influence to the model learning is weakened in the MIL-ULD algorithm. Based on the obtained relevance score rank list, SVR is used to learn a regression model for "Weather_News". This model is tested in the dataset ConceptFusion1, which includes 13 news videos with 5,037 shots. We get an average precision [11] of 0.6847 for "Weather_News". We trained and tested the two baseline algorithms in the same dataset. The results show that for "Weather_News", the average precision for SVM based supervised algorithm [9] which uses the same 512-bin color histogram feature is 0.4743, and for SVR based on audio confidence score rank list, the average precision is 0.5265.

For comparisons, we show the precision-recall curves. The beginning of the precision-recall is important because we are interested in the shots in the top of the rank list. Fig. 6 shows the P-R curves of the above mentioned models. We can see the good performance of the proposed algorithm.

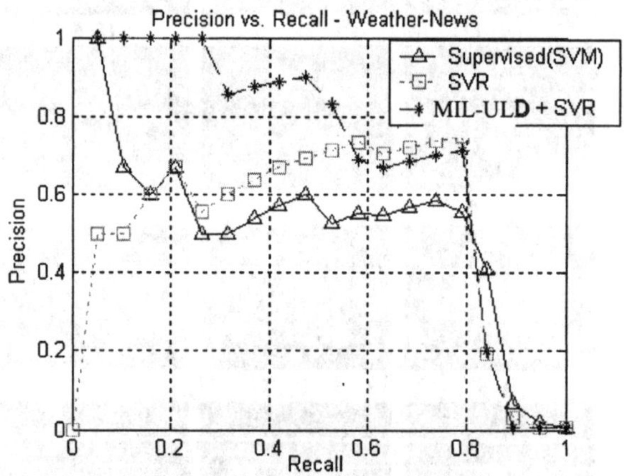

Fig. 6. A performance comparison of the visual models built by supervised learning (SVM), automatic learning by SVR, and automatic learning by (MIL-ULD+ SVR).

For the applications on training models from crawled images of Internet search engines, we applied our algorithm to learn models of four particular persons, Bill Clinton, Hillary Clinton, Newt Gingrich, and Madeleine Albright. Fig. 4 shows the dataflow in our scheme. First of all, a name is typed in Google Image Search Engine, such as "Bill Clinton". Then, an image crawler is applied to the resultant images from the search. These images were gathered in May 2004. The gathered images are in form of .jpg or .gif. Because most .gif images are just animation, we do not consider them in our data after image crawling. After that, faces are extracted from those images automatically and the faces from the same image constitute a Quasi-Positive bag. Then, the most informative example for that person is learned and a rank list is generated based on the distance from this example.

For the sake of copyright issues, we are not showing the figures in this chapter. Some of the results are shown in [18]. From our experiments, we can see that among those top ranked faces, our algorithm can find the correct face for the person we are interested in, while Google may not. Fig. 7 and Table 1 show the precision and recall comparisons. The images with profile faces and very small faces are all considered in the ground truth. We can see that even in our algorithm we just extract the big and frontal faces, which is not effective to those data with profile and very small faces, our algorithm still gets correct face models for those persons and improves the accuracy. For the case of "Bill Clinton", "Newt Gingrich", and "Hillary Clinton", we can get around 10% improvements on Average Precision [11] over the Google Image Search. For the case of "Madeleine Albright", where Google Search does a very good job and many profile and small faces occur, our average precision is still better.

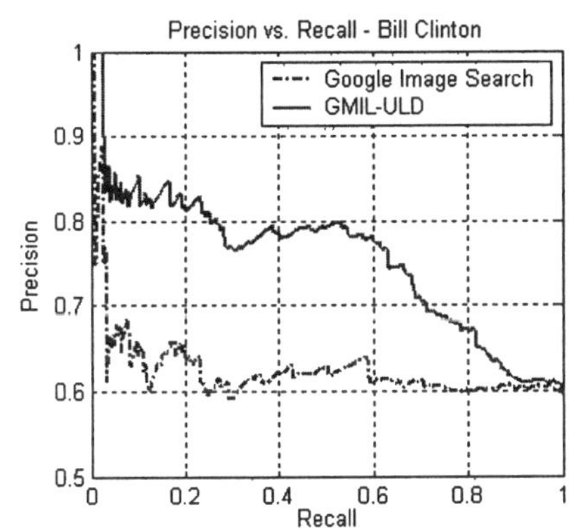

(a)

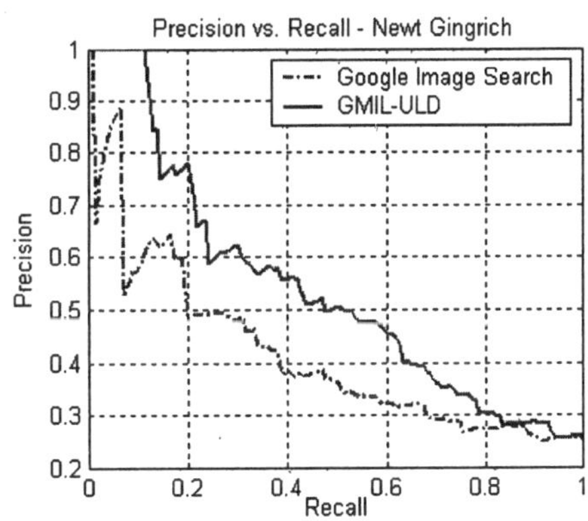

(b)

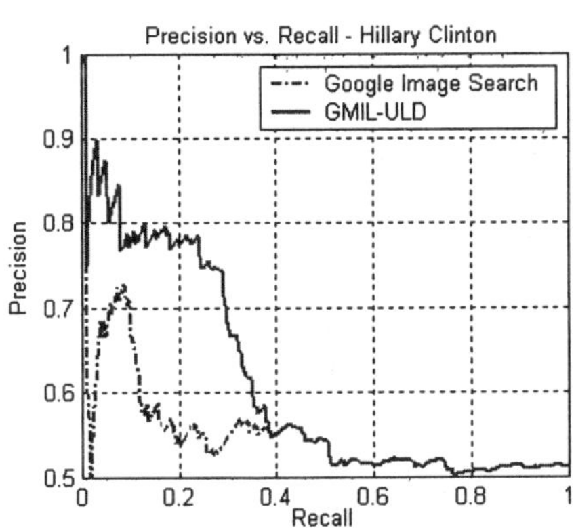

(c)

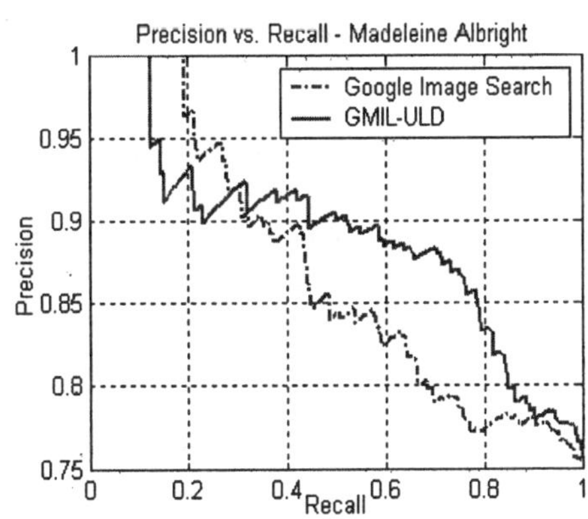

(d)

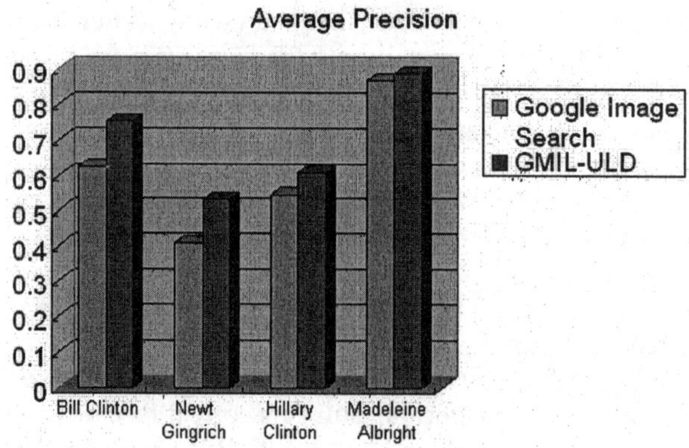

(e)

Fig. 7. Performance comparison of the results of Goolge Image search and the proposed generalized MIL-ULD algorithm

Table 1: Comparison of Average Precision

Average Precision	Bill Clinton	Newt Gingrich	Hillary Clinton	Madeleine Albright
Google Image Search	0.6250	0.4100	0.5467	0.8683
GMIL-ULD	0.7546	0.5339	0.6107	0.8899

6. CONCLUSIONS

We have presented a cross-modality autonomous learning algorithm to build models for visual concepts based on multi-modality videos or image crawling from the results provided by search engines. Generalized MIL is proposed by introducing "Quasi-Positive Bags", and "Fuzzy Diverse Density" is proposed to handle the Quasi-Positive Bags in order to find the most probable example for the concept we are interested in. Bag K-Means and Fuzzy Bag K-Means algorithms are proposed to find the maximum of DD and ULD respectively in an efficient way instead of the time-consuming gradient descent algorithm. The convergence of the algorithm is proved. Experiments are performed for learning the models for four persons. Comparing to Google Image Search results, our algorithm improves the accuracy and is able to build a correct model for a person. Ongoing works include applying this algorithm to learn more general concepts, e.g., outdoor and sports, as well as using these learned models for concept detection and search tasks on generic image/video concept detection benchmarking, e.g., NIST TRECVID corpus.

7. ACKNOWLEDGEMENT

We would like to thank Dr. Belle L. Tseng for her assistance on calculating average precision values in the experiments.

REFERENCES

1. Song, X., Lin, C.-Y., and Sun, M.-T. (2004) Cross-modality automatic face model training from large video databases, The First IEEE CVPR Workshop on Face Processing in Video (FPIV'04)
2. Maron, O. (1998) Learning from ambiguity, PhD dissertation, Department of Electrical Engineering and Computer Science, MIT
3. Maron, O., Lozano-Perez, T. (1998) A Framework for Multiple Instance Learning, Proc. of Neural Information Processing Systems
4. Maron, O., Ratan, A. L. (1998) Multiple-Instance Learning for Natural Scene Classification, Proc. of ICML 1998, 341-349
5. Dietterich, T. G., Lathrop, R. H., Lozano-Perez, T. (1997) Solving the multiple instance problem with axis-parallel rectangles, Artificial Intelligence Journal, **89**, 31-71
6. Amar, R. A., Dooly, D. R., Goldman, S. A., Zhang, Q. (2001) Multiple-instance learning of real-valued data, Proc. of the 18th International Conference on Machine Learning, Williamstown, MA, 3-10
7. Wang, J., Zucker, J. D. (2000) Solving Multiple-Instance Problem: A Lazy Learning Approach, Proc. of the 17th International Conference on Machine Learning, 1119-1125
8. Andrews, S., Hofmann, T., Tsochantaridis, I. (2002) Multiple instance learning with generalized support vector machines, Proc. of the eighteenth national conference on Artificial Intelligence, Edmonton, Alberta, Canada, 943-944
9. Schneider, A. (2000) Weighted possibilistic clustering algorithms, Proc. of the 9th IEEE International Conference on Fuzzy Systems. Texas, **1**, 176-180
10. Dave, R. N., Krishnapuram, R. (1997) Robust clustering methods: a unified view, IEEE Transactions on Fuzzy Systems, **5**(2) 270-293
11. Amir, A., Berg, M., Chang, S.-F., Iyengar, G., Lin, C.-Y., Natsev, A., Neti, C., Nock, H., Naphade, M., Hsu, W., Smith, J. R., Tseng, B., Wu, Y., Zhang, D. (2003) IBM Research TRECVID-2003 Video Retrieval System, Proc. of TRECVID 2003 Workshop
12. Viola P., Jones, M. J. (2002) Robust real-time object detection, Intl. J. Computer Vision
13. Lienhart, R., Kuranov, A., Pisarevsky, V. (2003) Empirical Analysis of Detection Cascades of Boosted Classifiers for Rapid Object Detection, DAGM-Symposium, 297-304
14. Jones, M. J., Rehg, J. M. (1999) Statistical color models with application to skin detection, Proc. of CVPR, 274-280

15. Zhang, Q., Goldman, S. A. (2002) EM-DD: an improved multi-instance learning technique, Proc. of Advances in Neural Information Processing Systems, Cambridge, MA, MIT Press, 1073-1080
16. Lin, C.-Y., Tseng B. L., Smith, J. R. (2003) Video Collaborative Annotation Forum: Establishing Ground-Truth Labels on Large Multimedia Datasets, Proc. of NIST Text Retrieval Conf. (TREC)
17. Lin, C.-Y., Tseng, B. L., Naphade, M., Natsev, A., Smith, J. R. (2003) VideoAL: A Novel End-to-End MPEG-7 Automatic Labeling System, IEEE Intl. Conf. on Image Processing, Barcelona
18. Song, X., Lin, C.-Y., Sun, M.-T. (2004) Autonomous visual model building based on image crawling through Internet Search Engines, submitted to ACM Workshop on Multimedia Information Retrieval, New York

Audio-Visual Event Recognition with Application in Sports Video

Ziyou Xiong[1], Regunathan Radhakrishnan[2], Ajay Divakaran[2], and Thomas S. Huang[1]

[1] Department of Electrical and Computer Engineering, University of Illinois at Urbana-Champaign, Urbana, IL, 61801, USA
{zxiong,huang}@ifp.uiuc.edu

[2] Mitsubishi Electric Research Laboratories, Cambridge, MA, USA
{regu,ajayd}@merl.com

Abstract. We summarize our recent work on "highlight" events detection and recognition in sports video. We have developed two different joint audio-visual fusion frameworks for this task, namely "audio-visual coupled hidden Markov model" and "audio classification then visual hidden Markov model verification". Our comparative study of these two frameworks shows that the second approach outperforms the first approach by a large margin. Our study also suggests the importance of modeling the so-called middle-level features such as audience reactions and camera patterns in sports video.

Keywords: sports highlights, event detection, Gaussian mixture models, hidden Markov models, coupled hidden Markov models

1 Introduction and Related Work

Sports highlights extraction is one of the most important applications of video analysis. Various approaches based on audio classification [12] [6], video feature extraction [7] and highlights modeling [13] [17] [4] have been reported. However, most of the current systems focus on a single modality when highlights are extracted. Rui et al. [12] detect the announcer's excited speech and ball-bat impact sound in baseball games using directional template matching based on the audio signal only. Kawashima et al. [7] try to extract bat-swing features based on the video signal. Hsu [6] uses frequency domain audio features and multi-variate Gaussian as classifiers to detect golf club-ball impact. Xie et al. [13] and Xu et al. [17] segment soccer videos into play and break segments using dominant color and motion information. Gong et al. [5] develop a soccer game parsing systems according to the field line pattern detection, ball detection and player position analysis. Ekin et al. [4] analyze soccer video based on video shot detection, classification and interesting shot selection with no usage of audio information. Although a simple, ad-hoc approach of weighted sum of likelihood has been used by Rui et al. [12] to fuse the excited speech likelihood and ball-bat impact likelihood, other information fusion techniques are seldom discussed in the sports highlights extraction literature.

In [16], we have reported an application of the coupled hidden Markov models (CHMMs) to fuse audio and video domain decisions for sports highlights extraction. Our experimental results on testing sports content show that CHMMs out-perform hidden Markov models (HMMs) trained on audio-only or video-only observations. However, overall the performance there is still not satisfactory because of the high false alarm rate.

In [14], we have presented an approach that makes considerable improvement on our earlier work that is built upon a foundation of audio classification framework [15] [16]. It is motivated by finding a solution to the following shortcoming of the Gaussian mixture models (GMMs). Traditionally the GMMs are assumed to have the same number of mixtures for a classification task. This single, "optimal" number of mixtures is usually chosen through cross validation. The practical problem is that for some class this number will lead to over-fitting of the training data if it is much less than the actual one or inversely, under-fitting of the data. Our solution is to use the MDL criterion in selecting the number of mixtures. MDL-GMMs fit the training data to the generative process as closely as possible, avoiding the problem of over-fitting or under-fitting. We have shown that the MDL-GMMs based approach out-performs those approaches in [16] by a large margin. For example, at 90% recall, the MDL-GMMs based approach [14] shows $\geq 70\%$ precision rate, while the CHMM based approach [16] shows only about 30% precision rate, suggesting that the false alarm rate is much lower using the MDL-GMMs based approach.

We report our further improvement on the audio-only MDL-GMMs based approach in [14] by introducing the modeling of visual features such as dominant color and motion activities. Here the fusion of audio and video domain decisions is sequential, i.e., audio first then video, quite different from that in [16].

2 Fusion 1: Coupled Hidden Markov Model based Fusion

2.1 Discrete-observations Coupled Hidden Markov Model (DCHMM)

We provide a brief introduction to DCHMM using the graphic model in Fig. 1. The two incoming arcs (a horizontal arc and a diagonal arc) ending at a square node represent the transition matrix of the CHMM:

$$\begin{aligned} a^1_{(i,j),k} &= Pr(S^1_{t+1} = k | S^1_t = i, S^2_t = j) \\ &1 \leq i, k \leq M; 1 \leq j \leq N \end{aligned} \quad (1)$$

i.e., the probability of transiting to state k in the first Markov chain at the next time instant given the current two hidden states are i and j, respectively. Here we assume the total number of states for two Markov chains are M and N, respectively. Similarly we can define $a^2_{(i,j),l}$:

$$\begin{aligned} a^2_{(i,j),l} &= Pr(S^2_{t+1} = l | S^1_t = i, S^2_t = j) \\ & 1 \leq i \leq M; 1 \leq j, l \leq N \end{aligned} \tag{2}$$

The parameters associated with the vertical arcs determine the probability of an observation given the current state.

For modeling a discrete-observations system with two state variables, we generate a single HMM from the Cartesian product of their states and similarly the Cartesian product of their observations [2], i.e., we can transform the coupling of two HMMs with M and N states respectively into a single HMM with $M \times N$ states with the following state transition matrix definition:

$$\begin{aligned} a_{(i,j),(k,l)} &= Pr(S^1_{t+1} = k, S^2_{t+1} = l | S^1_t = i, S^2_t = j) \\ & 1 \leq i, k \leq M; 1 \leq j, l \leq N \end{aligned} \tag{3}$$

This involves a "packing" and an "un-packing" stage of parameters from the two coupled HMMs to the single product HMM back and forth. The traditional forward-backward algorithm can be used to learn the parameters of the product HMM based on maximum likelihood estimation. The Viterbi algorithm can be used to determine the optimal state sequence given the observations and the model parameters.

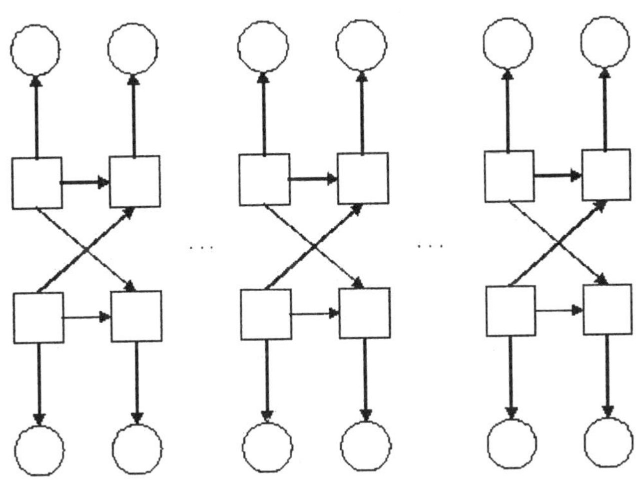

Fig. 1. The graphical model structure of the DCHMM. The two rows of squares are the coupled hidden state nodes. The circles are the observation nodes.

For more detail on the forward-backward algorithm and the Viterbi algorithm, please see [10]. For more detail on DCHMM, please refer to [8] and [2].

2.2 Our Approach

Our proposed approach is an extension of our work in [15] and [3] by introducing the CHMM-based information fusion. Since the performance of audio-based sports highlights extraction degrades drastically when the background noise increases from golf games to soccer games [15], the use of additional visual features is motivated by the complementary features provided by the visual information that are not corrupted by the acoustic noise of the audience or microphone, etc. Several key modules in our approach are described as follows.

Audio Classification

We are motivated to use audio classification because the audio labels are directly related to content semantics. During the training phase, we extract Mel-scale Frequency Cepstrum Coefficients (MFCC) from windowed audio frames. We then use Gaussian Mixture Models (GMMs) to learn to model 7 classes of sound individually. These 7 classes are: applause, ball-hit, female speech, male speech, music, music with speech and noise (audience noise, cheering, etc). We have used more than 3 hours of audio as the training data for these 7 classes. During the test phase, we apply the learned GMM classifiers to the audio track of the recorded sports games. we first use audio energy to detect silent segments. We then classify every second of non-silence audio into one of the above 7 classes. We list these classes together with the silence class in Table 1.

Table 1. Audio Labels and Class Names

Audio Label	Its Meaning
1	Silence
2	Applause
3	Ball-hit
4	Female Speech
5	Male Speech
6	Music
7	Music with Speech
8	Noise

Video Labels Generation

In this work, we use a modified version of the MPEG-7 motion activity descriptor to generate video labels. The MPEG-7 motion activity descriptor captures the intuitive notion of 'intensity of action' or 'pace of action' in a video segment [9]. It is extracted by quantizing the variance of the magnitude of the motion vectors from the video frames between two neighboring P-frames to one of 5 possible levels - very low, low, medium, high, very high. Since Peker et al. [9] have shown that the average motion vector magnitude also works well with lower computational complexity, we adopt this scheme and quantize the average of the magnitudes of motion vectors from those video frames between two neighboring P-frames to one of 4 levels - very low, low, medium, high. These labels are listed in Table 2.

Table 2. Video Labels and Class Names

Video Label	Its Meaning
1	Very Low Motion
2	Low Motion
3	Medium Motion
4	High Motion

Information Fusion with CHMM

We train an audio-visual highlight CHMM using the labels obtained by techniques described in the previous two sub-sections. The training data herein consists of video segments that are regarded as highlights such as golf club swings followed by audience applause etc. Our motivation of using discrete-time labels is that it is more computationally efficient to learn the discrete-observation CHMM than it is to learn the continuous-time CHMM. This is because it is not necessary to model the observations using the more complex Gaussian (or mixture of Gaussain) models.

We align the two sequences of labels by up-sampling the video labels to match the length of the audio label sequence for every highlight examples in the training set. We then carefully choose the number of states of the CHMMs by analyzing the semantic meaning of the labels corresponding to each state decoded by the Viterbi algorithm. More details can be found in Section 2.3.

Due to the inherently diverse nature of the non-highlight events in sports video, it is difficult to collect good negative training examples. So we don't attempt to learn a non-highlight CHMM.

During testing we adaptively threshold the likelihoods of the video segments, taken sequentially from the recorded sports games, using only the highlight CHMM. The intuition is that the highlight CHMM will produce higher likelihoods for highlight segments and lower values for non-highlight segments. This will be justified in the next subsection.

2.3 Experimental Results with DCHMM

In order to improve the capability of modeling the label sequences, we follow L. Rabiner's description of refinement on the model (e.g., more states, different code-book size, etc.) in [10] by segmenting each of the training label sequences into states, and then studying the properties of the observed labels occurring in each state. Note that the states are decoded via the Viterbi algorithm in an unsupervised fashion, i.e, unsupervised HMM.

In [16], We first show the refinement on the number of states for both the "Audio-alone" and the "Video-alone" approach respectively. With appropriate number of states, the physical meaning of the model states can be easily interpreted. We then build the CHMM using these refined states. We next compare the results of these three different approaches, i.e, "Audio-alone", "Video-alone" and CHMM-based approach.

Results of the CHMM Approach

After refining the states in the previous two single-modality HMMs, we build the CHMM with 2 states for the audio HMM and 2 states for the video HMM and introduce the coupling between the states of these two models.

The Precision-Recall (PR) curve of testing using the audio-visual CHMM is shown as the solid line curve in Fig. 2 where precision is the percentage of highlights that are correct of all those extracted and recall is the percentage of highlights that are in the ground-truth set.

Comparing the three PR curves in Fig. 2, we can make the following observations:

1. The CHMM based approach achieves twice as much precision than the other two approaches for recall rates that are greater than 0.2. This suggests a much smaller false alarm rate using CHMM approach.
2. For very small recall rates ($0 \sim 0.2$), the audio-alone HMM based approach is comparable with the CHMM based approach and their precision rates are much higher than those by the video-alone HMM based approach. This suggests the validity of the assumption that audio classification produces audio labels that are more closely related to content semantics (in this case, contiguous applause labels are likely to be related to highlights).
3. Overall the highlight extraction rates still need further improvement, as indicated by the low precision rates in Fig. 2. We have identified several factors related to the problem. The first is the uncertainty of the boundaries and duration of the highlight segments embedded in the entire broadcast sports content. We have avoided the boundary problem by using a slowly moving video chunk. Our way of dealing with the duration

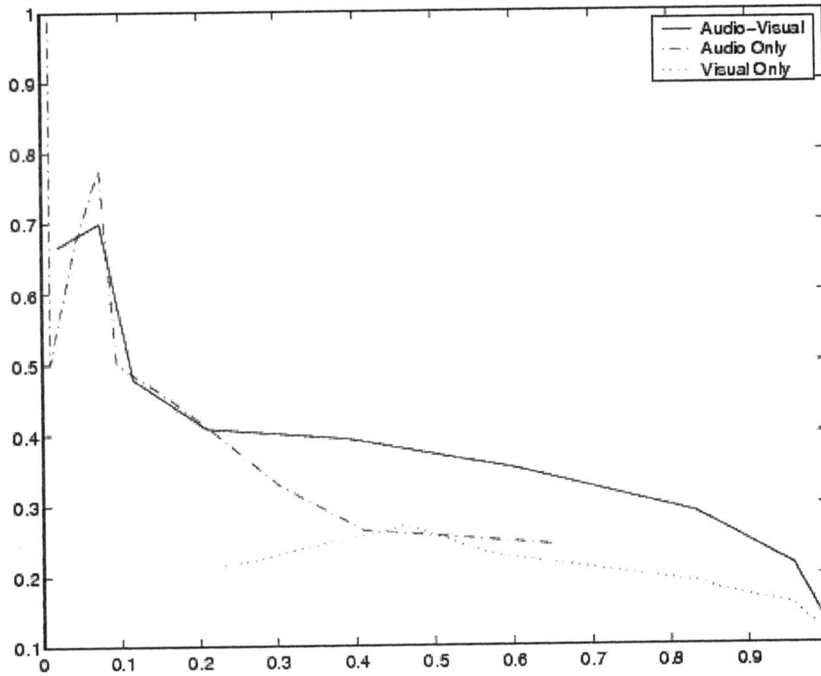

Fig. 2. Precision-Recall Curves for the Test Golf Game. X-axis: recall; Y-axis: Precision.

problem is even more ad-hoc, i.e., using fixed-length video chunks. The second factor is the choice of video features. In this work, we have only used motion activity descriptors which have been shown to be limited. We would introduce other video features such as dominant color, color histogram, etc.

3 Fusion 2: Audio Classification then Visual HMM Verification

3.1 GMM-MDL Audio Classification

Estimating the Number of Mixtures in GMMs Using MDL

The derivations here follow those in [1]. Let Y be an M dimensional random vector to be modeled using a Gaussian mixture distribution. Let K denote the number of Gaussian mixtures, and we use the notation π, μ, and R to denote the parameter sets $\{\pi_k\}_{k=1}^K$, $\{\mu_k\}_{k=1}^K$ and $\{R_k\}_{k=1}^K$ for mixture coefficients, means and variances. The complete set of parameters are then given by K and

$\theta = (\pi, \mu, R)$. The log of the probability of the entire sequence $Y = \{Y_n\}_{n=1}^N$ is then given by

$$\log p_y(y|K,\theta) = \sum_{n=1}^{N} \log \left(\sum_{k=1}^{K} p_{y_n|x_n}(y_n|k,\theta)\pi_k \right) . \tag{4}$$

The objective is then to estimate the parameters K and $\theta \in \Omega^{(K)}$. The maximum likelihood (ML) estimate is given by

$$\hat{\theta}_{ML} = \arg \max_{\theta \in \Omega^{(K)}} \log p_y(y|K,\theta)$$

, and the estimate of K is based on the minimization of the expression

$$MDL(K,\theta) = -\log p_y(y|K,\theta) + \frac{1}{2} L \log(NM) , \tag{5}$$

where L is the number of continuously valued real numbers required to specify the parameter θ. In this application,

$$L = K\left(1 + M + \frac{(M+1)M}{2}\right) - 1 .$$

Notice that this criterion has a penalty term on the total number of data values NM, suggested by Rissanen [11] called the minimum description length (MDL) estimator. Let us denote the parameter learning of GMMs using the MDL criterion MDL-GMM.

While the Expectation Maximization (EM) algorithm can be used to update the parameter θ, it does not provide a solution to the problem of how to change the model order K. Our approach starts with a large number of clusters, and then sequentially decrement the value of K. For each value of K, we apply the EM update until we converge to a local minimum of the MDL function. After we have done this for each value of K, we may simply select the value of K and corresponding parameters that resulted in the smallest value of the MDL criterion.

The question remains of how to decrement the number of clusters from K to $K-1$. We will do this by merging two closest clusters to form a single cluster. More specifically, the two clusters l and m are specified as a single cluster (l,m) with prior probability, mean and covariance given by

$$\pi^*_{(l,m)} = \bar{\pi}_l + \bar{\pi}_m \tag{6}$$

$$\mu^*_{(l,m)} = \frac{\bar{\pi}_l \bar{\mu}_l + \bar{\pi}_m \bar{\mu}_m}{\bar{\pi}_l + \bar{\pi}_m} \tag{7}$$

$$R^*_{(l,m)} = \frac{\bar{\pi}_l \left(\bar{R}_l + (\bar{\mu}_l - \mu_{(l,m)})(\bar{\mu}_l - \mu_{(l,m)})^t\right)}{\bar{\pi}_l + \bar{\pi}_m} + \frac{\bar{\pi}_m \left(\bar{R}_m + (\bar{\mu}_m - \mu_{(l,m)})(\bar{\mu}_m - \mu_{(l,m)})^t\right)}{\bar{\pi}_l + \bar{\pi}_m} . \tag{8}$$

Here the $\bar{\pi}$, $\bar{\mu}$, and $\bar{R}$ are given by the EM update of the two individual mixtures before they are merged.

An Example: MDL-GMM for Different Sound Classes

We've collected 679 audio clips from TV broadcasting of golf, baseball and soccer games. This database is a subset of that in [15]. Each of them is hand-labeled into one of the five classes as ground truth: applause, cheering, music, speech, "speech with music". Their corresponding numbers of clips are 105, 82, 185, 168, 139. Their duration differs from around 1 second to more than 10 seconds. The total duration is approximately 1 hour and 12 minutes. The audio signals are all mono-channel with a sampling rate of 16kHz.

We extract 100 12-dimensional MFCC parameter vectors per second using a 25 msec window. We also add the first- and second-order time derivatives to the basic MFCC parameters in order to enhance performance. For more details, please refer to [18].

For each class of sound data, we first assign a relative large number of mixtures to K, calculate the MDL score $MDL(K, \theta)$ using all the training sound files, then merge the two nearest Gaussian components to get the next MDL score $MDL(K-1, \theta)$, then iterate till $K = 1$. The "optimal" number K is chosen as the one that gives the minimum of the MDL scores. For the training database we have, the relationship between $MDL(K, \theta)$ and K for all five classes are shown in Fig. 3.

From Fig. 3 we observe that the optimal mixture numbers of the above five audio classes are 2, 2, 4, 18, 8 respectively. This observation can be intuitively interpreted as follows. Applause or cheering has a relatively simpler spectral structure, hence fewer Gaussian components can model the data well. In comparison, speech has a much more complex, variant spectral distribution, it needs much more components.

Also, we observe that the complexity of music is between that of applause or cheering and speech. For "speech with music", i.e., a mixture class of speech and music, its complexity is between the two classed that are in the mixture.

GMM-MDL Audio Classification for Sports Highlights Generation

In [14], we have shown that for the 90%/10% training/test split of the 5-class audio dataset, the overall classification accuracy has been improved by more than 8% by using the MDL-GMMs over the traditional GMMs based approach.

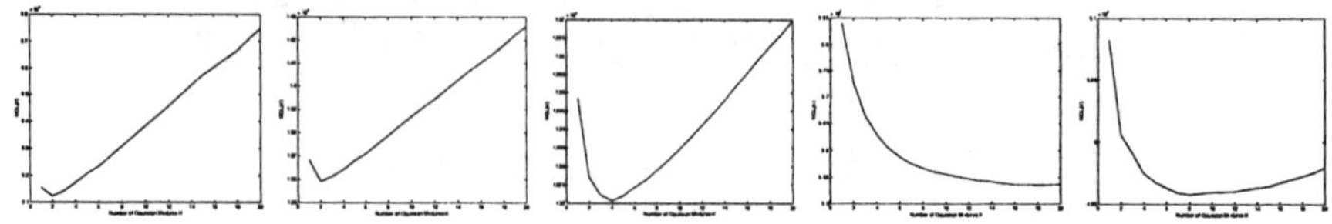

Fig. 3. $MDL(K, \theta)$(Y axis) with respect to different number of GMM mixtures K(X axis) to model Applause, Cheering, Music, Speech and "SpeechWithMusic" sound shown in the raster-scan order. $K = 1 \cdots 20$. The optimal mixture numbers at the lowest positions of the curves are 2, 2, 4, 18, 8 respectively.

With the trained MDL-GMMs, we ran audio classification on the audio sound track of a 3-hour golf game. The game took place on a rainy day so the existence of the sound of raining has corrupted our previous classification results in [15] to a great degree. Every second of the game audio is classified into one of the 5 classes. Those contiguous applause segments are sorted according to the duration of contiguity. The distribution of these contiguous applause segments is shown in Table 3. Note that the applause segments can be as long as 9 continuous seconds.

Table 3. Number of contiguous applause segments and highlights found by the MDL-GMMs in the golf game. These highlights are in the vicinity of the applause segments. These numbers are plotted in Fig. 4.

applause length	# of instances	# of highlights
$L \geq 9s$	1	1
$L \geq 8s$	3	3
$L \geq 7s$	6	5
$L \geq 6s$	11	9
$L \geq 5s$	19	15
$L \geq 4s$	35	28
$L \geq 3s$	61	43
$L \geq 2s$	101	70
$L \geq 1s$	255	95

Based on when the beginning of applause or cheering is, we choose to include a certain number of seconds of video before the beginning moment to include the play action (golf swing, par, etc.), then we compare these segments to those ground-truth highlights that are labeled by human viewers.

Performance and Comparison with Results in [16] in Terms of Precision-Recall Curves

We analyze the extracted highlights that are based on those segments in Table 3. For each length L of the contiguous applause segments, we calculate the precision and recall values. We then plot the precision vs. recall values for all different L into Fig. 4.

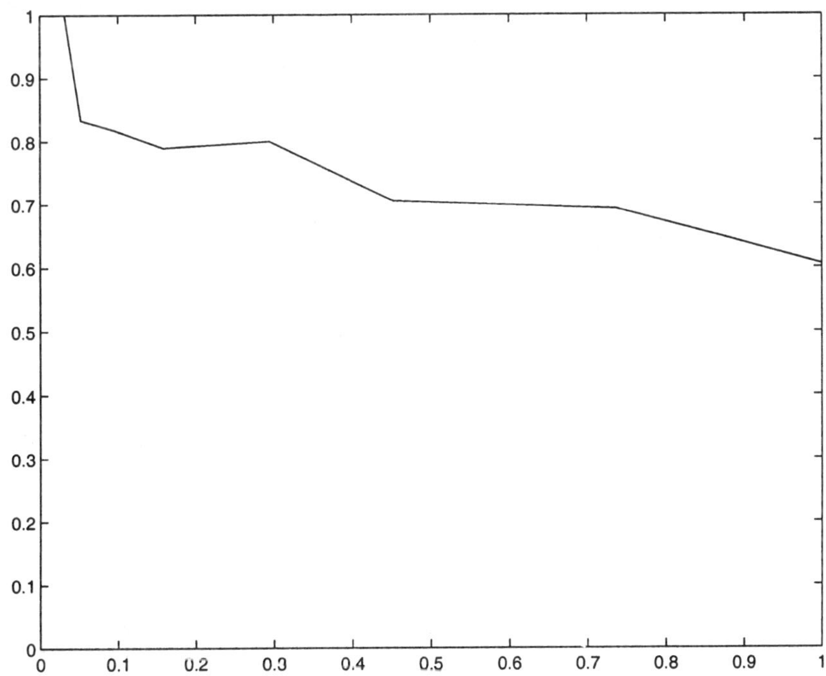

Fig. 4. Precision-recall curves for the test golf game by the " audio classification then visual HMM verification" approach. X-axis: recall; Y-axis: Precision.

From Fig. 2 and Fig. 4, we observe that the MDL-GMMs out-perform those approaches in [16] by a large margin. For example, at 90% recall, Fig. 4 shows $\geq$ 70% precision rate, while Fig. 2 shows only $\sim$ 30% precision rate, suggesting that the false alarm rate is much lower using the current approach.

System Interface

One important application of highlight generation from sports video is to provide the viewers the correct entry points to the video content so that they can adaptively choose other interesting contents that are not necessarily modeled by the training data. This requires a progressive highlight generation process. Depending on how long the sequence of highlights the viewers want to watch, the system should provide those most likely sequences. We thus use a content-adaptive threshold, the lowest of which being the smallest likelihood and the highest of which being the largest threshold over all the test sequences.

Then given such a time budget, we can calculate the value of the threshold above which the total length of highlight segments will be as close to the budget as possible. Then we can play those segments with likelihood greater than the threshold one after another until the budget is exhausted. This can be illustrated in Fig. 5 where a horizontal line is imposed on the likelihood curve so that only those segments with higher values than the threshold will be played for the users.

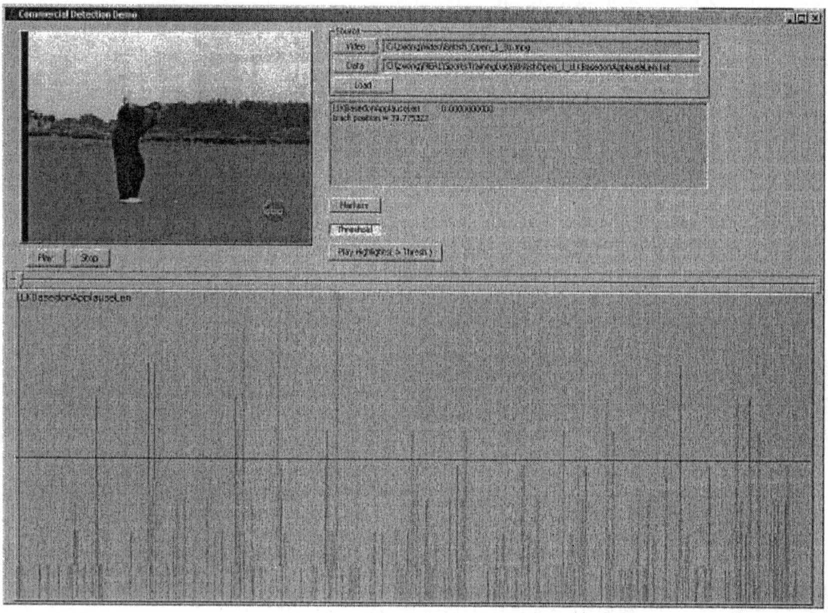

Fig. 5. The interface of our system displaying sports highlights. The horizontal line imposed on the curve is the threshold value the user can choose to display those segments with confidence level greater than the threshold.

3.2 Visual Verification with HMMs

Although some of the false alarm highlights returned by audio classification have long contiguous applause segments, they do not contain real highlight actions in play. For example, when a player is introduced to the audience, applause abounds. This shows the limit of the previous audio-based approach and calls for additional video domain techniques. We have noticed that the visual patterns in such segments are quite different from those in highlight segments such as "putt" or "swing" in golf. These visual patterns include the changes of dominant color and motion intensity. In "putt" segments, the player stands in the middle of the golf field that is usually green, which is the dominant color in the golf video. In contrast, when the announcer introduces a player to the audience, the camera focus usually is on the announcer, so there is not much green color of the golf field. In "swing" segments, the golf ball goes from the ground up, flies against the sky and comes down to the ground. In the process, there is a change of color from the color of the sky to the color of the play field. Note there are two different dominant colors in "swing" segments. Also, since the camera follows the ups and downs of the golf ball, there is the characteristic pan and zoom, both of which may be captured by the motion intensity features.

Modeling Highlights by Color Using HMM

We divide the 50 highlight segments we collected from a golf video into two categories, 18 "putt" and 32 "swing" video sequences. We use them to train a "putt" and a "swing" HMM respectively and test on another 95 highlight segments we collected from another golf video. Since we have the ground truth of these 95 highlight segments (i.e., whether they are "putt" or "swing"), we use the classification accuracy on these 95 highlight segments to guide us in search of the good color features.

First, we use the average hue value of all the pixels in an image frame as the frame feature. The color space here is the Hue-Saturation-Value(HSI) space. For each of the 18 "putt" training sequences, we model the average hue values of all the video frames using a 3-state HMM. In the HMM, the observations, i.e., the average hue values are modeled using a 3-mixture Gaussian Mixture Model. We model the "swing" HMM in a similar way. When we use the learned "putt" and "swing" HMMs to classify the 95 highlight segments from another golf video, the classification accuracy is quite low, $\sim$60% on average over many runs of experiments.

Next, noticing that the range of the average hue values is quite different between the segments from the two different golf videos, we use the following scaling scheme to make them comparable to each other: for each frame, divide its average hue value by the maximum of the average hue values of all the frames in each sequence. With proper scaling by another constant factor, we are able to improve the classification accuracy from $\sim$60% to $\sim$90%.

In Fig. 6, Fig. 7 and Fig. 8, we have plotted these average hue values of all the frames for the 18 "putt", 32 "swing" video sequences for training and the 95 video sequences for testing respectively. Note that the "putt" color pattern in Fig. 6 is quite different from that of "swing" in Fig. 7. This difference is also shown in the color pattern of those test sequences when we examine the features with the ground truth in the table in Fig. 8.

Further Verification by Dominant Color

The scaling scheme mentioned above does not perform well in differentiating "uniform" green color for "putt" from "uniform" color of an announcer's

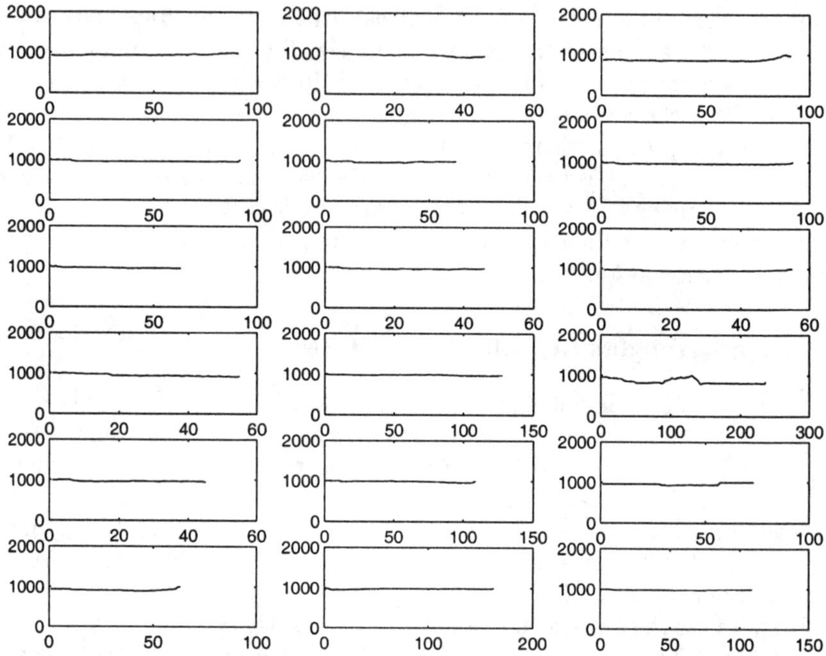

Fig. 6. The scaled version of each video frame's average hue value over time for the 18 training "putt" sequences. The scaling factor is 1000/MAX(·). X-axis: video frames; Y-axis: scaled average hue values.

clothes in a close video shot. To solve this confusion, we learn the dominant green color from those candidate highlight segments indicated by the GMM-MDL audio classification. The grass color of the golf field is the dominant color in this domain, since a televised golf game is bound to show the golf field most of the time, in order to correctly convey the game status. The appearance of the grass color however, ranges from dark green to yellowish green or olive, depending on the field condition and capturing device. Despite these factors, we have observed that within one game, the hue value in the HSI color space is relatively stable despite lighting variations, hence learning the hue value would yield a good definition of dominant color. The dominant color is adaptively learned from those candidate highlight segments using the following cumulative statistic: average the hue values of the pixels from all the video frames of those segments to be the center of the dominant color range; use twice of the variance of the hue values over all the frames as the bandwidth of the dominant color range.

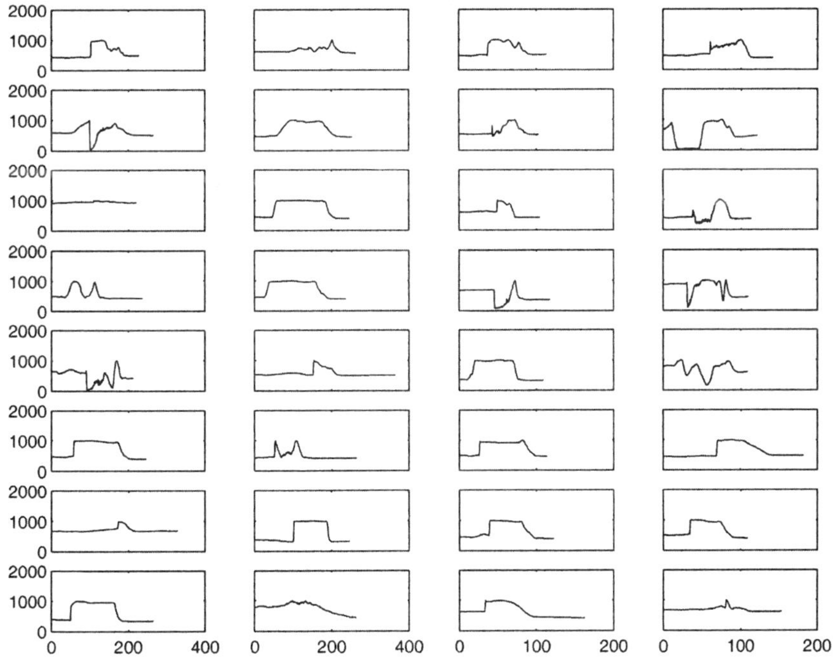

Fig. 7. The scaled version of each video frame's average hue value over time for the 32 training "swing" sequences. The scaling factor is 1000/MAX(·). X-axis: video frames; Y-axis: scaled average hue values.

Modeling Highlights by Motion Using HMM

Motion intensity m is computed as the average magnitude of the effective motion vectors in a frame:

$$m = \frac{1}{|\Phi|} \sum_{\Phi} \sqrt{v_x^2 + v_y^2}, \tag{9}$$

where $\Phi = \{\text{inter-coded macro-blocks}\}$ and $v = (v_x, v_y)$ is the motion vector for each macro-block. This measure of motion intensity gives an estimate of the gross motion in the whole frame, including object and camera motion. Moreover, motion intensity carries complementary information to the color feature, and it often indicates the semantics within a particular shot. For instance, a wide shot with high motion intensity often results from player motion and camera pan during a play; while a static wide shot usually occurs when the game has come to a pause. With the same scaling scheme as the one for color, we are able to achieve an classification accuracy of ~80% on the same 95 test sequences.

We have plotted these average motion intensity values of all the frames of all the sequences in Fig. 9, Fig. 10, and Fig. 11 for the 18 "putt", 32

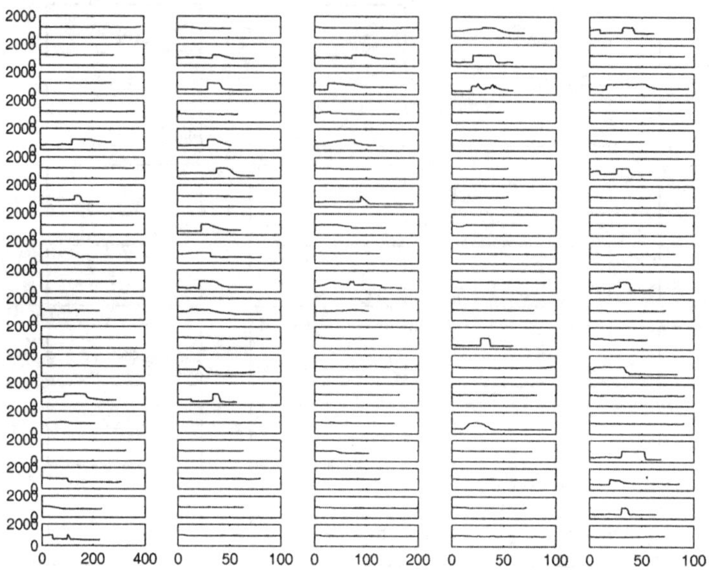

1	1	1	2	2
1	2	2	2	1
1	2	2	2	2
1	1	1	1	1
2	2	2	2	1
1	2	1	1	2
2	1	2	1	1
1	2	2	2	1
2	2	1	1	1
1	2	2	1	2
2	2	1	1	1
1	1	1	2	2
1	2	1	1	2
2	2	1	1	1
1	1	1	2	1
1	1	1	1	2
2	1	1	1	2
1	1	1	1	2
2	1	1	1	1

Fig. 8. Left: The scaled version of each video frame's average hue value over time for the 95 test sequences. Right: The ground truth of the corresponding video sequences where "1" stands for Putt and "2" stands for Swing.

"swing" video sequences for training and the 95 video sequences for testing respectively.

Proposed Audio + Visual Modeling Algorithm

Based on these observations, we model the color pattern and motion pattern using HMMs. We learn a "putt" HMM and a "swing" HMM of the color features. We also learn a "putt" HMM and a "swing" HMM of the motion intensity features.

Our algorithm can be summarized as follows:

1. Audio analysis for locating contiguous applause segments
   - Silence detection.
   - For non-silent segments, run the GMM-MDL classification algorithm using the trained GMM-MDL models.
2. Sort those contiguous applause segments based on the applause length.
3. Video analysis for verifying whether or not those applause segments follow correct color and motion pattern.
   - Take a certain number of video frames before the onset of each of the applause segments to estimate the dominant color range.
   - For a certain number of video frames before the onset of each of the applause segments, run the "putt" or "swing" HMM of the color features.

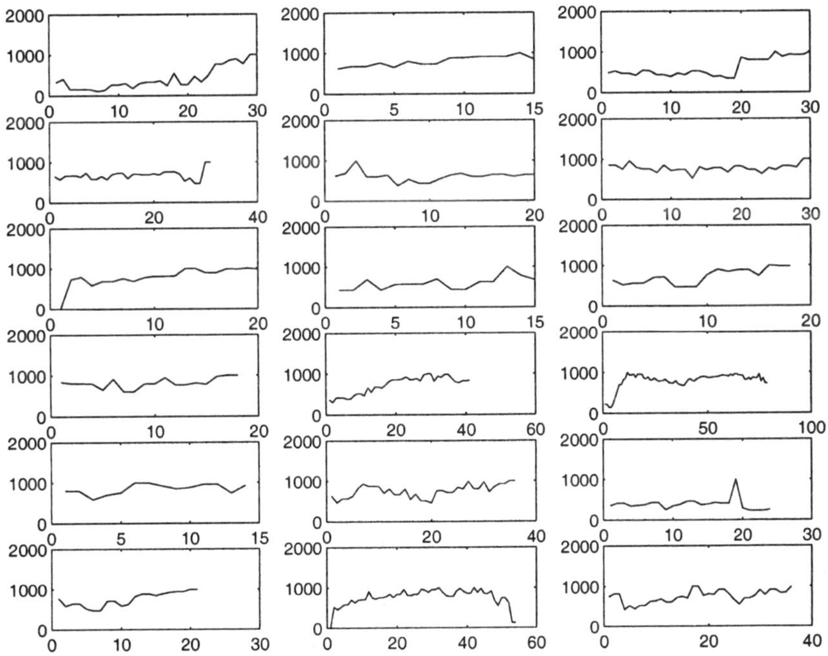

Fig. 9. The scaled version of each video frame's average motion intensity value over time for the 18 training "putt" sequences. The scaling factor is 1000/MAX(·). The scaling factor is 1000/MAX(·). X-axis: video P-frames; Y-axis: scaled average motion intensity values.

- If it is classified as "putt", then verify its dominant color is in the estimated dominant color range. If the color does not fit, then declare it as a false alarm and eliminate its candidacy.
- If it is classified as "swing", then run the "putt" or "swing" HMM of the motion intensity features, if it is classified again as "swing" we say it is "swing", otherwise declare it as a false alarm and eliminate its candidacy.

Experimental Results, Observations, and Comparisons

We further analyze the extracted highlights that are based on those segments in Table 3. For each contiguous applause segment, we extract a certain number of video frames before the onset of the detected applause. The number of the video frames is proportional to the average video frames of those "putt" or "swing" sequences in the training set. For these video frames, we verify whether they are of "putt" or "swing" using the proposed algorithm. To compare with the precision-recall curve in Fig. 4, we plot two more precision-recall curves, one being the "GMM-MDL audio classification + color HMM"

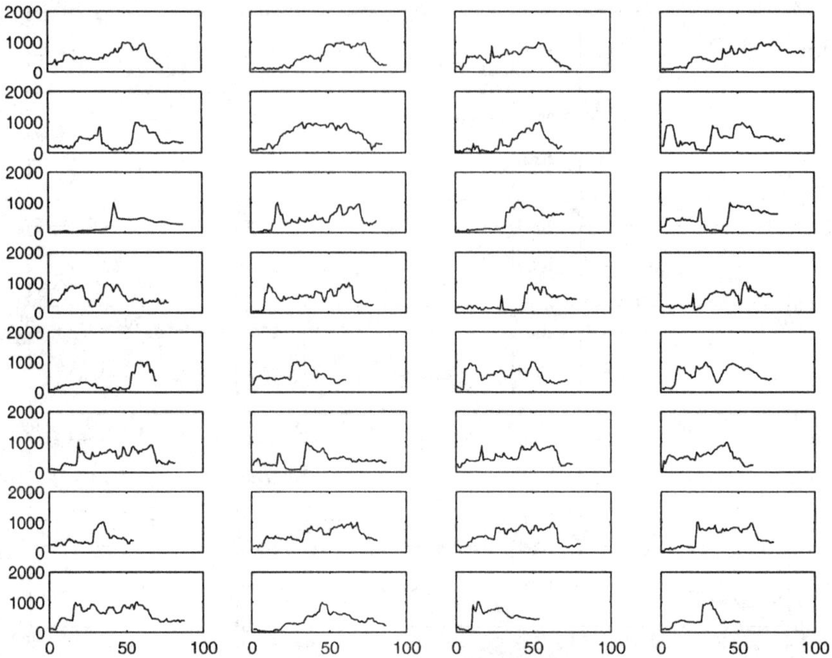

Fig. 10. The scaled version of each video frame's average motion intensity value over time for the 32 training "swing" sequences. The scaling factor is 1000/MAX(·). X-axis: video P-frames; Y-axis: scaled average motion intensity values.

approach and the other being the "GMM-MDL audio classification + color HMM + motion intensity HMM" approach in Fig. 12.

The following observations can be made from the precision-recall comparison in Fig. 12:

- Both the dashed curve and the dotted curve representing "audio modeling + visual modeling" show better precision-recall figures. By careful examining where the improvement comes from, we notice that the application of color and motion modeling has eliminated such false alarms as those involving the announcer or video sequences followed by non-applause audio. By jointly modeling audio and visual features for sports highlights, we have been able to eliminate these two kinds of false alarms: wrong video pattern followed by applause and video pattern followed by non-applause.
- Between the dashed curve and the dotted curve, the introduction of additional motion intensity modeling although improves performance over the "audio modeling + color modeling", the improvement is only marginal.

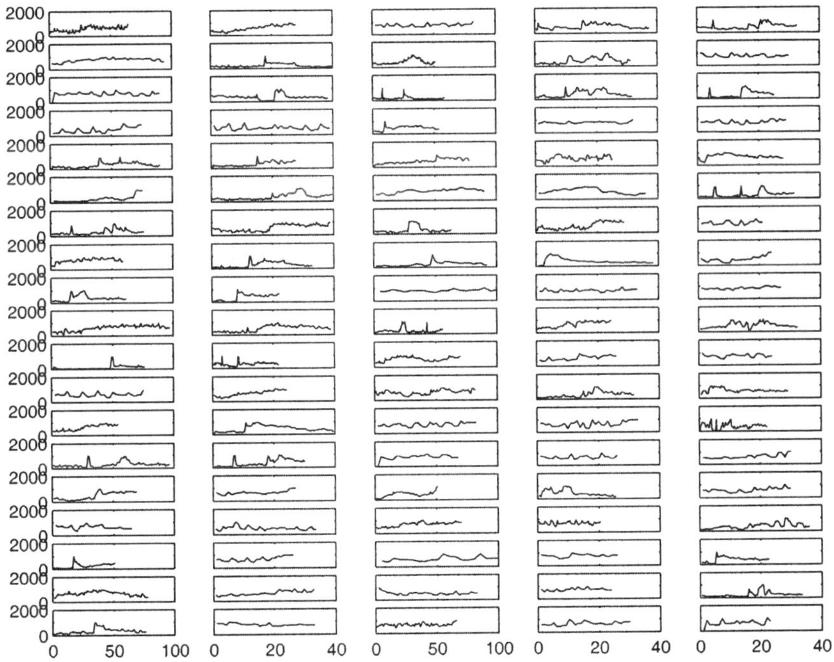

Fig. 11. The scaled version of each video frame's average motion intensity value over time for the 95 test sequences. The scaling factor is 1000/MAX(·). X-axis: video P-frames; Y-axis: scaled average motion intensity values.

4 Conclusions and Future Work

We have shown two different joint audio-visual event modeling methods, namely coupled hidden Markov models and sequential audio-visual modeling. The application of these two methods for the task of recognizing highlight events such as "putt" or "swing" in golf has shown that the second approach has its advantage over the first approach.

In the future, we will extend the framework to other kinds of sports such as baseball and soccer. Since the audio signal in baseball or soccer, in general, is much noisier, we will work on robust audio classification for these sports. We will also research on sport-specific audio or visual object detection, such as soccer ball, excited commentator's speech. Our future research will also cover fusion of these detection results with the current audio-visual features.

References

1. Bouman, C. A. CLUSTER: An unsupervised algorithm for modeling gaussian mixtures, http://www.ece.purdue.edu/~bouman, School of Electrical Engineering, Purdue University.

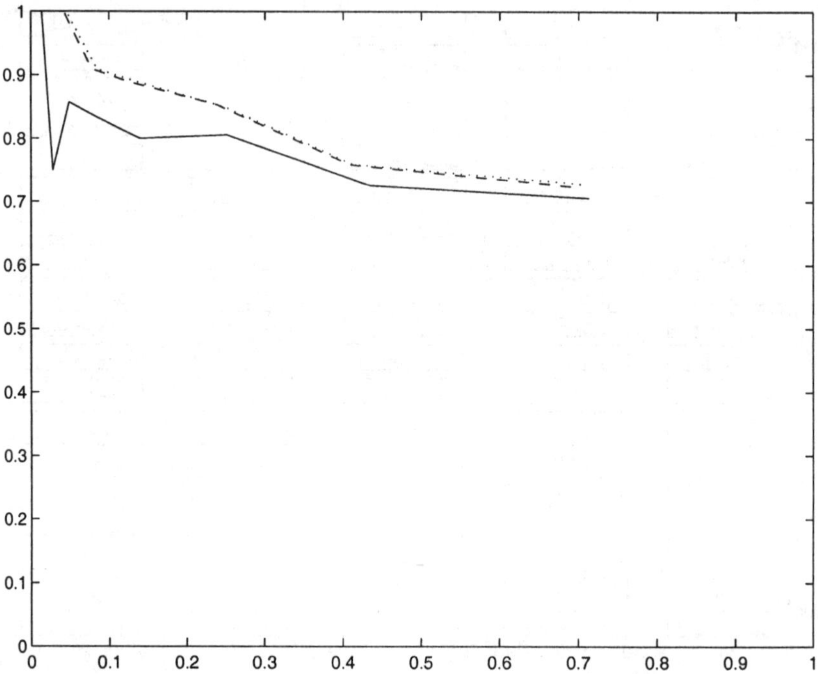

Fig. 12. Comparison Results of 3 different modeling approaches in terms of ROC curves. Solid line: audio modeling alone; Dashed line: audio + dominant color modeling, Dotted line: audio + dominant color + motion modeling.

2. Brand, M., Oliver, N., Pentland, A. (1996) Coupled hidden markov models for complex action recognition, Proceedings of IEEE CVPR97.
3. Divakaran, A., Peker, K., Radhakrishnan, R., Xiong, Z., Cabasson, R. (2003) Video summarization using MPEG-7 motion activity and audio descriptors, Video Mining, eds. A. Rosenfeld, D. Doermann and D. DeMenthon, Kluwer Academic Publishers.
4. Ekin, A., Tekalp, A. M. (2003) Automatic soccer video analysis and summarization, Symp. Electronic Imaging: Science and Technology: Storage and Retrieval for Image and Video Databases IV.
5. Gong, Y., Sin, L., Chuan, C., Zhang, H., Sakauchi, M. (1995) Automatic parsing of TV soccer programs, IEEE International Conference on Multimedia Computing and Systems, 167–174
6. Hsu, W. Speech audio project report, www.ee.columbia.edu/~winston.
7. Kawashima, T., Tateyama, K., Iijima, T., Aoki, Y. (1998) Indexing of baseball telecast for content-based video retrieval, International Conference on Image Processing, 871–874
8. Nefian, A. V., Liang, L., Liu, X., Pi, X., Mao, C., Murphy, K. (2002) A coupled HMM for audio-visual speech recognition, Proceedings of International Conference on Acoustics Speech and Signal Processing, II:2013–2016.

9. Peker, K. A., Cabasson, R., Divakaran, A. (2002) Rapid generation of sports highlights using the MPEG-7 motion activity descriptor, SPIE Conference on Storage and Retrieval from Media Databases.
10. Rabiner, L. (1989) A tutorial on hidden markov models and selected applications in speech recognition, Proceedings of the IEEE, **77(2)**, 257–286
11. Rissanen, J. (1983) A universal prior for integers and estimation by minimum description length, Annals of Statistics, **11(2)**, 417–431
12. Rui, Y., Gupta, A., Acero, A. (2000) Automatically extracting highlights for TV baseball programs, Eighth ACM International Conference on Multimedia, 105–115
13. Xie, L., Chang, S., Divakaran, A., Sun, H. (2002) Structure analysis of soccer video with hidden markov models, Proceedings of Intl. Conf. on Acoustic, Speech and Signal Processing, (ICASSP-2002).
14. Xiong, Z., Radhakrishnan, R., Divakaran, A. (2004) Effective and efficient sports highlights extraction using the minimum description length criterion in selecting gmm structures, Proceedings of Intl' Conf. on Multimedia and Expo (ICME).
15. Xiong, Z., Radhakrishnan, R., Divakaran, A., Huang, T. (2003) Audio-based highlights extraction from baseball, golf and soccer games in a unified framework, Proceedings of Intl. Conf. on Acoustic, Speech and Signal Processing (ICASSP), **5**, 628–631.
16. Xiong, Z., Radhakrishnan, R., Divakaran, A., Huang, T. (2004) Audio-visual sports highlights extraction using coupled hidden markov models, submitted to Pattern Analysis and Application Journal, Special Issue on Video Based Event Detection.
17. Xu, P., Xie, L., Chang, S., Divakaran, A., Vetro, A., Sun, H. (2001) Algorithms and system for segmentation and structure analysis in soccer video, Proceedings of IEEE Conference on Multimedia and Expo, 928–931
18. Young, S., Evermann, G., Kershaw, D., Moore, G., Odell, J., Ollason, D., Povey, D., Valtchev, V., Woodland, P. (2003) The HTK Book version 3.2, Cambridge University Press, Cambridge University Engineering Department.

Fuzzy Logic Methods for Video Shot Boundary Detection and Classification

Ralph M. Ford

School of Engineering and Engineering Technology, The Pennsylvania State University, The Behrend College, Erie, PA, 16563, USA

Abstract. A fuzzy logic system for the detection and classification of shot boundaries in uncompressed video sequences is presented. It integrates multiple sources of information and knowledge of editing procedures to detect shot boundaries. Furthermore, the system classifies the editing process employed to create the shot boundary into one of the following categories: abrupt cut, fade-in, fade-out, or dissolve. This system was tested on a database containing a wide variety of video classes. It achieved combined recall and precision rates that significantly exceed those of existing threshold-based techniques, and it correctly classified a high percentage of the detected boundaries.

Keywords: scene change detection, shot boundary detection, video indexing, video segmentation

1 Introduction

The need for shot boundary detection, also known as scene change detection or digital video segmentation, is well established and necessary for the identification of key frames in video. A shot is defined as one or more frames generated and recorded contiguously that represents a continuous action in time or space. A shot differs from a scene, in that a scene is a collection of shots that form a temporal, spatial, or perceptual natural unit [3]. Video editing procedures produce both abrupt and gradual shot transitions. An abrupt change is the result of splicing two dissimilar shots together, and this transition occurs over a single frame. Gradual transitions occur over multiple frames and are most commonly the product of fade-ins, fade-outs, and dissolves.

Shot boundary detection is a process that is carried out well by humans based on a number of rules, special cases, and subjective interpretation. However, the process is time consuming, tedious, and prone to error. This makes it a good candidate for analysis by a fuzzy logic system. For example, consider fade-outs where it is expected that the shot luminance will decrease by a large amount and that the shot structure will remain fairly constant. The terms that describe this edit, *a large amount* and *fairly constant*, have a degree of subjectivity, and this is handled well by a fuzzy logic system (FLS).

Two published works have been reported on the application of fuzzy logic to this problem. The first work applied fuzzy reasoning to shot boundary detection based upon established models of video editing [4]. This chapter extends that work further in terms of capabilities of the system and size of the database tested. The second work is similar, but proposes fuzzification of frame-to-frame differences using the Rayleigh distribution and uses a smaller feature set [10]. Both methods are applied to non-compressed data and report good detection and classification capabilities.

2 Related Work

The main approaches to shot boundary detection are based on histogram comparisons, statistic differences, pixel-differences, MPEG coefficients, and image features. Each is considered in this section. Further information can be found in [2, 5, 7] which provide surveys and comparisons of many algorithms and metrics that have been reported for shot boundary detection.

Histogram metrics are based upon intensity histograms of sequential images that are used to compute a value that is thresholded for detection. Nagasaka and Tanaka [15] experimented with histogram and pixel differences and concluded that histogram metrics are the most effective. Furthermore, they concluded that the Chi-Square (χ^2) test [16] is the best histogram metric. Nagasaka and Tanaka and Zhang *et al.* [24] both computed the sum of absolute value histogram differences. Zhang *et al.* concluded that the absolute value measure is a better metric than χ^2.

Swain and Ballard [18] introduced a metric, histogram intersection, where the objective was to discriminate between color objects in an image database. Gargi *et al.* [6] applied it to shot boundary detection and tested its efficacy under a variety of color spaces. Nakajima *et al.* [14] proposed a metric which is the inner product of chrominance histograms, and it was used in conjunction with Discrete Cosine Transform (DCT) differences to detect shot boundaries in MPEG sequences.

Sethi and Patel [17] utilized the Kolmogorov-Smirnov test [16], which is the maximum absolute value difference between Cumulative Distribution Functions (the integral of the histogram). They applied it to DCT coded images in MPEG sequences and employed a histogram of the first DCT coefficient of each block (that is the average gray level value of each 8x8 block). Tan *et al.* [20] have proposed a modified Komogorov-Smirnov statistic that is shown to have superior performance compared to other metrics.

Another approach is to compare sequential images based on first and second order intensity statistics in the form of a likelihood ratio [21] or a standard statistical hypothesis test. Jain [11] computed a likelihood ratio test based on the assumption of uniform second order statistics. Assuming a normal distribution, the likelihood ratio is known as the Yakimovsky Likelihood Ratio and it was used by Sethi and Patel [17]. Other related metrics that have been considered are the Student *t*-test, Snedecor's *F*-test, and several related metrics [5].

Pixel difference metrics compare images based on differences in the image intensity map. Nagasaka and Tanaka [15] computed a pixel-wise sum of absolute gray level differences. Jain [11] and Zhang *et al.* [24] employed a similar measure in which a binary difference picture is computed first, and the result summed. Pixel values in the binary picture are set to 1 if the original pixel differences exceed a threshold; otherwise they are set to zero. Then the number of pixels that exceed the first threshold is compared to a second threshold.

Image pixel values can be considered one-dimensional vectors, and one way to represent the similarity between vectors is to project one vector onto the other, computing the inner product. This led to the use of the inner product for comparing image pairs [5] in a manner similar to the MPEG method proposed by Arman *et al.* [1]. Hampapur *et al.* [8] used a pixel-difference metric based on a chromatic scaling model to detect fades and dissolves. However, as indicated in [2] and [5], this method performs poorly for shot boundaries that do not closely follow the model.

Shot boundary detection in the MPEG domain is attractive since compressed data can be directly processed. Arman [1] proposed an inner product metric using the DCT coefficients of MPEG sequences. Yeo and Liu [22] advocated the use of DC images for shot boundary detection in MPEG sequences. Each pixel in a DC image represents the average value from each transform block. This results in a significant data and processing time reduction. They then applied a combination of histogram and pixel-difference metrics to detect shot boundaries in DC images. An object-based method has been developed that is transition length independent and is well-suited to the MPEG-7 standard [9].

Zabih *et al.* [23] proposed an algorithm that relies on the number of edge pixels that change in neighboring images. The algorithm requires computing edges, registering the images, computing incoming and outgoing edges, and computing an edge change fraction. The algorithm is able to detect and classify shot boundaries. However, as the authors indicated, the computational complexity of this algorithm is high.

Many of the aforementioned works concentrate on a particular metric, or combination of several metrics for shot boundary detection, but not classification. Zabih's algorithm provides for both detection and classification in uncompressed sequences. The objective of this work is to describe a flexible, computationally fast technique for shot boundary detection and classification that intelligently integrates multiple sources of information. First, video editing models that characterize shot boundaries are presented. Then a fuzzy system implementation is developed based upon the models. The system classifies the editing process employed to create the shot boundary into one of the following categories: abrupt cut, fade-in, fade-out, or dissolve. This system was tested on a large database containing a wide variety of video classes. It achieved combined recall and precision rates that significantly exceed those of existing threshold-based techniques. It also correctly classifies a high percentage of the detected boundaries.

3 Shot Boundary Models

The processes employed by video editing tools to create shot boundaries are mathematically characterized to provide guidance for developing the FLS. The models come from the work by Hampapur [8]. Let the symbol S denote a single continuous shot that is a set of consecutive 2D images. The individual images of the set are denoted $I(x,y;k)$, where x and y are the pixel position and k is the discrete time index. A shot containing $N+1$ images is represented as

$$S = \{I(x,y;0), I(x,y;1),..., I(x,y;N)\}. \tag{1}$$

Abrupt cuts are formed by concatenating two shots as

$$S = S_1 \circ S_2, \tag{2}$$

where the symbol $\circ$ indicates concatenation. Due to the abrupt nature of this transition, it is expected to produce significant changes in the shot lighting and image structure if the two shots are dissimilar. Consequently, *large* histogram, pixel-difference, and statistic-based metric values are expected for abrupt cuts. Conversely, *small* values are expected for comparisons of frames from the same shot.

There are two fades to consider. The first is a fade-out, where the luminance of the shot is decreased over multiple frames, and the second is a fade-in, where the luminance of the shot is increased from some base level to full shot luminance. It is not assumed that fades must begin or end with a uniform black image, although this is often the case. A simple way to model a fade-out is to take a single frame in the shot, $I(x,y;k_1)$, and monotonically decrease the luminance. This is accomplished by scaling each frame in an $N+1$ (index $l = 0,\ldots,N$) frame edit sequence as

$$S(x,y;l) = I(x,y;k_1) \times \left(1 - \frac{l}{N}\right). \tag{3}$$

The shape of the intensity histogram remains fixed (ideally) for each frame in the sequence, but the width of the histogram is scaled by the multiplicative factor $\left(1 - \frac{l}{N}\right)$. The intensity mean (μ), median (*Med*), and standard deviation (σ) of each frame are scaled by this factor relative to their values in frame k_1. Another way to implement a fade-out is to shift the luminance level as

$$S(x,y;l) = I(x,y;k_1) - max_1 \times \left(\frac{l}{N}\right), \tag{4}$$

where max_1 is the maximum intensity value in the frame $I(x,y;k_1)$. In this model μ and *Med* are shifted downward in each consecutive frame, but σ remains constant. In practice, a non-linear limiting operation is applied to the results since intensity values are non-negative (the resulting negative intensity values are set equal to 0). The limiting operation decreases the width of the histogram and likewise the standard deviation. A general mathematical expression for the change in σ cannot be determined since it depends on the shape of the histogram and this is altered by the limiting operation. If the limiting operation is applied to any of the inputs, σ will decrease; otherwise it will remain constant.

Two analogous models for fade-ins are

$$S(x, y; l) = I(x, y; k_N) \times \left(\frac{l}{N} \right) \tag{5}$$

and

$$S(x, y; l) = I(x, y; k_N) - \max{}_N \times \left(\frac{l}{N} - 1 \right), \tag{6}$$

where max_N is the maximum intensity value in the frame $I(x, y; k_N)$. The scaling model ((3) and (5)) was employed by Hampapur *et al.* [8] to detect chromatic edits in video sequences. Experimental results indicate that some, but not all, fades follow this model and the level-shifting model ((4) and (6)) is proposed as an alternative. Both models are too simple because they model a sequence that is a single static image whose brightness is varied. In reality, this operation is applied to non-static sequences where inter-frame changes due to shot activity occur. Therefore, the image structure does not necessarily remain fixed.

During a fade it is assumed that the geometric structure of the shot remains *fairly constant* between frames, but that the lighting distribution changes. For example, during a fade-out that obeys (3) μ, *Med*, and σ all decrease at the same constant rate, but the structure of the shot remains fixed. If the fade obeys (4), μ and *Med* decrease at the same rate, but the standard deviation may not. The converse is true of fade-ins.

There is a special fade type, that we will refer to as a low light fade, that is common during fades of text on a dark background (particularly during movie credits). During low light fades *Med* remains constant at a low gray level value, and the overall illumination change is lower than an expected in a "regular" fade.

Dissolves are a combination of two or more shots. A dissolve is modeled as a combination of a fade-out of one shot (I_1), and a simultaneous fade-in of another (I_2) as follows

$$S(x, y; l) = I_1(x, y; k_1) \times \left(1 - \frac{l}{N} \right) + I_2(x, y; k_2) \times \left(\frac{l}{N} \right). \tag{7}$$

This is a reasonably accurate model, but there are several problems: the fade rates (in and out) do not have to be equal as modeled, there may be activity during the transition, and complex special effects may be applied during the transition. Dissolves are difficult to detect due to their gradual nature and lack of a reliable mathematical model. However, during dissolves μ, *Med*, and σ experience a sustained change from their starting values in I_1 to their ending values in I_2. This is also true of fades; however the migration of the statistics is not typically in the same direction for a dissolve, as it is for a fade. This "statistic migration" is utilized for dissolve detection. In order to detect the migration the following measure is used

$$\Gamma = \sqrt{(\mu_k - \mu_{k+N})^2 + (\sigma_k - \sigma_{k+N})^2 + (Med_k - Med_{k+N})^2}\ . \tag{8}$$

Dissolves experience a significant change in Γ and are a linear combination of I_1 and I_2, and typically last between 3 and 35 frames for the frame rates utilized.

The characteristics of the shot boundaries are summarized in Table 1 with the fuzzy descriptive terms shown in italics. These characteristics form the basis upon which the FLS is developed.

Table 1. Summary of shot boundary characteristics.

Shot Boundary	Characteristics
None (same shot)	• Small changes in all metrics (histogram, pixel-difference, and statistic).
Abrupt cut	• Large changes in all metrics (histogram, pixel-difference, and statistic).
Fades	• Large-positive (or negative) sustained increase/decrease in μ, Med, and possibly σ. • Rate of change of (μ and Med) or (μ and σ) is nearly the same. • Scene structure between consecutive frames is fairly constant.
Low light fades	• Medium-large-positive (or negative) sustained increase/decrease in μ, Med, and possibly σ. • Rate of change of (μ and Med) or (μ and σ) is nearly the same. • Scene structure between consecutive frames is fairly constant. • Med value remains nearly constant and small. • A large start-to-end change in Γ.
Dissolves	• Start and end frames are from different shots (I_1 and I_2). • A large start-to-end change in Γ. • Frames of the dissolve are a linear combination of the start and end frames.

4 The Fuzzy Logic System

A FLS was selected for shot boundary detection for the following reasons: *i)* the governing rules in Table 1 are based on expert knowledge of the process used to create the boundaries, *ii)* the rules can be modified without having to retrain the system, *iii)* the proposed FLS produces good results, much better than any single metric can achieve, and *iv)* the FLS is computationally inexpensive to implement. (Only a small number of mathematical and logical operations are required for the FLS itself. In addition, the metrics utilized by the FLS have relatively low computational complexity [5]).

Two general types of fuzzy systems can be implemented. The first is an expert system type where the system developer generates the membership functions and rules based on knowledge of the underlying process. The rules and membership functions are then adjusted until the desired performance is achieved. The second is the Sugeno-style [19] system where a semi-automated iterative approach to determining the membership functions is taken. It is more computationally efficient and lends itself better to mathematical analysis, but is less intuitive. The first approach was selected since a good knowledge of the shot boundary creation process is available from the editing models. The drawback of the selected approach is the tuning required for the membership functions.

To implement a fuzzy system five items are necessary [12,13] : i) the inputs and their ranges, ii) the outputs and their ranges, iii) fuzzy membership functions for each input and output, iv) a rule base, and v) a method to produce a crisp output or decision (a defuzzifier). These items are defined in the following sections.

4.1 System Inputs

A total of eleven inputs were selected - six metrics from those reported in Section 2 and five new ones. Of the first six, two are histogram-based, two are statistic-based, and two are pixel-difference metrics. The remaining five inputs are directly from the video edit models and were selected specifically for fade and dissolve detection. The metrics may be computed globally (for the entire image) or in non-overlapping blocks of the image. Based upon earlier work [5], it is clear that global comparisons are better for histogram and pixel-difference metrics, while blocks are better for statistic-based metrics. The two best performers from the histogram-based, statistic-based, and pixel-difference metrics were selected (best performers identified in [5]).

The histogram metrics selected are the Chi-Square and Kolmogorov-Smirnov tests which are

$$\chi^2 = \frac{1}{M}\sum_{i=1}^{M}\frac{\{h_j(i) - h_k(i)\}^2}{\{h_j(i) + h_k(i)\}}, \quad 0 \le \chi^2 \le 1, \tag{9}$$

$$ks = \max_i |\, CDF_j(i) - CDF_k(i)\,|, \qquad 0 \le ks \le 1, \tag{10}$$

where $h(\bullet)$ is the image histogram, $CDF(\bullet)$ is the Cumulative Distribution Function, (j,k) are the indices of two successive images, and M is the number of histogram bins. The statistic-based (likelihood ratio) metrics selected are

$$\lambda_1 = \frac{|\mu_j - \mu_k| * |\sigma_j - \sigma_k|}{\sigma_j\sigma_k\left(\dfrac{\mu_j + \mu_k}{2}\right)}, \; \lambda_1 \ge 0 \tag{11}$$

$$\lambda_2 = \left(\frac{\mu_j\sigma_j}{\mu_k\sigma_k}\right), \text{ where } \mu_j > \mu_k, \sigma_j > \sigma_k \text{ and } \lambda_2 \ge 1. \tag{12}$$

The first pixel-difference metric selected is the inner product of images. This is computed from DC images that are composed of the DC (average value) coefficients of 8x8 blocks [22]. It is computed as

$$\gamma = 1 - \frac{\vec{I}_{DC\,j} \bullet \vec{I}_{DC\,k}}{\|\vec{I}_{DC\,j}\| \|\vec{I}_{DC\,k}\|}, \quad 0 \le \gamma \le 1. \tag{13}$$

The second pixel-difference metric utilized is a modified inner product measure, where the input images (I') are normalized so that $\mu=0$ and $\sigma=1$

$$\gamma' = 1 - \frac{\vec{I}'_{DC\,j} \bullet \vec{I}'_{DC\,k}}{\|\vec{I}'_{DC\,j}\| \|\vec{I}'_{DC\,k}\|}, \quad 0 \le \gamma' \le 1. \tag{14}$$

Normalization aids in fade identification by removing lighting variations while maintaining the image structure. This allows identification of adjacent frames in fades where the images have similar structure but different lighting characteristics. All metrics are defined such that low values are indicative of the same shot and large values are indicative of shot boundaries.

The inputs derived from the video models are the inter-frame modulations of the gray level μ, σ, and Med, defined as

$$\Delta\mu = \frac{\mu_k - \mu_j}{\mu_k + \mu_j}, \quad \Delta\sigma = \frac{\sigma_k - \sigma_j}{\sigma_k + \sigma_j}, \text{ and } \Delta Med = \frac{Med_k - Med_j}{Med_k + Med_j} \tag{15}$$

and the ratios

$$r_1 = \frac{\Delta\mu}{\Delta\sigma} \quad \text{and} \quad r_2 = \frac{\Delta\mu}{\Delta Med}. \tag{16}$$

The modulation terms measure changes in μ, σ, and Med and the ratios determine how closely sequential frames match the fade models of (3)-(6). The models indicate that for fades μ and σ should change at the same rate, or μ and Med should change at the same rate, depending upon the model that the fade obeys. If two quantities change at the same rate, the ratio of the two modulation terms should be unity. In the fuzzy system this is measured by determining if the ratio is *close-to-1*.

The membership functions for all eleven inputs, shown in Fig. 1, were determined from statistical distributions and the bounds of the metrics. For example, the χ^2 metric lies in the region [0,1] and this determines the bounding values of x_1 and y_3. The values of x_2 and x_3 were determined from the statistical distribution of χ^2 for sequential images of the same shot; x_2 was selected as the point at which 50% of the population lies below and x_3 was selected as the point at which 95% of the population lies below. Likewise the values of y_1 and y_2 were determined by examining the distribution of χ^2 for sequential images representing abrupt shots; y_2 was selected as the point at which 50% of the population lies above and y_1 was selected as the point for which 95% of the population lies above. These values can be adjusted during training to improve the system performance (an option generally supplied in fuzzy system builders), but fuzzy systems are generally robust to small changes. As identified previously, this is one drawback to this approach to building fuzzy systems. Jadon *et al.* [10] utilized a Rayleigh distribution model of the metrics to select the boundaries for the membership functions. The membership functions for the modulation metrics in Fig. 1(b) were similarly determined from the distribution of these statistics during fades. The membership function in Fig. 1(c) is a simple way of representing the characteristic of *close-to-1* for the ratios.

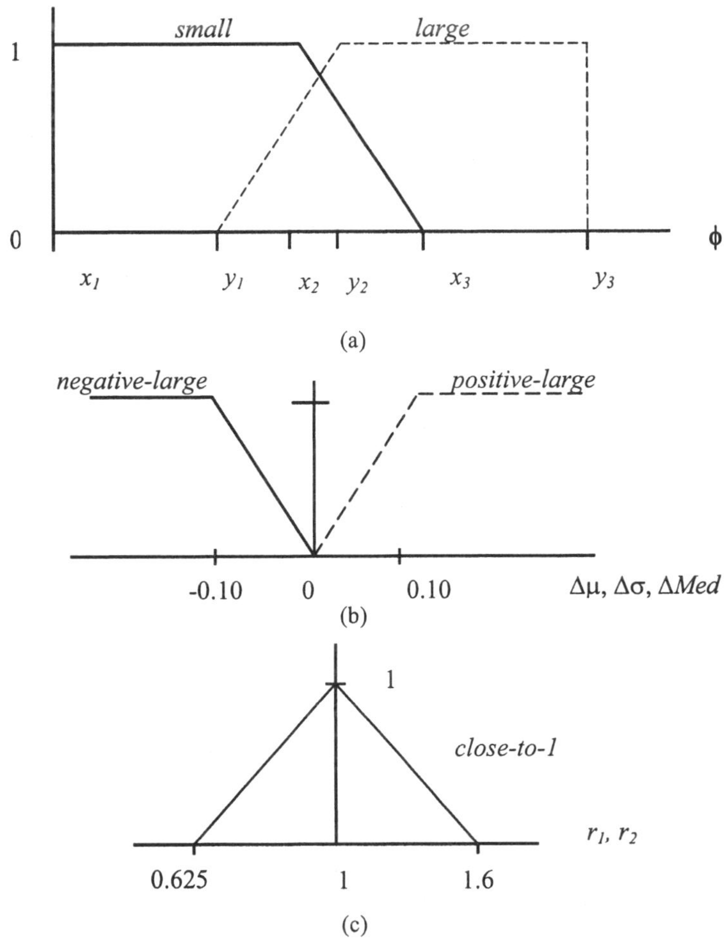

Fig. 1. Membership functions for the system inputs. (a) Histogram, statistic, and pixel-difference metrics in (9)-(14). (b) modulation inputs in (15). (c) ratio inputs in (16)

4.2 The Fuzzy System

The overall fuzzy system implementation is shown in Fig. 2. It is actually a two-level cascade of fuzzy systems as is explained shortly. Six system outputs are defined: same shot (O_{SS}), abrupt cut (O_{AC}), fade-out (O_{FO}), fade-in (O_{FI}), low-light fade-in (O_{LFI}), and low-light fade-out (O_{LFO}). The outputs were selected to range from 0 to 1, where 1 indicates the highest level of confidence that the frames compared are of that shot boundary type. No outputs are defined for dissolves because they are detected using the other six system outputs as described later.

A cascade of systems is implemented to reduce the number of possible combinations that must be considered and to group similar metrics to determine an aggregate characteristic. Each of the 11 input metrics is described by two fuzzy terms (*small* and *large*), producing 2^{11} possible rules to consider. To reduce this number, similar metrics are combined to produce intermediate outputs. This grouping also helps to better relate the inputs to the high-level knowledge governing the shot boundary types. For example, the histogram metrics are examined together to produce a crisp output that determines the degree to which their combined characteristic is *small*, *medium*, or *large*. This is also done for the statistic-based, pixel-difference, and modulation inputs. A simpler system implementation could be achieved by selecting only one input from each class, and circumventing the first level systems, but better discrimination power is achieved with the larger number of inputs. The ratio inputs are examined jointly to determine how *close-to-1* they are. As a result, the following intermediate outputs are created:

- OI_h - indicates the combined magnitude of histogram metrics.
- OI_s - indicates the combined magnitude of statistic-based metrics.
- OI_p - indicates the magnitude of pixel-difference metrics.
- $OI_{\Delta+}$, $OI_{\Delta-}$ - indicates the magnitude and sign of modulation values.
- OI_r - indicates whether ratios are *close-to-1*.

To illustrate how the input systems operate, consider the histogram case shown in Fig. 3. Here the inputs (χ^2 and *ks*) have two membership functions (*small* and *large*) and produce 3 outputs (*small*, *medium*, and *large*). Each row in the rule table is considered a series of AND ($\wedge$) operations. The first row is interpreted as the following rule: `IF` [*ks* is *small*] $\wedge$ [χ^2 is *small*] `THEN` [output (OI_h) is *small*]. A crisp output is computed using a centroid defuzzifier [13] and the output membership functions defined in Fig. 3. The five other fuzzy input systems operate analogously.

The intermediate outputs fall in the range [0,1] and are used as inputs to the second stage or output systems. Therefore, input membership functions are required for the $OI_\bullet$, which are defined in Fig. 4. The two membership functions defined are *small* and *large* since the objective is to determine the combined *small vs. large* characteristic for each group of metrics. A straight line relationship from 1 to 0 for *small* over the range, and vice versa for *large*, was selected.

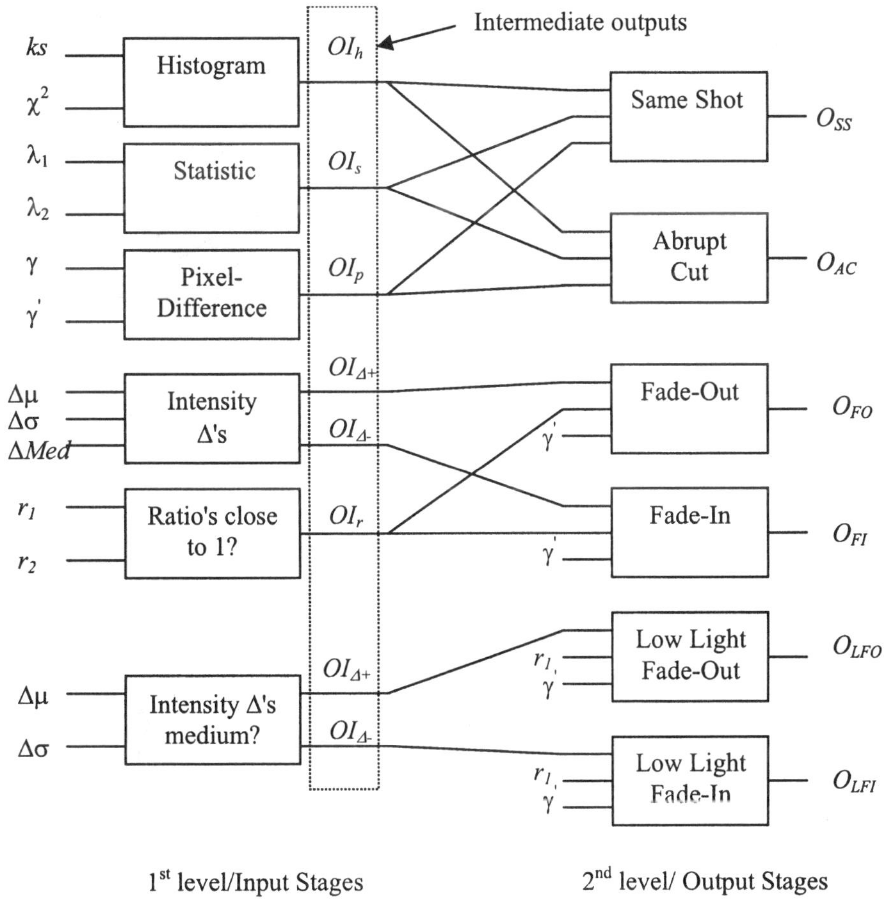

Fig. 2. System overview

Rules

ks	χ^2	OI_h
small	*small*	*small*
small	*large*	*medium*
large	*small*	*medium*
large	*large*	*large*

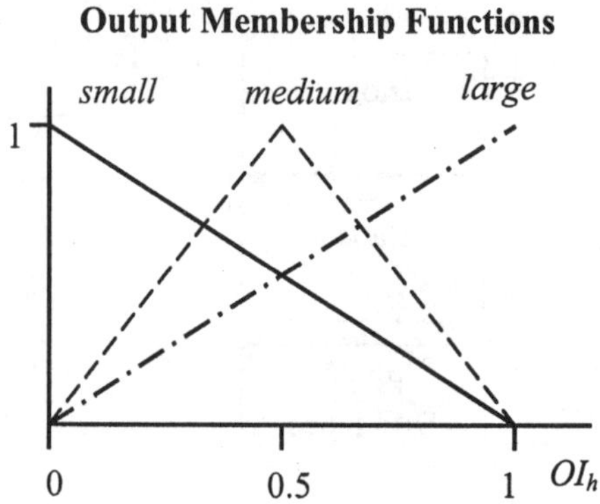

Fig. 3. Rules and output membership functions for centroid defuzzifier

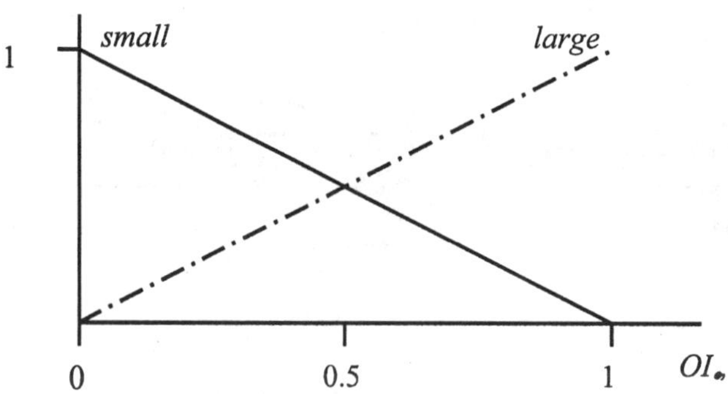

Fig. 4. Membership functions for 2nd stage inputs

Each of the 2nd stage output systems in Fig. 2 has 3 inputs, where each input has a characteristic of either *small* or *large* producing 8 total possibilities to consider for each. They operate in a manner similar to the previously defined first stage (input) systems. For example, consider the abrupt cut decision system shown in Fig. 5. The 8 possibilities are given in the rule table. Again, each rule in the table is interpreted as a series of AND operations. For example, The last line in the table is interpreted as: `IF` [OI_h is *large*] $\wedge$ [OI_s is *large*] $\wedge$ [OI_p is *large*] `THEN` [image pair is an abrupt cut]. This represents the characteristics of abrupt cuts developed earlier which indicated that an image pair is an abrupt cut if the histogram, pixel-difference, and statistic difference are simultaneously *large*. The output membership functions are given in Fig. 5 which are used by the centroid defuzzifier to produce a crisp output.

Rules

OI_h	OI_s	OI_p	O_{AC}
small	*small*	*small*	*same*
small	*small*	*large*	*likely-same*
small	*large*	*small*	*likely-same*
small	*large*	*large*	*likely-abrupt*
large	*small*	*small*	*likely-same*
large	*small*	*large*	*likely-abrupt*
large	*large*	*small*	*likely-abrupt*
large	*large*	*large*	*abrupt*

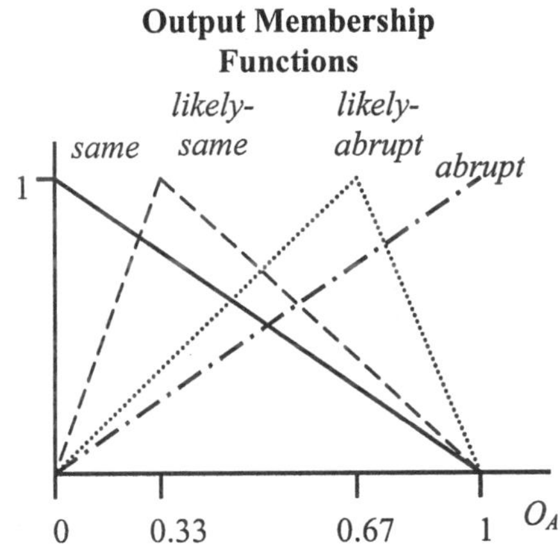

Fig. 5. Rules and output membership functions for abrupt cut output system

The remaining output systems operate analogously. For completeness, the rules (corresponding to the last row of the rule table in Fig. 5) for each output system are defined as follows (they follow the characteristics summarized in Table 1):

Same Shot: `IF` [OI_h is *small*] $\wedge$ [OI_s is *small*] $\wedge$ [OI_p is *small*] `THEN` [image pair is from same shot].
Justification: If two frames are from the same shot all metric values (histogram, pixel-difference, and statistic-based) should be *small*.

Fade Out: `IF` [$OI_{\Delta+}$ is *large*] $\wedge$ [OI_r is *large*] $\wedge$ [γ' is *small*] `THEN` [image pair is a fade-out] .
Justification: The fade models indicate that μ, σ, and *Med* decrease, therefore producing *large-positive* modulations. If the fade follows either mathematical fade model, r_1 and/or r_2 is *close-to-1*. γ' is *small* during a fade under the assumption that the structure of the shot remains *fairly constant.*

Fade-in: Same as fade out, except $OI_{\Delta-}$ must be *large.*

Low Light Fade-Out: `IF` [Δ_μ, and Δ_σ are *medium-large-positive*] $\wedge$ [r_1 is *close-to-1*] $\wedge$ [γ' is *small*] `THEN` [image pair is a low light fade-out].
Justification: In this fade μ and σ decrease and produce a *medium-large* positive modulation, while the medians are equal (Δ_{Med} =0). If the fade follows the mathematical fade model, r_1 is *close-to-1*. γ' is *small* during a fade under the assumption that the structure of the shot remains fairly constant.

Low Light Fade-in: Same as low light fade out, except Δ_μ, and Δ_σ must be negative.

Every pair of sequential frames in a video is compared, the six system outputs computed, and each pair labeled according to the highest output value. After this is complete, each resulting fade sequence is examined to ensure its length (*N*) is not too short or long in terms of number of frames.

4.3 Dissolve Detection

Dissolves are difficult to detect due to their gradual nature. Many metrics exhibit a slight sustained increase during dissolves, forming the basis of the twin comparison approach [24], but this increase is often difficult to detect. However, it is expected that the statistics (μ, σ, and *Med*) will slowly change (migrate) from their values in the start frame of the transition to their ending values, and therefore Γ is utilized to detect the start and end points of dissolves. This is generally superior to detection by a single metric as shown in the example in Fig. 6, where Γ and χ^2 are plotted for a dissolve sequence. The values (normalized) show that Γ has a stronger and more sustained response.

The leading and trailing edges of transitions in the Γ sequence are detected by applying a second-derivative-of-Gaussian edge detector. Leading and trailing edges are paired to represent *potential* or candidate dissolves. In order to constitute a potential start and end, there cannot be a shot boundary detected between the start and end points. Furthermore, the start and end frames are compared using the FLS and must be identified as an abrupt cut (meaning from different shots).

The potential dissolve sequences (start and end pairs) are then analyzed by the FLS to determine if they truly are dissolves. A synthesized dissolve sequence is created from the potential start and end frames using the dissolve model of (7) as

$$I_{synth}(x,y;l) = \left(1 - \frac{l}{end - start}\right) \times I(x,y;start) + \frac{l}{end - start} \times I(x,y;end)\,. \tag{16}$$

The synthesized images are then compared to the true sequence using the FLS. If the FLS determines that the synthesized and true images are from the same shot, the sequence is labeled as a dissolve.

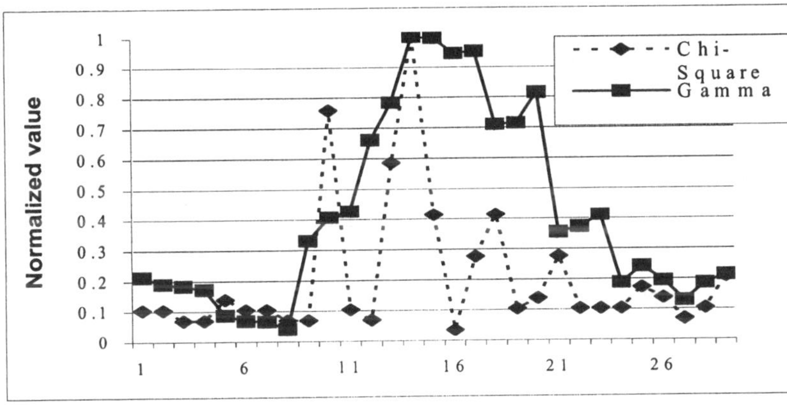

Fig. 6. Γ and χ^2 for a dissolve sequence. The dissolve begins at the 9th sample and ends at the 25th.

5 Results

The system was tested on a video database containing a total of 41,312 frames. The video clips were drawn mainly from the Internet, and included MPEG, QuickTime, AVI, and SGI movie formats and were decompressed prior to processing. The videos were categorized as one of the following: action, animation, comedy, commercial, drama, news, and sports. The categorized videos are listed in Appendix A. It is important to realize that this is one of the largest reported databases that have been reported for testing shot boundary techniques. Furthermore, the characteristics are challenging; many movie trailer videos were used which have a large number of shot boundaries relative to the length of the video, fast motion sequences, and special effects. Many of the trailers were also of fairly low-resolution (120x80). The frames were digitized at rates varying from 5 to 30 frames per second, and a range of image dimensions were used.

Two standard measures were used to quantify system performance

$$\text{recall} = \frac{\#\,\text{detected}}{\#\,\text{detected} + \#\,\text{missed}} \tag{18}$$

and

$$\text{precision} = \frac{\#\,\text{detected}}{\#\,\text{detected} + \#\,\text{false positives}}\,. \tag{19}$$

The results are summarized in Table 2 for the entire database. Caution is urged in comparing the rates to other published values. There is no standard database available at this time for comparing shot boundary detection techniques. A challenging dataset was purposely selected with many movie trailers that have fast motion sequences, explosions, credit fades, and special effects. More impressive numbers could have been achieved with a simpler database. To provide a quantitative perspective for these results, a single metric thresholding technique was applied to detect boundaries on the same database. A total of 16 different individual metrics were tested and it was found that the best rate that could be achieved on this database was a recall of 90% at a precision of 55%. Relative to the thresholding technique, the proposed FLS provides a significant performance improvement (90% recall with 84% precision). In addition, the fuzzy system correctly classified 93% of shot boundaries detected.

Table 2. Recall and precision rates for the FLS applied to the entire database

Shot boundary	# Boundaries in database	Recall (%)	Precision (%)
Abrupt Cut	1658	91.3	84.7
Fade-In	55	94.5	80.0
Fade-Out	95	91.6	93.5
Dissolve	127	73.2	71.5
Overall	1940	90.1	84.4

For abrupt cuts, the most common cause of errors is bright flashes of light due to phenomena such as explosions and fast action sequences. These problems sometimes manifest themselves as a series of abrupt cuts which are filtered out. The detection rates for fades are good, but fades of movie credits are the most difficult to detect because they have very small luminance changes, and attempts to detect them cause false positives. The integration of edge-based metrics could improve this performance, although at increased computation expense. Dissolve false alarms are most likely to be caused by fast action sequences. They are most commonly missed because their effects are too subtle to be detected. Most classification errors are caused when gradual transitions are labeled as abrupt cuts. For instance, this often occurs during fades when a black image appears or disappears.

The main objective of this work was to develop a fuzzy logic technique that performs well for shot boundary detection and classification. Therefore, a straightforward and practical procedure for fuzzy system implementation [12] was selected. Performance improvements can likely be made by developing an optimized fuzzy system and increasing the number of inputs to the system.

6 Conclusions

A fuzzy logic system for the detection and classification of shot boundaries in uncompressed video sequences was presented. This represents an effective method for shot boundary detection and classification. Use of a fuzzy logic system is advantageous since it allows straightforward system modification and is extensible to include new data sources without retraining. It integrates multiple information sources and knowledge of editing procedures to detect and classify shot boundaries into one of the following categories: abrupt cut, fade-in, fade-out, or dissolve.

It was developed based on models of video editing techniques. For the database tested, it achieved an overall recall rate of 90.1%, a precision rate of 84.4%, and correctly classified 93% of the boundaries detected. This significantly exceeded the performance of single metric, threshold-based approaches.

References

1. Arman F, Hsu A, Lee MY (1993) Image processing on compressed data for large video databases. In: Proceedings ACM International Conference on Multimedia, pp 267-272
2. Boreczky JS, Rowe LA (1996) Comparison of Shot Boundary Techniques. J of Electronic Imaging 5: 122-128
3. Davenport G, Smith TA, Pincever N (1991) Cinematic primitives for multimedia. IEEE Computer Graphics and Applications, 67-74
4. Ford RM (1998) A Fuzzy Logic Approach to Digital Video Segmentation. In: SPIE Proceedings on Storage and Retrieval in Image and Video Databases VII, pp 360-370
5. Ford RM, Robson C, Temple D, Gerlach M (2000) Metrics for shot boundary detection in digital video sequences. ACM Multimedia Systems Journal 8: 37-46
6. Gargi U, Oswald S, Kosiba D, Devadiga S, Kasturi R (1995) Evaluation of video sequence indexing and hierarchical video indexing. In: SPIE Proceedings on Storage and Retrieval in Image and Video Databases III, pp 144-151
7. Gargi U, Kasturi R, Strayer SH (2000) Performance characterization of video-shot-change detection methods. IEEE Transactions on Circuits and Systems for Video Technology, 10: 1-13
8. Hampapur A, Jain R, Weymouth TE (1995) Production model based digital video segmentation. Multimedia Tools and Applications, 1: 9-46
9. Heng WJ, Ngan KN (2002) Shot boundary refinement for long transition in digital video sequence. IEEE Transactions on Multimedia, 4: 434-445.
10. Jadon RS, Chaudury S, Biswas KK (2001) A fuzzy theoretic approach for video segmentation using syntactic features. Pattern Recognition Letters, 22: 1359-1369
11. Jain R, Kasturi R, Schunck BG (1995) Machine vision, McGraw Hill, New York
12. McNeill FM, Thro E (1994) Fuzzy logic: a practical approach, Academic Press, Boston
13. Mendel JM (1995) Fuzzy logic systems for engineering: a tutorial. IEEE Proceedings 83: 345-377
14. Nakajima Y, Uijhari K, Yoneyama A (1997) Universal scene change detection on MPEG-coded data domain. In: Visual Communications and Image Processing, Proc. SPIE 3024, pp 992-1003
15. Nagasaka A, Tanaka Y (1992) Automatic video indexing and full-video

search for object appearances. In: Visual Database Systems II, pp 113-127

16. Press WH, Flannery BP, Teukolsky SA, Vetterling WT (1993) Numerical recipes: the art of scientific computing, 2nd edn. Cambridge University Press, New York
17. Sethi IK, Patel N (1995) A statistical approach to scene change detection. In: SPIE Proceedings on Storage and Retrieval for Image and Video Databases III, pp 329-338
18. Swain MJ, Ballard DH (1991) Color indexing. International Journal of Computer Vision 7: 11-32
19. Takagi T, Sugeno M (1985) Fuzzy identification and its applications to modeling and control. IEEE Transactions on Systems, Man, and Cybernetics 15: 116-132
20. Tan YP, Nagamani J, Lu H (2003) Modified Kolmogorov-Smirnov metric for shot boundary detection. IEE Electronics Letters, 39: 1313-1315
21. Van Trees HL (1982) Detection estimation and modulation theory: part I, Wiley and Sons, New York
22. Yeo BL, Liu B (1995) Rapid scene analysis on compressed video. IEEE Transactions on Circuits and Systems for Video Technology 5: 533-544
23. Zabih R, Miller J, Mai K (1999) A feature-based algorithm for detecting and classifying scene breaks. ACM Journal Multimedia Systems Journal 7: 119-128
24. Zhang HJ, Kankanhalli A, Smoliar SW (1993) Automatic partitioning of full-motion video. ACM Multimedia Systems Journal, 1:10-28

Appendix – Video Database

Video Description	Frames	Shot Boundaries	Type
Airwolf	70	1	Action
Barbwire movie trailer	726	175	Action
Blade Runner	1112	21	Action
Dune movie	296	22	Action
Eraser movie trailer	997	115	Action
Independence Day movie trailer	2492	97	Action
Star Trek movie	1507	40	Action
Star Wars movie	602	23	Action
Star Wars movie trailer	318	29	Action
Terminator	564	4	Action
Anastasia movie trailer	1044	101	Animation
Comet Animation	524	0	Animation
Lion King movie	1390	22	Animation
Space animations	338	0	Animation
Space probe flight	1491	9	Animation
Star Wars animation	424	7	Animation
Terminator animation	331	0	Animation

Winnie the Pooh	1206	12	Animation
Friends sitcom	571	10	Comedy
Ghostbusters movie	147	5	Comedy
Mighty Aphrodite movie trailer	1841	38	Comedy
Rockey Horror movie	407	6	Comedy
Spacejam movie trailer	1079	157	Comedy
Apple "1984"	722	27	Commercial
Cartoon ad	95	3	Commercial
Rice Krispies	81	5	Commercial
A Few Good Men Movie	865	12	Drama
Alaska movie trailer	777	60	Drama
American President movie trailer	1375	58	Drama
Bed Time for Bonzo	436	15	Drama
Chung King movie trailer	1225	72	Drama
Close Encounters movie	566	9	Drama
Crossinguard move trailer	3038	110	Drama
Crow movie trailer	1560	122	Drama
First Knight movie trailer	271	15	Drama
Jamaica	115	2	Drama
My Left Foot movie trailer	449	14	Drama
Slingblade movie trailer	1704	101	Drama
Titanic movie	1067	14	Drama
Titanic movie trailer	1210	173	Drama
Truman movie trailer	166	8	Drama
Xfiles trailer	429	20	Drama
CNN news	169	7	News
Plane crash newsclip	96	0	News
Reuters newsclips	1126	11	News
Ron Brown's funeral	631	24	News
San Jose news	1377	6	News
Singer news clip	350	0	News
Space shuttle disaster	1411	13	News
Space shuttle Endeavor astronauts	1190	2	News
Space station Mir	588	5	News
Sunrise/sunset	286	2	News
Weather satellite clips	308	0	News
White House footage	131	5	News
Basketball	487	6	Sports
Hockey	205	11	Sports
Rodeo	146	3	Sports
Skateboarding	298	6	Sports
Sky surfing	74	0	Sports
Soccer	87	0	Sports

Rate-Distortion Optimal Video Summarization and Coding

[1,2]Zhu Li, [1]Aggelos K. Katsaggelos, and [3]Guido M. Schuster

[1]Department of Electrical & Computer Engineering, Northwestern University, Evanston, Illinois, USA
[2]Multimedia Communication Research Lab (MCRL), Motorola Labs, Schaumburg, Illinois, USA
[3]Hochschule fur Technik Rapperswil (HSR), Switzerland

Abstract. The demand for video summarization originates from a viewing time constraint as well as bit budget constraint from communication and storage limitations, in security, military, and entertainment applications. In this chapter we formulate and solve the video summarization problems as rate-distortion optimization problems. Effective new summarization distortion metric is developed. Several optimal algorithms are presented along with some effective heuristic solutions.

Keywords: Rate-distortion optimization, Lagrangian relaxation, video summarization, video coding.

1 Introduction

The demand for video summarization originates from a viewing time constraint as well as communication and storage limitations, in security, military, and entertainment applications. For example, in an entertainment application, a user may want to browse summaries of his/her personal video taken during several trips. In a security application, a supervisor may want to see a 2 minutes summary of what happened at airport gate B20, in the last 10 minutes. In a military situation, a soldier may need to communicate tactical information with video over a bandwidth-limited wireless channel, with a battery-energy-limited transmitter. Instead of sending all frames with severe frame SNR distortion, a better option is to transmit a subset of the frames with higher SNR quality. A video summary generator that can "optimally" select frames based on an optimality criterion is essential for these applications.

The solution to this problem is typically based on a two-step approach: first identifying video shots from the video sequence [13, 17, 21, 23], and then selecting "key frames" according to some criterion from each video shot. A comprehensive review of past video summarization results can be found in the introduction sections of [12, 36], and specific examples can be found in [4, 5, 9, 10, 13, 33, 37].

The approaches mentioned above are taking a vision-based approach, trying to establish certain semantic interpretation of the video sequence from visual features like color, motion and texture, and then generate summaries from this semantic interpretation. In general, such approaches require multiple passes of processing on the video sequence and are rather computationally involved. The resulting video summaries do not have smooth distortion degradation within a video shot and the performance metrics are heuristic in nature.

Since a video summary inevitably introduces distortion at the play back time and the amount of distortion is related to the "conciseness" of the summary, we formulate and solve this problem as a rate-distortion optimization problem. The optimality of the solution is established in the rate-distortion sense. The framework developed can accommodate various frame distortion metrics to reflect different user preferences in specific applications. The chapter is organized as follows: In section 2, we introduce the classical and operational rate-distortion theory and the rate-distortion optimization tools. In section 3, we give the rate-distortion formulation of the video summarization problem. In section 4, we present the algorithms that solve the various formulations of the summarization problem. In section 5, we present the simulation results and draw conclusions.

2 Rate-Distortion Optimization

The problem of coding a source with certain distortion measure can be formulated as a constrained optimization problem, i.e, coding the source with minimum distortion with certain coding rate (limited coding resource), or its dual problem of coding the source with minimum rate while satisfying certain distortion constraint. The study on the function that characterizes the relation between the rate and distortion is well established in information theory [1, 3]. In the following, we will give a brief introduction to the classical rate-distortion theory and then a more detailed discussion on the *operational* rate-distortion theory and optimization tools that are the bases of the formulation and solution to the summarization problem.

2.1 The Classical Rate-Distortion Theory

The minimum number of bits needed to encode a discrete random source X with n symbols is given by its entropy $H(X)$, given by

$$H(X) = -\sum_{j=1}^{n} \log(P(x_j)) \tag{1}$$

However the number of bits needed to encode a continuous source is infinite. In practice, to code a continuous source, the source must be quantized into discrete form $\hat{X}$, because the available bits are limited. Obviously, the quantization process introduces distortion between X and $\hat{X}$, which is described by a scalar function $d(X,\hat{X}): X \times \hat{X} \to R^+$. A typical distortion measure between symbols is the squared error function

$$d(x,\hat{x}) = (x-\hat{x})^2 \tag{2}$$

The rate-distortion (R-D) function is defined as the minimum mutual information between the source X and the reconstruction $\hat{X}$, for a given expected distortion constraint measure

$$R(D) = \min_{p(\hat{x}|x)} I(X;\hat{X}),\ s.t.\ \sum_{(x,\hat{x})\in X\times\hat{X}} p(x)p(\hat{x}\mid x)d(x,\hat{x}) \le D \tag{3}$$

The R-D function in (3) does not have closed form in most cases, but for the Gaussian source with distribution $X \sim N(0,\sigma^2)$, and squared distortion measure (2), the rate-distortion function is given by

$$R(D) = \begin{cases} (1/2)\log(\sigma^2/D), & 0 \le D \le \sigma^2 \\ 0, & D \ge \sigma^2 \end{cases} \tag{4}$$

Notice that this R-D function is convex and non-increasing. The R-D function establishes the lower bound on the achievable coding rate for a given expected distortion constraint.

2.2 The Operational Rate-Distortion Theory

The R-D function establishes the best theoretical performance bound in rate-distortion terms for any quantization-coding scheme. However it does not provide practical coding solutions to achieve the bound. In real applications like video sequence coding and shape coding, the number of combinations of quantization and coding schemes available to a source coder is limited. For each feasible quantization and coding solution, Q_j, called an "operating point", there is a rate-distortion pair $[R(Q_j), D(Q_j)]$ associated with it. The operational rate-distortion (ORD) function is defined as the minimum achievable rate for a given distortion threshold among all operating points, that is

$$R_{op}(D) = \min_{Q_j} R(Q_j),\ s.t.\ D(Q_j) \le D \tag{5}$$

The ORD is a non-increasing stair case function and the operating points associated with it are shown in an example plot in Fig. 1. Not all ORD operating points reside on the convex hull of the ORD function. This will have implication in optimization problem in later sections. All operating points are lower bounded by the convex hull of the ORD function, while the convex hull is also lower bounded by the RD function.

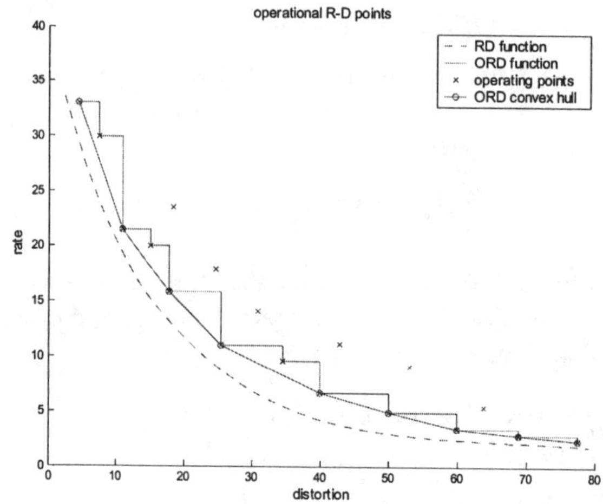

Fig. 1. Operational Rate-Distortion function and operating points

Hopefully, a good coding scheme will have most of its operating points close to the RD curve. Therefore, the rate-distortion optimal coding problem is to find the optimal operating point that will achieve minimum distortion for a given rate in the rate constrained case, or for a given distortion threshold, find the optimal operating point that will have the minimum rate in the distortion constrained case. Good references to research work in this area can be found in [27, 30, 32]. In the next sub-section, we will discuss mathematical tools, Dynamic Programming and Lagrangian Multiplier method that are essential for the task of finding the optimal operating point efficiently.

2.3 Rate-Distortion Optimization Tools

Dynamic Programming

Dynamic Programming (DP) is a powerful tool in solving optimization problems. A good reference for DP can be found in [2]. A well-known deterministic DP solution is the Viterbi algorithm [35] in communication engineering, while probably the most famous stochastic DP example is the Kalman filter in control engineering. In particular we are interested in the deterministic DP. If an optimization problem can be decomposed into sub-problems with a past, a current and a future state, and for the given current state, the future problem solution does not depend on the past problem solution, then DP can find the globally optimal solution efficiently. For the optimal video summarization/coding problem, we will employ the DP approach extensively.

In general, the quantization-coding process of the video summarization / coding problem comprises of multiple dependent decision stages $Q=[q_0, q_1, \ldots q_{m-1}]$. The optimal solution, or the optimal operating point can be expressed as

$$Q^* = \arg \min_{q_0, q_1, \cdots, q_{m-1}} J(q_0, q_1, \cdots, q_{m-1}) \tag{6}$$

in which J is the functional reflecting the goal of rate minimization under distortion constraint, or the distortion minimization under rate constraint. An exhaustive search on all feasible decisions can solve the problem in (6), but clearly, this is not an efficient solution and can be un-practical when the problem size is large. Fortunately for a large set of practical problems, the objective functional in (6) can be expressed as the summation of objective functionals for a set of dependent sub-problems J_k, as

$$J(q_0, q_1, \cdots, q_{m-1}) = \sum_{k=0}^{m-1} J_k(q_{k-a}, \cdots, q_{k+b}) \tag{7}$$

where a and b are the maximum numbers of decisions before and after decision q_k that the sub-problem J_k will depend on. Let J_t^* be the optimal solution to the summation of the sub-problem functionals up to and including the neighborhood of sub-problem t, that is

$$J_t^*(q_{t-a+1}, \cdots, q_{t+b}) = \min_{q_0, q_1, \cdots, q_{t-a}} \sum_{k=0}^{t} J_k(q_{k-a}, \cdots, q_{k+b}) \tag{8}$$

For $t+1$, from (8) we have

$$\begin{aligned} J_{t+1}^*(q_{t+1-a+1}, \cdots, q_{t+1+b}) &= \min_{q_0, q_1, \cdots, q_{t+1-a}} \sum_{k=0}^{t+1} J_k(q_{k-a}, \cdots, q_{k+b}) \\ &= \min_{q_{t+1-a}} \{ \min_{q_0, q_1, \cdots, q_{t-a}} \sum_{k=0}^{t} J_k(q_{k-a}, \cdots, q_{k+b}) + J_{t+1}(q_{t+1-a+1}, \cdots, q_{t+1+b}) \} \\ &= \min_{q_{t+1-a}} \{ J_t^*(q_{k-a}, \cdots, q_{k+b}) + J_{t+1}(q_{t+1-a+1}, \cdots, q_{t+1+b}) \} \end{aligned} \tag{9}$$

The minimization process can be split into two parts in (9) because the sub-problem objective functional $J_{t+1}(q_{t+1-a}, \cdots, q_{t+1+b})$ does not have dependency on decision processes $q_0, q_1, \ldots q_{t-a}$. The recursion established in (9) can be used to compute the optimal solution to the original problem as J_{m-1}^*. With (9) we can use DP to solve the original problem recursively and backtrack for the optimal decision. The process starts with the initial solution at J_0, and at each recursion stage, the optimal decision q_{t+1-a} is stored. When the final stage of the recursion J_{m-1}^* is reached, the backtracking process can select the optimal solution from the stored optimal decisions at previous stages.

Lagrangian Multiplier Method

Some optimization problems are like those in (9) and are "hard" to solve with DP. This is because the constraints cannot be decomposed to establish the recursion, then the Lagrangian multiplier method will be employed to relax the problem into an "easier" un-constrained problem for the DP formulation.

Lagrangian multiplier method is well-known in solving the constrained optimization problem in a continuous setting [8, 24]. For the discrete optimization problem, Lagrangian multiplier can also be used to relax the original constrained problem into an easier un-constrained problem, which can be solved efficiently, by DP for example. Then the optimal solution to the original problem is found by iteratively searching for the Lagrangian multiplier that achieves the tightest bound on the constraint [7].

In general, let the constrained optimization problem be

$$\min_{Q} D(Q),\ s.t.\, R(Q) \le R_{\max} \tag{10}$$

where Q is the decision vector, $D(Q)$ is the distortion objective functional we want to minimize and $R(Q)$ is the inequality constraint that the decision vector Q must satisfy. Instead of solving (10) directly, we relax the problem with a non-negative Lagrangian multiplier λ and try to minimize the Lagrangian functional

$$\min_{Q} J_{\lambda}(Q) = D(Q) + \lambda R(Q) \tag{11}$$

Clearly, as λ changes from zero to ∞, the un-constrained problem puts more and more emphasis on the minimization of rate $R(Q)$. For a given λ, let the optimal solution to the un-constrained problem be $Q_{\lambda}^{*} = \arg\min_{Q} J_{\lambda}(Q)$, and the resulting distortion and rate be $D(Q_{\lambda}^{*})$ and $R(Q_{\lambda}^{*})$ respectively. Notice that $R(Q_{\lambda}^{*})$ is a non-increasing function of λ while $D(Q_{\lambda}^{*})$ is a non-decreasing function of λ. The proof can be found in [30]. Also, for two multipliers $\lambda_1 < \lambda_2$, and the respective optimal solutions of the un-constrained problem, $Q_{\lambda_1}^{*}$ and $Q_{\lambda_2}^{*}$, the slope of the line between two operating points $Q_{\lambda_1}^{*}$ and $Q_{\lambda_2}^{*}$ is bounded between multipliers λ_1 and λ_2 as

$$\frac{-1}{\lambda_2} \ge \frac{R(Q_{\lambda_1}^{*}) - R(Q_{\lambda_2}^{*})}{D(Q_{\lambda_1}^{*}) - D(Q_{\lambda_2}^{*})} \ge \frac{-1}{\lambda_1} \tag{12}$$

It is known from [7, 29] that if there exists a λ^{*} such that $R(Q_{\lambda^{*}}^{*}) = R_{max}$, then $Q_{\lambda^{*}}^{*}$ is also the optimal solution to the original constrained problem in (10). In practical applications, if we can solve the un-constrained problem in (11) efficiently, the solution to the original problem in (10) can be found by searching for the optimal multiplier λ^{*} that results in the tightest bound to the rate constraint. The process can be viewed as finding the appropriate trade off between the distortion objective and rate constraint. Since $R(Q^*_\lambda)$ is a non-increasing function of λ, a bi-section search algorithm can be used to find λ^*.

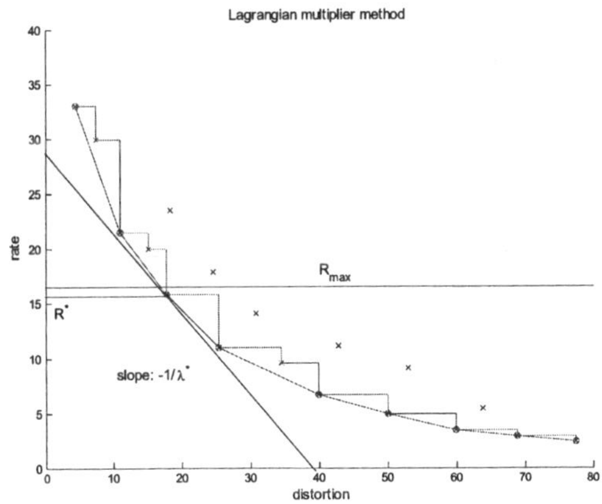

Fig. 2. Geometric interpretation of the Lagrangian multiplier method.

A geometric interpretation of the searching process can be found in [25]. As λ varies, the operating points on the convex hull of the ORD function are traced out by wave of lines with slope $-1/\lambda$. Since operating points set is discrete, after finite iterations, λ^* is found as the line that intercepts the convex hull and results in the rate $|R(Q^*_{\lambda^*}) - R_{\max}| \leq \varepsilon$, for some pre-determined ε. An example is shown in Fig. 2. The line with slope $-1/\lambda^*$ intercepts the optimal operating point on the convex hull of the ORD curve and results in rate R^*, which is the closest to the rate constraint R_{max}.

3 The problem formulation

With the operational rate-distortion theory and the numerical optimization tools introduced in the previous sections, we formulate and solve the video summarization problem as a rate-distortion optimization problem. A video summary is a shorter version of the original video sequence. Video summary frames are selected from the original video sequence and form a subset of it. The reconstructed video sequence is generated from the video summary by substituting the missing frames by the previous frames in the summary (zero-order hold). Clearly if we can afford more frames in the video summary, the distortion introduced by the missing frames will be less severe. On the other hand, more frames in the summary take longer time to view, require more bandwidth to communicate and more memory to store them. To express this trade off between the quality of the reconstructed sequences and the number of frames in the summary, we introduce next certain definitions and assumptions for our formulations.

3.1 Definitions and Assumptions

Let a video sequence of n frames be denoted by $V = \{f_0, f_1, ..., f_{n-1}\}$. Let its video summary of m frames be $S = \{f_{l_0}, f_{l_1}, \cdots f_{l_{m-1}}\}$, in which l_k denotes the k-th frame selected into the summary S. The summary S is completely determined by the frame selection process $L=\{l_0, l_1, ..., l_{m-1}\}$, which has an implicit constraint that $l_0 < l_1 < ... < l_{m-1}$.

The reconstructed sequence $V_S' = \{f_0', f_1', \cdots f_{n-1}'\}$ from the summary S is obtained by substituting missing frames with the most recent frame that belongs to the summary S, that is

$$f_k' = f_{i=\max(l):\ s.t.\ l \in \{l_0, l_1, \cdots, l_{m-1}\},\ i \le k} \qquad (13)$$

Let the distortion between two frames j and k be denoted by $d(f_j, f_k)$. We assume the distortion introduced by video coding is negligible under chosen quantization scheme, that is, if frame f_k is selected into S, then $d(f_k, f_k')=0$. Clearly there are various ways to define the frame distortion metric $d(f_j, f_k)$, and we will discuss this topic in more detail in section 4.6. However, the optimal solutions developed in this work are independent from the definition of this frame metric.

To characterize the sequence level summarization distortion, we can use the *average* frame distortion between the original sequence and the reconstruction, given by

$$D(S) = \frac{1}{n}\sum_{k=0}^{n-1} d(f_k, f_k') \qquad (14)$$

Or similarly, we can also characterize the sequence summarization distortion as the *maximum* frame distortion as

$$D(S) = \max_{k \in [0, n-1]} d(f_k, f_k') \qquad (15)$$

The temporal rate of the summarization process is defined as the ratio of the number of frames selected into the video summary m, over the total number of frames, in the original sequence, n, that is

$$R(S) = \frac{m}{n} \qquad (16)$$

Notice that the temporal rate $R(S)$ is in range (0, 1]. In our formulation we also assume that the first frame of the sequence is always selected into the summary, *i.e.*, $l_0=1$. Thus the rate $R(S)$ can only take values from the discrete set $\{1/n, 2/n, ..., n/n\}$. For example, for the video sequence $V=\{f_0, f_1, f_2, f_3, f_4\}$ and its video summary $S=\{f_0, f_2\}$, the reconstructed sequence is given by $V_S'=\{f_0, f_0, f_2, f_2, f_2\}$, the temporal rate is equal to $R(S)=2/5=0.4$, and the average temporal distortion computed from (14) is equal to $D(S) = (1/5)[d(f_0,f_1) + d(f_2,f_3) + d(f_2,f_4)]$. Similarly the maximum temporal distortion is computed as max $\{d(f_0,f_1), d(f_2,f_3), d(f_2,f_4)\}$.

3.2 MDOS Formulation

Video summarization can be viewed as a lossy temporal compression process and a rate-distortion framework is well suited for solving this problem. Using the definitions introduced in the previous section, we now formulate the video summarization problem as a temporal rate-distortion optimization problem. If a temporal rate constraint R_{max} is given, resulting from viewing time, or bandwidth and storage considerations, the optimal video summary is the one that minimizes the sumarization distortion. Thus we have:

Formulation I: Minimum Distortion Optimal Summarization (MDOS):

$$S^* = \arg\min_S D(S),\ s.t.\ R(S) \le R_{\max} \tag{17}$$

where $R(S)$ is defined by (16) and $D(S)$ can be either the average frame distortion (14) or the maximum distortion as defined in (15). The optimization is over all possible video summary frame selections $\{l_0, l_1, \ldots, l_{m-1}\}$, that contain no more than $m=nR_{max}$ frames. We call this an $(n\text{-}m)$ summarization problem.

In addition to the rate constraint, we may also impose a constraint on the maximum number of frames, K_{max}, that can be skipped between successive frames in the summary S. Such a constraint imposes a form of temporal smoothness and can be a useful feature in various applications, such as surveillance. We call this the $(n\text{-}m\text{-}K_{max})$ summarization problem, and its MDOS formulation can be written as

$$S^* = \min_S D(S),\ s.t.\ R(S) \le R_{\max},\ \text{and}\ l_k - l_{k-1} \le K_{\max} + 1,\ \forall k \tag{18}$$

The MDOS formulation is useful in many applications where the view time is constrained. The MDOS summary will provide minimum distortion summaries under this constraint.

3.3 MROS Formulation

Alternatively we can formulate the optimal summarization problem as a rate-minimization problem. For a given constraint on the maximum distortion D_{max}, the optimal summary is the one that satisfies this distortion constraint and contains the minimum number of frames. Thus we have:

Formulation II: Minimum Rate Optimal Summarization (MROS):

$$S^* = \arg\min_S R(S),\ s.t.\ D(S) \le D_{\max} \tag{19}$$

The optimization is over all possible frame selections $\{l_0, l_1, \ldots, l_{m-1}\}$ and the summary length m. We may also impose a skip constraint K_{max} on the MROS formulation, as given by

$$S^* = \arg\min_S R(S),\ s.t.\ D(S) \le D_{\max},\ \text{and}\ l_k - l_{k-1} \le K_{\max} + 1,\ \forall k \tag{20}$$

Clearly in both MDOS and MROS formulations, we can also use either the average or the maximum frame distortion as our summarization distortion criterion, and will lead to different solutions.

4 Optimal Summarization Solutions

With the optimization tools developed in section 2 and the formulations in section 3, we solve the summarization problems as rate-distortion problems. Since we have two different summarization distortion metrics, let the MDOS formulations with average frame distortion and maximum frame distortion metric be denoted by MINAVG-MDOS and MINMAX-MDOS respectively, and the MROS formulations be MINAVG-MROS and MINMAX-MROS respectively. The solutions will be given in the following sub-sections.

4.1 Solution to the MINAVG-MDOS problem

For the MDOS formulation in (17), if there are n frames in the original sequence, and can only have m frames in the summary, there are $\binom{n-1}{m-1} = \frac{(n-1)!}{(m-1)!(n-m)!}$ feasible solutions, assuming the first frame is always in the summary. When n and m are large the computational cost in exhaustively evaluating all these solutions becomes prohibitive. Clearly we need to find a smarter solution. To have an intuitive understanding of the problem, we discuss a heuristic greedy algorithm first before presenting the optimal solution.

Greedy Algorithm

Let us first consider a rather intuitive greedy algorithm. For the given rate constraint of allowable frames m, the algorithm selects the first frame into the summary and computes the frame distortions. It then identifies the current maximum frame distortion index as $k^* = \max_k \{d(f_k, f_k')\}$ and selects frame f_{k^*} into the summary. The process is repeated until the number of frames in the summary reaches m. The resulting solution is sub-optimal. The frames selected into the summary tend to cluster around the high activity regions where the frame-by-frame distortion $d(f_k, f_{k-1})$ is high. The video summary generated is "choppy" when viewed. Clearly we need to better understand the structure of the problem and search for an optimal solution.

MINAVG Distortion State Definition and Recursion

Consider the MINAVG-MDOS problem, which is MDOS problem with summarization distortion as the average frame distortion (14). We observe that this MDOS problem has a certain built-in structure and can be solved in stages. For a given current state of the problem, future solutions are independent from past solution. Exploiting this structure, a Dynamic Programming (DP) solution [19] is developed next.

Let the distortion state D_t^k be the minimum total distortion incurred by a summary that has t frames and ended with frame f_k ($l_{t-1}=k$), that is

$$D_t^k = \min_{l_1,l_2,\cdots,l_{t-2}} \sum_{j=0}^{n-1} d(f_j, f_{i=\max(l):s.t.\ l\in\{0,l_1,l_2,\cdots,l_{t-2},k\},i\le j}) \tag{21}$$

Notice that $l_0=0$ and $l_{t-1}=k$, and they are therefore removed from the optimization. Since $0<l_1<\ldots<l_{t-2}<k$, and $i \le j$, (21) can be re-written as

$$D_t^k = \min_{l_1,l_2,\cdots,l_{t-2}} \{\sum_{j=0}^{k-1} d(f_j, f_{i=\max(l):s.t.\ l\in\{0,l_1,l_2,\cdots,l_{t-2}\},i\le j})\} + \sum_{j=k}^{n-1} d(f_j, f_k) \tag{22}$$

in which the second part of the distortion depends on the last summary frame f_k only, and it is removed from the minimization operation. By adding and subtracting the same term in (22) we have

$$\begin{aligned} D_t^k = \min_{l_1,l_2,\cdots,l_{t-2}} & \{\sum_{j=0}^{k-1} d(f_j, f_{i=\max(l):s.t.\ l\in\{0,l_1,l_2,\cdots,l_{t-2}\},i\le j}) \\ & + \sum_{j=k}^{n-1} d(f_j, f_{i=\max(l):s.t.\ l\in\{0,l_1,l_2,\cdots,l_{t-2}\},i\le j}) - \\ & \sum_{j=k}^{n-1} d(f_j, f_{i=\max(l):s.t.\ l\in\{0,l_1,l_2,\cdots,l_{t-2}\},i\le j})\} \\ & + \sum_{j=k}^{n-1} d(f_j, f_k) \end{aligned} \tag{23}$$

We now observe that since $l_{t-2} < k$, we have

$$\sum_{j=k}^{n-1} d(f_j, f_{i=\max(l):s.t.\ l\in\{0,l_1,l_2,\cdots,l_{t-2}\},i\le j}) = \sum_{j=k}^{n-1} d(f_j, f_{l_{t-2}}) \tag{24}$$

Therefore the distortion state can be broken into two parts as

$$D_t^k = \min_{l_1,l_2,\cdots,l_{t-2}} \{\sum_{j=0}^{k-1} d(f_j, f_{i=\max(l):s.t.\ l\in\{0,l_1,l_2,\cdots,l_{t-2}\},i\le j}) +$$
$$\sum_{j=k}^{n-1} d(f_j, f_{i=\max(l):s.t.\ l\in\{0,l_1,l_2,\cdots,l_{t-2}\},i\le j}) - \sum_{j=k}^{n-1} d(f_j, f_{l_{t-2}})$$
$$+\sum_{j=k}^{n-1} d(f_j, f_k)\} \tag{25}$$
$$= \min_{l_1,l_2,\cdots,l_{t-2}} \{\sum_{j=0}^{n-1} d(f_j, f_{i=\max(l):s.t.\ l\in\{0,l_1,l_2,\cdots,l_{t-2}\},i\le j})$$
$$-\underbrace{\sum_{j=k}^{n-1}[d(f_j, f_{l_{t-2}}) - d(f_j, f_k)]}_{e^{l_{t-2},k}}\},$$

where the first part represents the problem of minimizing the distortion for the summaries with *t-1* frames and ending with frame l_{t-2}, and the second part represents the "edge cost" of the distortion reduction, if frame *k* is selected into the summary of *t-1* frames ending with frame l_{t-2}. Therefore we have

$$D_t^{l_{t-1}=k} = \min_{l_{t-2}}\{ \min_{l_1,l_2,\cdots,l_{t-3}} \{\sum_{j=0}^{n-1} d(f_j, f_{i=\max(l):s.t.\ l\in\{0,l_1,l_2,\cdots,l_{t-2}\},i\le j})\}$$
$$- e^{l_{t-2},k}\} \tag{26}$$
$$= \min_{l_{t-2}}\{D_{t-1}^{l_{t-2}} - e^{l_{t-2},k}\}$$

The relation in (26) establishes the distortion state recursion we need for a DP solution. The back pointer saves the optimal incoming node information from the previous stage. For state D_t^k, it is saved as

$$P_t^k = \begin{cases} 0, & t=2 \\ \arg\min_{l_{t-2}}\{D_{t-1}^{l_{t-2}} - e^{l_{t-2},k}\}, & t>2 \end{cases} \tag{27}$$

Since we assume that the first (0-th) frame is always selected into the summary, P_2^k is set to 0, and the initial state D_1^0 is given as

$$D_1^0 = \frac{1}{n}\sum_{j=1}^{n-1} d(f_0, f_j) \tag{28}$$

Now we can compute the minimum distortion D_t^k for any video summary of *t* frames and ending with frame *k* by the recursion in (26) with the initial state given by (28). This leads to the optimal DP solution of the MDOS problem.

Dynamic Programming Solution for the n-m Summarization Problem

Considering the *n-m* summarization problem case where the rate constraint is given as exactly *m* frames allowed for the summary out of *n* frames in the original sequence, the optimal solution has the minimum distortion of

$$D^* = \min_k \{D_m^k\}, \tag{29}$$

where *k* is chosen from all feasible frames for the *m*-th summary frame. The optimal summary frame selection $\{l_0, l_1, \ldots, l_{m-1}\}$ is therefore found by backtracking via the back pointers $\{P_t^k\}$

$$\begin{Bmatrix} l_{m-1} = \arg\min_k \{D_m^k\} \\ l_t = P_{t+2}^{l_{t+1}}, \text{ for } t \in [1, m-2] \\ l_0 = 1. \end{Bmatrix} \tag{30}$$

As an illustrative example, the distortion state trellis for $n=5$ and $m=3$ is shown in Fig. 3. Each node represents a distortion state D_t^k, and each edge $e^{j,k}$ represents the distortion reduction if frame f_k is selected into the summary which ends with frame f_j. Note that the trellis topology is completely determined by *n* and *m*. According to Fig. 3, node D_2^4 is not included, since *m*=3, therefore f_4 (the last frame in the sequence) cannot be the second frame in the summary.

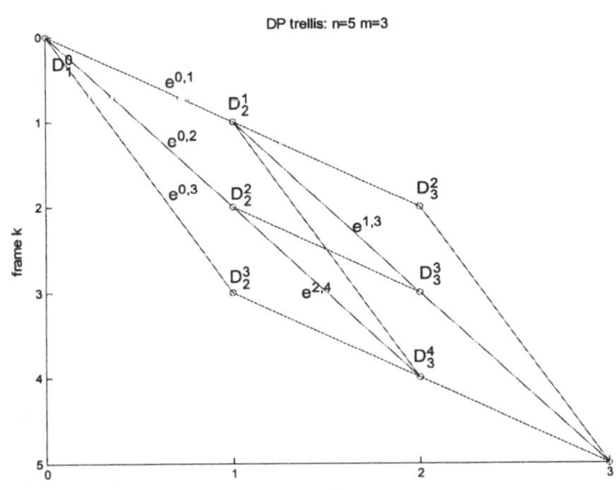

Fig. 3. MINAVG-MDOS DP trellis example for n=5 and m=3

Once the distortion state trellis and back pointers are computed recursively according to (26) and (27), the optimal frame selection can be found by (29) and (30). The number of nodes at every epoch $t>0$, or the depth of the trellis, is $n\text{-}m+1$, and we therefore have a total of $1+(m-1)(n-m+1)$ nodes in the n-m trellis that need to be evaluated.

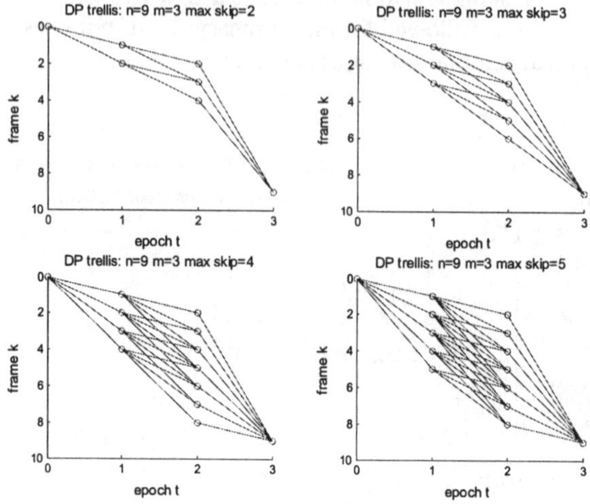

Fig. 4. Examples of frame-skip constrained DP trellises

The algorithm can also handle the frame skip constraint by eliminating edges in DP trellis that introduces frame skip larger than the constraint K_{max}. Examples of frame skip constrained trellises are shown in Fig. 4. Notice that the DP trellis for the same problem can have different topology with different skip constraints.

4.2 Solution to the MINAVG-MROS problem

For the MINAVG-MROS formulation, we minimize the temporal rate of the video summary, or select the smallest number of frames possible that satisfy the distortion constraint. There are two approaches to obtain the optimal solution. According to the first one, the optimal solution results from the modification of the DP algorithm for the MDOS problem. The DP "trellis" is not bounded by m (length or number of epochs), and its depth equals to $(n-m+1)$, anymore; it is actually a tree with root at D_1^0 and expands in the n x n grid. The only constraints for the frame selection process are the "no look back" and "no repeat" constraints. The algorithm performs a Breadth First Search (BFS) on this tree and stops at the first node that satisfies the distortion constraint, which therefore has the minimum depth, or the minimum temporal rate. The computational complexity of this algorithm grows exponentially and it is not practical for large-size problems.

To address the computational complexity issue of the first algorithm, we propose a second algorithm that is based on the DP algorithm for the solution of the MDOS formulation. Since we have the optimal solution to the MDOS problem, and we observe that feasible rates $\{1/n, 2/n, \ldots n/n\}$ are discrete and finite, we can solve the MROS problem by searching through all feasible rates, and for each feasible rate $R=m/n$, solve the MDOS problem to obtain the minimum distortion $D^*(R)$. Similar to the definition of the ORD function, the operational distortion-rate (ODR) function $D^*(R)$ resulting from the MDOS optimization is given by

$$D^*(R) = D^*(m/n) = \min_{l_1, l_2, \cdots, l_{m-1}} (1/n)\sum_{j=0}^{n-1} d(f_j, f_j'), \tag{31}$$

that is, it represents the minimum distortion corresponding to the rate m/n. An example of this ODR function is shown in Fig. 5.

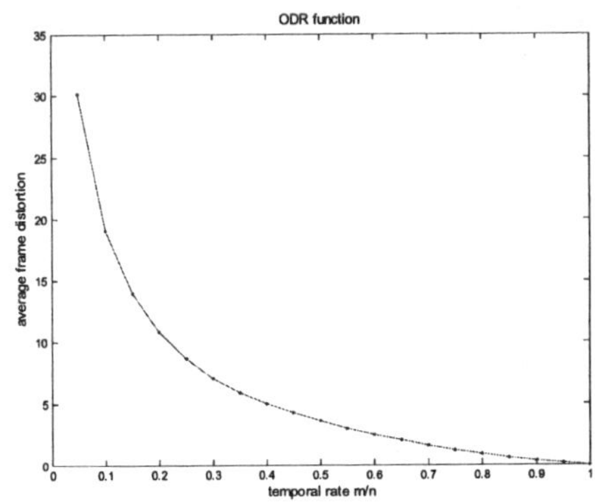

Fig. 5. An example of Operational Distortion-Rate (ODR) function

If the resulting distortion $D^*(R)$ satisfies the MROS distortion constraint, the rate R is labeled as "*admissible*". The optimal solution to the MROS problem is therefore the minimum rate among all admissible rates. Therefore, the MROS problem with distortion constraint D_{max} is solved by,

$$\min_{R \in \{\frac{1}{n}, \frac{2}{n}, \cdots, \frac{n}{n}\}} R, \ s.t. D^*(R) \le D_{\max} \tag{32}$$

The minimization process is over all feasible rates. The solution to (32) can be found in a more efficient way, since the rate-distortion function is a non-increasing function of m, that is,

Lemma 1: $D^*(m_1/n) \le D^*(m_2/n), \ if \ m_1 > m_2, \ \ for \ m_1, m_2 \in [1, n]$

Proof: If we prove that $D^*(m+1/n) \le D^*(m/n)$, then since we have $D^*(m/n) \le D^*(m-1/n) \cdots \le D^*(1/n)$, Lemma 1 is true. Let $D^*(m/n)$ be the minimum distortion introduced by the optimal m-frame summary solution $L^* = \{0, l_1, l_2, \ldots, l_{m-1}\}$, for some $1<m<n$. Since $m<n$, there exists an l_t such that the previous frame to frame f_{l_t}, i.e., f_{l_t-1} (clearly between frames $f_{l_{t-1}}$ and f_{l_t}) does not belong to the summary solution L^*. If frame f_{l_t-1} were to be included in the summary, a new summary with frame selection $L_N = L^* \cup \{f_{l_t-1}\}$ would be

generated with resulting distortion $D^{L_N} = D^*(m/n) - d(f_{l_{t-1}}, f_{l_t-1})$. Since $d(f_{l_{t-1}}, f_{l_t-1}) \geq 0$, we have $D^{L_N} \leq D^*(m/n)$. Since the so resulting *m+1* frame summary (with the inclusion of frame f_{l_t-1}) is not necessarily optimal, we have $D^*(m+1/n) \leq D^{L_N} \leq D^*(m/n)$.

Lemma 1 is quite intuitive, since adding a frame to the summary always reduces, or keeps the resulting distortion the same. Since the operational distortion-rate function $D^*(m/n)$ is a discrete and non-increasing function as established in Lemma 1, the MROS problem in (32) can be solved efficiently by a bi-section search on the $D^*(m/n)$ [30].

The algorithm starts with an initial rate bracket of $R_{lo}=1/n$ and $R_{hi}=n/n$, and computes its associated initial distortion bracket of $D_{lo}=D^*(R_{lo})$, and $D_{hi}=D^*(R_{hi})$. If the MROS distortion constraint $D_{max} > D_{lo}$, then the optimal rate is $1/n$. Otherwise we select a middle rate point $R_{new} = \lfloor (R_{hi} + R_{lo})/2 \rfloor$, compute its associated distortion $D^*(R_{new})$, and find the new rate and distortion bracket by replacing either the R_{lo} or the R_{hi} point with R_{new}, such that the distortion constraint D_{max} is within the new distortion bracket. The process is repeated until the rate bracket converges, i.e, $R_{hi}=m^*/n$, $R_{lo}=(m^*-1)/n$, for some m^*. At this point the optimal rate is found as $R^*=m^*/n$, and the optimal solution to the MROS problem is the solution of the n-m^* summarization problem as discussed in Section 4.1.

The complexity of the bi-section search algorithm is $O(\log(n))$ times the complexity of the DP *n-m* summarization algorithm, which is acceptable for off-line processing of video summaries.

4.3 Solution to the MINMAX-MROS problem

Now consider the MROS formulation with the max frame distortion for the summarization distortion metric. MINMAX is considered to be a better criterion in image/video compression for its better representation of subjective perception. As in the case of MINAVG-MDOS problem, exhaustive searching is not a practical solution. Instead we observe that MINMAX-MROS problem also has interesting structure and can also be solved by dynamic programming.

Dynamic Programming Solution

The MINMAX-MROS problem can be solved in stages. For a given current state of the problem, future solutions are independent from past solutions. Exploiting this structure, a Dynamic Programming (DP) solution based on [35, 30, 31] is developed. The initial result was reported in [20].

Let the distortion state for the video sequence segment starting with the frame selection l_t and ending with the frame $l_{t+1}-1$ be

$$D_{l_t}^{l_{t+1}} = \max_{j \in [l_t,\, l_{t+1}-1]} d(f_{l_t}, f_j) \tag{33}$$

Let the rate of this sequence segment be

$$R_{l_t}^{l_{t+1}} = \begin{cases} r(f_{l_t}) = 1, & if\ D_{l_t}^{l_{t+1}} \le D_{\max} \\ \infty, & otherwise \end{cases}, \tag{34}$$

which means that if the sequence segment distortion is larger than the maximum allowable distortion, there is no feasible rate solution for the segment. With this rate definition for the segment, the MROS problem in (19) is therefore equivalent to the unconstrained problem of

$$\min_{l_1, l_2, \cdots l_{m-1}} \{R_0^{l_1} + R_{l_1}^{l_2} + \cdots + R_{l_{m-1}}^{n}\} \tag{35}$$

The problem of (35) can be computed recursively. Let the minimum rate for the video segment starting with frame f_0 and ending with the summary frame choice l_t be

$$J_{l_t} = \min_{l_1, l_2, \cdots l_{t-1}} \{R_0^{l_1} + R_{l_1}^{l_2} + \cdots + R_{l_{t-1}}^{l_t}\}, \tag{36}$$

then for the video segment ending with the summary frame choice l_{t+1}, the minimum rate is given by,

$$\begin{aligned} J_{l_{t+1}} &= \min_{l_1, l_2, \cdots l_t} \{R_0^{l_1} + R_{l_1}^{l_2} + \cdots + R_{l_{t-1}}^{l_t} + R_{l_t}^{l_{t+1}}\} \\ &= \min_{l_t} \{J_{l_t} + R_{l_t}^{l_{t+1}}\} \end{aligned} \tag{37}$$

This gives us the recursion we need to compute the solution trellis for a Viterbi algorithm [35] like optimal solution. The initial condition is given by

$$J_{l_1} = \begin{cases} 1, & if\ D_0^{l_1} \le D_{\max} \\ \infty, & else \end{cases} \tag{38}$$

The recursion starts with the frame node f_0 and expands over all frames that introduce admissible segment distortion. A full trellis example for $n=6$ with all possible transition arcs is shown in Fig. 6.

There is a virtual final frame f_n for each possible summary frame selection in the trellis. The algorithm will stop at certain epoch t^*, if the virtual final frame is reached in the minimization process, that is, if we have $n \in \arg\min_{l_{t^*}} \{J_{l_{t^*}} + R_{l_{t^*}}^{n}\}$.

Notice that the edges in Fig. 6 between any frame pair f_j and f_{j+p} is admissible only if

$$\max_{i \in [0, p-1]} \{d(f_j, f_{j+i})\} \le D_{\max} \tag{39}$$

In addition we may also impose a constraint on the maximum number of frames, K_{max}, that can be skipped between two successive summary frames, that is

$$p \le K_{\max} + 1 \tag{40}$$

The skip constraint is useful in ensuing smooth play back as well as in certain security surveillance applications where the risk of missing certain events needs to be minimized.

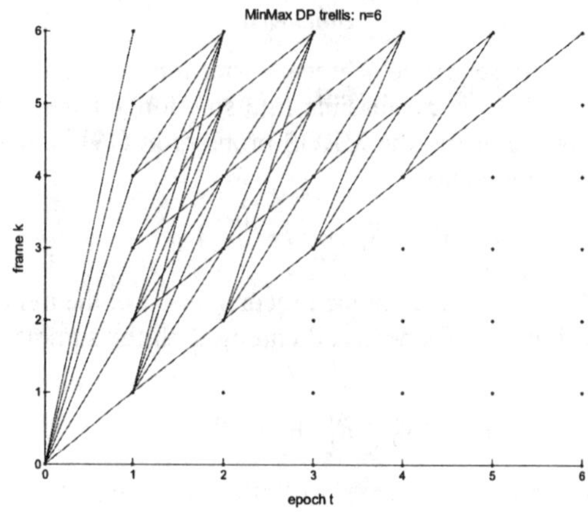

Fig. 6. MINMAX-MROS full DP trellis for n=6

The optimal solution to MINMAX-MROS formulation is not unique, as indicated in Fig. 7 by an example summary generation result for the "foreman" sequence, frames 150-157, with maximum skip constraint K_{max} = 6, and max distortion constraint $D_{max}=2.4$. The optimal rate in this case is $m=3$.

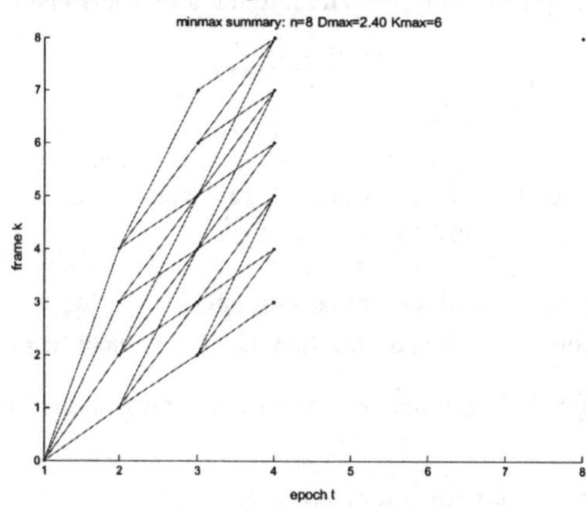

Fig. 7. MINMAX-MROS solution example, "foreman" sequence, n=8.

From Fig. 7 it is clear that multiple solutions like $\{f_0, f_4, f_7\}$, $\{f_0, f_4, f_6\}$ … $\{f_0, f_2, f_5\}$ are all optimal solutions to the MROS formulation. Additional constraint like minimum coding cost in bits can be applied to find the unique solution.

Greedy Algorithm for the MINMAX-MROS problem

A greedy Distortion Constrained Skip (DCS) solution [18] also exists for the example in Fig.7, that is the solution $\{f_0, f_4, f_7\}$, which is the inner most path of the trellis. The DCS algorithm starts with the selection of the first frame f_0, and skips all frames that do not introduce frame distortion exceeding the maximum distortion constraint D_{max}. A frame is selected into the summary if the distortion it introduces is greater than D_{max}. In summary the algorithm operates as follows,

```
Set L=0, add f_L to the summary S
FOR k=1 TO n
   IF d(f_L, f_k) > Dmax
       L=k,
       add f_L to the summary S
   END
END
```

It skips all frames that introduce acceptable distortion. The DCS algorithm is not optimal in general, but it is optimal if the following condition holds

$$D_{j+p}^{k} \le D_{j}^{k}, \; for\; j+p \le k \tag{41}$$

The condition in (41) requires that a shorter sub-segment of the sequences introduces smaller maximum distortion than the longer one with the same last frame. This is true for most natural video sequences within a video shot, but may not be true for sequences striding two video shots. The DCS algorithm is a much faster one-pass solution than the DP algorithm, and will be optimal if (41) holds. Even though this condition may not hold for some sequences, the performance penalty is acceptable. This makes the DCS algorithm an attractive practical alternative for one-pass, on-line applications like SDTV trans-coding for mobile users.

4.4 Solution to the MINMAX-MDOS problem

With the DP solution to the MINMAX-MROS problem, we investigate on the property of its *operational rate-distortion* (ORD) function, and solve the MINMAX-MDOS problem by bi-section searching on the distortion constraints, similar to the MINAVG-MROS case.

The operational rate-distortion characterizes the achievable rate-distortion performance with operating points under certain coding scheme. In the context of video summarization, the operational rate-distortion function is defined as

$$R^{*}(D) = m/n, \; s.t. \; \min_{l_1, l_2, \cdots, l_{m-1}} \{\max_{k}\{d(f_k, f_k')\}\} \le D, \tag{42}$$

which is the minimum rate achievable, m/n, for a given maximum distortion constraint, D. An example of this function is shown in Fig. 8.

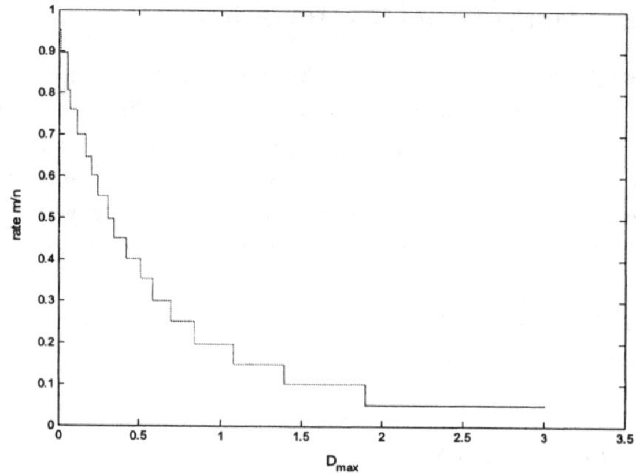

Fig. 8. An example of operational temporal rate-distortion (RD) function

The operational rate-distortion is not continuous, as the operating rate is a discrete set of $\{1/n, 2/n, ..., n/n\}$ and a range of D_{max} values can result in the same optimal rate. Similarly the operational distortion-rate function (ODR) for the max frame distortion criterion is defined as

$$D^*(R) = D^*(m/n) = \min_{l_1, l_2, \cdots, l_{m-1}} \{\max_k \{d(f_k, f_k')\}\}, \tag{43}$$

which is the minimum maximum frame distortion achievable for a given temporal rate of m/n. We also have,

Lemma 2: $D^*(R)$ is a non-increasing function.

Proof: Let the optimal frame selection with rate $R_1=m/n$ be $L_1^*=\{0, l_1, l_2, ..., l_{m-1}\}$, for some $1<m<n$, and the resulting minimum maximum frame distortion be D_1^*. Since $m<n$, there must exist a summary frame selection l_t in L_1^*, such that the previous frame f_{l_t-1} (clearly between frames $f_{l_{t-1}}$ and f_{l_t}) does not belong to the summary solution L_1^*, with the frame distortion $d(f_{l_t-1}, f_{l_t-1}') = d(f_{l_t-1}, f_{l_{t-1}}) \le D_1^*$. If frame f_{l_t-1} were to be included in the summary, a new summary with frame selection $L_2 = L_1^* \cup \{f_{l_t-1}\}$ would be generated with a new rate of $R_2=(m+1)/n$, and resulting in minimum maximum frame distortion D_2. If $d(f_{l_t-1}, f_{l_t-1}')$ is the only one equal to D_1^*, then $D_2<D_1^*$; otherwise $D_2=D_1^*$, that is $D_2 \le D_1^*$. Since L_2 is not necessarily the optimal solution with rate R_2, we have $D_2^* \le D_2$. Therefore we have, for $R_1=m/n$ and $R_2=(m+1)/n$, and $1<m<n$, $D^*(R_2) \le D^*(R_1)$. Since rates are discrete, by chain rule we have $D^*(1/n) \le D^*(2/n) \le \ldots \le D^*(n/n)$. And because $d(f_{l_{t-1}}, f_{l_t-1}) \ge 0$, we have $D^{L_N} \le D^*(m/n)$, and since the resulting $m+1$ frame

summary (with the inclusion of frame f_{l_t-1}) is not necessarily optimal, we have $D^*(m+1/n) \le D^{L_N} \le D^*(m/n)$.

Lemma 2 is quite intuitive, because adding a frame to the summary always reduces, or keeps the resulting maximum frame distortion the same. The ORD function in (42) is completely determined by the ODR function in (43). From Lemma 2 we know that the ORD function is also non-increasing with the distortion. Therefore, the problem of MDOS can be solved efficiently by a bi-section search on the ORD [30, 31].

For a given rate constraint of $R_0=m_0/n$, the algorithm starts with an initial maximum frame distortion bracket of $[D^{lo}, D^{hi}]$ and initial rate bracket of $[R^{lo}, R^{hi}]$, such that m_0/n is in the initial rate bracket. Then we compute a new distortion middle point as $D_{new}=(D^{lo}+D^{hi})/2$, solve for its optimal rate $R_{new}=m_{new}/n$ with the MROS algorithm, and find the new rate bracket by replacing either R^{lo} or R^{hi} with the R_{new}, such that the rate constraint R_0 is within the new rate bracket. Then we replace the distortion bracket with corresponding distortion pair $[D^{hi}, D^{lo}]$. The process will continue until the rate bracket boundaries converge to some R_0. At this point, the search may stop, and the final MROS distortion threshold is chosen as the solution to the MDOS problem. Since the ORD function is a piece-wise constant function with total n distinct rate values, the bi-section search will converge in a limited number of iterations. The complexity of the bi-section search algorithm is $O(\log(n))$ times the complexity of the MROS algorithm, which is acceptable for off-line processing of video summaries.

4.5 Bit Rate Constrained Summarization

In addition to the temporal rate constrained formulations, let us consider the bit rate constraint for the summarization problem. The summarization bit rate $R(S)$ is given by the total number of bits used to code the summary frames in S

$$R(S) = \sum_{t=0}^{m-1} b(f_{l_t}) = \begin{cases} \sum_{t=0}^{m-1} r^{l_t}, & \text{intra-coding} \\ r^{l_0} + \sum_{t=1}^{m-1} r^{l_t}_{l_{t-1}}, & \text{inter-coding} \end{cases}, \tag{44}$$

where r^{l_t} represents the number of bits spent to intra-code frame l_t, and $r^{l_t}_{l_{t-1}}$ the bits to inter-code frame l_t based on motion prediction from the frame l_{t-1}. We will discuss the solution to the MINAVG-MDOS and MINMAX-MROS problems. The MINAVG-MROS and MINMAX-MDOS can be solved similar to the temporal rate constrained cases.

MINAVG-MDOS problem with bit rate constraint

To solve the MINAVG-MDOS formulation with bit constraint, we use the Lagrangian multiplier method discussed in Section 2.3. We first relax the constrained MINAVG-MDOS minimization problem with a Lagrangian multiplier [7], that is

$$S_{\lambda}^{*} = \arg\min_{S}\{D(S) + \lambda R(S)\} \tag{45}$$

If there exists a λ^{*} such that $R(S_{\lambda^{*}}^{*}) = R_{\max}$, then the solution $S_{\lambda^{*}}^{*}$ is also the optimal solution to the original MDOS formulation.

We further observe that the relaxed MDOS problem in Eq. 4.25 has a certain built-in structure and can be solved in stages. For a given current state, the future solution is independent from the past solution. This structure will give us an efficient Dynamic Programming (DP) solution following [25, 26, 30].

Let the distortion state for the sequence segment starting with frame selection l_t and ending with the frame $l_{t+1}-1$ be

$$G_{l_t}^{l_{t+1}} = \sum_{j=l_t}^{l_{t+1}-1} d(f_{l_t}, f_j) \tag{46}$$

The summary then including t frames and ending with the last frame selection $l_{t-1}=k$ has minimum distortion

$$D_t^k = \min_{l_1,l_2,\cdots l_{t-2}} \{G_0^{l_1} + G_{l_1}^{l_2} + \cdots + G_{l_{t-2}}^{k} + G_k^n\}, \tag{47}$$

and associated bit rate $R_t^k = \sum_{j=0}^{t-1} b(f_{l_j})$. With Lagrangian relaxation, the objective becomes

$$J_{\lambda}^{t,k} = \min_{l_1,l_2,\cdots l_{t-2}} \{D_t^k + \lambda R_t^k\} \tag{48}$$

For the summary with $t+1$ frames and $l_t=k$, we have

$$
\begin{aligned}
J_\lambda^{t+1,k} &= \min_{l_1,l_2,\cdots l_{t-1}} \{D_{t+1}^k + \lambda R_{t+1}^k\} \\
&= \min_{l_1,l_2,\cdots l_{t-1}} \{G_0^{l_1} + \cdots + G_{l_{t-1}}^k + G_k^n + \lambda[b(f_0) + b(f_1) \\
&\qquad + \cdots b(f_{l_{t-1}}) + b(f_k)]\} \\
&= \min_{l_1,l_2,\cdots l_{t-1}} \{G_0^{l_1} + \cdots + G_{l_{t-2}}^{l_{t-1}} + G_{l_{t-1}}^n - G_{l_{t-1}}^n + G_{l_{t-1}}^k + G_k^n \\
&\qquad + \lambda[b(f_0) + b(f_1) + \cdots b(f_{l_{t-1}})] + \lambda b(f_k)\} \\
&= \min_{l_1,l_2,\cdots l_{t-1}} \{G_0^{l_1} + \cdots + G_{l_{t-1}}^n + \lambda[b(f_0) + \cdots b(f_{l_{t-1}})] \\
&\qquad - \underbrace{[G_{l_{t-1}}^n - (G_{l_{t-1}}^k + G_k^n)]}_{e^{l_{t-1},k}} + \lambda b(f_k)\} \\
&= \begin{Bmatrix} \min\limits_{l_{t-1}}\{J_\lambda^{t,l_{t-1}} - e^{l_{t-1},k} + \lambda r^k\}, & \text{if intra coding} \\ \min\limits_{l_{t-1}}\{J_\lambda^{t,l_{t-1}} - e^{l_{t-1},k} + \lambda r_{l_{t-1}}^k\}, & \text{if inter coding} \end{Bmatrix}
\end{aligned}
\tag{49}
$$

The "edge cost" $e^{l_{t-1},k}$ is the distortion difference if frame k is selected into the summary ending with frame l_{t-1}, given by

$$
e^{l_{t-1},k} = \sum_{j=k}^{n-1} [d(f_j, f_{l_{t-1}}) - d(f_j, f_k)] \tag{50}
$$

We can split the minimization in (49) because the quantities $e^{l_{t-1},k}$, r^k and $r_{l_{t-1}}^k$ do not depend on the previous frame selections $L_{t-2}= \{l_{t-2}, l_{t-3}, ...l_0\}$. This is true for $r_{l_{t-1}}^k$ only if frame f_k is predicted from the original frame $f_{l_{t-1}}$. But in video coder implementations like H.263 [11, 34] we use, the prediction is actually from the reconstructed frame $\hat{f}_{l_{t-1}}$, which can have multiple versions depending on L_{t-2}, and this introduces small variations in $r_{l_{t-1}}^k$. We can either force the prediction on $f_{l_{t-1}}$, or more practically, by using a constant PSNR rate profiler to allocate the number of bits, $r_{l_{t-1}}^k$, to each inter-coding frame pair. The goal is to have constant PSNR quality in the video summary sequence.

The initial condition for the recursion in (49) is given as

$$
J_\lambda^{1,0} = \{G_0^n + \lambda r^0\} \tag{51}
$$

From (49) and (50), we establish the recursion needed for the Dynamic Programming (DP) solution. The algorithm will build the trellis with this recursion starting from frame f_0, it will add more frames to the summary, and stop when the last (virtual) frame f_n is reached. For each epoch t, the final node is computed as

$$J_{\lambda}^{t,n} = \min_{k \in F_{t-1}} \{J_{\lambda}^{t-1,k}\}, \tag{52}$$

where F_{t-1} is the feasible frame set at epoch $t-1$ that can have transition to the last (virtual) frame f_n. The optimal solution for the relaxed MINAVG-MDOS problem (45) with a particular λ is therefore found by selecting the smallest $J_{\lambda}^{t,n}$ and backtracking for the optimal summary.

The operational rate-distortion function is non-increasing and actually convex in most cases, as shown in an example in Fig. 8. It is known that the Lagrangian multiplier λ is the inverse slope of the operational rate-distortion function convex hull. As λ goes from zero to infinity, the solution of the problem in (45) traces out the convex hull of the operational rate-distortion curve. The solution to the original MINAVG-MDOS problem, $S_{\lambda^*}^*$ is therefore found by a bi-section on λ.

The DP solution to the relaxed problem in (45) has complexity of O(n^2). The bi-section search on λ is efficient because the edge and bit costs in the recursion (49) do not change as λ changes, therefore needing only to be computed once in the bi-section search loop. An even faster searching based on Bezier curve search [30] is also available.

The MINAVG-MROS problem with an average frame distortion constraint can be solved by the same approach of a bi-section search on the hull of the operational rate-distortion (ORD) function. By varying the Lagrangian multiplier, we will be able to find the operating point on the convex hull that satisfies the distortion constraint yet achieves minimum bit rate. We will not discuss it in detail.

In the next sub-section, we will consider the MINMAX-MROS problem with bit constraint.

MINMAX-MROS Problem with Bit Constraint

For the MINMAX-MROS problem with bit rate constraint, the solution is similar to the temporal rate constrained formulation. Let us define the minimum number of bits needed to code the summary after t frames are selected and with the last frame selection $l_{t-1}=k$ be

$$B_t^k = \min_{l_1, l_2, \cdots l_{t-2}} \{b_0 + b_{l_1} + \cdots + b_{l_{t-2}} + b_k\}, \; s.t. \; D(S) \le D_{\max} \tag{53}$$

The minimization is over $\{l_1, l_2, \ldots l_{t-2}\}$, since $l_t=k$ is a given constant. Therefore the optimal solution with the minimum bit rate to the MINMAX-MROS problem is

$$\min_{l_1, l_2, \cdots l_{m-1}} B_{m+1}^n, s.t. D(S) \le D_{\max} \tag{54}$$

Let us define frame f_n as a virtual final frame, and its associated bits b_n be zero, since its value is not relevant to the minimization. Assuming the first frame is intra-coded and the rest of the summary frames are inter-coded in IPPP…P fashion, the minimization process in (53) can then be written as

$$
\begin{aligned}
B_t^k &= \min_{l_1, l_2, \cdots l_{t-2}} \{r^0 + r_0^{l_1} + \cdots + r_{l_{t-3}}^{l_{t-2}} + r_{l_{t-2}}^k\} \\
&= \min_{l_{t-2}}\{ \min_{l_1, l_2, \cdots l_{t-3} \in L^*} \{(r_0 + r_0^{l_1} \cdots + r_{l_{t-3}}^{l_{t-2}} + r_{l_{t-2}}^k\} \\
&= \min_{l_{t-2}}\{B_{l_{t-1}}^{l_{t-2}} + r_{l_{t-2}}^k\}
\end{aligned} \tag{55}
$$

This gives us the recursion for a dynamic programming solution similar to the MINMAX-MROS formulation with temporal rate constraint. The initial condition is given by $B_1^0 = r_0$. We can split the minimization in (55) because $r_{l_{t-2}}^k$ does not depend on the previous frame selections $\{l_1, l_2, \ldots l_{t-3}\}$.

Similarly, for the intra-coded case, the minimization process recursion is given as

$$
\begin{aligned}
B_t^k &= \min_{l_1, l_2, \cdots l_{t-2}} \{r_0 + r_{l_1} + \cdots + r_{l_{t-2}} + r_k\} \\
&= \min_{l_{t-2}}\{B_{l_{t-1}}^{l_{t-2}} + r_k\}
\end{aligned} \tag{56}
$$

The initial condition for intra-coding case is also given by $B_1^0 = r_0$. Notice that in MINMAX-MROS problem with temporal rate, the solution is typically not unique for a given distortion constraint D_{max}, as indicated by the previous example in Fig. 7. This solution to the bit constraint can also be used to break the tie in that case.

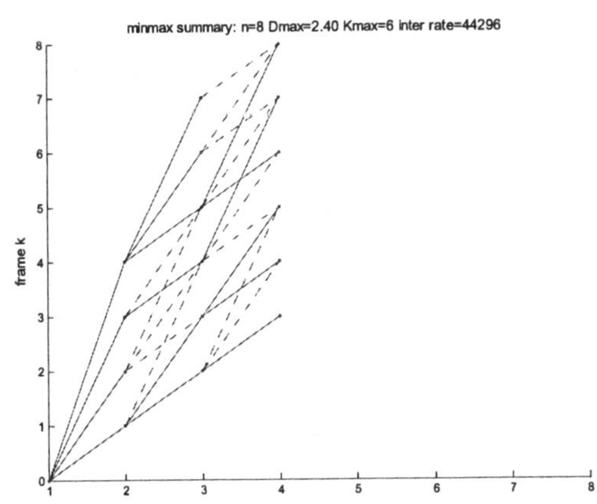

(a) Optimal path for the inter-coded summary

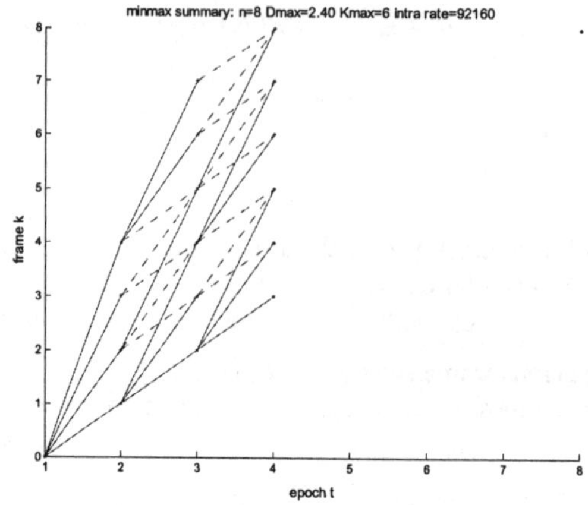

(b) Optimal path for the intra-coded summary

Fig. 9. MINMAX-MROS solution trellis example

In the bit rate constrained case, the solution to MINMAX-MROS is unique. Optimal coding solution for the example sequence of frames 150-157 for the "foreman" sequence is shown in Fig. 9a for the inter-coded case, and Fig. 9b for the intra-coded case, respectively. The solid lines are the solutions with optimal coding, while the dotted lines are the non-optimal solutions with the same temporal rates but not the minimum bit rate. In both cases, $D_{max} = 2.4$ and there is no effective skip constraint. For the inter-coding case, the optimal solution is S=$\{f_0 f_4 f_5\}$, the minimum bit rate achieved is 44296 bits. For the intra-coding case, the optimal solution is S=$\{f_0 f_2 f_5\}$, the minimum bit rate achieved is 92160 bits.

The MINMAX-MDOS problem with bit rate constraint can also be solved by a bi-section searching on the operational distortion-rate function, similar to the temporal rate constrained formulation. We will not discuss it in detail.

4.6 Frame Distortion Metric

The optimal MDOS and MROS formulations and solutions do not depend on a particular frame distortion metric, however, a good frame distortion metric will give satisfactory performance in subjective evaluation of the summaries. There are a number of ways to compute the frame distortion $d(f_j, f_k)$. The Mean Squared Error (MSE) has been widely used in image processing. However, it is well known that it does not represent well the visual quality of the results. For example, a simple one-pixel translation of a frame with complex texture will result in a large MSE, although the perceptual distortion is negligible. There is work in the literature addressing the perceptual quality issues, (for example, [14] and others), however such algorithms address primarily the distortion between an image and its quantized versions.

The color histogram-based distance is also a popular choice in many solutions, for example, [37], but it may not perform well either, since it does not reflect changes in the layout and orientation of images. For example, if a large red ball is moving in a green background, even though there are a lot of "changes", the color histogram will stay relatively constant. Motion activity [15] can also be used as a frame distortion metric, but it does not reflect the lighting changes well.

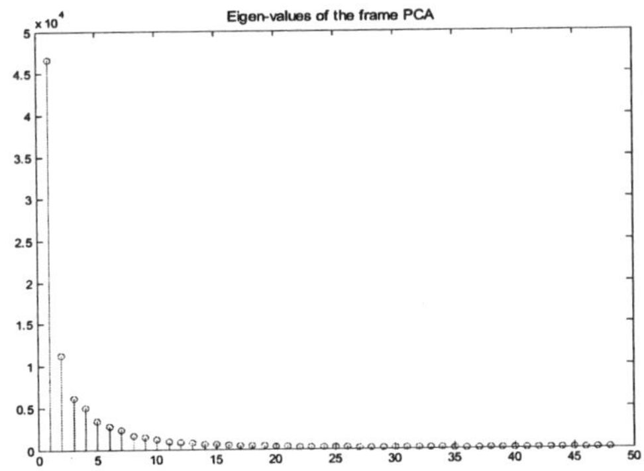

Fig. 10. Eigen-values of the proposed frame PCA

For a frame distortion metric that better reflects the subjective quality of an image perception, we use the Euclidean distance in the Principal Component (PC) space of the frames. Video frames are first scaled into smaller sizes (e.g., 8x6, 12x9 or 16x12). The benefit of this scaling process is to reduce noise and local variance such that the frame distance evaluation is performed at a spatial resolution scale that probably better matches human perception. This scaling process also benefits PCA by reducing the dimensionality of the data. The number of sample frames for PCA is limited and the reduced dimensionality makes the covariance matrix estimation from the limited data more accurate. The PCA transform T is found by diagonalizing the covariance matrix of the frames [6, 16, 22], and selecting the desired number of dimensions with the largest eigen-values. Therefore the frame distortion metric is given by

$$d(f_j, f_k) = \sqrt{\| T(D(f_j)) - T(D(f_k)) \|^2}\,, \tag{57}$$

where D denotes the scaling process, T is the PCA transform. In our experiment we collected 3200 frames from various video clips and scaled the frames to 8x6 pixels before performing PCA. The resulting eigenvalues are plotted in Fig. 10. Notice that most of the energy is captured by the bases corresponding to the 8 largest eigenvalues. Therefore our adopted PCA transform matrix T has dimension 8 by 48.

Other methods like Local Linear Embedding (LLE) [28] and Multiple Dimension Scaling (MDS) can also be used to identify the sub space and metric appropriate for frame differentiation. There is no solid "optimality" criterion to select the frame distortion metric, however, the experimental results with this PCA based frame distortion metric demonstrate that it is effective.

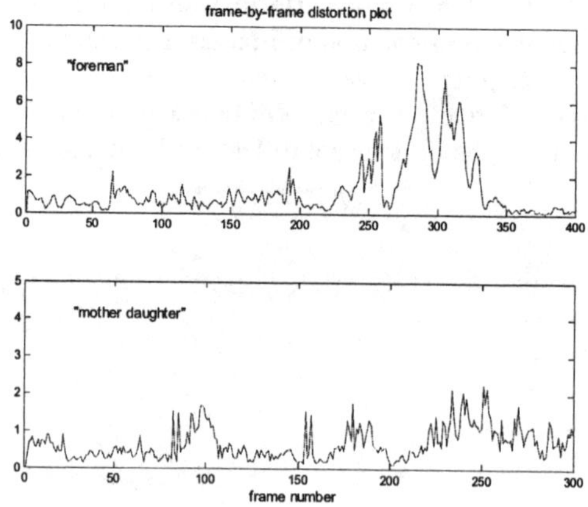

Fig. 11. Frame-by-frame distortion for the "foreman" and "mother-daughter" sequences

Examples for the "foreman" and the "mother daughter" sequences are shown as frame-by-frame distortion plot $d(f_k, f_{k-1})$ in Fig. 11 for the "foreman" (upper plot) and the "mother daughter" (lower plot) sequences. It seems to reflect well the perceptual quality of the sequence, since for the "foreman" sequence, frames 1-200 contain a talking head with little visual changes, therefore the frame-by-frame distortion remains low for this period. There is a hand waving occluding the face around frames 253-259, thus we have spikes corresponding to these frames. There is the camera panning motion around frames 274-320, thus we have high values in $d(f_k, f_{k-1})$ for this time period. The plot for the "mother daughter" sequence has similar interpretation. Comparing the plot between two sequences, it is also clear the "foreman" sequence contains more "changes" than the "mother daughter" sequence, as reflected by the much higher average frame-by-frame distortion in the "foreman" sequence. From this experiment it seems that the PCA based metric function in (57) is fairly accurate in depicting the distortion or the dissimilarity of frames, while at the same time keeping the computation at a moderate level.

5 Simulation Results and Conclusions

In previous section, we formulate and solve the video summarization problems as rate-distortion optimization problems with different rates and distortion definitions, as well as frame skip constraint. We performed test on real sequences and the results are reported in the following sub-sections.

5.1 Simulation Results

For the temporal rate based formulation, the MINAVG-MDOS summarization results for the "foreman" sequence frames 150~399 are shown in Fig. 12b for skip constrained cases and in Fig. 12a for not constrained cases.

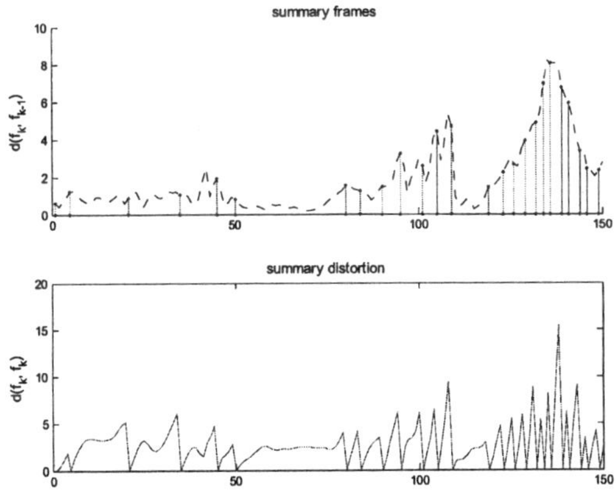

(a) Summarization results without the frame skip constraint

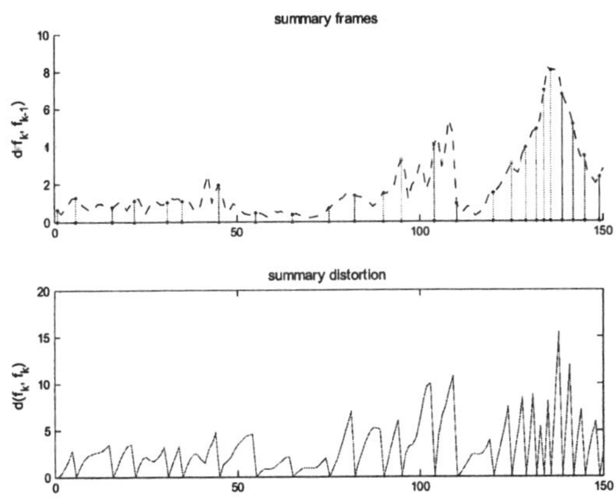

(b) Summarization results with the frame skip constraint $K_{max}=10$

Fig. 12. MINAVG-MDOS summarization results for the "foreman" sequence, frames 150-399

In both cases, in the upper plot, the summary frame selections are plotted as vertical lines against the dotted curve of the frame-by-frame distortion $d(f_k, f_{k-1})$, which gives an indication of the activity, or eventfulness of the sequence. The bottom plot is the per frame distortion, $d(f_k, f_k')$, between the original and the reconstructed sequence from the summary. The area under this d(f_k, f_k') function is the total distortion of the reconstruction. In both cases, the temporal rate is $R(S)=25/150$. The skip constrained version in Fig. 12b is very similar to the unconstrained case, except for a large skip around frame number 50 in the plot.

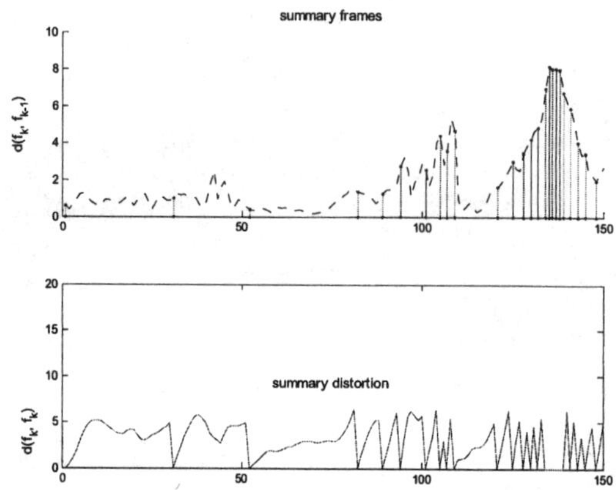

(a) Summarization results without the frame skip constraint, D_{max} = 6.4

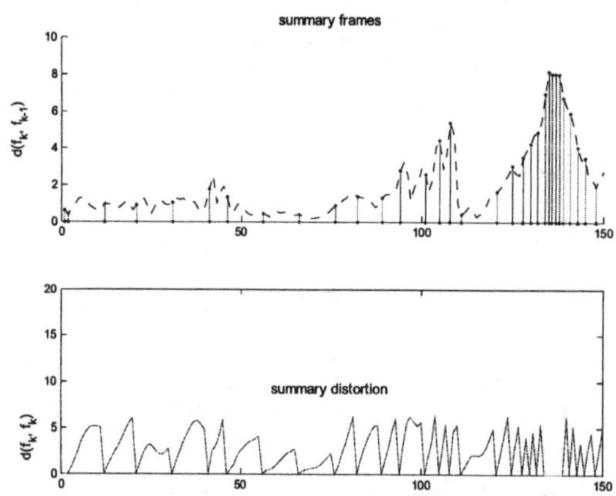

(b) Summarization results with the frame skip constraint K_{max}=10, D_{max}=6.4

Fig. 13. MINMAX-MROS summarization results for the "foreman" sequence, frames 150-399

For the MINMAX_MROS formulation, we set a distortion constraint of Dmax = 6.4 and also test out the skip constrained and non-constrained cases. The summarization results are similarly plotted in Fig. 13.

In both cases, the max frame distortion is 6.4, and in the no frame skip constraint case, the resulting temporal rate is $R(S)=25/150$, which matches the rate used in Fig. 12. When a skip constraint Kmax = 10 is applied, to achieve the same max distortion of 6.4, the temporal rate becomes $R(S)$=32/150.

We also generated summary for the "flower" sequence frames 150~299 with the same temporal rate setting of $R(S)=25/150$. The performances in both tests are summarized in the following table.

Table 1. MINAVG-MDOS and MINMAX-MDOS performance data

Alg/Sequence/Kmax	Avg Distortion	Max Distortion	Distortion Var
MAVG, "foreman", n/a	2.68	15.50	4.96
MAVG, "foreman, 10	2.90	15.50	7.64
MMAX,"foreman", n/a,	2.96	6.39	3.56
MAVG,"mo-dgtr", n/a	0.49	1.67	0.16
MAVG, "mo-dgtr", 10	0.53	2.50	0.27
MMAX,"mo-dgtr", n/a	0.71	1.39	0.20

Abbreviations: MAVG = MINAVG-MDOS, MMAX = MINMAX-MROS, „mo-dgtr", mother-daughter sequence.

Notice that for the same temporal rate, the average and maximum distortion achieved for the "mother daughter" sequence are much smaller than that of the "foreman" sequence, this is because the "foreman" sequence contains more information and is more "eventful" than the "mother-daughter" sequence.

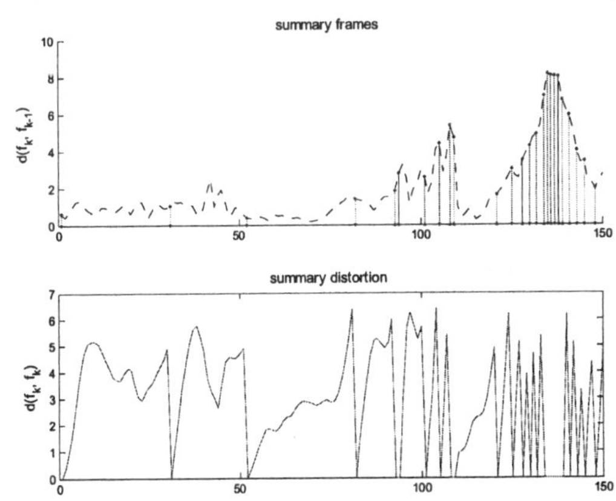

Fig. 14. Bit constrained MINMAX summarization results for "foreman" sequence, frames 150-299, with D_{max}=6.4

For the MINMAX-MROS algorithm, the average distortion performance is not that far behind the MINAVG-MDOS algorithm, while the maximum distortion and distortion variance performances are much better in the MINMAX-MROS case for the matched rate. Overall, MINMAX-MROS algorithm is the most satisfactory in subjective evaluation of the summary sequence. In fact, we developed a heuristic algorithm approximating the MINMAX solution, and the resulting performance was very close to the optimal solution, and was reported in [18].

For the MINMAX-MROS formulation with bit constraint, a summarization example with the "foreman" sequence, frames 150-299, is shown in Fig. 14. The distortion constraint is $D_{max} = 6.4$. Notice that the solution summary also contains 25 frames, thus the same temporal rate is the same as the example in Fig. 13a. The minimum bit rate achieved is 304496 bits for the constant PSNR quality coding at fixed QP=10.

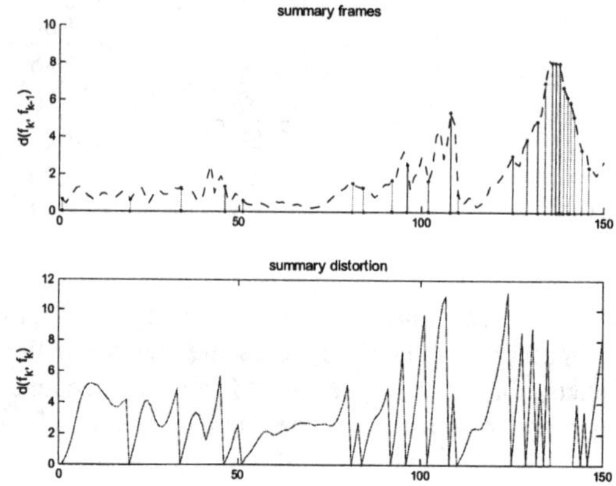

Fig. 15. Bit constrained MINAVG summarization results for "foreman" sequence, frames 150-299, with D_{max}=3.0

For the bit constrained MINMAX-MDOS formulation, our solution is based on Lagrangian relaxation and tracing out the convex hull of the ORD function. We assume a constant PSNR coding strategy for summary frames coding. An example is shown in Fig. 15 for the "foreman" sequence, frames 150-299, with an average frame distortion constraint of D_{max}=3.0. The resulting summary contains 25 frames, and the rate is 291112 bits. The optimal Lagrangian multiplier that achieves this rate is 0.00196.

For a subjective evaluation of MINMAX and MINAVG optimal video summarization results, please visit:

http://ivpl.ece.northwestern.edu/~zli/new_home/demo/minmax/minmax.html, and

http://ivpl.ece.northwestern.edu/~zli/new_home/demo/minavg/minavg.html.

Several video summary sequences in H.263 bit stream, along with a player are included for evaluation.

5.2 Conclusion and Future Work

In this work we formulated and solved the video summarization problems as rate-distortion problems. The optimal solutions and PCA based frame distortion metric, as well as several heuristic approximate solutions were demonstrated to be effective. Optimal summary coding with constant PSNR quality pictures was also solved under the same framework.

In the future, we will explore the application of local manifold embedding method in subspace learning and improve the frame distortion metric. We are also interested in exploring the joint summarization and coding problem as well as energy efficiency issues in summarization and summary transmission over wireless channels.

References

1. Berger, T. (1971) Rate Distortion Theory: A mathematical basis for data compression. Prentice-Hall.
2. Bertsekas, D. P. (1987) Dynamic Programming: Deterministic and stochastic models, Prentice-Hall.
3. Cover, T. M. (1991) Elements of Information Theory, John Wiley & Sons.
4. DeMenthon, D, Kobla, V., and Doermann, D., (1998) Video Summarization by Curve Simplification, Proceedings of ACM Multimedia Conference, Bristol, U.K.
5. Doulamis, N., Doulamis, A., Avrithis, Y., and Kollias, S. (1998) Video Content Representation Using Optimal Extraction of Frames and Scenes, Proc. of Int'l Conference on Image Processing, Chicago, Illinois.
6. Duda, R. O., Hart, P. E., and Stork, D. G. , (2001) Pattern Classification, 2nd ed. Wiley-Interscience Publication.
7. Everett, II. (1963) Generalized Lagrange multiplier method for solving problems of optimal allocation of resources. Operations Research, vol. 11, pp 399-417.
8. Gerald, C. F., and Wheatley, P. O.,(1990) Applied Numerical Analysis, 4th edition, Reading MA, Addision.
9. Girgenshohn, A., and Boreczky, J., (1999) Time-Constrained Key frame Selection Technique, Proc. of IEEE Multimedia Computing and Systems (ICMCS).
10. Gong, Y. and Liu, X., (2001) Video Summarization with Minimal Visual Content Redundancies. Proc. of Int'l Conference on Image Processing.
11. ITU-T Recommendation H.263, Video coding for low bit rate communication.
12. Hanjalic, A., and Zhang, H., (1999) An Integrated Scheme for Automated Video Abstraction Based on Unsupervised Cluster-Validity Analysis, IEEE Trans. on Circuits and Systems for Video Technology, vol.9.
13. Hanjalic, A., (2002) Shot-Boundary Detection: Unraveled and resolved ? IEEE Trans. on Circuits and Systems for Video Technology, vol.12.
14. Jayant, N., Johnston, J., and Safranek, R., (1993) Signal Compression Based on Models of Human Perception, Proceedings of IEEE, vol. 81, pp. 1385-1422.
15. Jeannin, S., and Divakaran, A. (2001) MPEG-7 Visual Motion Descriptors, IEEE Trans. on Circuits and Systems for Video Technology, vol.11.
16. Karhunen, H. (1960) On Linear Methods in Probability Theory. English translation, Doc. T-131, Rand Corp, Santa Monica, CA.
17. Koprinska, I., and Carrato, S. (2001) Temporal Video Segmentation: a survey. Signal Processing: Image Communication, vol.16, pp. 477-500.

18. Li, Z., Katsaggelos, A. K., and Gandhi, B., (2003) Temporal Rate-Distortion Optimal Video Summary Generation, Proceedings of Int'l Conference on Multimedia and Expo, Baltimore, USA.
19. Li, Z., Schuster, G., Katsaggelos, A. K., and Gandhi, B., (2004) Rate-Distortion Optimal Video Summarization: A Dynamic Programming Solution. Proceedings of Int'l Conference on Acoustics, Speech, and Signal Processing (ICASSP), Montreal, Canada.
20. Li, Z., Schuster, G., Katsaggelos, A. K., and Gandhi, B., (2004) MINMAX Optimal Video Summarization, Proceedings of Int'l Workshop on Image Analysis for Multimedia Interactive Services (WIAMIS), Lisboa, Portugal.
21. Lienhart, R. (2001) Reliable Transition Detection in Videos: A Survey and Practioner's Guide. International Journal of Image and Graphics, Vol.1, No.3, pp. 469-486.
22. Loeve, M. (1948) Fonctions aldatories de seconde ordre, Hermann, Paris.
23. Qi, Yanjun, Hauptmann, A., and Liu, T., (2003) Supervised Classification for Video Shot, Proceedings of Int'l Conference on Multimedia and Expo, Baltimore, USA
24. Luenberger, D. G. (1969) Optimization by Vector Space Methods, John Wiley and Sons, Inc., New York.
25. Ramchandran, K., and Vetterili, M., (1993) Best wavelet packet bases in a rate-distortion sense, IEEE Trans. Image Processing, vol. 2.
26. Ramchandran, K., Oretega, A., and Vetterili , M. (1994) Bit Allocation for dependent quantization with applications to multi-resolution and MPEG video coders, IEEE Trans. Image Processing, vol. 3.
27. Oretega, A., and Ramchandran K., (1998) Rate-distortion methods for image and video compression, IEEE Signal Processing Magazine, vol. 15 No. 6.
28. Saul, L. K., and Roweis, S. T., (2003) Think Globally, Fit Locally: Unsupervised Learning of Low Dimensional Manifolds. Journal of Machine Learning Research 4, pp 119-155.
29. Shoham, Y., and Gesho, A. (1988) Efficient bit allocation for an arbitrary set of quantizers, IEEE Trans. on Acoustics, Speech and Signal Processing, vol. 36, pp. 1445-1453.
30. Schuster, G. M., and Katsaggelos, A. K., (1997) Rate-Distortion Based Video Compression, Optimal Video Frame Compression and Object Boundary Encoding. Norwell, MA: Kluwer.
31. Schuster, G. M., Melnikov, G., and Katsaggelos, A. K., (1999) A Review of the Minimum Maximum Criterion for Optimal Bit Allocation Among Dependent Quantizers, IEEE Trans. on Multimedia, vol. 1.
32. Sullivan, G. J., and Wiegand, T., (1998) Rate-distortion optimization for video compression, IEEE Signal Processing Magazine, vol. 15.
33. Sundaram, H., and Chang, S.-F., (2001) Constrained Utility Maximization for Generating Visual Skims, IEEE Workshop on Content-Based Access of Image & Video Library.
34. University of British Columbia, H.263 Reference Software Model: TMN8.
35. Viterbi, A. J., (1967) Error Bounds for Convolutional Codes and an Asymptotically Optimum Decoding Algorithm, IEEE Trans. on Information Theory, April, vol. IT-13, pp. 260-269.
36. Wang, Y., Liu, Z., and Huang, J-C. (2000) Multimedia Content Analysis. IEEE Signal Processing Magazine, vol. 17.
37. Zhuang, Y., Rui, Y., Huang, T. S., and Mehrotra, S. (1998) Adaptive Key Frame Extracting Using Unsupervised Clustering, Proc. of Int'l Conference on Image Processing, Chicago, Illinois.

Video Compression by Neural Networks

Daniele Vigliano, Raffaele Parisi, and Aurelio Uncini

INFOCOM Department, University of Rome "La Sapienza" – Rome, Italy

Abstract. In this chapter a general overview of most common approaches to video compression is first provided. Standardization issues are briefly discussed and most recent neural compression techniques reviewed. In addition, a particularly effective novel neural paradigm is introduced and described. The new approach is based on a proper quad-tree segmentation of video frames and is capable to yield a considerable improvement with respect to existing standards in high quality video compression. Experimental tests are described to demonstrate the efficacy of the proposed solution.

Keywords: neural networks, cellular networks, fuzzy systems, MPEG standards, recurrent neural networks

1 Introduction

"A picture is worth a thousand words". This popular saying well synthesizes the different weight between visual and textual or linguistic information in everyday's life. As a matter of fact, visual information has reached a primary and undisputed role in modern Information and Communication Technology. In particular, the widespread diffusion of telecommunications and networking offers today new opportunities to the transmission and processing of multimedia data. Nevertheless, the transmission of highly informative video contents imposes strict requirements in terms of bandwidth occupancy. A trade-off between quality and compression is thus searched for.

Compression of video data aims at minimizing the number of bits required to represent each frame image in a video stream. Video compression has a huge number of applications in several fields, from telecommunications, to remote sensing, to medicine. Depending on the application, some distortion can be accepted in exchange for a higher compression ratio. This is the case of so-called lossy compression schemes. In other cases (e.g. biomedical applications), distortion is not allowed (lossless coding schemes).

Video compression techniques have been classified into four main classes: waveform, object-based, model-based and fractal coding techniques [45].

Waveform compression techniques use time as a third dimension. Into this class one can find all the applications working in the time domain (e.g. Discrete cosine transform, Wavelets and also Motion compensation techniques [58][53]). *Object-based techniques* consider video sequences as collections of different objects [62], which can be differently processed. Objects are typically extracted by a segmentation step [44]. *Model-based* approaches perform the analysis of the video input and the synthesis of a structural 2D or 3D model [66]. *Fractal-based techniques* extend to video applications the approaches successfully applied to image coding. In this framework images are expressed as the attractor of a contractive function system and then retrieved by iterating the set of functions [73]. Correspondingly, several standards have been also developed.

In recent years there has been a tremendous growth of interest in the use of neural networks (NNs) for video coding. This interest is justified by the well-known capabilities of NNs of performing complex input-output nonlinear mappings, in a *learning from examples* fashion. As a matter of fact, appropriate use of NNs can considerably improve the performance of all the four compression techniques above described.

This chapter is organized as follows. Section 2 provides a short description of most recent standards in video compression. Section 3 presents an overview of most popular neural approaches to video coding, while Section 4 describes two innovative and particularly effective solutions.

2 Review of Recent Standards

Compression of image and video data has been the object of intensive research in the past twenty years. The diffusion of a large number of compression algorithms has led to the definition of several standards. In particular, two international organizations (ISO/IEC and ITU-T) have been involved in the standardization of images, audio and video data. A complete overview of recent standards and trends in visual information compression is out of the scope of this work and can be found in [45][51][52]. A brief summary is provided here for convenience of description.

The standards proposed for general purpose compression of still images are JPEG [46][47], based on a block discrete cosine transform (DCT) followed by Huffman or Arithmetic coding, and the more recent JPEG2000 [48]-[50], based on discrete wavelet transform and EBCOT coding.

Concerning video compression, ITU H.261 suggests the use of hybrid schemes in order to reduce spatial redundancy by DCT and temporal correlation by motion compensated prediction coding [53]. This approach was designed and optimized for videoconference transmission over an ISDN channel, for a bit rate down to 64 kbit/sec.

H.263 [56] and H.263+ [54] have the same core architecture of H.261 but introduce improvements principally in the precision of motion compensation and in prediction. These standards allow for the transmission of audio video information at a very low bit rate (9.6 kbit/sec).

Most recent advances in video coding aim at developing improved standards by exploiting all the suitable features previously used in video compression. An example is H.26L [77][55].

The first studies of the Moving Picture Expert Group (MPEG) started in 1988. They aim at developing new standards for Audio-Video Coding. The main difference with respect to the other standards is that MPEGs are "open standards", in the sense that they are not oriented to a particular application.

MPEG-1 was developed to operate at bit rates of up to about 1.5Mbit/sec for the consumer video coding and video content storing on media like CD ROM, DAT. It provides important features including frame-based random access of video, fast forward/fast reverse (FF/FR) searches through compressed bit streams, reverse playback of video and editability of the compressed bit stream. MPEG-1 performs the compression by using several algorithms, such as the subsampling of video information to match the human visual system (HVS), variable length coding, motion compensation and DCT to reduce the temporal and spatial redundancy [57]-[59].

MPEG-2 is similar to MPEG-1 but it includes some extensions to cover a wider range of applications (e.g. HDTV and multi-channel audio coding). It was designed to operate at a bit rate between 1.5 and 35 Mb/sec. One of the main enhancements of MPEG-2 with respect to MPEG-1 is the introduction of syntactical rules for efficient coding of interlaced video. The Advanced Audio Coding (AAC) is one of the formats defined in the non back-compatible version of MPEG-2. It was developed to specifically perform multichannel audio coding. MPEG-2 AAC is based on the MPEG-2 layer III, where some aspects were improved (frequency resolution, joint stereo coding, Huffman coding) and some others (like spectral and time prediction) were introduced. The resulting standard is able to perform the coding of five audio channels [60][61].

Object-oriented techniques extensively developed in computer science have been successfully applied to video compression, leading to MPEG-4. In this standard the video signal can be considered as composed by different objects, each one with its own shape, motion and texture representation. Objects are coded independently, in order to allow for direct access and manipulation. The power of this coding approach is that different objects can be coded by different algorithms, with different compression rates. This approach is justified by the fact that in a video sequence different parts of the scene may accept different distortion levels. The original video is divided into streams: audio and video streams are separated and each object has its own stream, e.g. the information about object placement, scaling and motion (Binary Format of Scene).

Furthermore, in MPEG-4 synthetic and natural sounds are coded in a different way. In fact the Synthetic Natural Hybrid Coding (SNHC) performs the composition of natural compressed audio and of synthetic sounds (artificial sounds are created in real time by the decoder). In addition, MPEG-4 proposes also the distinction between speech and "non speech" sounds, since the former can be compressed by specific *ad hoc* techniques [62]-[65].

In modern information and communication technology, a fundamental issue is to guarantee that the information content of a message can be easily accessed and handled by the user. MPEG-7 (also named "Multimedia Content Description Tool") provides a rich set of tools performing the description of audio-video contents in a multimedia environment. The application areas that benefit from audio-video content description are multiple, from web search of multimedia contents to media broadcasting, from services in arts (e.g. in art galleries) to home entertainment, to database (of multimedia data) applications [67]-[70]. Descriptions provided by MPEG-7 are independent of the compression method and have to be meaningful just in the context of the considered application. For this reason different types of features perform different abstraction levels.

More specifically, the MPEG-7 standard consists of several parts. In this section Multimedia Description Schemes, the Visual description tool and the Audio description tool are detailed. Multimedia Description Schemes (DSs) are metadata structures used to describe audio-visual contents. It is defined by the Description Definition Language (DDL), based on XML. Resulting descriptions can be expressed in a text form (TeM) or in a binary compressed form (BiT). The former one allows for human reading and editing, the latter one improves the efficiency in storing and transmission. In this framework, tools are developed to provide DSs with information about the content and the creation of the multimedia document, and DSs to improve the browsing and the access to the audio-visual content. The Visual description tool performs the description of visual categories like colour, textures, motion, localization, shape and face recognition. The Audio description tool contains low level tools (e.g. spectral and temporal audio feature descriptions) and high-level specialized tools (like musical instrument timbre description, melody description, speech tools and those for the recognition and indexing of general sounds). The MPEG-7 standard provides also an application to represent the multimedia content description named "Terminal". It is important to underline that the Terminal takes care of both the ingoing and the outgoing transmissions, also taking into account specific queries from the end user.

MPEG standards aim at processing multimedia contents in a physical and in a semantic context (MPEG-7), but they do not address other issues like multimedia consumption, diffusion, copyright, access or management rights. MPEG-21 was introduced with the explicit goal of overcoming this limitation, by providing new solutions to access, consumption, delivery, management and protection processes of different types of contents. MPEG-21 is essentially based on two concepts: Digital Item and Users. The Digital Item (DI) represents the fundamental unit of distribution and transaction (e.g. video collections, music albums); it is modelled by Digital Item Declaration (DID), which is a set of abstract terms and concepts. A User is every entity (e.g. humans, communities, society) interacting with the MPEG-21 environment or making use of Digital Items. Management of Digital Items is permitted only to a restricted set of Users [71][72].

3 Neural Video Compression: Existing Approaches

The purpose of this section is to provide a summary of most popular neural approaches to video compression. In recent years, in fact, NNs have been successfully applied to video compression, for example in intra-frame coding schemes, object clustering, motion estimation and object segmentation. The power of NNs as learning systems has also been exploited to remove artifacts and in post processing.

An important issue in video compression is computational complexity, since more complex algorithms usually require more expensive hardware implementations. As a matter of fact, the parallel architecture of NNs allows one to considerably reduce the computational cost with respect to more conventional approaches. This is one of the reasons of the success of neural video coding techniques.

The following sections will focus on some of the most representative neural approaches to video compression, namely those based on vector quantization, singularity maps and human vision, motion compensation and fuzzy segmentation.

3.1 Vector Quantization

Vector quantization (VQ) is a very popular and efficient method for frame image (or still image) compression and it represents the natural extension of scalar quantization to n-dimensional spaces [17]-[19].

Fig. 1 shows a conceptual scheme of a VQ coder. Input vectors are quantized to the closest codeword of the codebook, so the coder's output is the index of the selected codeword. Codebooks are generated from a set of training images by using clustering algorithms. For example in [20] this optimization problem is approached by a Kohonen neural network having the same number of neurons as the number of pixels in a block (self organizing feature maps, SOFM). The number of clusters (output neurons) is set to the desired number of codewords.

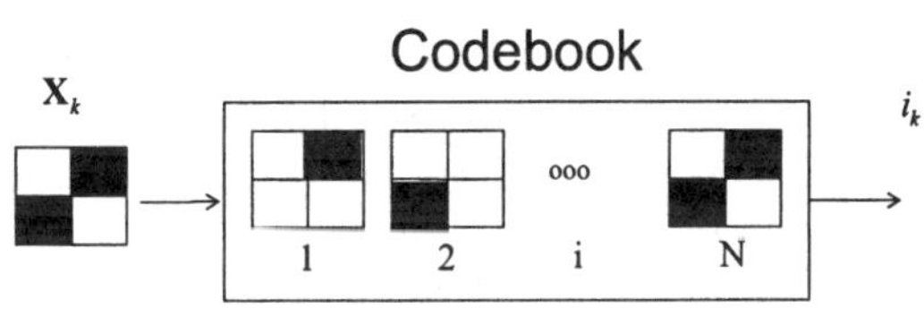

Fig. 1. Scheme of a VQ coder

Learning is based on evaluation of the minimum distance between outputs and inputs. The winner is the neuron having the smallest distance.

The advantages of using SOFM with respect to other clustering algorithms (k-means, LBG) include lower sensitivity to initialization, better performance in terms of rate distortion and faster convergence. In addition, during learning SOFM updates not only the winning class but also the neighboring one, since neurons unlikely to win are less frequently used.

For more details about general motivations justifying the use of SOFM in codebook design see [20]-[22]. Specific properties of SOFM can be used in performing more efficient codebook design, examples are APVQ (Adaptive Prediction VQ), FSVQ (Finite State VQ) and HVQ (Hierarchical VQ).

APVQ uses ordered codebooks where correlated inputs are quantized in adjacent codewords; an improvement in coding gain is obtained by encoding such codebook index with a DPCM (or some other neural predictor) [23].

FSVQ [24][27] introduces some form of memory in static VQ. It defines states by using previously encoded vectors. In each state the encoder selects a subset of codewords of the global codebook, the Side Match FSVQ [29], in which the current state of the coder is given by the closest side of the upper and left neighbouring vectors (i.e. the block of the frame image).

In order to reduce the computational cost, hierarchical structures can also be employed. In literature several techniques based on the cascade of multiple VQ encoders are described. Examples are two layer architectures or hierarchical structures [27] based on topological information [26].

Finally, in the VQ framework other neural approaches use a combination of different algorithms. As an example, [28] proposed neural principal component analysis (PCA) to generate the inputs to a SOFM.

3.2 Singularity Maps and Human Vision

Emulation of the human vision system (HVS) inspired several solutions to video compression, yielding low compression ratios (about 1000:1) [30]-[32]. Due to its physiological nature, human eye does not focus on each single pixel of an image or a video stream but more on aspects like edges or intensity changes.

The retina in the human eye has two kinds of receptors: rods and cones. Rods are used for monochromatic light and cones for colours (RGB). Each receptor fires when it receives light, at the same time inhibiting nearby receptors. This behaviour is known as "lateral inhibition" and inspired some artificial neural architectures. For this reason the eye is able to detect edges better than smooth surfaces. Transmission through the optical nerve suffers from dispersion, so edges are smoothed and borders are broadened.

A Singularity Map (SM) [30]-[32] is obtained by labelling, with topological index and greyscale correspondence, the singular point of the border of the frame image. By this way the whole edge can be transmitted as a sequence instead of as an image. In practice, an SM collects all the multiresolution edges of a frame image. The extraction process requires a special care since ordinary edge extractors (like Sobel) typically broaden edges.

A typical HVS-based algorithm is composed by two main parallel steps:

- very low bit rate compression performed with a method that does not produce artifacts;
- singularity map (SM) computed from the original video, before the compression.

The second step corresponds to the application of singularity map on compressed frames. A block scheme of the proposed technique is shown in Fig. 2. Application of SM improves the performance with respect to more conventional video compression techniques (upper path in Fig. 2).

The algorithm performs two types of singularity maps: hard SM for daylight video sequences and soft SM for nightlight video sequences. In addition this approach takes into account the presence of noise in the original video sequence, because it is able to perform a more difficult estimation of singularity map.

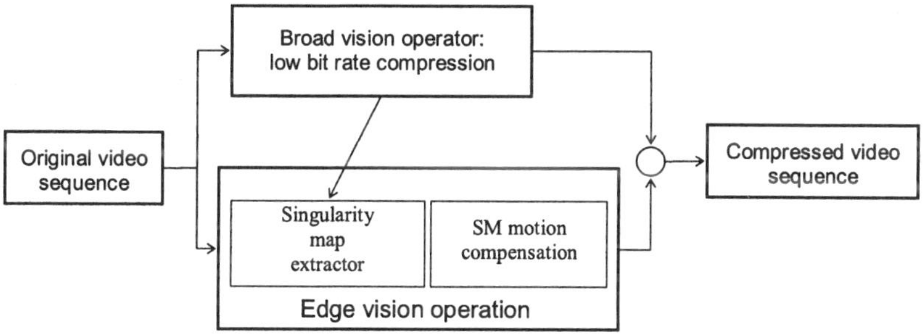

Fig. 2. Block scheme of HVS-based compressor

For hard SM iterative min-max was proposed, while soft SM can be performed by Cellular Neural Networks (CNNs), which can extract sharp edges in real time [31].

Once SM is computed, very low bit rate video compression is achieved by using Embedded Predictive Wavelet Image Coding (EPWIC [33]), Embedded Zerotrees of Wavelet coefficients (EZW [34]) or other wavelet-based compression techniques.

3.3 Motion Compensation

Motion compensation (MC) is one of the most powerful techniques that can be used to reduce temporal correlation between adjacent frames. It is based on the assumption that in a large number of applications adjacent frames are usually highly correlated. Temporal correlation can be reduced by coding a block in a frame as a translated version of a block in a preceding frame. Of course the motion vector has to be transmitted too. In the following only translational motion will be considered.

Frames are typically segmented in macroblocks of 16x16 pixels, made of 4 blocks of 8x8 pixels (a reduced block representation error is obtained with finer segmentation but it produces a computational overhead). Fig. 3 shows how in coding the block in frame *k*, the "best match block" of previous frame is computed and then the representation error is coded together with the information of the "motion vector".

Several methods have been investigated in order to reduce the estimation error and to speed up the search for the best match. In particular, predictive methods perform the matching only in the direction of previous frames, while bidirectional methods consider also future frames (bidirectional estimation).

In [35] a Hopfield neural algorithm is proposed to perform hierarchical motion estimation. It uses a classical best match method in order to reduce the number of possible macroblocks. Once obtained a subset of D candidates, a Hopfield network is used to obtain the best *vector of affinities* $\mathbf{v}$. The optimal affinity vector $\mathbf{v}$ is the one minimizing the function:

$$\frac{1}{2}\|\mathbf{f}-\mathbf{G}\mathbf{v}\|^2=\frac{1}{2}\sum_{p=1}^{L^2}\left(f_p-\sum_{i=1}^{D}g_{p,i}v_i\right) \tag{1}$$

In (1) **f** is the vector of the current block to be estimated, **G** is a matrix whose columns are the D candidate blocks, **v** is the affinity vector (i.e. the one selecting the best match block) and L^2 denotes the size of the search windows. The architecture of the neural network performing the vector optimization is shown in Fig. 4.

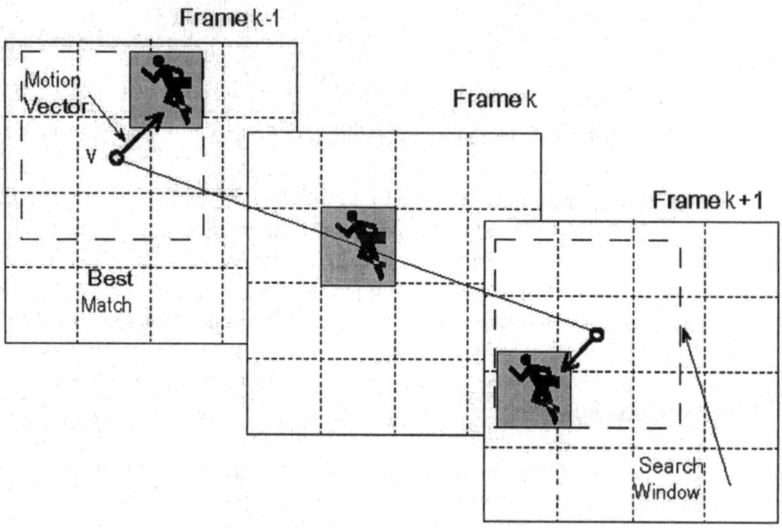

Fig. 3. Motion Compensation

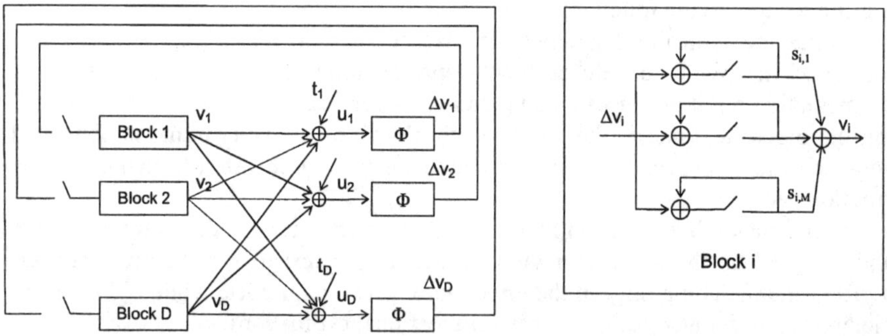

Fig. 4. Hopfield neural network for motion estimation

Other approaches to motion estimation include cellular neural networks (CNNs) [36]-[39][76]. These architectures can parallelize the computational flow required by both motion estimation and compensation, yielding faster and scalable computations. CNNs perform an optimization process based on their capacity to evolve toward a global minimum state.

Fig. 5 shows the cell architecture of the network described in [36]. Cells are located in a $N \times M$ array; the generic cell C_{ij} has a state x_{ij}, a constant external input u_{ij} and an output y_{ij} and has r neighbor cells.

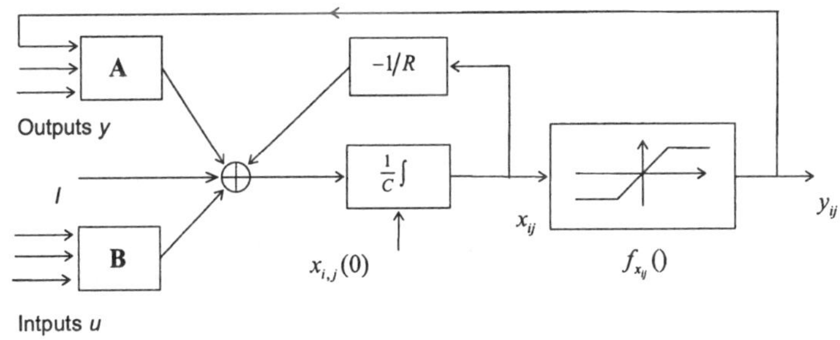

Fig. 5. Block diagram of cell C_{ij} of the Cellular Neural Network proposed in [36]

It is a graphical representation of the following difference equation:

$$C\dot{x}_{ij}(t) = -\frac{x_{ij}(t)}{R} + \sum_{k,l} A_{i,j;k,l}\, y_{kl}(t) + \sum_{k,l} B_{i,j;k,l}\, u_{kl}(t) + I \tag{2}$$

where C and R conform the integration time constant of the system, I is a constant scalar bias, **A** and **B** are $(2r+1)\times(2r+1)$ matrices; $A_{i,j;k,l}$ is the element k, l of the matrix **A** of the cell C_{ij}.

The dynamics of the CNN networks are described by a system of nonlinear ordinary differential equation (2) and by an energy function minimized during the computation process.

In [36] motion estimation is based on maximization of the *a-posteriori* probability (MAP) of the scene random field given the random motion field realization. It is possible to find similarity between MAP and CNN energy function.

For the scope of this section it is enough to consider that MAP may be interpreted in terms of CNN architecture: feedforward input terms originate from matrix **B**, and recurrent terms from the feedback matrix **A**. More details about the algorithm, stability and network design can be found in [36][37][40].

The capability of distributed computation, based on the parallel structure of CNNs, is exploited also in other contexts. For example, in [38][39] CNNs perform fast and distributed operation on frame images. The following mathematical formulation is used:

$$\begin{aligned}\dot{x}_{ij}(t) = x_{ij}(t) + \sum_{k,l} A_{i,j;k,l}\, y_{kl} + \sum_{k,l} B_{i,j;k,l}\, u_{kl} + \\ + \sum_{k,l} \hat{A}_{i,j;k,l}(y_{kl}) + \sum_{k,l} \hat{B}_{i,j;k,l}(u_{kl}) + I_{ij}\end{aligned} \tag{3}$$

The cell architecture is similar to the one described in Fig. 5 adding nonlinear feedforward and nonlinear feedback blocks represented respectively by $\hat{B}_{i,j;k,l}(y_{kl})$

and $\hat{A}_{i,j;k,l}(y_{kl})$. Motion compensation aims at determining what objects inside frame I_{n+k} are present also in frame I_n. Considering frame $n+k$, object positions in previous frame n are estimated by moving each object of frame n in a $p \times q$ -pixel window and comparing the result with the frame I_{n+k}.

Motion search is performed by following a "spiral" trajectory. All the processing is performed by the CNN, whose parameters (such as $\mathbf{A}$, $\mathbf{B}$, $\hat{\mathbf{A}}$, $\hat{\mathbf{B}}$, $\mathbf{x}$, $\mathbf{I}$, $\mathbf{u}$, $\mathbf{y}$) are preliminarily set to proper values in order to obtain the desired effect.

3.4 Neuro Fuzzy Segmentation of Human Image Sequences

In order to achieve better compression ratios, modern video coding techniques apply different schemes to different objects in the same video stream (*object-based compression*). The advantages of using different compression techniques for different objects are strictly tied to the capability of identifying and extracting the objects from the background. Classical tools for the generation of region-based representations are discussed in [44], where the state of art of this class of approaches is also described.

In [41] spatial and temporal information are combined to perform a neuro-fuzzy video segmentation of a videoconference video stream (one human speaker and background). The approach consists of three main steps: 1) clustering, 2) detection, and 3) refinement.

In the first step a fuzzy self-clustering algorithm is used to group into fuzzy clusters similar pixels in the base frame of the video stream. Each frame image is divided into 4x4 pixel blocks, which are grouped in segments by the clustering algorithm. Segments are then combined together in order to form larger clusters. Each cluster is represented by Gaussian membership functions (one for the luminance and one for each chrominance), with a given mean value and variance.

After fuzzy clustering is completed, the detection step starts. In this step human face and body (i.e. "human objects") are detected and extracted from the background. Face segments are easily identified since they are characterized by chrominance values within a restricted range and luminance values having consistent variations. Once the area containing the face has been identified, the rest of body is assumed to lay in the area below the face.

On the basis of such analysis, clusters can be divided into foreground, background and ambiguous regions. A fuzzy neural network is employed to identify the ambiguous regions. The architecture of the network is shown in Fig. 6. Its operations are explained as follows.

Each pixel of each cluster yields three inputs x_1, x_2, x_3, which are the values of luminance and chrominances. The output of the network will be 1 if the cluster (or the pixel) is completely contained in the human object and 0 otherwise. The network layers are designed in the following way:

- *Layer 1*. The *input layer* contains the three inputs, which are directly transmitted to the next layer.

- *Layer 2*. The *fuzzification layer* contains *N* groups of three neurons each, where *N* is the number of fuzzy clusters. The output is computed as a Gaussian function: $o_{ij}^{(2)} = \exp\left[-\left(\frac{o_i^{(1)} - m_{ij}}{\sigma_{ij}}\right)^2\right]$ where m_{ij}, and σ_{ij} are proper learning parameters.
- *Layer 3*. The *inference layer* contains *N* neurons. The output of each neuron is $o_j^{(3)} = \prod_{i=1}^{3} o_{ij}^{(2)}$.
- *Layer 4*. The *output layer* contains only one neuron, which performs the centroid *defuzzification*. Its output is: $o^{(4)} = \frac{\sum_{j=1}^{N} c_j o_j^{(3)}}{\sum_{j=1}^{N} o_j^{(3)}}$.

Parameters (m_{ij}, σ_{ij}, c_i) are trained from foreground and background blocks. The training algorithm is a combination of an SVD-based least-squares estimator and gradient-based optimization (hybrid learning).

Other approaches to fuzzy neural segmentation are based on fuzzy clustering of more complex data structures. Data include both intra-frame information such as colour, shape, texture and contour, and inter-frame information, such as motion and object temporal shape.

In [42] good segmentation results are obtained by a two-step decomposition. The first step splits the image in subsets by using an unsupervised neural network. The frame image is then divided into clusters. The hierarchical clustering phase reduces the complexity of the object structure. Finally a PCA-based processing performs the refinement step, providing the final foreground-background segmentation.

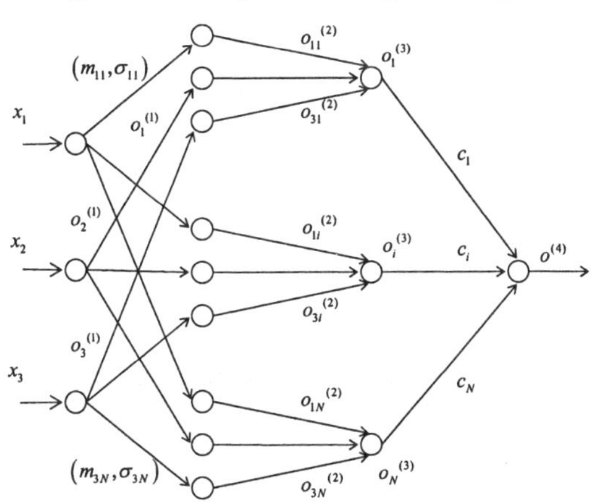

Fig. 6. Architecture of the fuzzy neural network for human object refinement

Other approaches are based on a subspace representation of the video sequence [43]. In this case video sequences are described by the minimum set of maximally distant frames that are able to describe the video sequence (*key frames*), selected on the basis of their semantic content. These frames are collected in a codebook. The core of the coding system is the video keyframe codebook (VKC) definition, which is based on video analysis in the *vector space*. This definition is performed by an unsupervised neural network, through a *storyboarding* of the recorded sequence. Image feature vectors are used to represent images into the vector space. Clustering of all images in the feature vector space is employed to select the smaller set of video key frames for VKC definition.

4 Quad-tree Segmentation and Neural Compression

The following sections describe in detail two *waveform* video compression algorithms, based on the use of feedforward and locally recurrent neural networks.

Techniques described so far were based on generalization of methods used for the compression of still images [75]. In particular, *transform coding* techniques achieve the desired compression by introducing proper transformations of images [51]. More specifically, given the set of coefficients representing a portion of an image or a video frame, transform coding produces a reduced set of coefficients such that reconstruction of the original image produces the minimum possible distortion. This reduction is possible since most of the initial block energy is concentrated in a reduced number of coefficients.

The optimal transform coder, in the sense of the minimum mean square error, is the one minimizing the mean-square distortion of the reconstructed data for a fixed quantization. In particular, the well-known Karhunen-Loève transform fulfils this constraint.

In the framework of video compression, techniques used for still images can be applied jointly with a temporal decomposition, thus calling for proper space-time processing. The following sections describe an effective video preprocessing technique and a feasible and particularly attractive solution to the design of neural transform coders.

4.1 Video preprocessing

Still images usually contain uniformly coloured areas, with poor informative content, and highly detailed areas. Different compression schemes can be adopted on areas with different activity levels, thus providing a better quality on detailed areas, and higher compression ratios on more uniform areas.

Frame images are decomposed in blocks that are individually processed. In particular, higher activity blocks can be extracted on the basis of their orientation: horizontal, vertical, diagonal. Blocks are then divided into subclasses and coded with different coders, in order to improve the performance of the compression [14]-[16].

Several papers described this kind of approach. Very good performance were obtained in [15], where blocks were grouped according to nine possible orientations: two horizontal (one darker on the left, one darker on the right), two vertical, four diagonal and the last shaded.

Fig. 7 shows a picture splitted in blocks of different size by means of a *quad-tree* approach, based on a measure of the pixels' variance: the bigger is the dimension of the block, the lower is the content detail, and vice versa.

Blocks having the same mask size carry about the same information and are processed by the same neural network, requiring specific training sets.

In video sequences, areas can be segmented also on the basis of changes in images, thus identifying sub-sequences where limited action takes place. Useful video representation can be obtained by identifying adjacent frames with reduced dissimilarities (group of frames, GOF). Each GOF collects frames having the same Depth of Activity (*DA*), by comparison of a pre-set threshold *th* with the variance between pixels of several adjacent frames. These frames have the same quad-tree segmentation structure.

The choice of the proper threshold is a critical issue in determining the *DA*. Higher values of the threshold yield lower quality of the reconstructed video, since frames are not represented by their own quad-tree structure. On the other hand, too low values of the threshold yield better quality but higher bit rate.

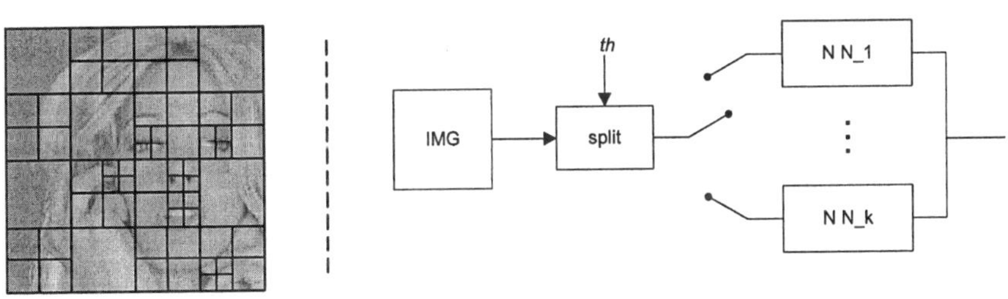

a) b)

Fig. 7. a) Quad-tree segmentation; b) Adaptive size mask splitting block

The GOF generation algorithm consists of the following steps (Fig. 8):

1. the first frame (keyframe) is selected as a reference image of the *i*-th GOF;
2. a subsequent frame *n* belongs to the *i*-th GOF if the variance of the image difference between frame *n* and the keyframe is below *th*. The number of frames for which this condition is verified gives the *DA*, i.e. the length of the identified sub-sequence;
3. the final extracted sub-sequence consists of the keyframe *I* and the frames obtained by subtracting each subsequent frame to the keyframe (*D*-frames).

Images contained in every GOF are coded by a set of properly trained neural networks. The keyframe *I* and the last frame of the GOF *D1* will be coded with a fitted *quad-tree* structure, as shown in Fig. 9. For each sub-block of the keyframe *I* and of the frame *D1* in addition to the compressed data it is necessary to code also the quad-tree segmentation, the network used for coding the sub-block, the sub-block mean value, the quantization and finally the number of frames internal to the GOF.

Sub-blocks of *D2* (the residual frames of the GOF) only require information about the compressed data, since they have the same segmentation of *D1*.

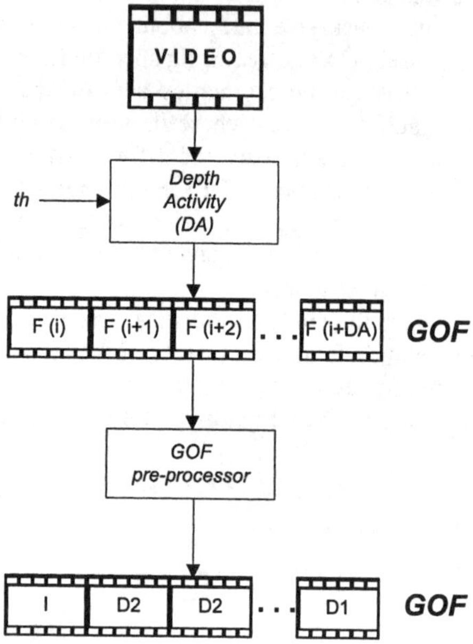

Fig. 8. Group of frames generation

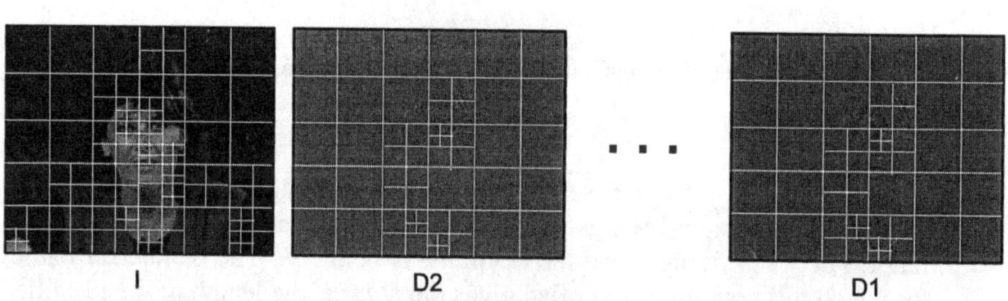

Fig. 9. Quad-tree schemes applied to frames within the GOF

The advantage of using the *D2* frames lies in the fact that frames near to *D1* have the same quad-tree segmentation structure (Fig. 9). In addition, these images are mostly made of uniform areas, so that the mask applied will be principally constituted by large blocks (e.g. 16×16), thus reducing the bit rate. Fig. 10 presents an overall scheme of the proposed approach.

The video preprocessor, given the original video stream, establishes the value of the *DA*. The GOF preprocessor computes the differences between frames, while the controller selects the keyframe and frames *D1* and *D2*, to be segmented in different ways.

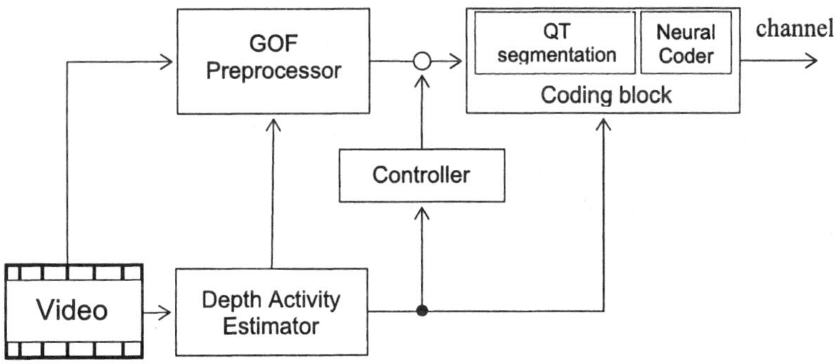

Fig. 10. Scheme of the proposed neural quad-tree video coding

4.2 Feed-forward Neural Compressor

Once segmentation has been performed, the next step is compression of each image block. In the transform coding framework, the Karhunen-Loève transform is commonly exploited to represent signals on the basis of their *principal components*.

In particular, it is possible to use a reduced set of principal components (reduced rank approximation), then obtaining a reconstruction error which depends on the variance of the eigenvalues of discarded eigenvectors. In more detail, given an N-dimensional vector signal $\mathbf{x}$, the Karhunen-Loève transform represents it by using a basis $\mathbf{W}$ formed by the eigenvectors of its autocovariance matrix:

$$\mathbf{y} = \mathbf{W}\mathbf{x} \tag{4}$$

In this case no compression is performed [21]. A reduced rank (i.e. compressed) approximation of $\mathbf{y}$ is obtained by using the M eigenvectors corresponding to the M larger eigenvalues:

$$\hat{\mathbf{y}}=\hat{\mathbf{W}}\mathbf{x} = \sum_{i=1}^{M<N} w_i x \tag{5}$$

The representation error is bounded by the sum of the squared eigenvalues corresponding to the discarded eigenvectors [1]. It can be shown that the output vector coefficients are uncorrelated and therefore the redundancy due to correlation between neighbouring pixels is removed. Unfortunately application of KLT to video compression is not fully effective since it exploits second order statistics only.

The calculation of the estimate of the covariance of an image may be unwieldy and may require a large amount of memory; moreover the eigendecomposition implies a high additional computational cost due to the often large image size. These issues are important since KLT basis must be updated continuously during the video sequence.

A possible alternative to KLT is the discrete cosine transform (performed via FFT), which yields performance similar to KLT [51][45].

Another possible alternative to avoid these problems is the use of iterative neural techniques. Neural approaches require a reduced storage overhead giving a faster and computationally more convenient solution to the compression problem. Moreover neural networks are able to adapt over long-term variations in the frame image statistics 3. In the following, linear and nonlinear PCA are described.

Linear PCA: Hebbian learning

Linear PCA is an efficient solution to eigendecomposition computation. In [2] a mechanism inspired to neurobiology was proposed, where synaptic connections between neurons are modified by learning. Hebb's assumption consists in reinforcing the synaptic connection between two neurons if they are both active at the same time. Fig. 11 shows the architecture of the artificial neuron used to perform the principal component extraction by Hebbian learning .

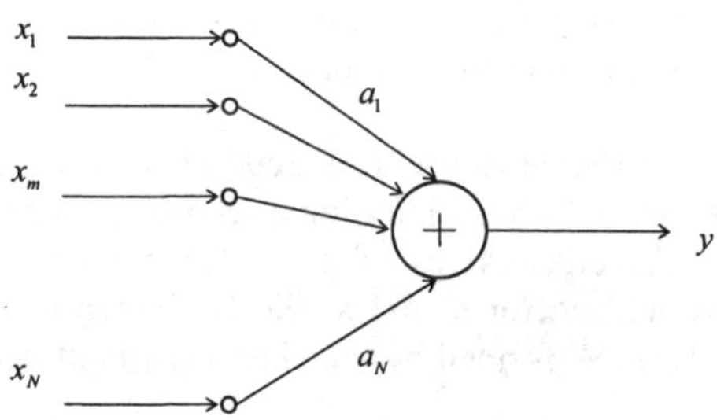

Fig. 11. Hebbian Neuron

The neuron's output is:

$$y = \mathbf{a}\mathbf{x} \tag{6}$$

The Hebbian learning rule is given by the following recursive equation:

$$\mathbf{a}[n+1] = \frac{\mathbf{a}[n] + \mu\mathbf{a}[n]\mathbf{x}[n]}{\left\|\mathbf{a}[n] + \mu\mathbf{a}[n]\mathbf{x}[n]\right\|} \tag{7}$$

where μ is the learning rate and $\|\cdot\|$ is the Euclidean norm. Eq. (7) has been shown to converge to the first principal component.

Hebbian learning can be generalized to find the first M principal components. More specifically, the second principal component can be obtained by removing the first principal component from original data and performing PCA on updated data, and so on. The generalized Hebbian Algorithm includes also orthogonalization:

$$\mathbf{A}[n+1]=\mathbf{A}[n]+\mu\left[\mathbf{y}\mathbf{x}^T-LT\left[\mathbf{y}\mathbf{y}^T\right]\mathbf{A}[n]\right] \quad (8)$$

In (8) LT (i.e. lower triangular) is the matrix operator that sets to zero all the elements above the matrix diagonal. After convergence, matrix **A** contains the first M principal directions. An alternative is the APEX (*Adaptive Principal Component Extraction*) network, where hebbian synapses are used together with anti-hebbian ones.

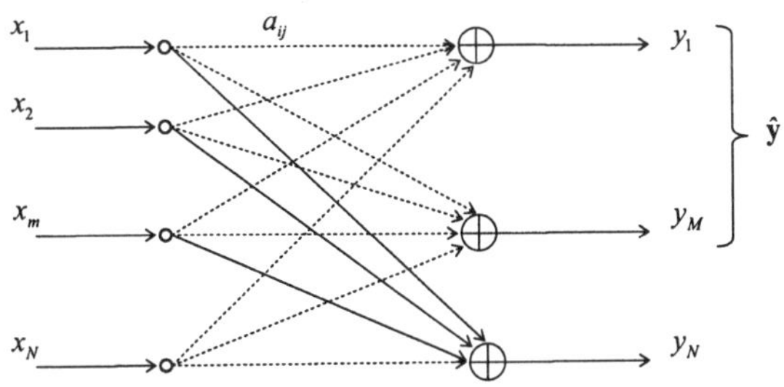

Fig. 12. Linear network for principal component extraction

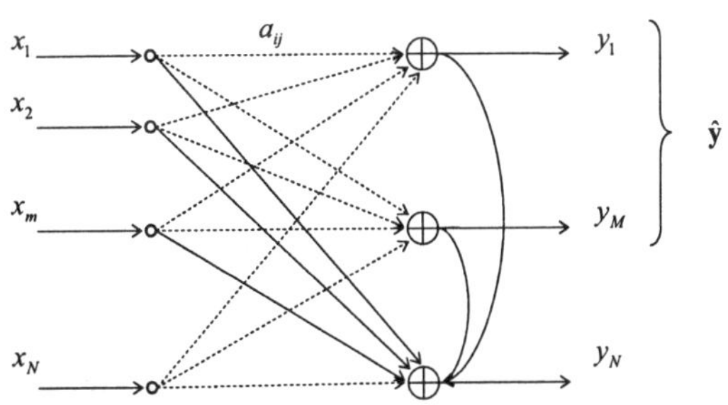

Fig. 13. The APEX network

Also this architecture has a biological justification. The m-th principal component can be computed on the basis of the previous m-1. More details can be found in [74].

Nonlinear PCA: Multilayer Perceptron

In 1988, Cottrel, Murno and Zipper applied a two-layer perceptron to the PCA problem [5]. The net was trained with the so called *autoassociative backpropagation*. This work opened the way to a large number of future developments.

Fig. 14 shows the proposed architecture. In a first formulation a *linear neuron* was used. Its output is:

$$\hat{y}_i = \mathbf{a}^T{}_i\mathbf{x} \tag{9}$$

In matrix formulation:

$$\begin{aligned}\hat{\mathbf{y}} &= \mathbf{A}^T\mathbf{x}\\ \hat{\mathbf{x}} &= \mathbf{A}\hat{\mathbf{y}} = \mathbf{A}\mathbf{A}^T\mathbf{x}\end{aligned} \tag{10}$$

Linear neural networks can achieve the same compression ratio as KLT without necessarily obtaining the same weight matrices of the PCA transform: according to (10) given the optimum PCA solution **A=W**, different optimal solutions can be obtained by $\mathbf{A}=\mathbf{W}\mathbf{Q}^{\mathrm{T}}$, where **Q** is an orthogonal matrix.

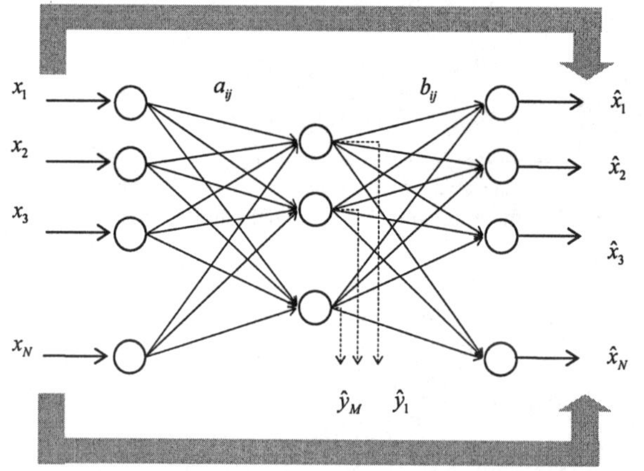

Fig. 14. Multilayer perceptron trained by autoassociative backpropagation

Other approaches developed neural networks with sigmoidal activation functions, yielding better results with respect to the linear network [3][4].

A critical issue in neural PCA is the fixed compression ratio of each processed block: the network performs the compression with a low distortion on uniform blocks but produces higher distortion on less uniform ones.

In order to overcome this problem, size-adaptive networks [6] can be employed to perform compression depending on block activity. This allows for higher compression of blocks with low activity level and good reconstruction of blocks with higher activity level.

As already described, the quad-tree algorithm segments images into several blocks of different size, on the basis of the activity level. An example of segmentation is shown in Fig. 15, where blocks of size 4x4, 8x8 and 16x16 are used.

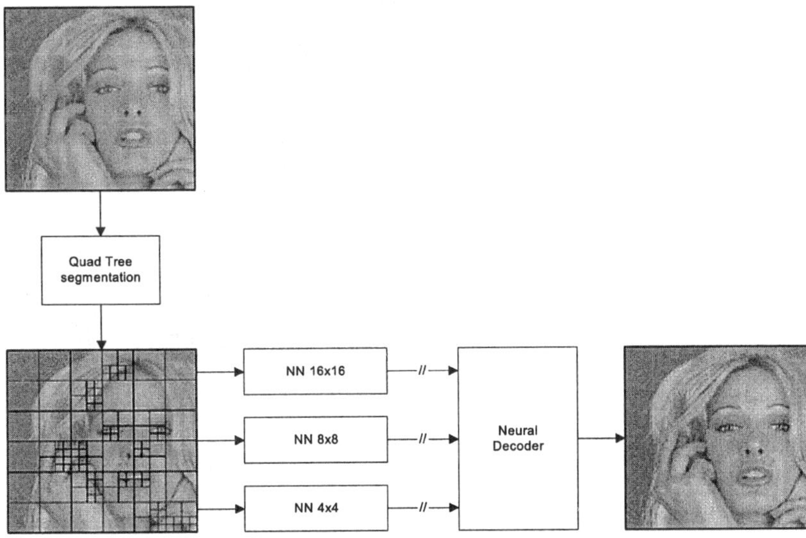

Fig. 15. Adaptive size mask compression of visual information

Three neural architectures were developed. They all have eight hidden neurons, while the number of inputs is equal to the number of pixels in a block. The output of each neuron is quantized with 4 bits.

Learning capabilities were improved by use of adaptable sigmoidal functions. In alternative, spline adaptive models were fruitfully employed [8].

Performance in video compression is usually evaluated on the basis of the peak signal-to-noise ratio (*PSNR*), defined as:

$$PSNR = 10 \cdot \log_{10}\left(\frac{256^2}{\frac{1}{M \times N} \cdot \sum_{m=1}^{M}\sum_{n=1}^{N}\left[pix_{org}(m,n) - pix_{comp}(m,n)\right]^2}\right) \tag{11}$$

where $pix_{org}(m,n)$ is the pixel of the current frame, and $pix_{comp}(m,n)$ is the compressed one and M and N are the frame dimension.

Fig. 16 shows the PSNR values obtained on the 'Missa.avi' benchmark file by processing GOFs with different thresholds.

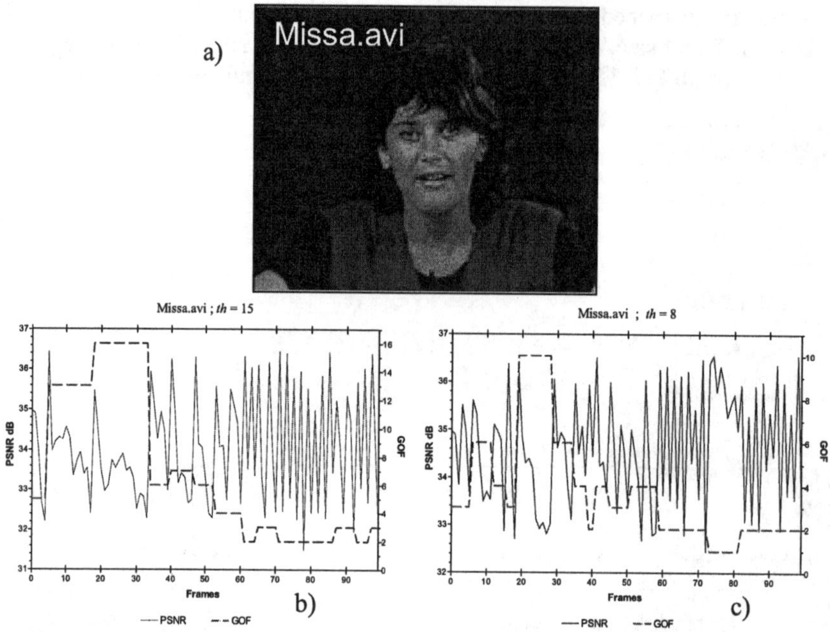

Fig. 16. a) Missa.avi movie segmented and compressed; b-c) PSNR and GOF evolution with two different thresholds

Table 1 shows different PSNR and bit rate values for different thresholds, for the Missa and Susi benchmark movies. It is easy to see that higher thresholds produce a gain in compression but decrease the quality of video reconstruction.

Table 1. Peak signal-to-noise ratio (PSNR) and bit rate (br) for different thresholds in Missa and Susi videos

	th = 8		th = 15		th = 30	
	PSNR (dB)	br (kbps)	PSNR (dB)	br (kbps)	PSNR (dB)	br (kbps)
Missa	34,62	205,63	34,02	166,05	33,02	152,85
Susi	31,11	469,53	30,91	422,31	30,38	361,52

Hierarchical neural networks

As described, multilayer neural nets offer an attractive solution to video compression. Their success is due to several advantages, like short time encoding-decoding and no explicit use of codebooks. Nevertheless only information carried by contiguous pixels within the same segmented block is exploited. Better performance can be obtained by considering information on contiguous blocks.

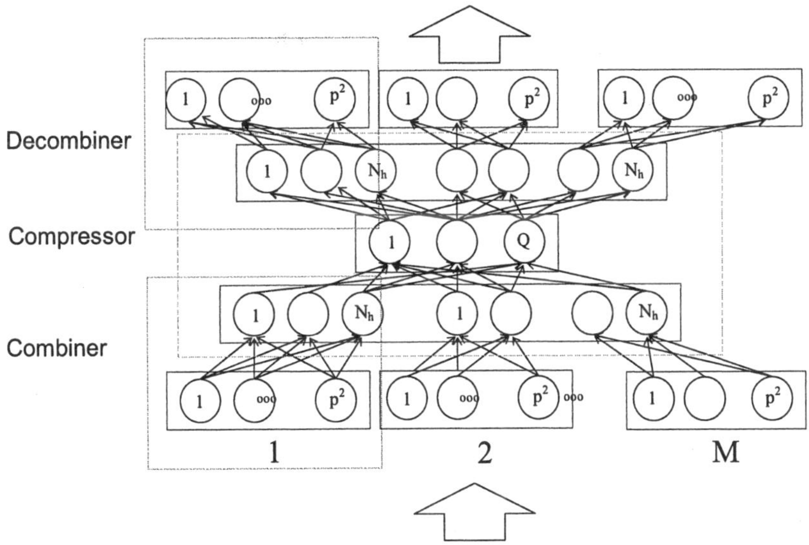

Fig. 17. Multilayer neural network for high order data compression-decompression

Hierarchical neural networks (HNNs) take into account the information about block contiguity [7]. The idea is to divide a scene into N disjoint sub-scenes, each one segmented in $n \times n$ pixels blocks. Blocks are processed together by the hierarchical structure shown in Fig. 17.

The HNN consists of input, hidden and output layers and it is not fully connected. The input and the output layers are single layers, composed by N input blocks (one for each section of the image), where each block has n^2 neurons. The hidden-layer section consists instead of three layers: combiner, compressor and decombiner layer. The connections between the input and combiner layers and between the decombiner and the output layers are not full.

Although learning in HNN could be performed by the classical back propagation algorithm, the so called *nested training algorithm* (NTA) provides better performances. NTA is a three phase training, one for each part of the architecture:

- *OLNN* (outer loop neural network). It performs the training of each fully connected network obtained by the corresponding sub-blocks of input, combiner and output layer. Standard back propagation is applied. The target output is equal to the input. The training set is given by segmented blocks.
- *ILNN* (inner loop neural network). It performs the training of the hidden fully connected layers: combiner, compressor and decombiner.
- Once the *OLNN* and the *ILNN* have been separately trained, their weights are used to construct the overall network.

It is important to note that this hierarchical structure performs inter-block decorrelation in order to achieve a better compression level. About the same performance in terms of image quality and compression level was reached by use of adaptive spline activation functions, yielding a simpler structure.

4.3 Recurrent Neural Compressor

Multilayer neural networks can be properly adapted by introducing topological recurrency, in order to take into account the temporal dependence of video sequences. This allows either to improve the quality of the reconstructed video, for a fixed bit rate, or to further reduce the compression level [78].

Dynamic behavior in multilayer perceptrons can be obtained by two different approaches:

- *Local approach*: a dynamical (e.g. ARMA) model of the neuron is employed.
- *Non local Approach*: external feedback is introduced.

In both cases the dynamical model is such that the input at time *n:* $x[n]$ may influence the output at time *n-h:* $y[n-h]$. In the case of asymptotic stability, the derivative $\partial y[n-h]/\partial x[n]$ goes to zero when h goes to infinity. The value of h for which the derivative becomes negligible is called *temporal depth*, whereas the number of adaptable parameters divided by the temporal depth is named *temporal resolution*.

An example of architecture used in this context is the IIR-MLP proposed in [10][11], where static synapses are replaced by conventional IIR adaptive filters, as depicted in Fig. 18.

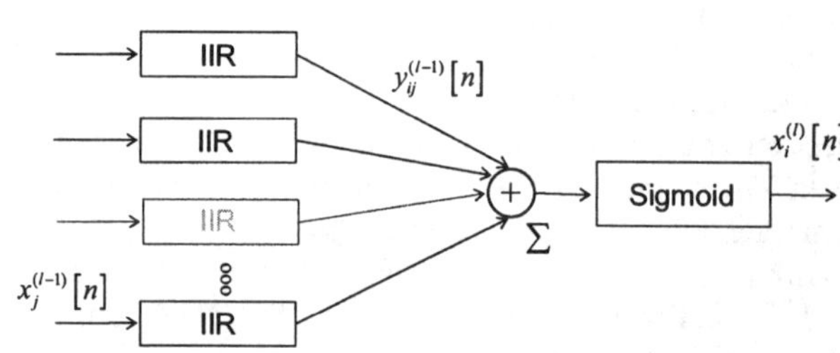

Fig. 18. Locally recurrent neuron for multilayer neural networks

Several learning algorithms for recurrent architectures exist in literature, although a comprehensive framework is still missing. In [9] a very effective algorithm was introduced for learning of locally recurrent neural networks. Learning is performed by a new gradient-based on-line algorithm [9], called causal recursive back-propagation (CRBP). It yields some advantages with respect to known online training methods and the well-known recursive back propagation. CRBP includes backpropagation as a particular case [12][13]. This approach is based on the introduction of an ARMA model of synapses (Fig. 19). The forward phase at time *n* is described by the following equations, evaluated for layers $l = 1,\ldots,M$ and neurons $m = 1,..,N_l$:

$$y_{km}^{(l)}[n] = \sum_{p=0}^{L_{km}^{(l)}-1} w_{km(p)}^{(l)} x_m^{(l-1)}[n-p] + \sum_{p=1}^{I_{km}^{(l)}} v_{km(p)}^{(l)} y_{km}^{(l)}[n-p] \tag{12}$$

$$x_k^{(l)}[n] = sgm\left(\sum_{m=0}^{N_{l-1}} y_{km}^{(l)}[n]\right) \tag{13}$$

where *sgm(.)* is the sigmoidal function. If $\Phi^{(l)}[n]$ is the set of weights of layer *l* at time *n*, the updating rule is:

$$\Phi^{(l)}[n+1] = \Phi^{(l)}[n] + \Delta\Phi^{(l)}[n+1-D_l] \tag{14}$$

where:

$$D_l = \begin{cases} 0 & \text{if } l = M \\ \sum_{i=l+1}^{M} \max_{n,m}\left(L_{nm}^{(i)} - 1\right) & \text{if } 1 \le l \le M \end{cases} \tag{15}$$

and $\left(L_{nm}^{(i)} - 1\right)$ is the order of the moving average part of the synapse of the *n*-th neuron of the *l*-th layer, relative to the *m*-th output of the (*l*-1)-th layer.

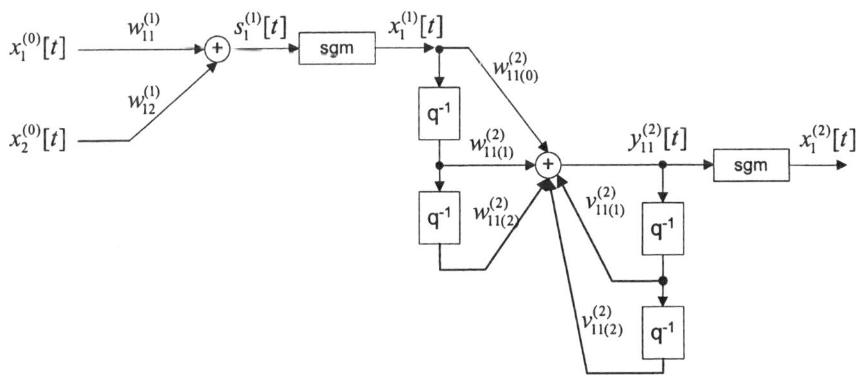

Fig. 19. Locally recurrent ARMA model for multilayer perceptrons

Referring to symbols in Fig. 19, the CRBP learning rules are:

$$\Delta\Phi_{km(p)}^{(l)}[n+1] = \mu e_k^{(l)}[n] sgm\left[s_k^{(l)}[n]\right] \frac{\partial s_k^{(l)}[n]}{\partial \Phi_{km(p)}^{(l)}} \tag{16}$$

$$e_k^{(l)}[n] = \begin{cases} e_k[n] & l = M \\ \sum_{q=1}^{N_{l+1}} \sum_{p=0}^{Q_{l+1}} \delta_q^{(l+1)}[n+p] \frac{\partial y_{qk}^{(l+1)}[n+p]}{\partial x_k^{(l)}[n]} & l = (M-1),...,1 \end{cases} \tag{17}$$

The CRBP algorithm is computationally simple and can be fruitfully applied to the video compression problem. In particular, the proposed architecture was applied as neural coder in the coding block of Fig. 10.

Learning of locally recurrent neural networks for video compression is a critical issue since recurrent networks are typically sensitive to factors like choice of the proper training set, video length, or order by which the examples are presented. An inappropriate choice of these factors might compromise the correct learning of the network, typically producing artifacts in the reconstructed video. Most common artifacts are the so called "*regularities*" and "*memory effect*". An example of "*regularities*" is shown in Fig. 20. They can be avoided by reducing the length of the video training set.

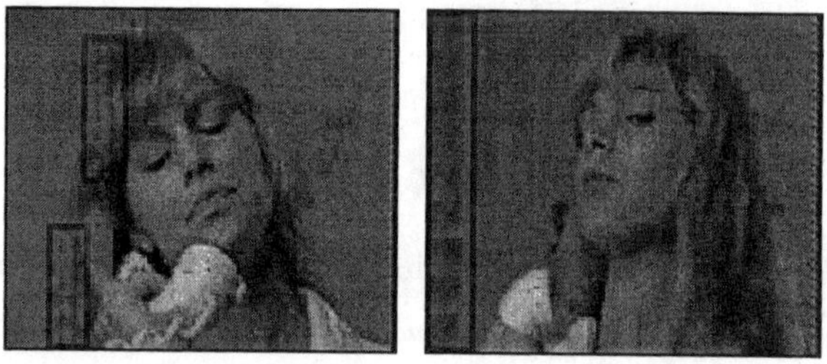

Fig. 20. Regularity effects in two frames of a video sequence

The "*memory effect*" is due to the delay lines in the synapse. It is typically detected by the presence in the reconstructed video of objects that are no longer present in the scene, especially on uniform color backgrounds (Fig. 21). This artifact can be avoided by carefully dimensioning the neuron dynamics and the number of taps of the ARMA filter.

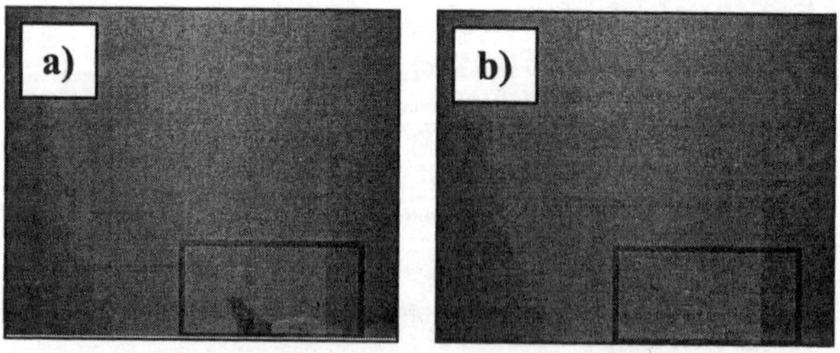

Fig. 21. Memory effect in two frames of a video sequence

Regularities and memory effects can be actually reduced if locally recurrent neurons only in the second layer of the structure of Fig. 14 are used.

It has been observed that most of the artifacts are actually in the "background" of the scene. As a matter of fact, recurrent neural networks perform quite well on dynamical parts while they are not always effective on static background sections.

In order to overcome this limitation, an hybrid approach could be used after the scene segmentation. The idea is to use static neural networks on more static sub-scenes (the ones with the lowest activity), and to employ recurrent neural networks to code blocks with higher levels of detail. This solution requires a different processing for lower and higher activity blocks, in terms of network size, architecture and learning. Table 2 shows the performance typically obtained by a hybrid approach, where IIR synapses are used.

Table 2. Average bit rate and peak signal-to-noise ratio obtained with three different neural architectures

Reconstructed video	Susi_02	Susi_03	Susi_04
No. of hidden neurons	6	5	4
br (kbs)	433,38	372,51	319,32
PSNR (dB)	28,92	28,45	28,01

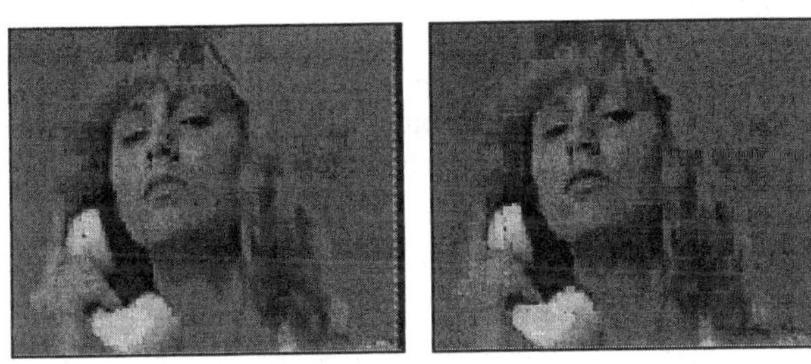

Fig. 22. Frames of the Susi video compressed and recovered. Left: Susi_02 (no block effect), right: Suzi_04 (block effect).

The improvement obtained by use of recurrent neural networks is not completely clear from a straight comparison between Tables 1 and 2, but it could be easily verified when watching at the reconstructed video sequence, where smoother and more natural motions and transitions among frames are actually performed.

5 References

1. Jiang J (1999) Image compression with neural network – A survey. In: Signal Processing and image communications, vol 14, 1999, pp 737-760.
2. Hebb D O (1949) The organizazion of behaviour. New York, Wiley, 1949
3. Dony R D, Hykin S (1995) Neural network approach to image compression. Proc. IEEE 83, vol 2, February 1995, pp 288-303.
4. Kohno R, Arai M, Imai H (1990), Image compression using neural network with learning capability of variable function of a neural unit. In: SPIE vol 1360, Visual Communication and Image processing '90, pp 69-75, 1990.
5. Cottrel G W, Munro P, Zipser D (1988), Image Compression by back propagation and examples of extensional programming. In: Sharkey. N. E. (Ed.) Advances in cognition science (Ablex norwood, NJ 1988).
6. Parodi G, Passaggio F (1994), Size-Adaptive Neural Network for Image Compression. International Conference on Image Processing, ICIP '94, Austin, TX, USA.
7. Namphon A, Chin S H, Azrozullah M (1996), Image compression with a Hierarchical Neural Network, IEEE Transaction on Aereospace and electronic System, vol 32, No.1 January 1996.
8. Guarnirei S, Piazza F, Uncini A, (1999) Multilayer Feedforward Networks with Adaptive Spline Activation Function, IEEE Trans. On Neural Network, vol 10, No. 3, pp. 672-683.
9. Campolucci P, Uncini A, Piazza F, Rao B D (1999), On-Line Learning Algorithms for Locally Recurrent Neural Networks. IEEE Trans. on Neural Network, vol 10, No. 2, pp 253-271 March 1999.
10. Back A D, Tsoi A C (1991) FIR and IIR synapses, a new neural network architecture for time series modelling. Neural Computation, vol 3, pp. 375-385.
11. Back A D, Tsoi A C (1994) Locally recurrent globally feedforward networks: a critical review of architectures, IEEE Trans. Neural Networks, vol 5, pp 229-239.
12. Rumelhart D E, Ton G E, Williams R J, (1986) Learning internal representations by error propagation, Parallel Distributed Processing: Explorations in the Microstructure of Cognition, vol 1, D. E. Rumelhart, J. L. McClelland, and the PDP Research Group, Eds. Cambridge, MA: MIT Press.
13. Widrow B, Lehr M A, (Sept 1990) 30 years of adaptive neural networks: perceptron, madaline and backpropagation, Proc. IEEE, vol 78, pp 1415-1442.
14. Cramer C (1998) Neural Network for image and video compression: A review. European Journal of Operational research pp 266-282.
15. Marsi S, Ramponi G, Sicuranza L (1991) Improved neural structure for image compression. In: Proceedings of the international conference on acoustic speech and signal processing Toronto, Ont., IEEE Piscataway, NJ, 1991 pp.2821-2824.
16. Zheng Z, Nakajiama M, Agui T (1992) Study on image data compression by using neural network. In: Visual communication and image processing'92, SPIE 1992, pp 1425-1433.
17. Gray R M (1984) Vector quantization. In: IEEE Acoustic and Speech Signal Processing. Apr. 1984, pp 4-29.
18. Goldberg M, Boucher P R, Shliner S (1988) Image compression using adaptive vector quantization. In: IEEE Trans. Communication, vol 36, 1988, pp 957-971.

19. Nasrabadi N M, King R A (1988) Image coding using vector quantization: A review. In: IEEE Transaction on communication, vol 36, 1988, pp 957-971.
20. Nasrabadi N M, Feng Y (1988) Vector quantization of images based upon Kohonen self organizing feature maps. In: IEEE Proceeding of international conference of Neural Networks, S.Diego, CA, 1988, pp.101-108.
21. Haykin S (1998) Neural Networks: A Comprehensive Foundation. In: Prentice Hall, 06 July, 1998
22. Kohonen T (1990) The self organizing map. In: Proc. IEEE, vol 78, pp. 1464-1480, Sept 1990.
23. Poggi G, Sasso E (1993) Codebook ordering technique for address predictive VQ. In: Proc. IEEE Int. Conf. Acoustic and Speech and Signal Processing '93, pp. V 586-589, Minneapolis, MN Apr. 1993.
24. Liu H, Yum D J J (1993) Self organizing finite state vector quantization for image coding. In: Proc. of international Workshop on Application of neural networks in telecommunications, Hillsdale, NJ: Lawrence Erlbrume Assoc., 1993.
25. Forster J, Gray R M, Dunham M O (1985) Finite state vector quantization of waveform coding. In: IEEE transaction on information Theory, vol 31, 1985, pp 348-359.
26. Luttrel S P(1989) Hierarchical vector quantization. In : IEE Proc. (London), vol 136 (Part I), pp 405-413, 1989
27. Li J, Manicopulos C N (1989) Multi stage vector quantization based on self organizing feature map. In: SPIE vol 1199, visual Communic and Image Processing IV (1989), pp. 1046-1055.
28. Weingessel A, Bishof H, Jornik K, Leish F (1997) Adaptive Combination of PCA and VQ neural networks. In: Letters on IEEE Transaction on Neural Network, vol.8 no. 5, Sept 1997.
29. Huang Y L, Chang R F (2002) A new Side-Match Finite State Vetor Quantization Using Neural Network for image coding. In: Journal of visual Communication and image reppresentation vol 13, pp 335-347.
30. Noel S, Szu H, Tzeng N F, Chu C H H, Tanchatchawal S (1999) Video Compression with Embedded Wavelet Coding and Singularity Maps. In: 13th Annual International Symposium on Aerospace/Defense Sensing, Simulation, and Controls, Orlando, Florida, April 1999.
31. Szu H, Wang H, Chanyagorn P (2000) Human visual system singularity map analyses. In: Proc. of SPIE: Wavelet Applications VII, vol 4056, pp 525-538, Apr. 26-28, 2000.
32. Hsu C, Szu H (May 2002) Video Compression by Means of Singularity Maps of Human Vision System. In: Proceedings of World Congress of Computational Intelligence, May 2002, Hawaii, USA.
33. Buccigrossi R, Simoncelli E (Dec. 1999) Image Compression via Joint Statistical Characterization in the Wavelet Domain. In: IEEE Trans. Image Processing, vol 8, no 12, pp 1688-1700, Dec. 1999.
34. Shapiro J M (1993) Embedded Image Coding Using Zerotrees of Wavelet Coefficients. In: IEEE Trans. Signal Processing, vol. 41, no. 12, pp 3445-3462, Dec. 1993.
35. Skrzypkowiak S S, Jain V K (2001) Hierarchical video motion estimation using a neural network. In: Proceedings, Second International Workshop on Digital and Computational Video 2001, 8-9 Feb. 2001 pp 202-208.

36. Milanova M G, Campilho A C, Correia M V (2000) Cellular neural networks for motion estimation. In: International Conference on Pattern Recognition, Barcelona, Spain, Sept 3-7, 2000. pp 827-830.
37. Toffels A, Roska A, Chua L O (1996) An object-oriented approach to video coding via the CNN Universal Machine. In: Fourth IEEE International Workshop on Cellular Neural Networks and their Applications, 1996, CNNA-96, 24-26 June 1996, pp 13-18.
38. Grassi G, Greco L A (2002) Object-oriented image analysis via analogical CNN algorithms - part I: Motion estimation. In: 7th IEEE International Workshop Frankfurt, Germany 22 - 24 July 2002.
39. Grassi G, Grieco L A (2003) Object-oriented image analysis using the CNN universal machine: new analogic CNN algorithms for motion compensation, image synthesis, and consistency observation. In: IEEE Transactions on Circuits and Systems I, vol 50, no 4 , April 2003, pp 488 – 499.
40. Luthon F, Dragomirescu D (1999) A cellular analog network for MRF-based video motion detection. In: IEEE Transactions on Circuits and Systems, vol 46, no 2, Feb 1999 pp 281-293.
41. Lee S J, Ouyang C S, Du S H (2003) A neuro-fuzzy approach for segmentation of human objects in image sequences. In: IEEE Transactions on Systems, Man and Cybernetics, Part B vol 33, no3, pp 420-437.
42. Acciani G, Guaragnella C (2002) Unsupervised NN approach and PCA for background-foreground video segmentation. In: Proc. ISCAS 2002, 26-29 May 2002, Scottsdale, Arizona, USA
43. Acciani G, Girimonte D, Guaragnella C (2002) Extension of the forward-backward motion compensation scheme for MPEG coded sequences: a sub-space approach. In: 14th International Conference on Digital Signal Processing, 2002. DSP 2002 vol 1, 1-3 July 2002 pp 191 - 194.
44. Salembier P, Marqués F (1999) Region-based representations of image and video: Segmentation tools for multimedia services. In: IEEE Trans. on Circuits and Systems for Video Technology, vol 9, no 8, pp 1147-1169, December 1999.
45. Ebrahimi T, Kunt M (1988) Visual data compression for multimedia applications. In: Proceedings of the IEEE, vol 86, no 6, June 1998, pp 1109- 1125.
46. The International telegraph and telephone Consultative Committee (CCITT) (1992) Information technology - Digital Compression and coding of continuous – tone Still Image Requirements and guidelines. Rec T.81, 1992.
47. Pennebaker W, Mitchell J (1992) JPEG Still Image Data Compression Standard. Van Nostrand Reinhold, USA, 1992.
48. Christopoulos C, Skodras A, Ebrahimi T (2000) The JPEG2000 still image coding system: an overview. In: IEEE Transactions on Consumer Electronics, vol 46, no. 4, pp. 1103-1127, November 2000.
49. ISO/IEC FDIS15444-1:2000 Information Technology – JPEG 2000 Image Coding System. Aug. 2000.
50. ISO/IEC FCD15444-2:2000 Information Technology – JPEG 2000 Image Coding System: Extensions. Dec. 2000.
51. Egger O, Fleury P, Ebrahimi T, Kunt M (1999) High-Performance Compression of Visual Information-A Tutorial Review-Part I: Still Pictures. In: Proceedings of the IEEE, vol. 87, no 6, June 1999.

52. Torres L, Delp E (2000) New Trends in Image and Video Compression. In: EUSIPCO '2000: 10th European Signal Processing Conference, 5-8 September, Tampere, Finland,2000.
53. CCITT SG 15, COM 15 R-16E (1993), ITU-T Recommendation H.261 Video Codec for audiovisual services at p x 64 kbit/s. March 1993.
54. Côtè G, Erol B, Gallant M, Kossentini F (1998) H.263+: Video Coding at Low Bit Rates. In: IEEE Transaction on Circuits and Systems for video technology, vol 8, no 7, Nov 1998.
55. Côtè G, Winger L (2002) Recent Advances in Video Compression Standards. In: IEEE Canadian Review, Spring 2002.
56. CCITT SG 15 ITU-T Recommendation H.263 Version 2 (1998) Video coding for lowbitrate communication. Geneve. 1998.
57. Noll P (1997) MPEG digital audio coding. In: IEEE Signal processing Magazine vol 14, no 5, pp 59-81, Sept 1997.
58. ISO/IEC 11172-2:1993 Information Technology (1993) Coding of moving pictures and Associated Audio for digital Storage media at up to 1.5 Mbits/s. Part 2.
59. Sikora T (1997) MPEG Digital Video coding Standard. In: IEEE Signal Processing Magazine, vol 14, no 5, Sept 1997 pp.82-100.
60. ISO/IEC 13818-2, Information Technology (2000) Generic coding of Moving Pictures and Associated Audio Information. Part 2.
61. Haskell G B, Puri A, Netravali A N (1997) Digital video: an introduction to MPEG-2. Digital Multimedia, standard Series. In: Chapman & Hall 1997.
62. ISO/IEC 14496-2:2001 Information Technology. Coding of audio-visual objects. Part 2.
63. Grill B (1999) The MPEG-4 General Audio Coder. In: Proc. AES 17th International Conference, Set 1999.
64. Scheirer E D (1998) The MPEG-4 structured audio Standard. In: IEEE Proc. On ICASSP, 1998.
65. Koenen R (2002) Overview of the MPEG-4 Standard (V.21-Jeju Version). ISO/IEC JTC1/SC29/WG11 N4668, March 2002.
66. Aizawa K, T. S. Huang, Model Based Image Coding: Advanced Video Coding techniques for low bit-rate applications. In: Proc. IEEE, vol 83, no 2, Feb. 95.
67. Avaro O, Salembier P (2001) MPEG-7 systems: Overview. In: IEEE Transaction on circuit and system for video Tecnology, vol 2. no 6, June 2001.
68. ISO/IEC JTC1/SC29/WG11 N3933, Jan 2001. MPEG-7 Requiremens document.
69. Manjunath B S, Salambier P, Sikora T (2002) Introduction to MPEG-7: multimedia content description language. In: Jhon Wiley & Sons 2002.
70. Martínez J M, MPEG-7 Overview (version 9), ISO/IEC JTC1/SC29/WG11N5525, March 2003
71. Burnett I, Walle R W, Hill K, Bormans J, Pereira F (2003) MPEG-21: Goals and Achievements. In: IEEE Computer Society, 2003
72. Bormans J, Hill K (2002) MPEG-21 Overview v5, ISO/IEC JTC1/SC29/WG11 N5231, October 2002
73. Saupe D, Hamzaoui R, Hartenstein H (1996) Fractal image compression: An introductory overview. In: Technical report, Institut für Informatik, University of Freiburg, 1996.
74. Kung S Y, Diamantaras K I, Taur J S (1994) Adaptive Principal component extraction (APEX) and application. In: IEEE Trans. Signal. Processing vol 42 (May 1994) pp 1202-1217.

75. Piazza F, Smerilli S, Uncini A, Griffo M, Zumino R, (1996) Fast Spline Neural Networks for Image Compression. In: WIRN-96, Proc. Of the 8th Italian Workshop on Neural Nets, Vietri sul Mare, Salerno, Italy.
76. Skrzypkowiak S S, Jain V K (1997) Formative motion estimation using affinity cells neural network for application to MPEG-2. In: Proc. International Conference on Communications, pp 1649-1653, June 1997.
77. ISO/IEC JTC1/SC29/WG11, ITU-T VCEG: working draft number 2 of Joint Video team standard".
78. Topi L, Parisi R, Uncini A (2002) Spline Recurrent Neural Networks for Quad-Tree Video Coding. In: WIRN-2002, Proc. Of the 13th Italian Workshop on Neural Nets, Vietri sul Mare, Salerno, Italy, 29-31 May 2002.

Knowledge Extraction in Stereo Video Sequences Using Adaptive Neural Networks

Anastasios Doulamis

National Technical University of Athens
Electrical and Computer Engineering Department
9, Heroon Polytechniou str.
Zografou 15773, Athens, Greece
E-mail: adoulam@cs.ntua.gr

Abstract. In this chapter, an adaptive neural network architecture is proposed for efficient knowledge extraction in video sequences. The system is focused on video object segmentation and tracking in stereoscopic video sequences. The proposed scheme includes: (a) a retraining algorithm for adapting the network weights to current conditions, (b) a semantically meaningful object extraction module for creating a retraining set and (c) a decision mechanism, which detects the time instances when a new network retraining is activated. The retraining algorithm optimally adapts network weights by exploiting information of the current conditions with a minimal deviation of the network weights. The algorithm results in the minimization of a convex function subject to linear constraints, and thus, one minimum exists. Description of current conditions is provided by a segmentation fusion scheme, which appropriately combines color and depth information. Experimental results on real-life video sequences are presented to indicate the promising performance of the proposed adaptive neural network-based scheme.

Keywords: knowledge modeling, knowledge discovering, semantic segmentation, content analysis, adaptive neural networks

1 Introduction

The success of the new emerging multimedia applications, such as video editing, content-based image retrieval, video summarization, object-based video transmission and video surveillance depends on the development of new sophisticated algorithms for efficient description, segmentation and representation of the image visual content (knowledge modeling & extraction). To address these needs, the MPEG-4 standard has introduced the concept of Video Objects (VOs) for content-oriented coding of video sequences [17]. Usually, a VO is an arbitrarily shaped region with different color, texture or motion characteristics, such as a human, a chair, an airplane and so on [26]. Such a VO-representation a) provides *high compression ratios* by allowing the encoder to place more emphasis on objects of interest [26]. b) It offers *multimedia capabilities and enables content interactivity,* since a video object can be handled and manipulated independently. c) It facilitates sophisticated *video queries* and *content-based retrieval operations* on image/video databases.

Although VOs and their functionalities are well described within the MPEG-4 standard, the techniques to generate them are out of the standard scope, and left to content developer. Generally, identifying semantic entities remains a very interesting but difficult problem to solve, except for some special cases, such as video games or graphics applications, where video objects are a priori available or the case of video sequences produced in a studio environment using the chroma-key technology. Currently, most schemes describe visual content by applying image segmentation of low-level homogeneity criteria, such as color or motion.

Some typical works for color segmentation include the k-nearest neighbor algorithm [7], the morphological watershed [22], pyramidal linking [5], split and merge techniques, or the Recursive Shortest Spanning Tree algorithm (RSST) [22] [23]. However, video objects usually consist of regions with totally different color characteristics and consequently the main problem of any color-oriented segmentation scheme is that it oversegments a video object into multiple color regions. A more meaningful content representation than color information is provided by a motion-based segmentation algorithm, like the algorithms proposed in [27] and [29]. However, object boundaries cannot be identified with high accuracy by a motion segmentation scheme mainly due to erroneous estimation of motion vectors. For this reason, hybrid schemes have been recently proposed in the literature to combine color and motion information so as to improve the knowledge description of the visual content.

In particular, in [28] a multiscale gradient algorithm followed by a watershed approach is used for color segmentation, while motion parameters of each region are estimated and regions with coherent motion are merged together to extract the final video object. In [21], a binary model of the objects of interest is derived, consisting of edge pixels detected by the Canny operator. The model is initialized and updated using motion information criteria, which incorporate Change Detection Masks (CDMs) or morphological filtering. Another scheme is presented in [18], where temporal and spatial segmentation are performed. The temporal segmentation method is based on intensity differences between successive frames including a statistical hypothesis test of variance comparison, while spatial segmentation is carried out by the watershed algorithm. However, the aforementioned techniques can produce sufficient results when 1) background and foreground objects present different motion characteristics, and 2) color segments of foreground objects follow coherent motion. Nevertheless, in real-life sequences, there are several cases where motion information is not adequate for semantic segmentation. This is, for example, the case of scenes with no motion or when parts of an object present different motion properties, such as a news-speaker who moves his/her head or hands, while keeping the rest of his/her body still.

Better description of the image visual content can be achieved by exploiting depth information due to the fact that video objects are usually located on the same depth plane. Depth information can be straightforwardly estimated by a two-camera system, where two different views of an object are available. However, as in motion segmentation, object boundaries are not accurately estimated by a depth segmentation algorithm due to rough calculation of the disparity field and occlusion issues.

To overcome this difficulty, in this chapter, depth information is efficiently combined with color properties resulting in a constrained *color-depth* segmentation fusion scheme. This is due to the fact that color information contains the most reliable object boundaries, while depth provides a more semantic description of the image visual content [12]. However, application of this scheme to each video frame of a sequence is computationally demanding. For this reason, *tracking algorithms* are incorporated to enable object segmentation through time by exploiting information of an initial segmentation mask.

Several tracking algorithms have been presented in the literature in recent years, such as the works reported in [4], [6], [16], [30] and [31]. These techniques are usually boundary-based schemes, which start from an initial curve (provided either by the user or by a segmentation algorithm) and then track the variation of object boundaries by exploiting motion information. Although these approaches provide good results for slow varying object boundaries, they are not suitable in case that abrupt changes of an object occur. In addition, they present lack of global shape information of the object due to their inherently local nature. Consequently, they latch onto strong edges in the scene rather than tracking the boundary correctly. To overcome this problem, constraints on the objects to be tracked are imposed resulting in a general class of object descriptors known as deformable models. Although these models present sufficient results for objects of specific geometry, such as eyes or mouths, they still present difficulties arising from inaccuracies in motion estimation, especially in case of object of unknown and abruptly time varying geometry. This is, for example, the case of a news speaker who opens and closes his/her hands.

To handle the aforementioned difficulties, a new approach is presented in this chapter, which considers the tracking problem as a classification problem. Consequently, no motion information is exploited. In particular, each video object is represented by a class and then, tracking is performed by assigning each image region to the class (i.e., video object) of the highest probability. To perform the classification task (i.e., object tracking), object modeling is required to describe object properties with high efficiency. In this chapter, *neural networks* are used for object modeling mainly due to their highly non-linear capabilities which permit efficient description of complicated object properties. In this way, the network weights can be seen as model parameters estimated through a training algorithm to fit a specific object type. However, since video object properties change through time, the model parameters (i.e., the network weights) cannot be considered constant, as it happens in conventional neural network architectures. For this reason, a dynamic modification of the network weights (object model parameters) is required at each change of object properties resulting in an *adaptable neural network architecture*.

In this chapter, an effective and computationally efficient *retraining algorithm* is proposed to perform the weight adaptation. The algorithm estimates network weights a) by exploiting information derived from the current conditions and simultaneously b) a minimum modification of the obtained network knowledge is achieved. The first condition is expressed by analyzing the input-output relationship of the network using Taylor series expansion. As provided in this chapter, this results in a set of linear equations (linear constraints) of the weight increments. The second condition is satisfied by the perpendicular from the origins to the constraint hyper-plane so that the minimum weight increment is accomplished. Combining the two above-mentioned conditions, the optimal weight increments are uniquely estimated in an efficient and cost effective manner.

For the weight modification, description of the current object properties is required as indicated by a *retraining set.* Thus, the retraining algorithm updates networks weights (model parameters) with respect to the information of the retraining set (current object properties). In our case, a combined color-depth segmentation fusion algorithm is proposed for the retraining set construction. This is due to the fact that depth provides good object localization (usually a video object is located on the same depth plane), while color extracts object boundaries very precisely. As a result, the retraining set gives an initial representation of the current conditions, while the aforementioned retraining algorithm is then applied to the following frames of the sequence to track video objects through time. Finally, *a decision mechanism* is included to detect the time instances when a new retraining is required. In particular, for every change of the environment, the decision mechanism activates the retraining set extraction module and then the retraining algorithm so that the network weights are updated to the new conditions. Otherwise, the same network weights are used for the object tracking.

Since the initial segmentation and object tracking are automatically performed, the scheme is fully unsupervised and the extraction of video objects is performed without user's interaction. It should be mentioned that the proposed architecture could also be applied to semi-automatic segmentation schemes. In this case, the retraining set is created by the user in an interactive framework, while video object tracking is implemented similarly. A block diagram of the proposed scheme is shown in Fig. 1.

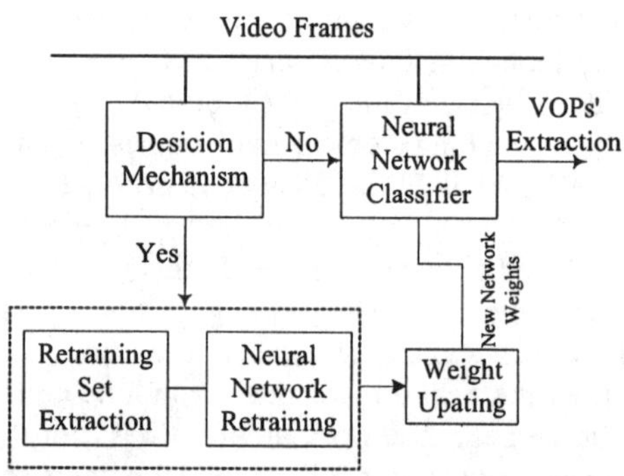

Fig. 1. Block diagram of the proposed scheme

This chapter is organized as follows: Section 2 presents the problem formulation of network retraining while Section 3 describes the retraining strategy used for updating the network weights to current conditions. Section 4 explains the decision mechanism, which activates a new retraining phase. Finally, experimental results are presented in Section 5, while Section 6 concludes the chapter.

2 Adaptable Neural Networks for Unsupervised Tracking of Video Objects

In our case, video object tracking is handled as a classification problem. This means that each video object is assigned to one class, say ω_i out of Q available. Thus Q is the number of video objects in an image. In this framework, each region of the image (e.g., an image block) is assigned to the jth object (class), if this region presents higher likelihood of belonging to the class ω_j, than to the other classes $\omega_i, i \neq j$, with i=1,2,…,Q.

2.1 Problem Formulation

Let us also assume that a neural network architecture is used to perform the classification task, i.e., video object tracking. Then, for each image region, a Q-dimensional network output $\mathbf{z}(\mathbf{x}_i)$ will be estimated of the form

$$\mathbf{z}(\mathbf{x}_i) = \left[\, p^i_{\omega_1} \; p^i_{\omega_2} \cdots p^i_{\omega_p} \, \right]^T \tag{1}$$

where $\mathbf{x}_i$ is a feature vector which describes the content of the ith image region while $p^i_{\omega_j}$ denotes the likelihood that the ith image region belongs to the jth class ω_j, i.e., the jth video object. Usually, image blocks of 8×8 pixels are used as image regions and all the extracted features are obtained by exploiting information of the blocks.

Let us first consider that the neural network has been initially trained using the training set, $S_b = \{(\mathbf{x}_1^b, \mathbf{d}_1^b), \cdots, (\mathbf{x}_M^b, \mathbf{d}_M^b)\}$, where vector $\mathbf{x}_i^b$, $i = 1,2,\cdots,M$, denotes the ith input training vector of a block, while $\mathbf{d}_i^b$ corresponds to the respective desired output vector. Vector $\mathbf{d}_i^b$ is of the same form as vector of (1). Let us also denote as $\mathbf{w}_b$ the network weights, which have been estimated using the set S_b.

Let us now consider that the decision mechanism activates a new retraining phase for the network and let us denote as $\mathbf{w}_a$ the weights estimated *after* the retraining phase. In this case, the following tasks are involved: Initially, a segmentation algorithm is applied by exploiting color and depth information. Then, a new training set, say $S_c = \{(\mathbf{x}_1, \mathbf{d}_1), \cdots (\mathbf{x}_N, \mathbf{d}_N)\}$ is created from the initial segmentation mask to describe more efficiently the current network knowledge. Vectors $\mathbf{x}_i$ and $\mathbf{d}_i$, with $i = 1,2,\cdots,N$, are of the same forms as vectors $\mathbf{x}_i^b$ and $\mathbf{d}_i^b$ and are estimated from the regions of the initial segmentation. To formulate the weight adaptation algorithm, we impose the constraint that the actual network outputs should equal the desired ones; that is

$$\mathbf{z}_a(\mathbf{x}_i) = \mathbf{d}_i \qquad i = 1,...,N, \quad \text{for all data in } S_c, \tag{2}$$

where $\mathbf{z}_a(\mathbf{x}_i)$ indicates the network output when the new weights $\mathbf{w}_a$ are used and vectors $\mathbf{x}_i$ of set S_c are fed as network inputs.

2.2 The Retraining Strategy

Let us consider, for simplicity, a) a two-class classification problem, where classes ω_1 and ω_2 refer, for example, to the foreground and background objects and b) a feedforward neural network classifier, which includes a single output neuron and one hidden layer consisting of R neurons, each of which is fed with a feature vector of J elements. Let us also ignore neuron biases. Extension to problems with more than one class or network with higher complexity can be performed in a similar way. Let $\mathbf{w}^1_{\{a,b\}}$ denote a vector containing the $R \times 1$ weights between the output and the hidden layer neurons and $\mathbf{w}^0_{k,\{a,b\}}$, k=1,2,..,R , denote the $J \times 1$ vector of weights between the kth hidden neuron and the network inputs, where subscripts $\{a,b\}$ refer to the state "after" and "before" retraining, respectively. Similarly, we can define as

$$\mathbf{w}_{\{a,b\}} = \left[(\mathbf{w}^0_{1,\{a,b\}})^{\mathrm{T}} ...(\mathbf{w}^0_{R,\{a,b\}})^{\mathrm{T}} \; (\mathbf{w}^1_{\{a,b\}})^T \right]^T \tag{3}$$

the vector of all network weights. For a given input $\mathbf{x}_j$, corresponding to the jth image block, the output of the final neural network classifier is given by

$$z_{\{a,b\}}(\mathbf{x}_j) = \Phi\left((\mathbf{w}^1_{\{a,b\}})^T \cdot \mathbf{u}_{\{a,b\}}(\mathbf{x}_j) \right) \tag{4}$$

In (4), the network output is scalar since we have assumed one output neuron. Values close to one correspond to the class ω_1 (e.g., the foreground object) while values close to zero to the class ω_2 (the background object). z_b expresses the network output in the case of the old network weights $\mathbf{w}_b$. Function $\Phi(\cdot)$ is the sigmoidal function and

$$\mathbf{u}_{\{a,b\}}(\underline{\mathbf{x}}_j) = \left[u_{1,\{a,b\}}(\mathbf{x}_j) ... u_{R,\{a,b\}}(\mathbf{x}_j) \right]^T \tag{5}$$

is a vector containing the hidden neuron outputs when the network weights are $\mathbf{w}_b$ (before retraining) or $\mathbf{w}_a$ (after retraining).

The output of the ith neuron of the hidden layer can be expressed in terms of the input vector and the weights $\mathbf{w}^0_{i,\{a,b\}}$

$$u_{i,\{a,b\}}(\mathbf{x}_j) = \Phi\left((\mathbf{w}^0_{i,\{a,b\}})^T \cdot \mathbf{x}_j\right) \tag{6}$$

Gathering u_i over all hidden neurons $i = 1,2,\ldots,R$, and taking into account (4) and (5), we conclude that

$$\mathbf{u}_{\{a,b\}}(\mathbf{x}_j) = \mathbf{\Phi}\left((\mathbf{W}^0_{\{a,b\}})^T \cdot \mathbf{x}_j\right) \tag{7}$$

where $\mathbf{W}^0_{\{a,b\}}$ is a $J \times R$ matrix defined as $\mathbf{W}^0_{\{a,b\}} = \left[\mathbf{w}^0_{1,\{a,b\}} \ldots \mathbf{w}^0_{R,\{a,b\}}\right]$ and $\mathbf{\Phi} = [\underbrace{\Phi(\cdot)\cdots\Phi(\cdot)}_{R-times}]^T$ is a vector-valued function, the elements of which represent the activation function of one hidden neuron.

Let us assume in the following that a small weight perturbation is sufficient to perform the weight adaptation. In this case, the network weights before and after the adaptation are related as

$$\mathbf{W}^0_a = \mathbf{W}^0_b + \Delta\mathbf{W}^0 \qquad \text{and} \qquad \mathbf{w}^1_a = \mathbf{w}^1_b + \Delta\mathbf{w}^1 \tag{8}$$

where $\Delta\mathbf{W}^0$ and $\Delta\mathbf{w}^1$ correspond to small weight increments. Then, vector $\Delta\mathbf{w}$ denotes the perturbation of all network weights and is related as follows

$$\Delta\mathbf{w} = \left[(\Delta\mathbf{w}^0)^T (\Delta\mathbf{w}^1)^T\right]^T \tag{9}$$

where $\Delta\mathbf{w}^0 = \text{vec}\left\{\Delta\mathbf{W}^0\right\}$, with $\text{vec}\left\{\Delta\mathbf{W}^0\right\}$ denoting a vector formed by stacking up all columns of $\Delta\mathbf{W}^0$. Therefore, vector $\Delta\mathbf{w}^0$ includes the perturbation of all weights between the input–hidden neurons.

Equation (9) permits the linearization of the network activation functions using a first order Taylor series expansion. Then, the constraint expressed in (2) can be decomposed in a system of linear equations as [8]

$$\mathbf{c} = \mathbf{A} \cdot \Delta\mathbf{w} \tag{10}$$

Vector $\mathbf{c}$ and matrix $\mathbf{A}$ are related to the previous network weights $\mathbf{w}_b$. In particular, let us define as $\mathbf{D}$ a diagonal matrix, which contains the derivatives of the activation function of the neurons of the first hidden layer.

Vector $\mathbf{c}$ of (10) expresses the output difference of the network before and after weight updating and is given as

$$\mathbf{c} = \left[\mathbf{c}(\mathbf{x}_1)\ \mathbf{c}(\mathbf{x}_2) \cdots \mathbf{c}(\mathbf{x}_{m_c})\right]^T \quad \text{with}$$

$$c(\mathbf{x}_j) = z_a(\mathbf{x}_j) - z_b(\mathbf{x}_j) = \mathbf{w}^1_b \cdot \mathbf{D} \cdot \Delta\mathbf{W}^T \cdot \mathbf{x}_j + \Delta\mathbf{w}^1 \cdot \mathbf{u}_b, j=1,2,\ldots,m_c \tag{11}$$

while matrix $\mathbf{A}$ is expressed with respect to the previous weights as follows:

$$\mathbf{A}^T = \left[\, \mathbf{a}(\mathbf{x}_1)\ \mathbf{a}(\mathbf{x}_2) \cdots \mathbf{a}(\mathbf{x}_{m_c})\, \right]$$

$$\text{with } \mathbf{a} = [\text{vec}\{\mathbf{x}_j \cdot (\mathbf{D} \cdot \mathbf{w}_b^1)^T\}\ \ \mathbf{u}_b(\mathbf{x}_j)\ \ 1]^T \qquad (12)$$

2.3 Problem Minimization

The dimension of vector $\mathbf{c}$ is usually smaller than the number of unknown weights $\Delta\mathbf{w}$, since a small number of retraining data M is chosen. As a result, many $\Delta\mathbf{w}$ can satisfy the system $\mathbf{c} = \mathbf{A} \cdot \Delta\mathbf{w}$. To achieve uniqueness in the solution, an additional requirement is imposed, which takes into consideration the variation of the network weights. In particular, among all solutions, the one which provides a minimal modification of the network weights is chosen as most appropriate one. As a result, the following constraint minimization problem is defined

$$\text{minimize } \|\Delta\mathbf{w}\|_2 \text{ or equivalently } (\Delta\mathbf{w})^T \cdot \Delta\mathbf{w} \qquad (13a)$$

$$\text{subject to } \mathbf{c} - \mathbf{A} \cdot \Delta\mathbf{w} = \mathbf{0} \qquad (13b)$$

The above constraint minimization concludes to a unique optimal solution for the weight increment, say $\Delta\hat{\mathbf{w}}$, which is given by the following equation

$$\Delta\hat{\mathbf{w}} \equiv \mathbf{A}^T \cdot (\mathbf{A} \cdot \mathbf{A}^T)^{-1} \cdot \mathbf{c} = \mathbf{Q} \cdot \mathbf{c}. \qquad (14)$$

3 Retraining Set Extraction

The aforementioned retraining algorithm requires the estimation of the retraining set S_c, which provides information about the current conditions that the neural network is applied to. This is due to the fact that this set defines the actual value of vector $\mathbf{c}$. The retraining set extraction module is responsible for constructing the set S_c, as mentioned in Section 2. In our approach, the construction of the set S_c is provided using a combined color-depth segmentation fusion algorithm as described next.

3.1 Depth Map Estimation

Depth information provides a more efficient description of the image visual content compared to color and/or motion since video objects are usually located on the same depth plane [9]. For a reliable estimation of depth information, multiview (e.g., stereoscopic) video sequences are used, where more than one separate image view of the same plane is available [15].

To estimate the depth map, we should first calculate the correspondence between the 2-D image plane points (x_1,y_1) and (x_2,y_2). This correspondence is expressed by the disparity vector between two points (x_1,y_1) and (x_2,y_2). If the disparity vectors for all points (x_1, y_1) are known, the depth field can be computed as a least-squares solution of the disparity field. As a result, the first step for calculating the depth map is to determine the disparity field.

In our case, the disparity field is calculated by minimizing a two-term error criterion. The first term indicates the displaced frame difference (DFD), while the second corresponds to a spatial consistency criterion in order to provide a smooth disparity field. In particular,

$$\mathbf{d}(x_l, y_l) = \arg\min_{\mathbf{u}\in\Gamma} C(\mathbf{v}, x_l, y_l) = \arg\min_{\mathbf{u}\in\Gamma} \{B(\mathbf{v}, x_l, y_l) + F(\mathbf{v}, x_l, y_l)\}, \quad (15)$$

where $\mathbf{d}(x_l \; y_l)^T$ denotes the disparity vector of a point $\mathbf{p}$ with projected coordinates onto the left camera I_l as (x_l, y_l). Similarly, the projected coordinates onto the right camera I_r are (x_r, y_r). Vector $\mathbf{v} = [v_x \; v_y]^T$ is an arbitrary vector taking values in a searching area Γ (e.g., 8x2 searching area).

The term $B(\mathbf{v}, x_l, y_l)$ of (15) refers to the displaced frame difference and in our case it is expressed as:

$$D(\mathbf{v}, x_l, y_l) = \frac{1}{w^2} \sum_{m,n\in W} \left| I_r(x_l + v_x + m, y_l + v_y + n) - I_l(x_l + m, y_l + n) \right| \quad (16)$$

where W corresponds to the rectangular window or block in which the displaced frame difference is evaluated, while w^2 is the area of window W.

The term $F(\mathbf{v}, x_l, y_l)$ of (15) refers to a smoothing function,

$$F(\mathbf{v}, x_l, y_l) = G(x_l, y_l) \sum_{\mathbf{y}\in\Pi(x_l, y_l)} \|\mathbf{v} - \mathbf{y}\|^2 \quad (17)$$

where $\Pi(x_l, y_l) = \{\ \mathbf{d}(x_l-1, y_l), \mathbf{d}(x_l-1, y_l-1), \mathbf{d}(x_l, y_l-1), \mathbf{d}(x_l+1, y_l-1)\ \}$ contains all disparity vectors of pixels neighboring to (x_l, y_l) that have already been calculated, and $\|\cdot\|$ denotes the Euclidean norm. A *smoothing weight function* $G(x_l, y_l)$ has been added in (16) to regulate the strength of the smoothness criterion. In particular, $G(x_l, y_l)$ takes low values in regions where the disparity field can be estimated with high accuracy, such as edges or highly textured areas and high values in homogeneous regions of uniform intensity, in which the disparity field cannot be reliably estimated since many points of similar pixel values exist. The local variance of the image intensity is adopted in this chapter as the *smoothing weight function* $G(x_l, y_l)$ since this function satisfies all the aforementioned properties.

3.2 Color/Depth Segmentation

For color/depth segmentation, a multiresolution implementation of the *Recursive Shortest Spanning Tree* (RSST) algorithm [23], called *M-RSST*, is adopted. In particular, the M-RSST recursively applies the conventional RSST to images of increasing resolution by creating a truncating image pyramid, each layer of which contains a quarter of the pixels of the layer below [10].

The main advantage of the M-RSST algorithm compared with the conventional RSST is that the overall computation complexity remains very low, specially for images of large size while simultaneously keeping almost the same effective performance [1, 24]. In particular, comparison of the computational complexity of both algorithms indicates that the M-RSST is up to 400 times faster than the conventional RSST for images of size 720×576 pixels (PAL system) [3]. Further reduction of the cost complexity can be achieved by selecting blocks of 8x8 pixels as the initial resolution of the M-RSST algorithm. In this way, information directly available in the MPEG stream is exploited and no decoding of the compressed video stream at the initial level is required [10]. At higher resolution levels, however, only the "boundary" blocks are decoded, which constitute a very small percentage of the total image blocks. Furthermore, depth segmentation can be performed only to the initial resolution level, (i.e., at blocks of 8x8 pixels), since the depth map does not extract accurate object boundaries even in higher resolution levels due to erroneous estimation of the disparity field and occlusion issues.

3.3 Color and Depth Information Fusion

Although depth information is an important element towards content segmentation, since video objects are usually composed of regions located on the same depth plane, it does not provide accurate object boundaries (contours), due to erroneous estimation of disparity field and/or occlusion issues. On the contrary, segmentation based on color homogeneity criteria contains the most reliable object boundaries, but usually oversegments a video object into multiple regions [1]. For this reason, the retraining set S_c is estimated based on a depth-color segmentation fusion method as described next.

Let us assume that K^c color segments and K^d depth segments have been extracted by the aforementioned M-RSST algorithm, denoted as CS_i, $i=1,2,\dots,K^c$ and DS_i, $i=1,2,\dots,K^d$, respectively. The segments CS_i and DS_i are mutually exclusive.

Let us also denote by M^c and M^d the output masks of color and depth segmentation, which are defined as the sets of all color and depth segments, respectively:

$$\begin{aligned} M^c &= \{CS_i\,, i=1,2,\dots,K^c\}, \\ M^d &= \{DS_i\,, i=1,2,\dots,K^d\} \end{aligned} \tag{18}$$

Color segments are projected onto depth segments so that video objects provided by the depth segmentation are retained and, at the same time, object boundaries given by the color segmentation are accurately extracted. For this reason, each color segment CS_i is associated with a depth segment, so that the area of intersection between the two segments is maximized. This is accomplished by means of a *projection function*:

$$P(C_i, M^d) = \arg\max_{g \in M^d} \{a(g \cap C_i)\}, i = 1,2,\ldots,K^c \,, \tag{19}$$

where $a(\cdot)$ is the area, i.e., the number of pixels, of a segment. Based on the previous equation, K^d sets of *fused color segment classes*, say FC_i, $i = 1,2,\ldots,K^d$, are created, each of which contains all color segments that are projected onto the same depth segment DS_i :

$$FC_i = \{g \in M^c : P(g, M^d) = DS_i\}, i = 1,2,\ldots,K^d \tag{20}$$

The final segmentation mask, M, consists of $K = K^d$ segments FS_i, $i = 1,2,\ldots,K$, each of which is generated as the union of all elements of the corresponding set FC_i:

$$FS_i = \bigcup_{g \in FC_i} g \,, \quad i = 1,2,\ldots,K \tag{21}$$

$$M = \{FS_i, i = 1,2,\ldots,K\} \tag{22}$$

In other words, color segments are merged together into $K = K^d$ new segments according to depth similarity. The final segmentation consists of these segments that contain the same image regions as the corresponding depth segments, but with accurate contours obtained from color segments.

3.4 Retraining Set Construction

The number K of segments FS_i defines the number of video objects that should be tracked by the neural network architecture. This number remains constant until the decision mechanism activates a new retraining process. For the estimation of the retraining set S_c, K different sets are created, say E_i, $i = 1,\ldots,K$, each of which is associated to a video object.

$$E_i = \{(\mathbf{x}_j, \gamma_i) : P(\beta_j, M) = FS_i\} \tag{23}$$

with

$$\gamma_i = [\cdots 0 \quad \underset{i-position}{1} \quad 0 \cdots]^T \tag{24}$$

where $\mathbf{x}_j$ is the feature vector corresponding to the jth image region (in our case image block), say β_j, and $P(\cdot)$ indicates the projection function defined in (19), while M is the final segmentation mask, provided by the segmentation fusion algorithm. Equation (23) indicates that the image regions (e.g., image blocks) β_j, which mainly belong to segments FS_i, are selected as appropriate regions to describe the content of the *i*th video object. Vector γ_i represents the respective desired output and is of similar form as in (1).

The retraining set S_c is constructed by merging together the sets E_i,

$$S_c = \bigcup_{i=1}^{K} E_i \tag{25}$$

Since there are a large number of similar training blocks associated with a specific video object, a distance measure is used to reduce their number before using them for the network weight updating (see Section 2). Therefore, a small number of training blocks is finally included in the retraining set S_c (by using, for example, a Principal Component Analysis (PCA) of the set S_c).

4 The Decision Mechanism

The purpose of this mechanism is to detect when a change of the environment occurs and consequently to activate the retraining algorithm.

Let us index images or video frames in time, denoting by $V(k,T)$ the *k*th image or image frame following the image at which the *T*th network retraining occurred. Index *k* is therefore reset each time retraining takes place, with $V(0,T)$ corresponding to the first image of the *T*th retraining. Fig. 2 indicates a scenario with two retraining phases (at frames 3 and 6 respectively of a video sequence composed of 8 frames) and the corresponding values of indices *k* and *T*.

In the framework of this chapter, retraining is performed every time the beginning of a new scene is detected. For this reason, a shot cut detection algorithm is applied so that frames or stereo pairs of similar visual characteristics are gathered together. Several algorithms have been reported in literature for scene change detection of 2-D video sequences, which deal with the detection of cut, fading or dissolve changes either in compressed or in uncompressed domain [32].

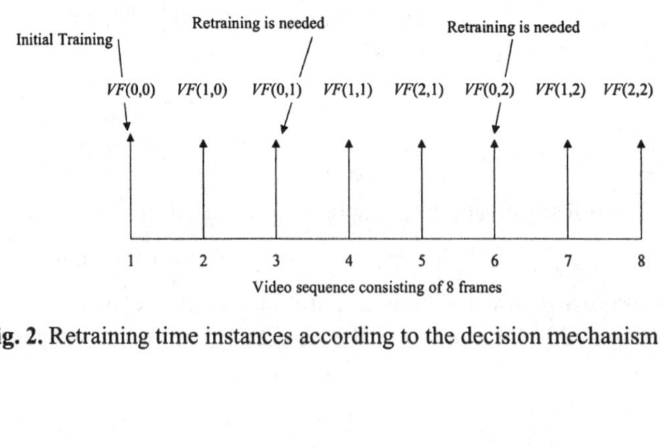

Fig. 2. Retraining time instances according to the decision mechanism

In our approach, the algorithm proposed in [32] has been adopted for shot detection due to its efficiency and low computational complexity, since it is based on the DC coefficients of the DCT transform of each frame. These coefficients are directly available in the case of intracoded frames (I frames) of MPEG compressed video sequences, while for the intercoded ones (P and B frames), they can be estimated by the motion compensated error with a minimal decoding effort [35]. The adoption of the above-described algorithm results in significant reduction of the computational complexity, compared to other algorithms, which require a full resolution search of the video data.

5 Experimental Results

In this section the performance of the proposed adaptive neural network scheme for unsupervised tracking of stereo video objects is investigated. In particular, a stereoscopic sequence consisting of 10 shots was formed. The shots of this sequence were obtained from the stereoscopic television program "Eye to Eye". This program has been produced in the framework of the ACTS MIRAGE project [14] in collaboration with AEA Technology and ITC.

Each stereo frame was in QCIF format, i.e., each image channel consisted of 144x176 pixels per color image component. In the following each image frame is separated into blocks of size 8x8 pixels. Therefore 396 blocks per color component are available. The DC coefficient and the first 8 AC coefficients of the zig-zag scanned Discrete Cosine Transform (DCT) for each color component of a block (i.e., 27 elements in total) are used as feature vector $\mathbf{x}_i$ of the respective block. In the performed experiment we assumed, without loss of generality, that the maximum number of video objects is 3, i.e., two foreground objects and the background. The neural network architecture is selected to consist of q=15 hidden neurons and 3 outputs, each of which is associated with a specific video object. Therefore the network has 450 network weights. Initially, a set of approximately 1000 image blocks is used to train the neural network.

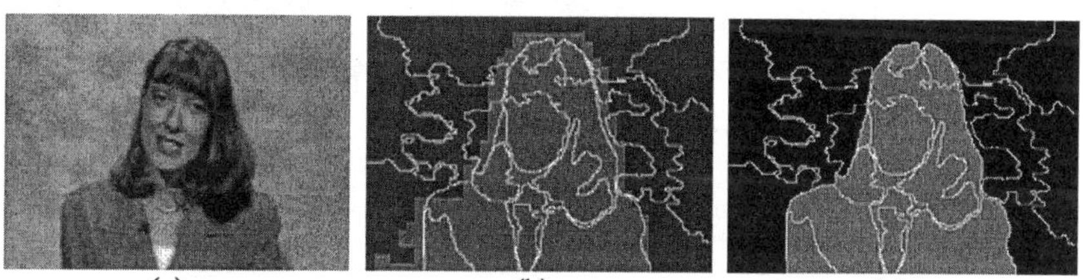

(a) (b) (c)

Fig. 3. (a) An original frame of the shot. (b) Segmentation fusion results for the image of Fig. 3(a). Depth segmentation overlaid with color segment contours (in white). (c) Fused segments overlaid with color segment contours

The decision mechanism activates the first retraining process at the stereo frame, which is depicted in Fig. 3(a). Then, this stereo frame is analyzed and a color and depth segmentation mask is constructed. After the creation of color and depth segmentation maps, the information fusion scheme is incorporated to extract the retraining set. More specifically, color segments are projected onto the depth map and fused according to depth similarity. Fig. 3 describes the proposed segmentation fusion method in case of the image in Fig. 3(a). In Fig. 3(b), depth segmentation, shown with two different gray levels as in Fig. 3(a), is overlaid with the white contours of the color segments. It is apparent that the person in the foreground (speaker) corresponds only to one depth segment but to several color segments. The same happens to the background object. Fig. 3(c) shows the fused segments of both segmentations. Although, color-depth segmentation fusion technique accurately detects video objects, its computational complexity is high for being applied to each video frame. For this reason, tracking of the initial video objects is required.

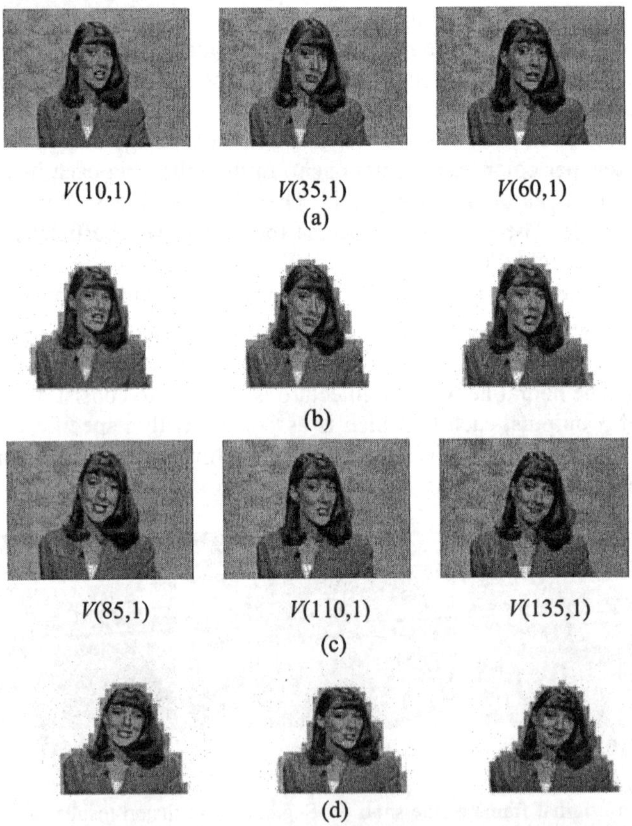

Fig. 4. The tracking performance of the proposed adaptive neural network architecture for several frames at different time instances within the first retraining phase. (a,c) The original frames. (b,d) The respective tracking results of the foreground object

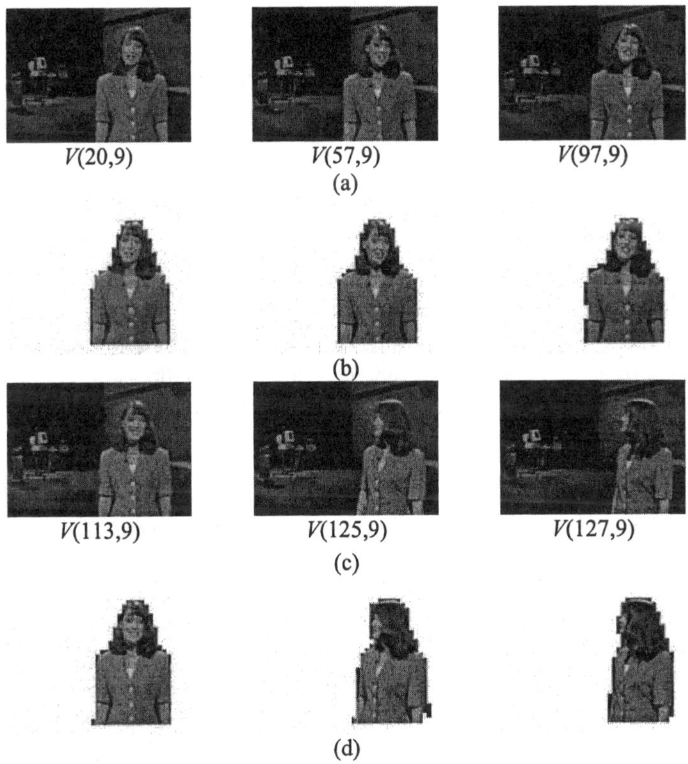

Fig. 5. The tracking performance of the proposed adaptive neural network architecture for several frames at different time instances within the 9th retraining phase. (a,c) The original frames. (b,d) The respective tracking of the foreground object

Based on the color-depth segmentation fusion, the retraining set S_c is constructed as mentioned in Section 3.4. Since there are a large number of similar retraining blocks, Principal Component Analysis (PCA) is used to reduce their number. More specifically the number of selected retraining blocks was reduced to 20. Afterwards, adaptation of the network weights is accomplished based on the algorithm described in Section 2. Then the retrained *neural networks* perform video object tracking, until a new retraining process is activated. In order to evaluate the tracking efficiency of the network, in Figs. 4(b,d) we present the tracking results of six different frames belonging to the same retraining process with the frame of Fig. 3(a). In this phase, only two video objects are tracked since the final segmentation mask, provided by the color-depth segmentation fusion consists of two segments [see Figs. 3(b,c)]. In order to present the visual content of the frame where tracking is performed, we also depict the original left-channel stereo frames in Figs. 4(a,c). It should be also mentioned that the video object is extracted in block resolution (8x8 pixels) since each block is classified only to one class.

The ninth retraining phase is activated for the stereo scene of Fig. 5. The respective original frames are depicted in Figs. 5(a,c), while the tracking performance in Figs 5(b,d). From the above experimental results we can observe a very accurate tracking performance, although complex or rapid motion exists in the frames within a retraining phase.

6 Conclusions

New multimedia applications addressing content-based image retrieval, video editing and processing, video summarization and content-based transmission require an efficient representation of the image visual information and extraction of the visual knowledge. This is due to the fact that efficient content characterization provides a new range of capabilities in terms of accessing, transmitting, manipulating and processing of the visual information. For this reason, video object extraction has received a great attention in the recent years, both in the academic society and the industry. However, segmentation and tracking of video objects in real-life video sequences is in general a difficult task, due to the fact that object characteristics frequently change through time. Furthermore, video objects usually consist of regions with different color, motion or texture properties, making their extraction and tracking an arduous process.

In this chapter, the problem of content segmentation and tracking is addressed using an adaptive neural network model, implemented through a retraining algorithm. The adaptive behavior of the network is very important in such dynamically changing environments, where object properties frequently vary through time. The proposed algorithm updates network weights so that a) the network response after adaptation satisfies the current conditions and b) the obtained network knowledge is minimally deteriorated. The two aforementioned conditions result in the minimization of a convex function subject to linear constraints. Thus, the optimization problem guarantees that only one minimum exists, which is the global one. Furthermore, in this chapter, a color-depth segmentation fusion approach is adopted to describe the current conditions. This is due to the fact that color segmentation provides accurate object boundaries but it oversegments an object into multiple regions. On the contrary, depth segmentation efficiently describes the objects but usually blurs their boundaries. Since depth information can be estimated more reliably in stereoscopic sequences, where two views of the same scene are available, our study is focused on this type of sequences. Based on this approach, a retraining set is created, which is then used to adapt the network (i.e., to update the network weights).

The proposed adaptive neural network-based tracking algorithm is fully automatic and no user-interaction is required. Moreover, weight adaptation is performed in an efficient and cost effective manner in contrast to other conventional training schemes, which usually induce high computational load. This is an important issue, especially for video sequence applications where many frames should be processed. In addition, the proposed approach a) cannot be trapped to local minima, which may deteriorate the network performance, b) guarantees that the network response to the current conditions is satisfactory, and c) prevents the network from a catastrophic forgetting of the obtained knowledge. Another advantage of the proposed adaptive neural network scheme is that it does not require the tracking results obtained at the previous frames, to perform the segmentation of the current frame like most of the existing tracking algorithms. This can lead to a fully paralleled system with respect to frame number, which also yields a significant reduction of the computational cost.

Experimental results on real-life stereoscopic video sequences indicate the reliable and promising performance of the proposed scheme, even in cases of complex background, video objects with complicated non-rigid motion or in shots with multiple objects.

References

1. Alatan, A., Onural, L., Wollborn, M., Mech, R., Tuncel E., Sikora, T. (1998) Image sequence analysis for emerging interactive multimedia services-The European cost 211 framework. IEEE Trans. Circuits and Systems for Video Technology, **8**, 802- 813
2. Avid, G. (1985) Determining three-dimensional motion and structure from optical flow generated by several moving objects. IEEE Trans. Pattern Anal. Machine Intel. **7**, 384-401
3. Avrithis, Y., Doulamis, N., Doulamis, A., Kollias, S. (1999) Optimization Methods for Key Frames and Scenes Extraction. Journal of Computer Vision and Image Understanding, Academic Press, **75**, 3-24
4. Bremond, F., Thonnat, M. (1998) Tracking multiple nonrigid objects in video sequences. IEEE Trans. Circuits and Systems for Video Technology, **8**, 585-591
5. Burt, P, Hong, T.H., Rosenfield, A. (1981) Segmentation and estimation of image region through cooperative hierarchical computation. IEEE Trans. Syst. Man, Cybern., **11**,802-809
6. Castagno, R., Ebrahimi, T., Kunt, M. (1998) Video segmentation based on multiple features for interactive multimedia applications. IEEE Trans. Circuits and Systems for Video Technology, **8**, 562-571
7. Cover, T.M., Hart, P.,E. (1967) Nearest neighbor pattern classification. IEEE Trans. on Information Theory, **13**, 21-27
8. Doulamis, A., Doulamis, N., Kollias, S. (2000) On line retrainable neural networks: Improving the performance of neural networks in image analysis problems. IEEE Trans. on Neural Networks, **11**, 137-155
9. Doulamis, A., Doulamis, N., Ntalianis, K., Kollias, S. (2000) Efficient unsupervised content-based segmentation in stereoscopic video sequences. Journal of Artificial Intelligence Tools, World Scientific Press, **9**, 277-303
10. Doulamis, A., Doulamis, N., Kollias, S. (2000) A fuzzy video content representation for video summarization and content-based retrieval. Signal Processing, **80**, 1049-1067
11. Doulamis, N., Doulamis, A., Kalogeras D., Kollias, S. (1998) Very low bit-rate coding of image sequences using adaptive regions of interest. IEEE Trans. Circuits and Systems for Video Technology, **8**,928-934

12. Doulamis, N., Doulamis, A., Avrithis, Y., Ntalianis K., Kollias, S. (2000) Efficient summarization of stereoscopic video sequences. IEEE Trans. Circuits and Systems for Video Technology, **10,** 501-517
13. Doulamis, N., Doulamis, A., Kollias, S. (2000) Low bit rate coding of image sequence using adaptive neural networks and regions of interest, Real Time Imaging, **6**, 327-345
14. Girdwood, C., Chiwy, P. (1996) MIRAGE: An ACTS Project in Virtual Production and Stereoscopy. IBC Conference Publication, **428**, 155-160
15. Gonzalez, R.C., Woods, R. E. (1992) Digital Image Processing. Addison-Wesley.
16. Gu, C., Lee, M.-C. (1998) Semiautomatic segmentation and tracking of semantic video objects. IEEE Tran. Circuits, Syst. Video Techn., **8**, 572-584
17. ISO/IEC JTC1/SC29/WG11 N3156, (1999) MPEG-4 Overview. Doc. N3156, Maui, Hawaii.
18. Kim, M., Choi, J.G., Kim, D., Lee, H., Lee, M.-H., Ahn, C., Ho, Y.-S. (1990) A VOP generation tool: Automatic segmentation of moving objects in image sequences based on spatio-temporal information. IEEE Tran. Circuits and Systems for Video Technology, **9**, 1216-1226
19. Kunt, M., Ikonomopoulos, A., Kocher, M. (1985) Second Generation Image Coding Techniques," Proc. IEEE, **73**, 549-574
20. Luenberger, J. (1984) Linear and Non-Linear Programming, Addison-Wesley.
21. Meier, T., Ngan, K. (1999) Video segmentation for content-Based coding. IEEE Tran. Circuits and Systems for Video Technology, **9,** 1190-1203
22. Meyer, T., Beucher, S. (1990) Morphological segmentation. Journal of Visual Communication on Image Representation, **1**, 21-46
23. Morris, J. Lee, M. J., Constantinides, A.G. (1986) Graph theory for image analysis: an approach based on the shortest spanning tree. IEE Proceedings, **133**, 146-152
24. Mulroy, P.J. (1997) Video content extraction: review of current automatic segmentation algorithms. Proc. of Workshop on Image Analysis and Multimedia Interactive Systems (WIAMIS)
25. Patel, V., Sethi, I. K. (1997) Video shot detection and characterization for video databases. Pattern Recognition, **30**, 583-592
26. Sikora, T. (1997) The MPEG-4 video standard verification model. IEEE Trans. Circuits and Systems for Video Technology, **7**, 19-31
27. Thompson, W. B., Pong, T. G. (1990) Detecting moving objects. Int. J. Comput. Vision, **4**, 39-57
28. Wang, D., (1998) Unsupervised video segmentation based on watersheds and temporal tracking. IEEE Tran. Circuits and Systems for Video Technology, **8**,539-546
29. Wang, J., Adelson, E., (1994) Representing moving images with layers. IEEE Trans. Image Processing, **3**, 625-638
30. Xu, C., Prince, J. L. (1998) Snakes, shapes, and gradient vector flow. IEEE Trans. Image Processing, **7**, 359-369
31. Yao, Y. S., Chellappa, R. (1995) Tracking a dynamic set of feature points. IEEE Trans. Image Processing, **4(10)**, 1382-1395
32. Yeo, L., Liu, B. (1995) Rapid scene analysis on compressed videos. IEEE Trans. Circuits and Systems for Video Technology, **5**, 533-544

An Efficient Genetic Algorithm for Small Search Range Problems and Its Applications

Ja-Ling Wu, Chun-Hung Lin, and Chun-Hsiang Huang

Communication and Multimedia Laboratory,
Department of Computer Science and Information Engineering,
National Taiwan University

Abstract. Genetic algorithms have been applied to many optimization and search problems and shown to be very efficient. However, the efficiency of genetic algorithms is not guaranteed in those applications where the search space is small, such as the block motion estimation in video coding applications, or equivalently the chromosome length is relatively short, less than 5 for example. Since the characteristics of these small search space applications are far away from that of the conventional search problems in which the common genetic algorithms worked well, new treatments of genetic algorithms for dealing with the small range search problems are therefore of interest. In this paper, the efficiency of the genetic operations of common genetic algorithms, such as crossover and mutation, is analyzed for this special situation. As expected, the so-obtained efficiency/performance of the genetic operations is quite different from that of their traditional counterparts. To fill this gap, a lightweight genetic search algorithm is presented to provide an efficient way for generating near optimal solutions for these kinds of applications. The control overheads of the lightweight genetic search algorithm are very low as compared with that of the conventional genetic algorithms. It is shown by simulations that many computations can be saved by applying the newly proposed algorithm while the search results are still well acceptable.

Keywords: genetic algorithms, small search range problems, lightweight genetic search algorithms

1 Introduction

Genetic algorithms (GAs) based on the laws of natural selection and genetics have been developed since 1975 [1] and been applied to a variety of optimization and search problems [2]-[5]. In each iteration of the genetic evolution, a population of search points are maintained. The points of the population are evaluated by means of an objective function. The points with smaller objective values are expected to be replaced by other points in the search space.

In the applications with large amounts of search points, it is impossible, due to execution time and storage space, to perform the full search by visiting all the points in the search space. GAs can help to find the global optima although a few computational overheads of the genetic evolution are unavoidable. While compared with the computational complexity of the full search, the evolution overheads are small and worthwhile.

Nevertheless, when the search space is very small, the genetic algorithm overhead might overtake the computational complexity of applying the full search. This implies in this situation that it would be better to perform the full search directly. However, the time constraint for these small search range applications is usually very tight. For example, in the motion estimation stage of video coding [6] (which is also a search problem), the ideal execution time for each 16×16 block search is less than 3.95×10^{-8} second. The computational complexity of the full search is still too high to satisfy the above requirement. The evolution overheads of GAs have to be reduced, so as to meet the embedded strict time constraint in the above applications.

GAs have been applied to these kinds of applications in the literature [7,8]. The huge computational complexity of traditional GA-based search algorithms has made them become handicaps in real video coding applications. In this chapter, a lightweight genetic search algorithm (LGSA) will be presented. When GAs are applied to search related applications, the computational complexity comes mainly from the following two parts: (1) the computations of evaluating the similarity between the search points and the reference template; (2) the computations of the genetic evolution. The first part is dominated by the number of evaluated search points. Fewer computations would be required if the number of evaluated points is reduced. But, this reduction involves the risk of finding a bad solution. The second part is controlled by the structure of the genetic evolution. Low control overhead brings less computational complexity. In LGSA, both the number of evaluated points and the control overheads of genetic evolution are reduced to meet the time constraint of video coding. The structure and the evolution strategy of LGSA are amended several times after performing many simulations to approve the performance with limited iterations. The proposed LGSA has successfully been applied to three different small search range applications: the block matching of video coding [9], the automatic facial feature extraction (AFFE) [10], and the performance optimization of digital watermark schemes [11].

Block matching has been proved to be very efficient in reducing the temporal redundancy of video data [6], and therefore, has become a critical component of many video coding standards, such as ITU-T recommendation H.261 [12] and H.263 [13], and ISO MPEG-1 [14] , MPEG-2 [15] and MPEG-4 [16]. AFFE plays an important role in human face identification [17] and very low bit-rate video coding [18, 19]. That is, in these applications, the facial features of each face image have to be extracted automatically. Either the extracted feature regions can be used to identify a human face or a feature-based coding algorithms can be applied to process the video data based on the extracted information. High fidelity, strong robustness and large data capacity are the three goals of most existing watermark schemes [20] expected to achieve. However, the above requirements are conflicting with each other, and optimal watermarking for a specific application scenario is still a difficult and challenging problem. In this chapter, the fidelity enhancement of a block-based private digital watermarking scheme [21] is also modeled as an optimization problem with a limited search range and solved by using LGSA. Simulation results show that LGSA saves about half of the required computations while retains nearly the same visual fidelity as compared to the conventional GA-based approach.

This chapter is organized as follows. In Section 2, a brief survey of GAs is presented. Furthermore, the efficiency of the crossover operation(with different chromosome lengths) is analyzed by both mathematical derivation and simulations. Then, the efficiency of the conventional mutation operation is derived and its profile is plotted with respect to different numbers of generations. The efficiency of the modified mutation operation, which is used in LGSA, is also provided for comparison. LGSA is detailed in Section 3. The comparisons of LGSA with conventional GAs are also included in this section. In Section 4, the convergence property of LGSA is addressed. Section 5 presents three successful applications of the LGSA. Finally, Section 6 concludes this chapter.

2 A Brief Survey of Genetic Algorithms

In traditional search-based optimization algorithm, such as the well-known gradient based search, the search trajectory is always based on a deterministic rule. The search results are usually trapped to local optima in many applications whenever the search-cost space is multimodal in nature. Fig. 1(a) shows one example of the heuristic search methods (the well-known three-step search [22]). In the first-step search, the point with the maximum functional value is selected and its neighboring points are probed in the succeeding steps. It can be seen that the local maximum located on the same hill with the initially selected point was found. An alternative approach is the random search, where different search points are probed at random. The selection of probed points in different steps is irrelevant to the locations of the previously searched points. As shown in Fig. 1(b), this approach is inefficient although the search will not be trapped to local maxima. GAs, which could be classified as one kind of the guided random search methods, are a compromise between these two extremes. The next-step search points in GAs are selected according to the fitness values of the previous-step search points. As shown in Fig. 1(c), the two resultant points of the first-step search, with similar functional values, will have similar probabilities to generate the next-step search points. This explains why the probability of finding the global maximum is reasonably high in GAs. It is this characteristic of GAs which contributes to the robustness and the advantageousness over other search methods.

In other words, in GAs, the points with larger functional values will have higher probability to derive the next-step search points. Whereas, in the

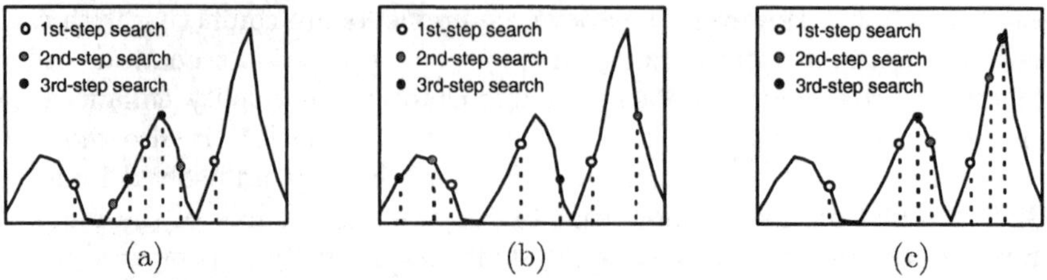

Fig. 1. Comparisons of different search methods: (a) a heuristic search method, (b) a random search method, and (c) a genetic search method.

heuristic search methods, only the best point can derive the next-step search points. Besides, in the random search approach, each point has the same probability to derive the next-step search points.

In GAs, each search point in the search space can be represented as a data string which is usually called a chromosome. A cluster of chromosomes are gathered to form a population. Each chromosome in the population is considered as a candidate for the final solution. Let P_k represent the population of the kth iteration step. There will be a list of chromosomes contained in P_k. That is, $P_k = \{C_0, C_1, C_2, \ldots, C_{N-1}\}$, where N is the population size.

For each chromosome, there is an associated fitness value, i.e., $f_i = f(C_i), i = 0, 1, \cdots, N-1$, where f is an objective function. In each iteration, the chromosomes with smaller fitness values will be replaced by some other new chromosomes with larger fitness values, whereas the chromosomes with acceptable fitness values would be retained in the population. All those chromosomes with better fitness values form a new population and go through the iteration procedures again.

Fig. 2 shows the elementary structure of a simple GA. The initial population P_0 consists of initial chromosomes. The fitness value for each initial chromosome should be evaluated. Then, the genetic system will check the termination conditions. If it is time to terminate the iteration, the chromosome with the best fitness value will be selected from the final population as the solution. Otherwise, the iteration will go on and the improper chromosomes will be replaced by the new ones as follows.

The chromosomes in the population P_{k-1} with better fitness values are selected as the seeds for generating the new chromosomes of the population P_k. This process is known as reproduction or selection. In this stage, the individual chromosome is duplicated according to its fitness value. The chromosomes with larger fitness values will have higher probability to be selected as seeds. For example, if we have a population $P_{k-1} = \{C_0, C_1, C_2, C_3\}$, and the associated fitness values are $\{1, 10, 2, 30\}$. Under perfect conditions, the seeds for generating the new population will be $\{C_1, C_3, C_3, C_3\}$.

After the embryonic chromosomes are formed in the reproduction stage, the initial chromosomes must be recombined to turn into the new chromosomes of the next generation. Two commonly used recombination operations

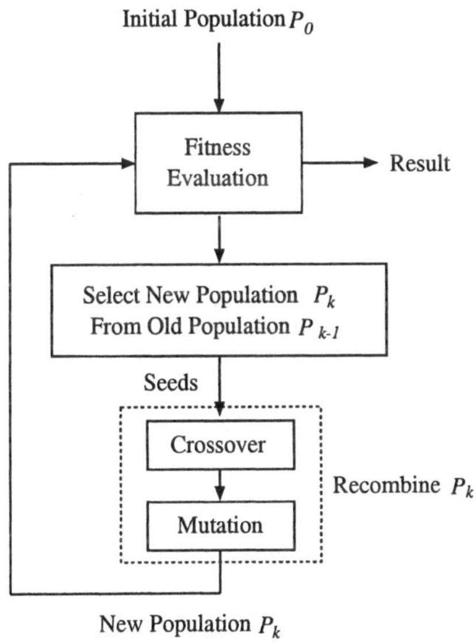

Fig. 2. The basic structure of a simple GA.

are crossover and mutation. As shown in Fig. 3, single-point crossover is usually used in a simple GA. A crossover point is determined randomly among two consecutive genes of the two randomly selected chromosomes from the population. The corresponding parts of genes in the two chromosomes are then exchanged to generate two new chromosomes. Each gene of chromosomes has its own probability to be mutated from 0 to 1 or 1 to 0. The mutation probability is usually a constant and is called the mutation probability in GAs.

The chromosomes of different generations will gradually cover the search points of the whole search space via the prescribed recombination process. The fitness values of the new chromosomes must be evaluated, and the evolution process is performed again and again until the termination conditions are satisfied.

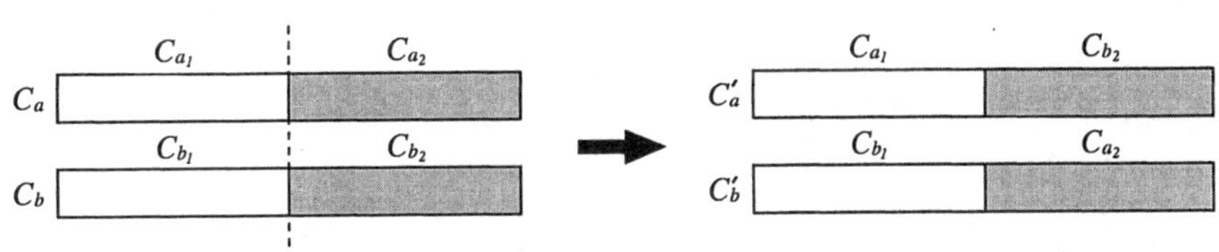

Fig. 3. The single-point crossover.

2.1 Analysis of Crossover Efficiency

In conventional GAs, the evolution is analyzed based on schema theory [2]. The schemata with better fitness are expected to be more prosperous. The disruption of crossover is therefore analyzed based on a provided schema. The crossover disruption rate is defined as the probability that the schema is disrupted by crossover. For a good genetic algorithm, it is hoped that the crossover disruption rate of a highly fit schema will be very low. In [2], an upper bound for the crossover disruption rate of a schema was given.

Based on the primitive results of the schema theory, a further analysis was provided in [23]. It concludes that at least in two situations where disruption is advantageous: (1) when the population is quite homogeneous, and (2) when the population size is too small to provide the necessary sampling accuracy for complex search spaces. It is also known that smaller population sizes tend to become homogeneous more quickly. Because population sizes are small when the search space is not large [24], the disruption will also be favorite in a small search space. The crossover productivity rate (i.e. disruption rate) will be denoted as P_{eff}. It is hoped that the crossover productivity rate will be large enough when the population becomes homogeneous. In [23], a rough estimation of P_{eff} was given based on a provided schema.

Except the above two situations, disruption is also advantageous when real-time constraint is a must. In this situation, the number of generations of genetic evolution is not allowed to be large. In order to probe more search points, the crossover productivity rate should be high, especially when an elitist selection is applied in the reproduction stage.

In the previous analysis, the crossover disruption rates are discussed based on schemata (chromosome patterns) while applying conventional GAs. However, it is difficult to determine the fitness of a schema in applications with various kinds of search spaces. An analysis of the crossover productivity rates based on a randomly given chromosome will be provided in the following sections.

(a) Single-point crossover and two-point crossover

Assume the search space can be represented by chromosomes of length k, the probabilities for a chromosome to be mated with the other chromosomes in the search space are all equal, and the crossover points are selected between any two consecutive genes with equal probabilities. As shown in Fig. 3, for the single-point crossover, the two chromosomes C_a and C_b are each divided into two segments. Let P_i represent the probability that the two corresponding segments C_{a_i} and C_{b_i} are equal. The probability of producing two new chromosomes (i.e. $C'_a \neq C_a$ and $C'_b \neq C_b$) is equal to $\bar{P}_1 \cap \bar{P}_2$ (i.e. $C_{a_1} \neq C_{b_1}$ and $C_{a_2} \neq C_{b_2}$), where $\bar{P}_i = 1 - P_i$. The crossover productivity rate $P^{(1)}_{eff}$ for the single-point crossover is

$$P_{eff}^{(1)} = 1 - P_{inv}^{(1)}, \tag{1}$$

$$P_{inv}^{(1)} = P_1 \cup P_2 = \frac{1}{C_1^{k-1}} \sum_{i=1}^{k-1} \left(\frac{1}{2^i} + \frac{1}{2^{k-i}} - \frac{1}{2^k}\right) = \frac{2^{k+1} - (k+3)}{(k-1)2^k}. \tag{2}$$

For the two-point crossover, to retain chromosomes unchanged, the probability is $(P_1 \cap P_3) \cup P_2$, as shown in Fig. 4(a). The crossover productivity rate of the two-point crossover becomes

$$P_{eff}^{(2)} = 1 - P_{inv}^{(2)}, \tag{3}$$

$$\begin{aligned} P_{inv}^{(2)} &= (P_1 \cap P_3) \cup P_2 \\ &= \frac{1}{C_2^{k-1}} \sum_{i=1}^{k-2} \sum_{j=i+1}^{k-1} \left(\frac{1}{2^{i+k-j}} + \frac{1}{2^{j-i}} - \frac{1}{2^k}\right) \\ &= \frac{2^{k+1} - (k+3)}{(k-1)2^k}. \end{aligned} \tag{4}$$

By comparing (4) with (2), it follows that $P_{eff}^{(2)} = P_{eff}^{(1)}$. As shown in Fig. 4(b), the two-point crossover can be denoted by the single-point crossover.

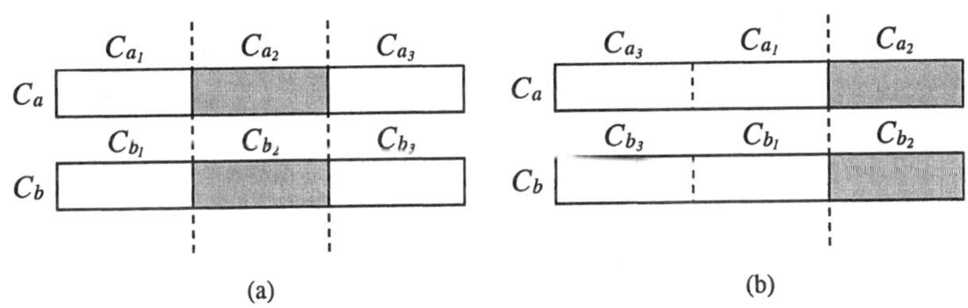

Fig. 4. (a) The two-point crossover, (b) the equivalent representation of a two-point crossover as a single-point crossover.

(b) General case of crossover productivity

For an n-point crossover, the crossover productivity rate can be derived as follows. The n crossover points divide each chromosome into $(n+1)$ segments, i.e., $C_a = C_{a_1} + C_{a_2} + \cdots + C_{a_{n+1}}$ and $C_b = C_{b_1} + C_{b_2} + \cdots + C_{b_{n+1}}$. At the initial derivation, n is assumed to be an odd number. An n-point crossover can be identically represented as shown in Fig. 5(b). The corresponding crossover productivity rate can then be calculated as

$$P_{eff}^{(n)} = 1 - P_{inv}^{(n)}, \tag{5}$$

$$\begin{aligned} P_{inv}^{(n)} &= (P_1 \cap P_3 \cap \cdots \cap P_n) \cup (P_2 \cap P_4 \cap \cdots \cap P_{n+1}) \\ &= P_1 P_3 \cdots P_n + P_2 P_4 \cdots P_{n+1} - \prod_{i=1}^{n+1} P_i \\ &= \frac{1}{C_n^{k-1}} \sum_{i=\frac{n+1}{2}}^{k-\frac{n+1}{2}} [C_{\frac{n-1}{2}}^{i-1} C_{\frac{n-1}{2}}^{k-1-i} (\frac{1}{2^i} + \frac{1}{2^{k-i}} - \frac{1}{2^k})] \\ &= \frac{2}{C_n^{k-1}} \sum_{i=\frac{n+1}{2}}^{k-\frac{n+1}{2}} [C_{\frac{n-1}{2}}^{i-1} C_{\frac{n-1}{2}}^{k-1-i} \frac{1}{2^i}] - \frac{1}{2^k}. \end{aligned} \tag{6}$$

It has been shown in Section 2.1 that the crossover productivity rates of the single-point crossover and the two-point crossover are the same. Here we show that for an even-number-point crossover, the productivity rate $P_{eff}^{(n)}$ is equal to $P_{eff}^{(n-1)}$. This result introduces the following lemma.

Lemma 1: $P_{eff}^{(n)} = P_{eff}^{(n-1)}$, for n is even.

Moreover, for the uniform crossover operation [25], the crossover productivity rate becomes

$$P_{eff}^{(u)} = 1 - P_{inv}^{(u)}, \tag{7}$$

and

$$P_{inv}^{(u)} = \frac{1}{2^{k-1}} [C_0^{k-1} \cdot 0 + C_1^{k-1} \cdot P_{inv}^{(1)} + \cdots + C_{k-1}^{k-1} \cdot P_{inv}^{(k-1)}], \tag{8}$$

where $(C_n^{k-1}/2^{k-1})$ is the probability of performing an n-point crossover in the uniform crossover situation.The proof of Lemma 1 can be found in [26]. This equivalence simplifies analysis and simulations in the next section.

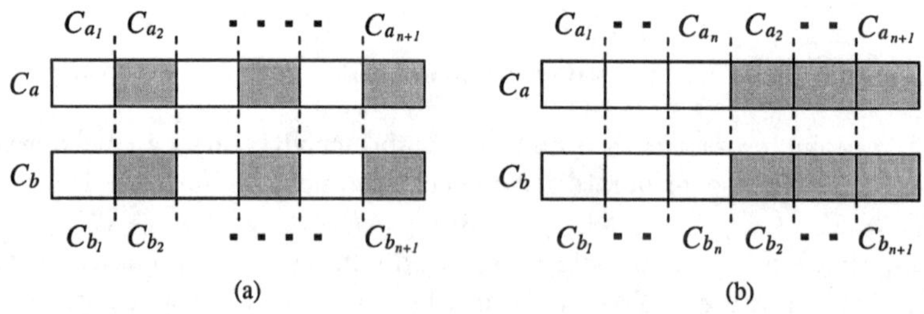

Fig. 5. (a) The N-point crossover, (b) an equivalent representation of an n-point crossover.

(c) Simulations

According to Section 3.2 and Eq.(8), the crossover productivity rates of single- to seven-point crossovers and the uniform crossover with different chromosome lengths are plotted in Fig. 6. Without loss of generality, in this simulation, the crossover probability is assumed to be 1. (the maximum value). It can be seen from Fig. 6 that higher crossover productivity rates can be reached if the number of crossover points is increased. The crossover productivity rates will approach 1 if the chromosome length is large enough. For a small search space situation, i.e., with a short chromosome length (e.g. $k \leq 5$), the crossover productivity rate is very low even if the crossover probability equals 1.

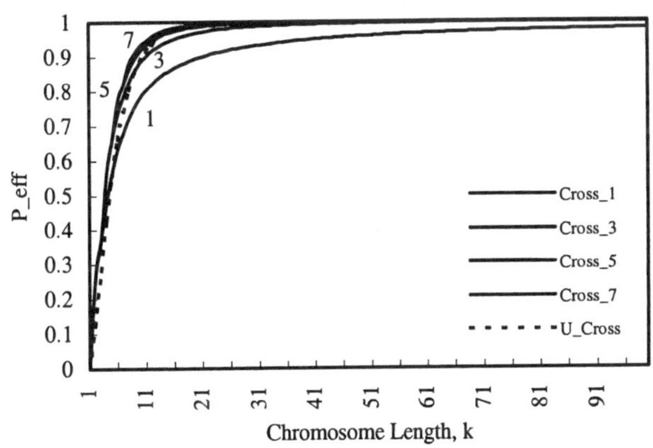

Fig. 6. The plot of the crossover productivity rates according to pure theoretical derivations.

The previous derivation of the crossover productivity rates is based on the ideal assumption that the probabilities of any chromosomes mated with the other chromosomes are all equal. In real applications, the homogeneity of chromosomes in a population increases with the number of generations. Therefore, the real crossover productivity rates will be inferior to the theoretical ones derived above. In the following simulations, a more precise plot for the crossover productivity rates will be drawn, where a whole genetic evolution system is applied and the crossover probability is, again, set to be 1. For the ease of reproduction, the genetic algorithm depicted in [27] is adopted in our simulation.

In the simulations, the fitness function is defined as

$$f(x) = \frac{c}{b-a+1}(V(x) - b + 1), \tag{9}$$

where c is a constant and

$$V(x) = -x \prod_{i=1}^{2\delta-1} (x - \rho_i), \tag{10}$$

$$a = max\{V(x)|x \in S\}, \tag{11}$$

$$b = min\{V(x)|x \in S\}, \tag{12}$$

where ρ_i ($\rho_1 \neq \rho_2 \neq \cdots \neq \rho_{2\delta-1}$) are random integers selected from 1 to $2^k - 1$ and δ denotes the number of existing peaks in the search space S. Different number of peaks (i.e. different number of local maxima), from 1 to 7, are tested in our simulations. The results of the simulations are not quite stable because most components of the genetic evolution are largely affected by the behavior of the adopted random number generator. It is quite common that different results are obtained although the same genetic algorithm and the identical conditions are input. To get more stable results, the same genetic system is performed one hundred times and the average values are calculated as the results.

Fig. 7(a) shows the average crossover productivity rates for different crossover points. It is approved that more crossover points produce higher productivity rates. Moreover, the productivity rates of even-number-point crossovers are very close to that of their odd-number-point counterparts, as was claimed in Lemma 1.

Fig. 8 shows the plot of the crossover productivity rates acquired from the simulations. From Fig. 6 and Fig. 8, we found that the more the crossover points are, the higher the productivity rates are reached; moreover, the real (simulated) productivity rates are smaller than their theoretical counterparts due to the homogeneity of chromosomes in the population.

The average crossover productivity rates for small chromosome lengths ($1 \leq k \leq 7$) are shown in Fig. 7(b). It is clear that the productivity rates are very low (< 0.35) although the maximum crossover probability was set. While applying genetic evolution to small search space problems, an inefficient crossover operation will spend lots of computations but get only tiny gains. When the efficiency of crossover is poor, a larger number of generations is required to reach a good solution. Under this circumstance, the computational complexity of applying genetic evolution might be very close to that of the full search (brute force) approach. Crossover is therefore not included in LGSA for saving computations. The role of crossover will be taken over by more efficient mutation operations, as will be described in the next section.

2.2 Analysis of Mutation Efficiency

In conventional GAs, mutation is applied to probe the search points that can not be reached by crossover operations. The mutation probability is usually small so as not to spoil the population and ruin the chromosomes with good fitness. The mutation efficiency is therefore not so important, traditionally.

When crossover operations are taken out from the genetic evolution, due to their inefficiency in a small search space situation, the task of probing new

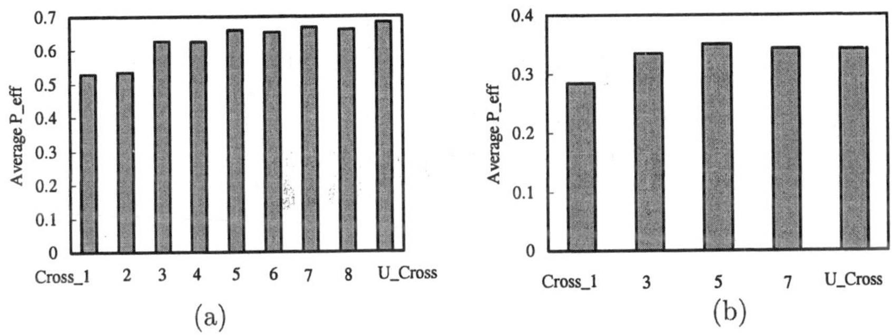

Fig. 7. The average crossover productivity rates of (a) different chromosome lengths, (b) smaller chromosome lengths.

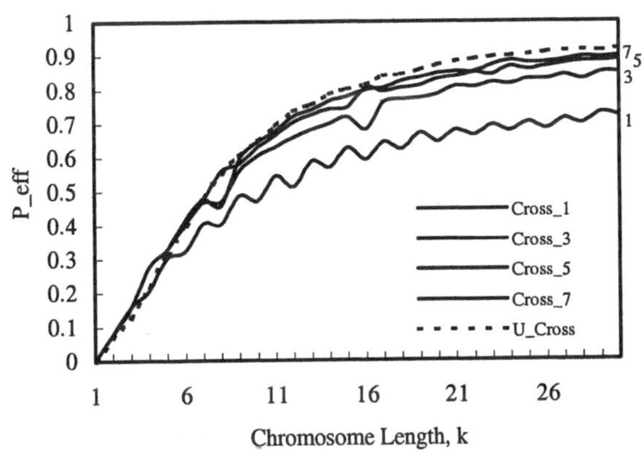

Fig. 8. The plot of the crossover productivity rates according to experimental results.

search points must be done by mutation operations. It should be guaranteed that every legal search point can be reached by mutating any selected chromosomes. The necessary number of generations for a selected chromosome to be mutated into any other chromosomes should also be small if the time constraint is an important issue. Therefore, the mutation efficiency becomes a very important issue for small search space applications.

For a selected chromosome, it is hoped that the chromosome can change to any other chromosomes with high probability. If an efficient mutation operation is applied, the probability of transferring any given chromosome to other chromosomes should be identical after a small number of iterations, such that there is not any search point which is hard to be reached from the selected chromosome.

To improve the mutation efficiency, the mutation probability has to be increased; however, the accumulated evolution information will also be destroyed which makes the genetic search somewhat like the random search.

Unless an elitist selection is applied in the reproduction stage to maintain the evolution information, the genetic search will degrade to the random search if the mutation probability is high. When an elitist selection is applied to avoid the disruption of population by mutation, the mutation invariance (or unchanged) rate for a selected chromosome would be very low. The probability of transferring one chromosome to other different chromosomes is proportional to the mutation efficiency.

The probability for a chromosome C_i to be mutated into another chromosome C_j is

$$P_{eff}(i,j) = P_m^{H(C_i,C_j)}(1-P_m)^{k-H(C_i,C_j)}, \tag{13}$$

where P_m is the mutation probability, k the chromosome length, and $H(i,j)$ the Hamming distance between C_i and C_j. A mutation efficiency matrix can then be formed as

$$M^t = [m_{ij}^{(t)}], \tag{14}$$

where t is the number of generations and

$$m_{ij}^{(1)} = P_{eff}(i,j). \tag{15}$$

Assume the selected chromosome is strong (i.e., with a high fitness value), such that it and its offsprings will always be selected in the reproduction stage. When the crossover stage is disabled, the mutation efficiency can be calculated according to M^t.

Fig. 9 shows the mutation efficiency for the case of chromosome length $k = 2$. In Fig. 9(a), the average mutation disruption rates with three different mutation probabilities $P_m = 0.01$, 0.5, and 0.99 are depicted, where the mutation disruption rate is defined to be the mean value of the probabilities for a selected chromosome being mutated into distinct chromosomes in the search space. The variances of the probabilities of being mutated into various chromosomes are shown in Fig. 9(b).

In conventional GAs, a small mutation probability is usually adopted, for example, $P_m = 0.01$ is suggested in [28]. It can be seen from Fig. 9(a) that the average mutation disruption rate is very low in the early generations. The average disruption rate increases slowly while the number of generations increases. The average disruption rate will reach the upper bound 0.25 after more than one hundred generations. In order to promote the mutation efficiency, the mutation probability is increased. If the mutation probability approaches 1, e.g. $P_m = 0.99$, it is found that the average disruption rate will bounce between two extreme values. Moreover, by comparing Fig. 9(a) and (b), it is found that the variance of the disruption rates is very large when the average disruption rate is high. The probabilities of transferring each chromosome to all other chromosomes are still very low. Hence, increasing the mutation probability will not improve the mutation efficiency well. If a compromised value is used, e.g. $P_m = 0.5$, the average disruption rate will be retained to 0.25. Under this condition, the mutation efficiency will be better than that of the previous two cases; however, the invariance rate will still be $1 - 0.25 \times (2^2 - 1) = 0.25$. This invariance rate is still too high to improve the mutation efficiency for each chromosome.

Fig. 10 shows the mutation efficiency for the case of $k = 5$. The results are very similar to that of the case of $k = 2$. Because, when the search space is getting large, i.e. there are more and more chromosomes, the average disruption rates are therefore becoming smaller since the disruption rates should be always less than 1. Since the chromosome length is larger in this case, so that the mutation efficiency is better $(0.03 \times (2^5 - 1) > 0.25 \times (2^2 - 1))$. A smaller generation number is required for the curves of different mutation probabilities to converge to the value $2^{-k} = 1/32$. Although the mutation efficiency is better when the chromosome length is larger, the resultant efficiency is still not high enough.

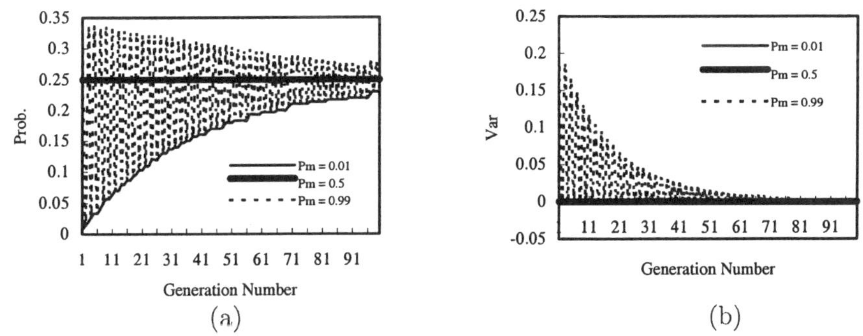

Fig. 9. Mutation efficiency of chromosome length $k = 2$: (a) the average mutation disruption rates, (b) the variances of the disruption rates for different chromosomes.

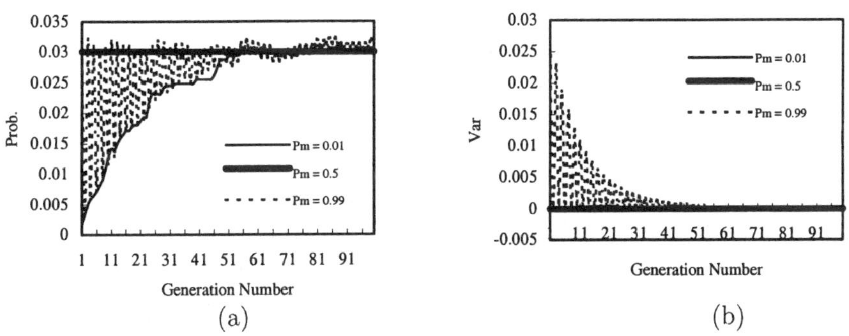

Fig. 10. Mutation efficiency of chromosome length $k = 5$: (a) the average mutation disruption rates, (b) the variances of the disruption rates for different chromosomes.

3 The Lightweight Genetic Search Algorithm

In LGSA, each gene of a chromosome is altered by adding one of the following three values, $0, 1, -1$, with identical probabilities, to improve the corresponding mutation efficiency. In the kth generation, the original mutation invariance rate is equal to $1/2^k$. Fig. 11 shows an example of the prescribed alternation of the mutation process, where $k = 2$ and, without loss of generality, the selected chromosome is assumed to be "00". The mutation efficiency of LGSA, in the kth generation, is shown in Table. 1, where four kinds of chromosome lengths are tested. It is found that, within a small number of generations, the mutation efficiency of LGSA will be better than that of the conventional ones. Moreover, the corresponding average mutation disruption rates will be higher and the variances of the disruption rates will be smaller. Notice that the mutation invariance rates of LGSA are reasonably small as compared to that of the conventional mutation approach, as shown in Figs. 9 and 10.

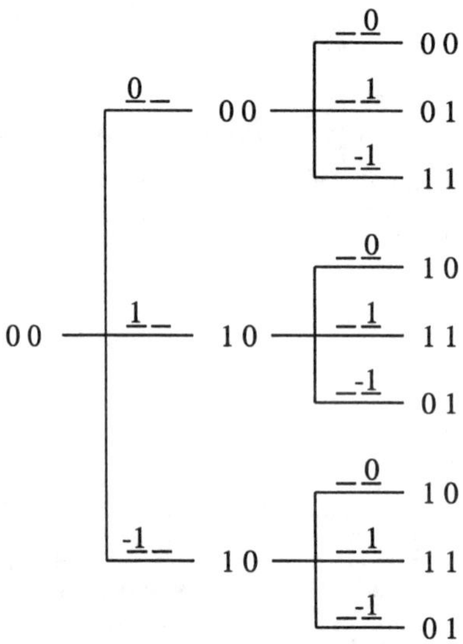

(a)

	00	01	10	11
Prob.	1/9	3/9	2/9	3/9

(b)

Fig. 11. An example of the modified mutation evolution adopted in LGSA: (a) the mutation evolution, (b) the associated probability of transferring from the selected chromosome to all possible chromosomes (after two generations of mutation evolution).

Assume the central point of the two-dimensional search space S locates at $(\hat{x}, \hat{y})$. The ith chromosome, C_i for $i = 0, 1, \cdots, N-1$, of the population set is defined as

Table 1. Mutation efficiency of the LGSA.

Chromosome Leng.	Mut. Disrup. Rate	Var. of Mut. Disrup.	Mut. Invariance Mut. Rate
2	0.2963	0.0027	0.1111
3	0.1376	0.0017	0.0370
4	0.0661	0.0006	0.0123
5	0.0321	0.0002	0.0041

$$C_i = \begin{bmatrix} m_i \\ n_i \end{bmatrix} = \begin{bmatrix} a_{i,k-1} \; a_{i,k-2} \cdots a_{i,1} \; a_{i,0} \\ b_{i,k-1} \; b_{i,k-2} \cdots b_{i,1} \; b_{i,0} \end{bmatrix}, \tag{16}$$

and the relative location is

$$(m_i, n_i) = (x_i - \hat{x}, y_i - \hat{y}), \tag{17}$$

where (x_i, y_i) denotes the location of the search point associated with the chromosome and the codeword size k depends on the size of the search space. If the search space is $\{(i,j)| -w \leq i, j \leq w-1\}$, the value of k will be $\lceil \log_2(2w) \rceil$, where $\lceil \cdot \rceil$ is the ceiling function. The values of the genes are derived from the associated relative location; that is

$$a_{i,j} = \lfloor \frac{m_i + 2w}{2^j} \rfloor \;\; mod \;\; 2, \tag{18}$$

$$b_{i,j} = \lfloor \frac{n_i + 2w}{2^j} \rfloor \;\; mod \;\; 2, \qquad j = 0, 1, \cdots, k-1, \tag{19}$$

where *mod* denotes the modulus operation and $\lfloor \cdot \rfloor$ is the floor function. The relative location can be one-to-one encoded into a series of genes with values of 0 and 1. And the relative location (m_i, n_i) can be calculated from the values of the genes by

$$m_i = \sum_{j=0}^{k-1} a_{i,j} \cdot 2^j - 2a_{i,k-1}w, \tag{20}$$

$$n_i = \sum_{j=0}^{k-1} b_{i,j} \cdot 2^j - 2b_{i,k-1}w. \tag{21}$$

Although the values of the genes might not equal 0 or 1 after mutation; however, they can be transferred to a relative location without any ambiguity.

The block diagram of genetic evolution in LGSA is shown in Fig. 12. It is well-known that when GAs are applied to search for the global optimum in the solution space S, a population set P composed of N chromosomes will be maintained, where N is the population size. Each chromosome (composed of a list of genes) in P represents a search point in S. The population P will evolve into another population P' by performing some genetic operations.

The chromosomes with higher fitness values will have higher probability to be kept in the population set of the next generation and to propagate their offspring. On the other hand, the weak chromosomes whose fitness values are small will be replaced by other stronger chromosomes. By this way, the quality of the chromosomes in the population set will get better and better. After a certain number of generations, the global optimum is expected in the mature population set.

As shown in Fig. 12, an initial population is created before the evolution. In most GA-based applications, the initial population is created by randomly selecting points from the solution space. To reduce the iteration number, in LGSA, the proper initial chromosomes can be selected from the solution space at some fixed locations if some knowledge about the application was known before hand. For example, if $N = 18$, the proper locations of the initial chromosomes for the block motion estimation, in video coding applications [9], can be selected as shown in Fig. 13. The coordinate (x_i, y_i) of the ith initial chromosome is [29]

$$x_i = \hat{x} + \Delta \cdot \tilde{x}_i, \tag{22}$$

$$y_i = \hat{y} + \Delta \cdot \tilde{y}_i, \tag{23}$$

$$\Delta = \lceil \frac{w}{2max(\tilde{x}_{N-1}, \tilde{y}_{N-1})} \rceil, \tag{24}$$

$$\tilde{x}_i = (-1)^l([i - l(l+1)] \cdot [1 - (\lfloor 2\sqrt{i} \rfloor \ mod \ 2)] + \lceil \frac{1}{2} l \rceil), \tag{25}$$

$$\tilde{y}_i = (-1)^l([i - l(l+1)] \cdot [\lfloor 2\sqrt{i} \rfloor \ mod \ 2] - \lceil \frac{1}{2} l \rceil), \tag{26}$$

$$l = \lfloor \sqrt{i} \rfloor. \tag{27}$$

The above selection comes from the observation that the global optimum of the prescribed applications locates much probably near the center of the search area. Therefore, the average number of iterations of genetic evolution will be largely reduced if the initial chromosomes are scattered around the central point.

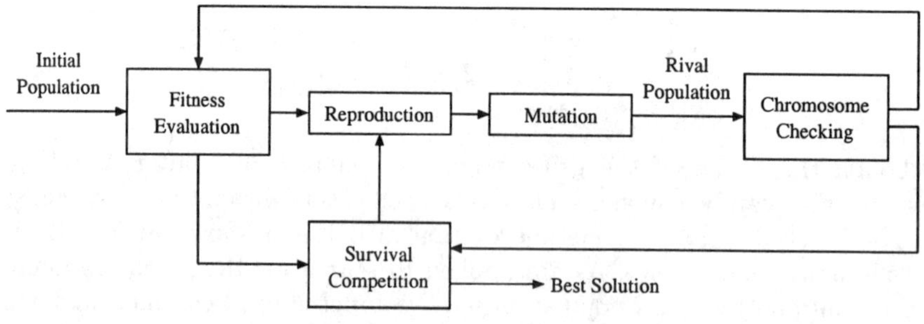

Fig. 12. The block diagram of the lightweight genetic search algorithm.

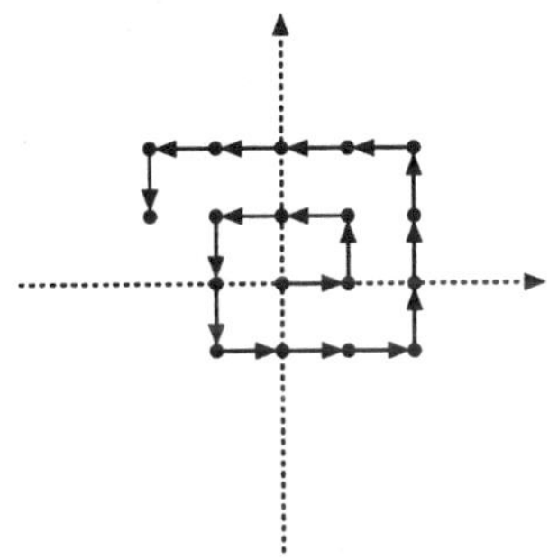

Fig. 13. The initial chromosomes distribute equally on the search space.

3.1 Fitness Values

Each chromosome has an associated fitness value which is defined as

$$f_i = U_{D(d_i,\hat{d}_\tau)} \cdot D(d_i, \hat{d}_\tau) + \delta_{D(d_i,\hat{d}_\tau)}, \tag{28}$$

where d_i is the matching value of the search point represented by the ith chromosome, D is a distance function, and U and δ are the unit step function and the delta function, respectively. When the target of the search problem is to find a point with the minimum matching value, the distance function is defined as

$$D(d_i, \hat{d}_\tau) = \hat{d}_\tau - d_i, \tag{29}$$

where $\hat{d}_\tau$ is the τth minimum matching value among the N values, $\{d_i | i = 0, 1, \cdots, N-1\}$. If the target is the global maximum, the distance function is defined as

$$D(d_i, \hat{d}_\tau) = d_i - \hat{d}_\tau, \tag{30}$$

where $\hat{d}_\tau$ is the τth maximum matching value. The constant τ determines how many chromosomes, at most, should be selected as seeds in the reproduction stage for producing a rival population. The chromosomes with larger fitness values, in the current population set, will have higher probability to be selected as seeds for generating the rival population. This probabilistic scheme of selecting seeds of the new generation is known as the probabilistic reproduction. Because the value of $U_{D(d_i,\hat{d}_\tau)}$ is either 0 or 1, there needs no multiplication for computing the fitness values.

3.2 Reproduction

The reproduction method used in this work is similar to the weighted roulette wheel method [1]. For each chromosome C_i, an incidence range r_i is calculated as

$$r_i = \left[\frac{\sum_{k=0}^{i-1} f_k}{\sum_{k=0}^{N-1} f_k}, \frac{\sum_{k=0}^{i} f_k}{\sum_{k=0}^{N-1} f_k} \right), \tag{31}$$

where f_k is the fitness value of the kth chromosome in the population, and '[' and ')' denote closing and opening boundaries, respectively. When the incidence range of each chromosome has been determined, N real numbers α_i for $i = 0, 1, \cdots, N-1$, are randomly generated, where $0 \leq \alpha_i < 1$. The value of α_i will be bounded by some incidence range r_j, that is, $\alpha_i \in r_j$. The jth chromosome C_j is then selected as a seed to generate the rival population. It is possible that one chromosome can be selected twice or more. Because N real random numbers are generated, N seeds will be selected and placed in the mating pool.

As comparing with the traditional implementation [3], the advantage of this approach is that the seeds can be directly indexed so that the control overhead is small. On the other hand, the disadvantage is that N divisions are required to calculate the incidence ranges. The computational complexity of this stage might be a little higher than that of the traditional approaches.

3.3 Mutation

After the reproduction stage, the seeds in the mating pool are transferred into candidate chromosomes of the new population set by mutation. Assuming the current chromosome to be processed is $[m_i \; n_i]^t$, where $m_i = [a_{i,k-1} a_{i,k-2} \ldots a_{i,0}]$ and $n_i = [b_{i,k-1} b_{i,k-2} \ldots b_{i,0}]$. In the jth generation, two genes $a_{i,z}$ and $b_{i,z}$ are varied, where $z = k - 1 - (j \bmod k)$.

There are eight mutation operators, $\{(\zeta_p, \eta_p) | p = 0, 1, \cdots, 7\}$, which can be adopted in our implementation, that is

$$a'_{i,z} = a_{i,z} + \zeta_p, \tag{32}$$

$$b'_{i,z} = b_{i,z} + \eta_p, \tag{33}$$

where p is a random integer whose value is between 0 and 7. Because the chromosomes are randomly selected and put on the mating pool, it is not necessary to generate a random number for determining the value of p. We simply set p to be $(i \; mod \; 8)$. The mutation operators are therefore defined as,

$$\zeta_p = (-1)^l ([p + 1 - l(l+1)] \cdot [1 - (\lfloor 2\sqrt{p+1} \rfloor \; mod \; 2)] + \lceil \frac{1}{2} l \rceil), \tag{34}$$

$$\eta_p = (-1)^l ([p + 1 - l(l+1)] \cdot [\lfloor 2\sqrt{p+1} \rfloor \; mod \; 2] - \lceil \frac{1}{2} l \rceil), \tag{35}$$

$$l = \lfloor \sqrt{p+1} \rfloor. \tag{36}$$

By applying these mutation operators, the neighboring points of the seeds are included in the rival population to be evaluated for their fitness values. The chromosomes with larger fitness values will have more copies in the mating pool, so more neighboring points of them will be included. On the contrary, less neighboring points will be included for those chromosomes with smaller fitness values. In other words, the number of the included neighboring points are determined by the fitness values. This explains the superiority of LGSA over the multiple candidate search (MCS) algorithm [30] in terms of the flexibility for search point selection.

Notice that when the mutation operators are performed on the most significant genes of the chromosomes (e.g., a_{k-2}, b_{k-2}, etc.), the chromosomes which are far from the original ones in the search space are generated. Whereas, the nearby chromosomes are generated when the mutation operators are performed on the least significant genes.

3.4 Termination Conditions

There are N chromosomes in the rival population set after performing the genetic operations in the mating pool. The rival population set is examined. For the chromosomes that have appeared in previous generations, that is the associated fitness values have been calculated and stored, it is not necessary to manipulate them again. Only the fitness values of the new born chromosomes have to be computed.

N chromosomes are selected from the union of the original population set and the rival population set ($2N$ chromosomes in total) according to the fitness values. Each chromosome can only be selected once. The chromosomes with larger fitness values will be picked up as the members of the new population set and go through the next iteration of the genetic evolution. Although the chromosomes have to be sorted in this survival competition stage, the overhead is not high because the population size is usually not large in LGSA. In GA, the new chromosomes generated from the original ones are not guaranteed to have larger fitness values. A survival competition stage is therefore included in LGSA to prevent the chromosomes from being replaced by the new ones with poorer fitness values, because the maximum number of generations will be restricted to be quite small so as to cope with the tight time constraint.

The chromosome with the maximum fitness value is selected from the current population as a possible solution. The possible solution might be replaced by others from one generation to the others. The iteration will be terminated when the termination conditions are satisfied. There are three termination conditions in LGSA: (1) the possible solution is not updated for a predetermined period of generations; (2) the matching value of the possible solution is better than a predefined threshold; (3) the number of iterations reaches the given maximum generation bound.

3.5 Comparisons of LGSA with Conventional GAs

As comparing LGSA with conventional GAs, Table 2 lists their main differences. These features make LGSA more suitable for the small search space optimization problems than conventional GAs do.

Table 2. The main differences of the LGSA and the conventional GAs.

	LGSA	Conventional GAs
Probability of calling random no. generator	Low	High
Crossover	No	Yes
Survival competition stage	Yes	No
Mutation probability	High	Low
Maximum generation number	Small	Large

The computational cost of generating random numbers is not low. In conventional GA-based applications, the search space is usually large and the time constraint is not an important issue; hence, the computational cost required to generate random numbers is tolerable. However, when GAs are applied to time critical applications, such as the block matching of video coding, the cost of generating random numbers becomes a critical issue because the search space is relatively small and the time constraint is extremely tight. The on-line cost of generating random numbers can be somewhat reduced by generating and storing them ahead of time. However, in conventional GAs, random numbers have to be generated in the reproduction, the crossover, and the mutation stages; nevertheless, in LGSA, the random number generator is only called in the reproduction stage.

In conventional GAs, crossover is usually applied. The purpose of performing crossover is to randomly exploit new search points. Because the search space is not large in LGSA, there are no large amounts of local optima in the search space. The effectiveness of crossover is not prominent (as prescribed in Section 3); therefore, the crossover stage is not included in LGSA for complexity reduction.

Because weaker chromosomes might propagate stronger chromosomes, they are not excluded in the new population set of the conventional GAs. The population will be gradually mature after a long period of generations. That is, weaker chromosomes will not hinder the population from being mature; however, they will reduce the effectiveness of LGSA in which the number of generations of evolution is restricted to be small. To solve this problem, in LGSA, a survival competition stage is included. It ensures that the quality of each chromosome in the current population set is better than that of the old ones.

There are two kinds of mutation operators used in traditional GA-based implementation: changing a gene's value (i) from 0 to 1, or (ii) from 1 to 0. Generally, the mutation probability is very low so as not to impair the overall quality of a given population. In LGSA, the mutation probability is relatively high so the evolution of chromosomes is relatively violent. Fortunately, the bad effect of high mutation rate will be totally controlled by the survival competition. Interestingly, lots of search points will be explored due to high mutation rate although there is no crossover stage in LGSA.

Because the evolution of chromosomes is slow, the maximum and the average number of generations are large in conventional GAs, and so are the required average computations for finding the extreme value. Therefore, both the control overheads and the cost of performing extreme value finding are tremendous. In LGSA, the evolution is relatively violent and the quality of chromosomes is well controlled by the survival competition stage, so the maximum number of generations is small and the control overheads of chromosome evolution are also reduced. Moreover, the cost for extreme value finding in LGSA is relatively small because most of the irrelevant search points have been removed beforehand.

4 Convergence Analysis of LGSA

It has been proven that conventional GAs do not converge to global optima unless an elitist selection is applied [31]. In this section, the convergence property of LGSA will be investigated. It follows from Section 3 that LGSA is one kind of elitist selection methods.

Let n denote the population size, k the chromosome length, and $S = \{0,1\}^k$ the solution space. The target of LGSA is to find

$$\max_{b}\{f(b)|b \in S\}, \tag{37}$$

where f is a fitness evaluation function. The derivation will be carried out by means of finite Markov chain processes presented in [31]. The following important theorem which founds the basis of our derivation is quoted from [31].

Theorem 1: [31] Let $P = \begin{bmatrix} P_{11} & 0 \\ P_{21} & P_{22} \end{bmatrix}$ be a reducible stochastic matrix, where P_{11} of size $m \times m$ is a primitive stochastic matrix and $P_{21}, P_{22} \neq 0$. Then

$$P^{\infty} = \lim_{t \to \infty} P^t = \begin{bmatrix} P_{11}^{\infty} & 0 \\ P_{21}^{\infty} & 0 \end{bmatrix} \tag{38}$$

is a stable stochastic matrix, where $p^{\infty} = p^0 P^{\infty}$ is unique regardless of the initial distribution, and p^{∞} satisfies: $p_i^{\infty} > 0$ for $1 \le i \le m$ and $p_i^{\infty} = 0$ for $m < i \le n$.

Lemma 2: The LGSA will converge to the global optimum with probability one after infinite number of iterations.The proof of Lemma 2 can be found in [26].

Although the theoretical convergence property of LGSA has been provided in Lemma 2, the above derivation only shows that the solution will converge to the global maximum after infinite iterations. When a lower computational load is required, the maximum number of iterations is usually restricted. To see the performance of LGSA and conventional GAs under the circumstances of finite generation evolution, several simulations have been performed. In the simulations, the genetic algorithm depicted in [27] is implemented for comparison. Different peak (local optimum) numbers, from 1 to 7, are tested.

Table 3 shows the average difference between the global optima and the search results obtained in LGSA and the chosen conventional GA with different sizes of the search space, where k represents the chromosome length used to encode the whole search space. From the table, it is observed that the average difference between the obtained results and the global maxima is less than 0.1 in LGSA when the chromosome length is less than 10. This fact coincides with our claim that LGSA is an efficient genetic algorithm for dealing with the small size and time critical search problems.

Table 3. Average difference between the global optima and the search results obtained by LGSA and a conventional genetic algorithm. (Where the population size $N = 10$, the GA's crossover and mutation probabilities are 0.6 and 0.5, respectively, the LGSA's mutation rate is 0.5, and the maximum number of generations is 50.)

k	1	2	3	4	5	6	7	8
GA	0.07	0.34	0.72	0.79	0.94	1.7	3.12	6.16
LGSA	0	0	0.14	0.07	0.01	0.01	0.01	0.01

k	9	10	11	12	13	14	15	16
GA	14.28	27.8	59.78	91.34	248.91	461.47	821.15	1715.54
LGSA	0.01	0.14	0.5	1.09	2.1	4.38	10.6	18.55

5 Three Applications of LGSA

We have applied LGSA to three kinds of applications: the block-based motion estimation [9], the automatic facial feature extraction [10] and the watermarking performance optimization. Since methods of embedding LGSA into the first two applications have been addressed in detail in [9] and [10], only their simulation results are demonstrated in this section.

Digital watermarking has been regarded as an effective solution against media piracy. Digital contents are invisibly embedded with watermark data, which can be extracted later to prove copyrights or identities of creators. Watermarking schemes designed for different application scenarios may have different application-specific requirements. But in general, higher fidelity, better robustness, and larger data capacity are the three goals that most watermarking or data-hiding applications would like to achieve. However, since these requirements are conflicting with each other, optimal watermarking has become an inherently difficult and interesting problem. For example, the fidelity requirement limits the strength of embedded signals, which consequently constraints the robustness of a watermarking scheme against common or malicious manipulations. As another example, the higher the embedded data capacity is, the lower the perceptually quality is observed, since more noise is embedded into the original media. A comprehensive introduction to digital watermarking can be found in [20].

To optimize the performance of watermarking schemes, as specified in [11], the block-DCT-based image-watermarking scheme given in [21] is used to prove the enhancing effectiveness of the proposed optimization. Since the fidelity of watermarked image is selected as our objective function representing the fitness of each candidate chromosome, objective visual quality indexes, such as peak signal-to-noise ratio(PSNR), are adopted as the fitness values that guide the optimizing procedure. The optimization procedures are done in a block-by-block sense, and all the possible embedding positions in each DCT transformed block are treated as chromosomes. Embedding in repeated positions or the DC coefficient is forbidden, and illegal chromosomes will be labeled with extremely low fitness values to avoid being selected as parents of the next generation. The fidelity enhancement is obvious; however, for certain watermarking applications, such as copy-control of video clips, the time complexity of watermark embedding is as important as other watermarking requirements such as fidelity after watermark embedding or robustness against attacks. In order to reduce the required complexity and demonstrate the efficiency of LGSA, the conventional GA optimization procedures specified in [11] are replaced by LGSA in this work.

The target of motion estimation is to find the magnitudes of movement for one or several objects in a video sequence. Block matching algorithms (BMAs) [32, 33] are usually applied to reduce the complexity of estimating object motion. In the block matching algorithm, the image block is matched with the candidate blocks within the search area in the referenced image frame, and the block with the minimum summed absolute difference is selected as the solution block. The offset between the image block and the solution block is declared as the motion of the block.

In order to see the performance of the LGSA, the full search algorithm (FSA), the three-step search method (TSS) [22], and the multi-candidate search method (MCS) [30] are all implemented in our simulations for comparison. In our simulations, the image block size is 16×16 pixels, and the search area is from -16 to 16 pixels.

Fig. 14 shows the motion estimated frames selected from the experimental results by applying different block matching algorithms. It can be found that the quality of the estimated frame by applying the LGSA is very similar to that of the FSA. As it can be seen, the edge of the table and the racket cannot be well estimated by using the other two fast search algorithms. The average numbers of block matching in different BMAs are shown in Table 4. The LGSA has similar estimation accuracy to the FSA, but its average block matching number is only 4.6% of that of the FSA. As comparing with MCS, LGSA has better estimation accuracy, and its average block matching number is just 84.4% of that of the MCS.

The main target of automatic facial feature extraction is to extract the important facial feature regions from an image. In the previous works [34]–[39], searching all the candidate regions in the image is a must. In order to reduce the computational complexity of extracting the facial feature regions, LGSA is applied. The face region is first extracted from the image. We define a feature template and use the feature template to match with the candidate feature regions. The most suitable candidate is found based on the defined evaluation function.

Fig. 15 shows some results selected from our simulations. Although the materials are originally color images, only the luminance components are shown because the chrominance components are not utilized in this work.

In Fig. 15, three images captured by a normal V8 camera are shown. These images are all in SIF format (352 $\times$ 240 pixels). Each image was processed by applying the proposed algorithm and as expected the facial features could be extracted correctly.

Table 5 shows the ratios of the average number of searched points to the total number of candidate points. According to the table, it is known that most of the unnecessary point evaluations can be avoided by applying the LGSA.

Table 6 shows the required generation numbers to obtain embedded Lena images with different visual qualities, respectively. Other experimental parameters and settings are specified in the table caption. According to this table, it is clear that LGSA can save about half the unnecessary computations while optimizing the watermarking performance, in terms of PSNR, at the same time. To show the results subjectively, Fig. 16 shows the enlarged versions of the embedded Lena image before and after LGSA optimization.

Therefore, in all three applications, the computational complexity is largely reduced, although overhead is needed for the evolution of genetic search.

Table 4. Average block matching number for each block in the block motion estimation applications.

Algorithm	FSA	TSS	MCS	LGSA
Block matching	973.70	30.61	53.10	44.84

6 Conclusion

Much research has been done on the properties and the applications of various genetic algorithms. However, very few works focus on the applications with a small search space. In this kind of applications, the control overheads of the genetic evolution have to be well adjusted, such that the efficiency of the

Table 5. The ratios of the averaged number of searched points to the total number of candidate points for different video sequences in the AFFE application.

Sequence	Ratio
Tseng	0.11
Chou	0.12
Chuan	0.21
Miss America	0.22
Claire	0.43

Table 6. The average generation numbers required to improve an embedded Lena image to certain image fidelity by conventional GA and LGSA are listed. The experimental results are obtained by embedding 4 bits of watermark signals into each block of the original image. The PSNR of the original watermarked image without optimization is 35.33 dB.

PSNR	36	38	40	42
Generation number of GA	20.46	49.46	87.92	134.40
Generation number of LGSA	10.17	22.66	45.28	73.04
Saving percentage	50.29	54.19	48.50	45.66

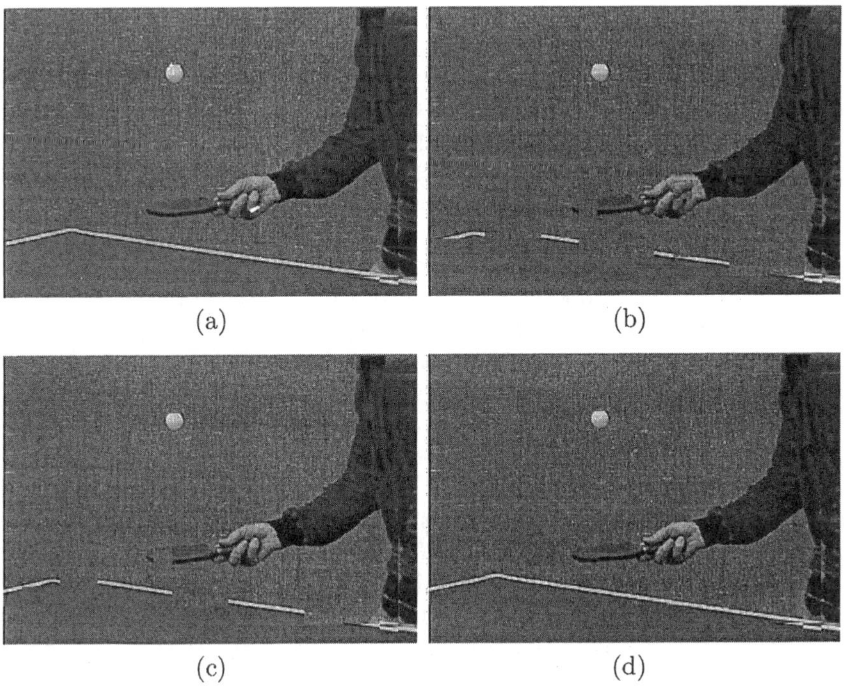

(a) (b) (c) (d)

Fig. 14. The predicted images selected from the "Table Tennis" sequence by using different search algorithms: (a) FSA, (b) TSS, (c) MCS, (d) LGSA.

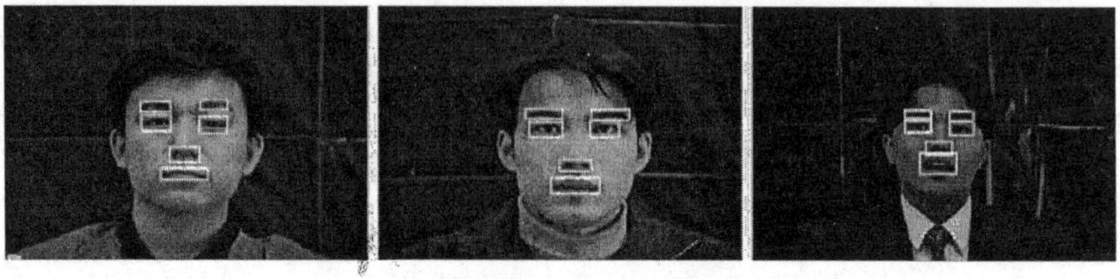

Fig. 15. Experimental results of the AFFE applications by applying the LGSA.

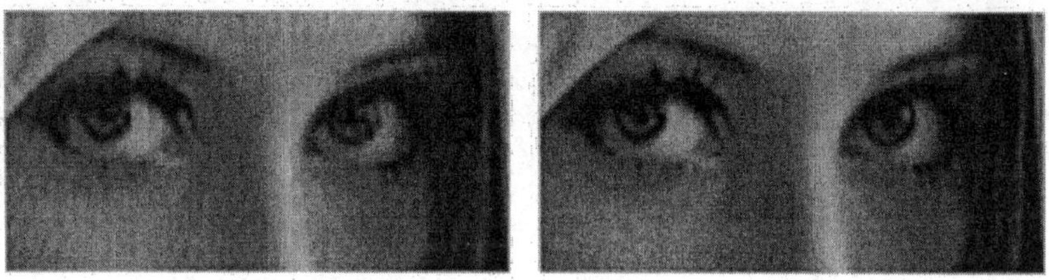

(a) (b)

Fig. 16. Snapshots of the watermark-embedded Lena image (a) before and (b) after applying the LGSA optimization procedures.

applied genetic algorithm can be approved. In this chapter, some important issues of genetic evolution, such as the efficiency of crossover and mutation operations and the global convergence property were analyzed. It follows from the analysis, when the search space is small, the efficiency of the crossover operation is not good enough for deserving the required computations. It is also hard to adjust the mutation probability to promote the efficiency of the conventional mutation operations. A modified mutation operator is therefore applied in the newly proposed genetic algorithm.

In the proposed LGSA, the computational complexity is well controlled by taking the characteristics of a smaller search space into account. The convergence property of the proposed algorithm is also provided. By adding a survival competition stage, it is shown that a small number of generations will be enough to find a good solution. The algorithm has been applied to three kinds of applications: the block motion estimation, the automatic facial feature extraction and the watermarking performance optimization. It is shown by experimental results that LGSA can find the near optimal solutions with quite low computational complexity. It is believed that LGSA will work well for other kinds of applications where the search space is small and low computational complexity is a must.

References

1. Holland, J. H. (1975) Adaptation in Natural and Artificial Systems. AnnArbor: University Michigan Press.
2. Goldberg, D. E. (1989) Genetic Algorithms in Search, Optimization Machine Learning. Reading: Addison-Wesley.
3. Srinivas M., Patnaik, L. M. (1994) Genetic algorithms: a survey. IEEE Computer Magazine. June, 17-26.
4. Tang, K. S., Man, K. F., Kwong, S., He, Q. (1996) Genetic algorithms and their applications. IEEE Signal Processing Magazine. 13, 22-37.
5. Ng, S. C., Leung, S. H., Chung, C. Y., Luk, A., Lau, W. H. (1996) The genetic search approach. IEEE Signal Processing Magazine. 13, 38-46.
6. Jain, J. R., Jain A. K. (1981) Displacement measurement and its application in interframe image coding. IEEE Transactions on Communication. COM-29, 1799-1808.
7. Chow, H. K. K., Liou, M. L. (1993) Genetic motion search algorithm for video compression. IEEE Transactions on Circuits and Systems for Video Technology. 3(6), 440-445.
8. Kim, I. K., Park R. H. (1995) Block matching algorithm using a genetic algorithm. SPIE Symposium on Visual Communications and Image Processing. Taipei, 1545-1552.
9. Lin, C. H., Wu,J. L. (1998) A lightweight genetic block matching algorithm for video coding. IEEE Transactions on Circuits and Systems for Video Technology. 8(4), 386-392.
10. Lin, C. H., Wu, J. L. (1999) Automatic facial feature extraction by genetic algorithms. IEEE Transactions on Image Processing. 8(6), 834-845.
11. Huang, C. H., Wu, J. L. (2000) A watermark optimization technique based on genetic algorithms. Proc. of SPIE Electronic Imaging.
12. ITU-T SGXV Recommendation H.261. (1990) Video codec for audio visual services at p×64 Kbits/s.
13. Draft ITU-T Recommendation H.263. (1995) Video coding for low bitrate communication.
14. ISO/IEC MPEG.. (1991) Coding of moving pictures and associated audio. Committee Draft of Standard ISO11172.
15. ITU-T Recommendation H.262, ISO/IEC 13818-2 (1995) Generic coding of moving pictures and associated audio information. Draft International Standard.
16. MPEG-4 Video Group (1998) Generic Coding of Audio-Visual Objects: Part 2-Visual, ISO/IEC JTC1/SC29/WG11 N1902, FDIS of ISO/IEC 14496-2, Atlantic City.
17. Samal A., Iyengar, P. A. (1992) Automatic recognition and analysis of human faces and facial expressions: a survey. Pattern Recognition, 25(1), 65-77.
18. Aizawa K., Huang, T. S. (1995) Model-based image coding: advanced video coding techniques for very low bit-rate applications. Proceedings of the IEEE, 83(2), 259-271.
19. Wollborn, M. (1994) Prototype prediction for colour update in object-based analysis-synthesis coding. IEEE Trans. Circuits and Systems for Video Technology, 4(3), 236-245.
20. Cox, I., Bloom, J., Miller, M. (2001) Digital Watermarking, Morgan Kaufmann Publishers, 1st Edition.

21. Hsu, C. T., Wu, J. L. (1999) Hidden Digital Watermarks in Images. IEEE Transactions on Image Processing, 8(1), 58-68.
22. Koga, T., Iinuma, K., Hirano, A., Iijima,Y., Ishiguro, T. (1981) Motion compensated interframe coding for video conferencing. Proc. Nat. Telecommun. Conf., New Orleans, LA, 5.3.1-5.3.5.
23. DeJong, K. A., Spears, W. M. (1991) An analysis of the interacting roles of population size and crossover in genetic algorithms. Parallel Problem Solving from Nature, H. P. Schwefel and R. Männer, Eds. Springer, Berlin and Heidelberg, 38-47.
24. Goldberg, D. E. (1989) Sizing populations for serial and parallel genetic algorithms. Proc. 3rd Int. Conf. Genetic Algorithms and Applications, San Mateo, CA.
25. Syswerda, G. (1989) Uniform crossover in genetic algorithms. Proc. 3rd Int. Conf. Genetic Algorithms and Applications, San Mateo, CA, 2-9.
26. Lin, C. H., Wu, J. L. (2004) The lightweight genetic search algorithm: an efficient genetic algorithm for small search range problems. to appear in International Journal of Computational Engineering Science.
27. Filho, J. L. R., Treleaven, P. C., (1994) Genetic-algorithm programming environments. IEEE Computer Magazine, June, 28-43.
28. Greffenstette, J. J. (1986) Optimization of control parameters for genetic algorithms. IEEE Trans. Systems Man and Cybernetics, 16(1), 122-128.
29. Graham, R. L., Knuth, D. E., Patashnik, O. (1994) Concrete Mathematics, 2nd edition. Addison-Wesley Publishing Company, Inc..
30. Jong, H. M., Chen, L. G., Chiueh, T. D. (1994) Accuracy improvement and cost reduction of 3-step search block matching algorithm for video coding. IEEE Trans. Circuits and Systems for Video Technology, 4(1), 88-90.
31. Rudolph, G. (1994) Convergence analysis of canonical genetic algorithms. IEEE Transactions on Neural Networks, 5(1), 96-101.
32. Wang, Q., Clarke, R. J., (1992) Motion estimation and compensation for image sequence coding. Signal Processing: Image Communication, 4(2), 161-174.
33. Dufaux, F., Moscheni, F. (1995) Motion estimation techniques for digital TV: a review and a new contribution. Proceedings of the IEEE, 83(6), 858-875.
34. Yuille, A. L., Hallinan, P. W., and Cohen, D. S. (1992) Feature extraction from faces using deformable templates. Int. Journal of Computer Vision, 8(2), 99-111.
35. Huang, H. C., Ouhyoung, M., Wu, J. L. (1993) Automatic feature point extraction on a human face in model-based image coding. Optical Engineering, 32(7), 1571-1580.
36. Lavagetto, F., Curinga, S. (1994) Object-oriented scene modeling for interpersonal video communication at very low bit-rate.Signal Processing: Image Communication, 6, 379-395.
37. Yang, G., Huang, T. S. (1994) Human face detection in a complex background. Pattern Recognition, 27(1), 53-63.
38. Desilva, L. C., Aizawa, K., Hatori, M. (1995) Detection and tracking of facial features. SPIE Symposium on Visual Communications and Image Processing, Taipei. May, 1161-1172.
39. Eleftheriadis, A., Jacquin, A. (1995) Automatic face location detection for model-assisted rate control in H.261-compatible coding of video. Signal Processing: Image Communication, 7, 435-455.

Manifold Learning and Applications in Recognition

Junping Zhang[1], Stan Z. Li[2], and Jue Wang[3]

[1] Intelligent Information Processing Laboratory, Fudan University, 200433, Shanghai, China
jpzhang@fudan.edu.cn
[2] Face Group, Microsoft Research Asia
100080, Beijing, China
szli@microsoft.com
[3] The Key Lab of Complex Systems and Intelligent Science, Institute of Automation, Chinese Academy of Sciences, 100080, Beijing, China
jue.wang@mail.ia.ac.cn

Abstract. Great amount of data under varying intrinsic features are empirically thought of as high-dimensional nonlinear manifold in the observation space. With respect to different categories, we present two recognition approaches, i.e. the combination of manifold learning algorithm and linear discriminant analysis (MLA+LDA), and nonlinear auto-associative modeling (NAM). For similar object recognition, e.g. face recognition, MLA + LDA is used. Otherwise, NAM is employed for objects from largely different categories. Experimental results on different benchmark databases show the advantages of the proposed approaches.

Keywords: manifold learning algorithm, nonlinear auto-associative modelling, linear discriminant analysis, object recognition, face recognition

1 Introduction

A large number of data such as images and characters under varying intrinsic principal features are thought of as constituting highly nonlinear manifolds in the high-dimensional observation space. Visualization and exploration of high-dimensional vector data are therefore the focus of much current machine learning research. However, most recognition systems using linear method are bound to ignore subtleties of manifolds such as concavities and protrusions, and this is a bottleneck for achieving highly accurate recognition. This problem has to be solved before we can make a high performance recognition system.

During these years progresses have been achieved in modeling nonlinear subspaces or manifolds. Rich literature exists on manifold learning. On the basis of different representations of manifold learning, it can be roughly divided into four major classes: projection methods, generative methods, embedding methods, and mutual information methods.

1. The first is to find principal surfaces passing through the middle of data, such as the principal curves [1][2]. Though geometrically intuitive, the first one has difficulty on how to generalize the global variable–arc-length parameter– into higher-dimensional surface.
2. The second adopts generative topology models [3] [4] [5], and hypothesizes that observed data are generated from the evenly spaced low-dimensional latent nodes. And then the mapping relationship between the observation space and the latent space can be modeled. Resulting from the inherent insufficiency of the adopted EM (Expectation-Maximization) algorithms, nevertheless, the generative models fall into local minimum easily and have slow convergence rates.
3. The third is generally divided into global and local embedding algorithms. ISOMAP [6], as a global algorithm, presumes that isometric properties should be preserved in both the observation space and the intrinsic embedding space in the affine sense. And extensions to conformal mappings are also discussed in [7]. On the other hand, Locally Linear Embedding (LLE) [8] and Laplacian Eigenamp [9] focus on the preservation of local neighbor structure.
4. In the fourth category, it is assumed that the mutual information is a measurement of the differences of probability distribution between the observed space and the embedded space, as in stochastic nearest neighborhood (henceforth SNE) [10] and manifold charting [11].

While there are many impressive results about how to discover the intrinsical features of the manifold, there have been few reports on the practical applications in manifold-learning, especially on object recognition. Some literature even makes negative conclusion that LLE is only useful for small numbers of dimensions, whereas the classifiers perform better for large numbers of dimensions on PCA-mapped data [12]. A possible explanation is that the practical data include a large number of intrinsic features and have high curvature both in the observation space and in the embedded space, whereas present manifold learning methods strongly depend on the selection of parameters. Furthermore, we also find that if data of different classes belong to similar category, for example, face images, recognition can be implemented under the same subspace with manifold learning approaches. Otherwise, data (for example, character) should be mapped into the different subspace for further recognition.

Assuming that data are drawn independentlly and identically distributed from the underlying unknown distribution, we propose two recognition algorithms for processing the above-mentioned two cases in section 2. Experiments on image and character data show the advantages of the proposed recognition approaches. Finally, we discuss potential problems and further research.

2 Manifold Learning Algorithm

2.1 Dimensionality Reduction

To establish the mapping relationship between the observed data and the corresponding low-dimensional one, the locally linear embedding (LLE) algorithm [8] is used to obtain the corresponding low-dimensional data Y ($Y \subset \mathbb{R}^d$) of the training set X ($X \subset \mathbb{R}^N, N \gg d$). And then the dataset (X, Y) is used for modeling the subsequent mapping relationship.

The main principle of LLE algorithm is to preserve local neighborhood relation of data in both the embedding space and the intrinsic one. Each sample in the observation space is a linearly weighted average of its neighbors. The basic LLE algorithm is described as follows:

Step 1: define

$$\psi(W) = \| x_i - \sum_{j=1}^{K} W_{ij} x_{ij} \|^2 \tag{1}$$

where samples x_{ij} are the neighbors of x_i. Considering the constraint term $\sum_{j=1} W_{ij} = 1$, and if x_i and x_{ij} are not in the same neighbor, $W_{ij} = 0$, compute the weighted matrix W according to the least square.

Step 2: define

$$\varphi(Y) = \| y_i - \sum_{j=1}^{K} W_{ij}^* y_{ij} \|^2 \tag{2}$$

where $W^* = arg\min_w \psi(W)$. Considering the constraint $\sum_i y_i = 0$ and $\sum_i y_i y_i^T / n = I$, where n is the number of local covering set, calculate $Y^* = arg\min_Y \varphi(Y)$.

Step 2 of the algorithm is to approximate the nonlinear manifold around sample x_i with the linear hyperplane that passes through its neighbors $\{x_{i1}, \ldots, x_{ik}\}$. Considering that the objective $\varphi(Y)$ is invariant to translation in Y, constraint term $\sum_i y_i = 0$ is added in the step 2. Moreover, the other term $\sum_i y_i y_i^T / n = I$ is to avoid the degenerate solution of $Y = 0$. Hence, step 2 is transformed to the solution of eigenvector decomposition which can be seen as follows:

$$\begin{aligned} Y^* &= arg\min_Y \phi(Y) \\ &= \| y_i - \sum_{j=1}^{K} W_{ij}^* y_{ij} \|^2 \\ &= arg\min_Y \| (I - W)Y \|^2 \\ &= arg\min_Y Y^T (I - W)^T (I - W) Y \end{aligned} \tag{3}$$

The optimal solution of Y^* in Formula (3) is the smallest eigenvectors of matrix $(I - W)^T (I - W)$. With respect to the constraint conditions, the eigenvalue which is zero needs to be removed. So we need to compute the bottom $(d+1)$ eigenvectors of the matrix and discard the smallest eigenvector considering constraint term.

Thus, we obtain the corresponding low-dimensional dataset Y in embedding space. And the completed set (X, Y) is used for the subsequent modeling of the mapping relationship.

A disadvantage of LLE algorithm is that it is difficult to compute the mapping of test samples due to the computational cost of eigenmatrix. With respect to weierstrass approximation theorem, we use the following gaussian RBF kernel to approximate the relationship:

$$y_i = \sum_{j=1}^{n} \alpha_j k(x_i, x_j) \tag{4}$$

where y_i is the corresponding low-dimensional point of sample x_i. And $k(x_i, x_j)$ is:

$$k(x_i, x_j) = \exp(-\frac{\|x_i - x_j\|^2}{2\sigma^2}) \tag{5}$$

The parameter σ^2 can be predefined or computed with respect to data distribution. We assume that the selection of parameter σ^2 may have close relationship with the intrinsic dimensions of manifold. For simplicity, the corresponding matrix form of Eq. (4) is:

$$Y = \mathcal{A}K \tag{6}$$

where $\mathcal{A} \in M_{d,n}, K \in M_{n,n}$. $M_{s,t}$ means that the matrix has s rows and t columns, and $\mathcal{A}$ and K are formulated as follows:

$$\mathcal{A} = (\alpha_1, \cdots, \alpha_n) \quad K = \begin{pmatrix} k(x_1, x_1) & \cdots & k(x_1, x_n) \\ \cdots & \cdots & \cdots \\ k(x_n, x_1) & \cdots & k(x_n, x_n) \end{pmatrix} \tag{7}$$

Because the completed data (X, Y) has been obtained by mentioned LLE algorithm, given gaussian kernel, the matrix $\mathcal{A}$ is calculated as follows:

$$\mathcal{A} = YK^{-1} \tag{8}$$

where K^{-1} is the Moore-Penrose inverse matrix of K. As a result, the corresponding low-dimensional vector y' of the unknown sample x' is calculated:

$$y' = \sum_{i=1}^{n} \alpha_i k(x_i, x') \tag{9}$$

We name the procedure manifold learning algorithm (MLA), which means most manifold learning approaches can be employed for reducing high dimensional data into low-dimensional space.

3 Linear Discriminant Analysis

Assuming the data of different classes have the same or similar categories, for instance, facial images sampled from difference persons are generally thought of owning the same cognitive concept. So data of different classes can be reduced into the same subspace with manifold learning approaches. While MLA is capable of recovering the intrinsic low-dimensional space, it may not be optimal for recognition. When the two highly nonlinear manifolds are mapped into the same low-dimensional subspace through MLA, for example, there is no reason to believe that the optimal classification hyperplane also exists between the two unravelled manifolds. If the principal axes of the two low-dimensional mapping classes of manifolds have an acute angle, the classification ability may be impaired [13]. Therefore, Linear Discriminant Analysis (LDA) is introduced to maximize the separability of data among different classes.

Suppose that each class has equal probability of event, Within-class scatter matrix is therefore defined as: $S_w = \sum_{i=1}^{L} \sum_{j=1}^{n_i} (y_j - m_i)(y_j - m_i)^T$ for n_i samples from class i with class means m_i, $i = 1, 2, \ldots, L$. For the overall mean m for all samples from all classes, meanwhile, the between-class scatter matrix is defined as $S_b = \sum_{i=1}^{L} (m_i - m)(m_i - m)^T$ [13].

To maximize the between-class distances while minimizing the within-class distances of manifolds, the column vectors of discriminant matrix W are the eigenvectors of $S_b^{-1} S_w$ associated with the largest eigenvalues. Projection matrix W plays a role that projects a vector in the low-dimensional face subspace into discriminatory feature space.

With the combination of MLA and LDA (MLA+LDA), we therefore avoid the problem of dimensionality curse and recognition task can be realized on the basis of reduced dimensions.

4 Nonlinear Auto-Associative Model

If data to be classified have remarkable different categories (for example, characters), MLA+LDA will be inefficient for recognition as these data cannot be commonly mapped into a single subspace with MLA. A corresponding strategy is to extract the intrinsical principal features of these manifolds with some dimensionality reduction methods separately, and then the unknown sample can be auto-associated in light of the intrinsical principal features.

In light of Eq. (9), the reconstruction of low-dimensional data can be formulated as follows:

$$x' = \sum_{j=1}^{n_i} \beta_j k'(y_j, y') \quad y_j \in Z, y' \in R^d \tag{10}$$

$$k'(y_j, y') = \exp(- \parallel y_j - y' \parallel^2 / 2(\sigma')^2) \tag{11}$$

where $\mathcal{B} = \{\beta_j\}$ is the $N \times n$ weighted inverse mapping matrix or reconstruction matrix.

By choosing Eq. (5) and (11), the data can be effectively reconstructed. In this paper, the Frey face database (20*28 pixels, 1956 examples) [8] is used to explain the proposed method. Firstly, the 491 cluster centers are extracted using vector quantization and mapped into 2-D space using LLE. Then all the 1956 face examples are mapped into the 2-D space (where $\sigma^2 = 100$) as shown in Figure 1(a). Thirdly, we randomly sample two points and use them as the upper-left and lower-right corner points for a rectangle, and then sample 11 evenly spaced points along each of the boundary and diagonal lines of the rectangle, and these points are reconstructed with Eq.(10) and (11), as displayed in Figure 1(b). We observe that a continuous expressional change in the vertical axes and pose change from the right side to the left side. Therefore, we have approximately recovered 2 intrinsic principal features, those of expression and pose, for the FREY database using the proposed method. To compare

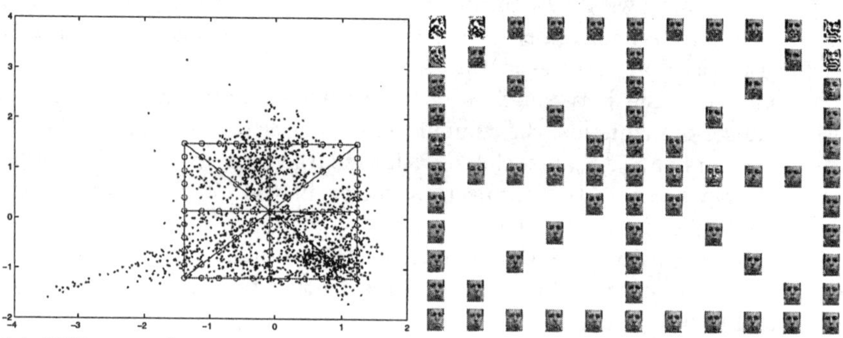

(a) 1956 examples mapped to the 2-D MLA subspace. (b) The corresponding reconstruct faces

Fig. 1. 2-dimensional mapping and reconstruction of Frey Face data

the difference between the original images and the reconstructed images, 10 points from 2-dim reduced data as in Figure 2(a) are randomly sampled and then reconstructed via the proposed method where $(\sigma')^2 = 1$. The original facial images are shown on the top of Figure 2(b), while the corresponding reconstructed facial images at the bottom of Figure 2(b). It can be seen that the proposed method effectively reconstructs these images.

The procedure has the foundation of cognitive sciences, namely, auto-association, which argues that recalling objects or concepts is achieved through preserving the underlying principal features of objects or concepts. Therefore, we call the proposed model "Nonlinear Auto-Associative Modeling" (NAM).

It is obvious that the Frey data belong to one class. To implement recognition with NAM, we assume that each NAM_i represents the ith NAM of

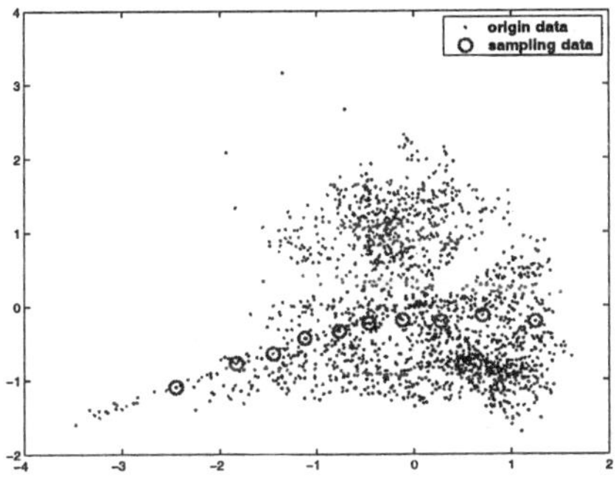

(a) Two-dimensional samples

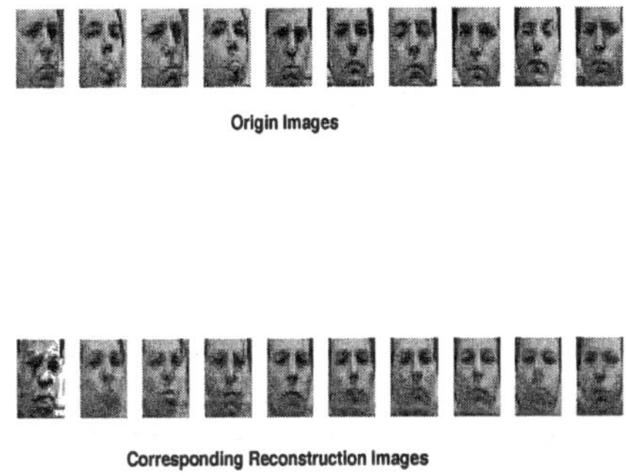

(b) The corresponding reconstruct faces

Fig. 2. 2-dimensional mapping and reconstruction of Frey Face data

the ith class so that we can model a total of L different NAMs, for example, character 'a' corresponds to the 1-th NAM, and 'b' 2-th NAM, and so on. Under the assumption, the data of different classes can be represented as

$$(X(1), Y(1)), (X(2), Y(2)), \cdots, (X(L), Y(L))$$

Different from the MLD+LDA, each completed data $(X(i), Y(i)), i = 1, \cdots, L$ is realized with MLA separately. Considering auto-associative properties of NAMs, corresponding auto-associative sample through the NAM of the same class than through those of the different class would have higher similarity with the original sample. It is obvious that a variety of similarity measure techniques can be adopted. In this paper, recognition can be achieved by comparing the probability metric between each unknown sample and corresponding auto-associative sample with different NAMs. Without loss of generality, the probability metric (in this paper, we use Gaussian function) between each sample x' and auto-associative sample $x'(i)$ of the ith NAM is given by:

$$P(x'(i)|x', NAM_i) = \exp^{(-\|x'-x'(i)\|^2)}, x', x'(i) \in R^N, i = 1, \cdots, L \quad (12)$$

where x'_i means the auto-associative sample through the ith NAM given unknown sample x'. It is not difficult to see that when the reconstructed sample is the same as the original sample, $P(x'(i)|x', NAM(i))$ is equal to 1, whereas if the reconstructed sample is far away from the original sample, $P(x'(i)|x', NAM_i)$ will decrease to zero rapidly with respect to the properties of Gaussian function.

To guarantee the consistency of probability metric, normalization is performed. The corresponding equation is given by:

$$\begin{aligned} P(x'(i)|x') &= \frac{P(x'(i)|x', NAM_i)}{\sum_{j=1}^{L} P(x'(j)|x', NAM_j)} \\ &= \frac{\exp(-||x' - x'(i)||^2)}{\sum_{j=1}^{L} \exp(-||x' - x'(j)||^2)} \end{aligned} \quad (13)$$

Considering Formula (13), the NAM where probability metric between auto-associative samples and original sample is the highest can be viewed as a criterion of recognition. Hence, the recognition criterion is given by:

$$Cl(x') = arg\max_{i} P(x'(i)|x'), i = 1, \cdots, L \tag{14}$$

The proposed NAM has several obvious merits: Firstly, the proposed NAM avoids the problems of local minimum and low convergence rate. Secondly, the proposed NAM is constructive, and geometrically intuitive. Thirdly, it can find unlabeled sample through predefined threshold. This suggests "semi-supervised learning" characteristics where only partially labelled data are needed for the learning. Finally, it can add new NAMs without redesigning original NAMs.

5 Experiments

Experiments are performed using three object (face) databases (namely the Olivetti database [14], UMIST database [15] and JAFFE database [16]) and two character databases ((UCI character database [17] and OCR (optical character recognition) database [18])), to evaluate the feasibility of the proposed nonlinear dimension reduction (MLA+LDA) method and NAM method, respectively.

5.1 Face Recognition

The first object database provided by AT&T Cambridge Laboratories (formerly known as the Olivetti database) consists of 10 different images for 40 people each (four female and 36 male subjects). The images are taken at different time, varying lighting, facial expressions (open/closed eyes, smiling/non-smiling), and facial details(glasses/no-glasses). All the images are taken against a dark homogeneous background and the people are in up-right, frontal position. There are unstructured intermediate changes ($\pm$ 20 degrees) in head pose. Examples of ORL database are shown in Figure 3. We crop images into 112*96 pixels (namely 10304 dimensions).

The training set and test set are divided in the same way as in [19]: The 10 images of each of the 40 persons are randomly partitioned into two sets, that is, 200 training images and 200 test images, without overlapping between the two sets.

The second one, UMIST database consists of 575 images of 20 people with varied poses. The images of each subject cover a range of poses from right profile (-90 degree) to frontal (0 degree)[15]. Examples of the UMIST database are shown in Figure 4(a). All these images of UMIST database are cropped to the size of 112 $\times$ 94, namely 10304 dimensions.

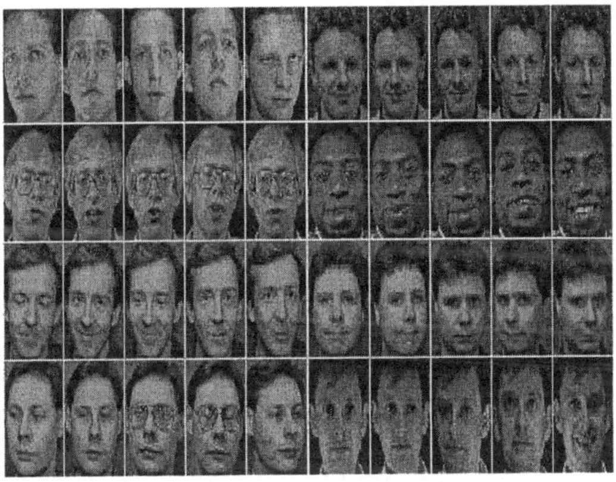

Fig. 3. Examples of ORL Face Database

The main difficulty of UMIST database is that face data in the observation space may have higher curvature and stronger nonlinearity in multiple views than in frontal views. From the aspect of computer vision, meanwhile, "the variations between the images of the same face due to illumination and viewing direction are almost always larger than image variations due to change in face identity"[20]. This makes multi-view face recognition a great challenge.

In this experiment, we randomly select 10 images of each person as the training set, and the remaining 375 images as the test set.

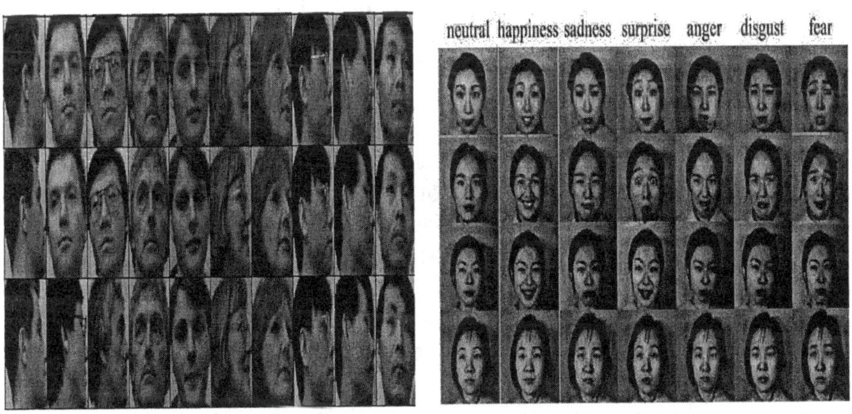

(a) Examples of UMIST Face Database (b) Examples of JAFFE Face Database

Fig. 4. Examples of Face Databases

The JAFFE database, which has been used in facial expression recognition, consists of 213 images of 10 Japanese females. The head is almost in frontal pose. The number of each image represents one of the 7 categories of expressions (neutral, happiness, sadness, surprise, anger, disgust and fear). In our experiment, the database is used for both oriental face recognition and expression recognition. All these images of JAFFE database are cropped to the size of 146×111 pixels.

When being used for face recognition, the JAFFE database is partitioned into two sets: 6 images of each of the 10 persons are randomly extracted to make 60 training set and the remaining 153 images are used as the test images. Meanwhile, in expression recognition, 24 images of each expressional categories are randomly extracted to make 168 training set and the remaining 45 images are used as the test set. Examples of JAFFE database are shown in Figure 4(b).

The dimensions of LLE-reduced data are set to be 150 except for JAFFE face recognition (where the dimension is 50 as in Figure 5(c)). For the 2nd mapping, LDA based reduction, the reduced dimension is generally no more than $L - 1$. otherwise eigenvalues and eigenvectors will have complex values. Actually, we remain the real-value part of complex values when the 2th reduced dimensions are higher than $L - 1$.

In order to compare the performance of MLA+LDA in dimensionality reduction, classical linear dimensionality reduction algorithm–PCA (principal component analysis) [21] is introduced, and then four combinational algorithms are conducted on face recognition: the combination of 1-nearest neighborhood classifiers with PCA+LDA (PCA+LDA+NN), the combination of means classifiers with PCA+LDA (PCA+LDA+M), the combination of 1-nearest neighborhood with MLA+LDA (MLA+LDA+NN) and the combination of means classifiers with MLA+LDA (MLA+LDA+M). All the experimental data have been normalized. The experimental results are the average of 100 runs.

In our experiments, two parameters (neighbor factor K of LLE algorithm and σ^2 of kernel function) need to be predefined. Without loss of generality, we set K be 40 for ORL , UMIST and Jaffe expression database, 20 for JAFFE Face database, and set σ^2 be 10000 for ORL and UMIST databases, 80000 for JAFFE expression and face database.

The experimental results are illustrated as in Figure 5(a), Figure 5(b), Figure 5(c), and Figure 5(d), respectively. The error rates (ER) of several face recognitions are also tabulated in Table 1. Where 1 means MLA+LDA+NN, 2 MLA+LDA+M, 3 PCA+LDA+NN, and 4 PCA+LDA+M in Table 1, respectively.

From the Figures and Table 1, it can be seen that dimension of face manifolds has been remarkablely reduced based on the proposed MLA+LDA methods. For example, the ratio between original dimensions and the 2th biggest reduced dimension of ORL database is about 264. Compared with PCA+LDA, recognition obtains better results in the reduced dimensions of three face databases except for UMIST database. For example, in 150 reduced dimensions, the error rates of MLA+LDA+M algorithm are about 93.6%

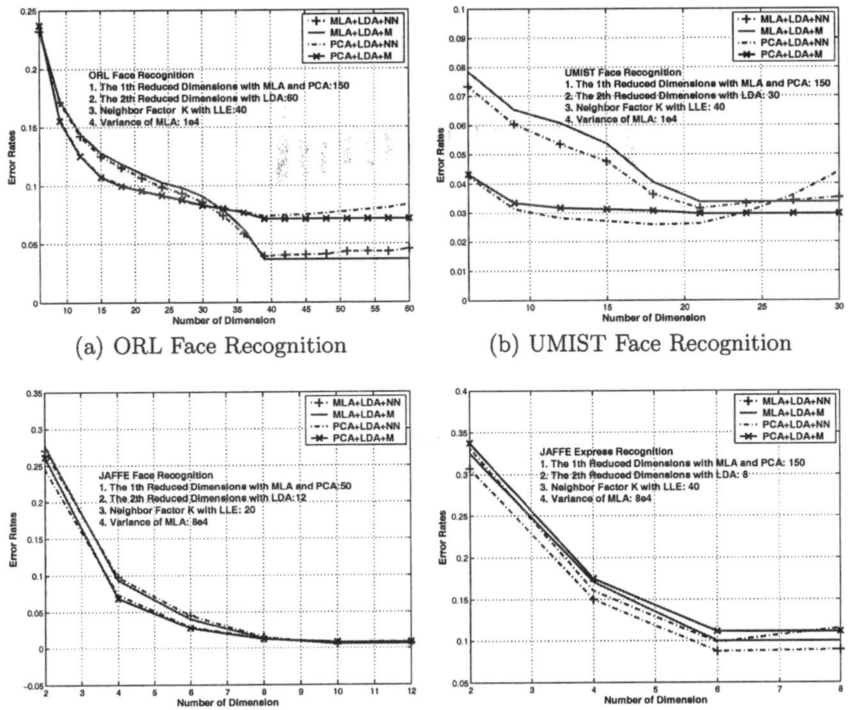

(a) ORL Face Recognition

(b) UMIST Face Recognition

(c) JAFFE Face Recognition

(d) JAFFE Express Recognition

Fig. 5. Recognition Comparison

Table 1. Error rates with the MLA+LDA

Database(Dim)	MLA+LDA+NN	MLA+LDA+M	PCA+LDA+NN	PCA+LDA+M
ORL (39)	3.93%	3.68%	7.37%	7.13%
UMIST (21)	3.16%	3.38%	2.62%	2.98%
JAFFE (10)	0.57%	0.58%	0.78%	0.82%
EXPRESS(6)	8.73%	10%	9.82%	11.16%

of the MLA+LDA+NN, 49.9% of the PCA+LDA+NN, and 51.6% of the PCA+LDA+M on the ORL face database.

It is worth noting that several parameters influence final experimental results. For example, thc influences of variance σ^2 of Gaussian RBF kernel, and training samples on ORL face recognition are illustrated as in Figure 6(a) and Figure 6(b), respectively. When training sample is 9 each person, meanwhile, the proposed MLA+LDA+M than the other three methods has the lowest error rates and is about 1.32%. And the influences of parameter σ^2 will be explained in the subsection 5.3.

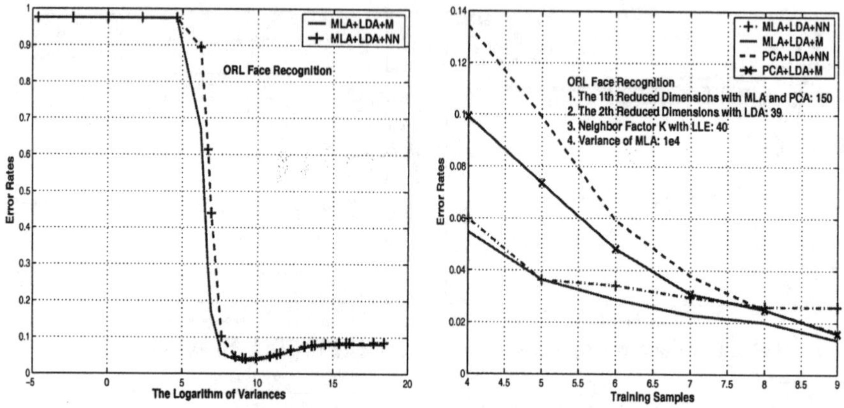

(a) Variance Influences (b) Influences of Training Samples

Fig. 6. Influences of Parameters

For comparing the recognition performance between the proposed approach (MLA+LDA) and MLA, we cite the recent experimental results from literature [22] as in Table 2.

Table 2. Error rates with MLA

Database(Dim)	MLA+NM	MLA+NN	PCA+NM	PCA+NN
UMIST(150)	3.73%	5.71%	4.83%	8.11%
ORL(120)	3.83%	7.75%	8.13%	9.86%
JAFFE (50)	2.99%	8.86%	8.76%	11.12%
EXPRESS(150)	12.39%	13.73%	16.63%	32.94%

Where NM means nearest manifold approach. The detail of NM approach can be seen in [22]. It is not difficult to see that the proposed MLA+LDA has greater reduced dimensions that MLA (Note: The reason is that the total number of classes of these mentioned data is less than the reduced dimensions of the data). And also with comparison of the recognition ability, the recognition results of MLA+LDA are better than that of MLA in the average sense.

5.2 Exception

While the proposed MLA+LDA approach obtains better recognition rate in three of four databases than PCA+LDA. In Table 1, experimental results on UMIST database show that the performance is even worse while using MLA + LDA. The reason is that the UMIST database contains faces with more pose variations, and intrinsic pose information of faces may therefore be damaged by LDA which is a linear dimensionality reduction method because faces of the same person with different poses are regarded as the same class.

If data contain different categories like digit or character, furthermore, recognition performance would be impaired. The exception using the proposed MLA+NM algorithm in digit recognition is shown as follows[23]:

The digit database includes digits from '0' to '9' and each digit has 39 images with 16*20 pixels [4]. Examples of the database are illustrated in Figure 7(a).

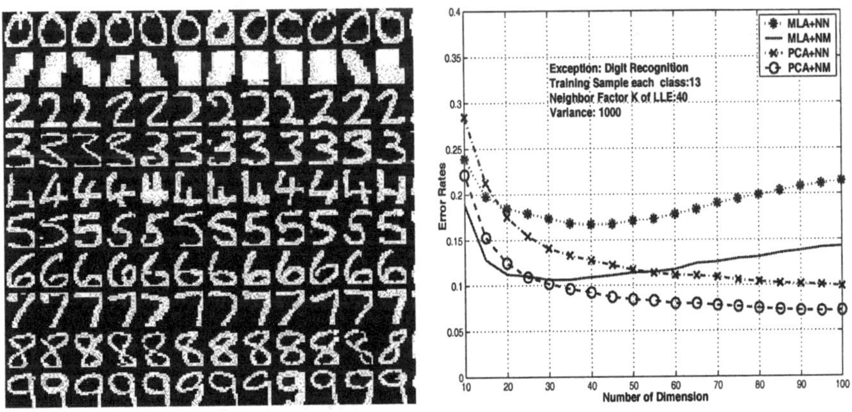

(a) Example of digit database   (b) Digit Recognition

Fig. 7. Exception of MLA+NM

In our experiments, the 10 images of each of the 10 digits are extracted to make 100 training images randomly and the remaining 290 digits are used as the test images. The other experimental way is the same as the experiments mentioned above.

From Figure 7(b) we can see that when the reduced dimensions are less than 20, the error rates of MLA are lower than that of the PCA methods; meanwhile, the error rates of MLA+NM are lower than that of the PCA+NM methods if reduced dimensions are less than 25. As the reduced dimensions increase, PCA or PCA+NM has better recognition performance than MLA or MLA+NM. It is obvious that the experiments using the proposed method in digit recognition have not obtained the same effects as in face and expression recognitions.

A possible explanations about the exception is that when data are made up of obviously different categories, extracting intrinsical principal features of different categories in different embedding subspaces rather than the same

[4]http://www.cs.toronto.edu/ roweis/data.html

embedding subspace may result in better recognition performance and geometrical explanation. Therefore, we perform experiments in the two character databases to verify our assumption.

5.3 Character Recognition

The first character dataset from the UCI repository, comprises of a total of 20,000 labelled samples of, on an average, 770 examples per class. The total number of classes is 26. The character images were based on 20 different fonts and each character within these fonts was randomly distorted to produce a file of 20,000 unique stimuli. The fonts imply five different strokes (simplexduplextriplexcomplex and Gothic) and six different styles(blocksscriptitalicEnglishItalian and German). Each stimulus was converted into 16 numerical attributes (statistical moments and edge counts), which were then scaled to fit into a range of integer values from 0 through 15. Examples of the character images are illustrated in Figure 8. Because of the wide diversity among the different fonts and the primitive nature of the attributes, the recognition task was especially challenging [17]. The database

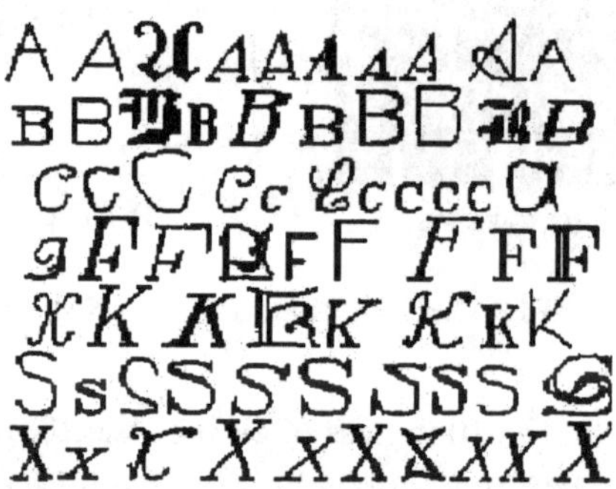

Fig. 8. Examples of UCI character databases

is randomly partitioned into two disjointing sets, that is , 350 training samples of each of the 26 classes as the training set, and the remaining samples as the test set.

The second database was created by National Institute of Standards and Technology (NIST) and contains 16,280 handwritten characters. There are, on an average, 600 characters per class (26 classes). Each character is represented by a 30 dimensional feature vector of edge tangents. In this experiment, we randomly select 300 samples of each character concept as the training set, and the remaining samples as the test set. Each dimension in both datasets was linearly scaled to [0,1] interval.

The biggest reduced dimensions are extracted in terms of the spectral properties of LLE algorithm [8](where the biggest reduced dimensions are 12

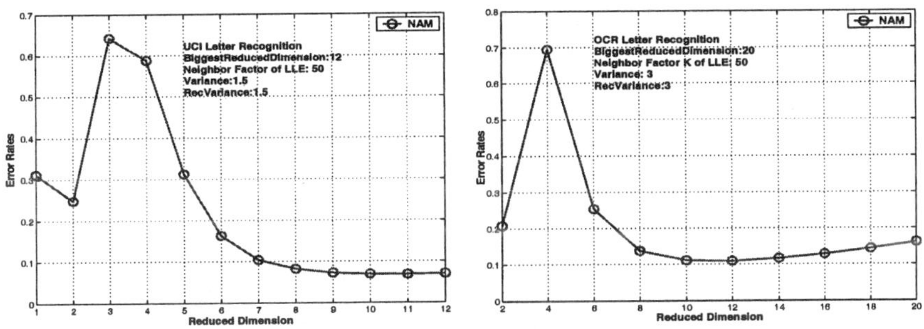

(a) UCI Database (b) OCR Database

Fig. 9. Character Recognition

for UCI and 20 for OCR, respectively), and then the dimensions are gradually decreased according to the non-increasing order of eigenvalues used by LLE algorithm.

Furthermore, several parameters need to be predefined. Without loss of generality, neighbor factor K of LLE is set to 50. Considering the dimensionality difference of the two mentioned databases, parameters σ^2 and $(\sigma')^2$ are equal to 1.5 in UCI character database while being equal to 3 in OCR database. And then 26 independent NAMs are established for 26 different classes. The experimental results are the average of 100 runs.

The experimental results of two databases are illustrated as in Figure 9. From Figure 9 it can be seen that when intrinsical principal dimensions are equal to 12, the lowest error rates of two character databases are obtained. We therefore assume that the possible number of principal features of character manifolds should be extracted is 12 or so.

For comparing the recognition performance between the proposed NAMs and other known state-of-the-art algorithms, we cite the recent experimental results from literature [18] as in Table 3. . As in Table 3, the proposed NAM than other classifiers has better recognition rates. For instances, in UCI character database, the error rates of NAMs are about 67.13% of the K-NN, 32.8% of the MLP; while in OCR character database, the error rates of NAMs are about 98.6% of the K-NN, 43.52% of the MLP. Furthermore, the proposed NAMs for two character databases use fewer features (12) to model intrinsical feature spaces. It is also noticeable that our experimental results are the average of 100 runs, whereas other results are the average of 10 runs. We also investigate the error rates of character recognition in the top n matches with the proposed NAM. This lets one know how many characters have to be examined to get a desired level of performance. The performance statistics are reported as cumulative error rates, which are plotted on Figure 10. The horizontal axis of the graph is rank and the vertical axis the percentage of error rates. For example, when in the top 3 matches, the error rate of NAM for UCI

Table 3. The Average Error Rates of sevaral algorithms on the two character databases for NAM, K-nearest Neighbor (K-NN, K=3), Maximum Likelihood Classifier (MLC), Bayesian pairwise classifier with single Gaussian with voting combination method (BPC(1,V)), and MAP estimate combination (BPC(1,M)), and Bayesian pairwise classifier with mixture of Gaussian for voting (BPC(n,v)) and MAP estimate (BPC(n,M)) combination

CLASSIFIER	UCI %	OCR %
NAM	6.78 (12-DIM)	10.358 (12-DIM)
K-NN	10.10	10.5
MLP	20.7	23.8
MLC	17.3	20.5
BPC(1,V)	14.6	17.9
BPC(1,M)	14.7	16.7
BPC(N,V)	13.8	16.9
BPC (N,M)	12.4	13.7

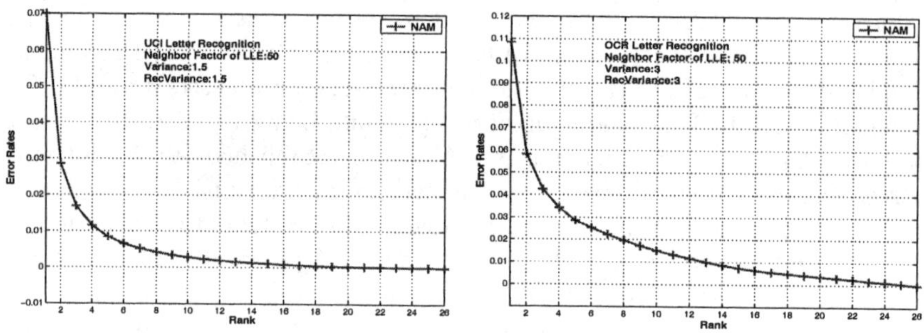

(a) UCI Database

(b) OCR Database

Fig. 10. Rank Performance

is 1.7%, and the error rate of NAM for OCR database is about 4.25%. Meanwhile, when in the top 6 matches, the error rate of NAM for UCI database is 0.65%, and the error rate of NAM for OCR database is about 2.5%.

It is worth noting that several parameters, such as neighbor factor K of LLE algorithm, variance σ^2, reconstructed variance $(\sigma')^2$, and the number of training sample, influence recognition results. We observe that the curve of error rates about parameter σ^2 will appear a 'valley' which is corresponding to the lowest error rates when adjusting parameter σ^2. For example, the influences of variance σ^2 on several databases are illustrated as in Figure 6(a), Figure 11(a) and Figure 11(b). The lowest error rates are obtained when σ^2 is equal to 1.5 for UCI and 3 for OCR, respectively. On the basis of experiments, we observe that the recognition ability of the proposed approach would be impaired seriously when σ^2 tends to infinitesimal, whereas the recognition ability would first reach saturation and then be impaired seriously if σ^2 tends to infinity. The reason is that when σ^2 tends to infinitesimal, the metric from sample to be classified to the training samples tends to zero so that the information of manifold structure can not be recovered. Further, when σ^2 tends to infinity, the metric from sample to training samples tends to one. Consequently, the rank of kernel matrix is less than the number of training samples so that the solution is ill-posed. The another reason is that kernel matrix tends to unit matrix when σ^2 tends to infinitesimal, whereas the rank of kernel matrix tends to 1 when σ^2 tends to infinity. Meanwhile, we observe that parameter $(\sigma')^2$, independent of the selection of parameter σ^2, has similar phenomenon on the curve of error rates. With respect to these properties, we assume that parameter σ^2 and $(\sigma')^2$ may be selected automatically in further work.

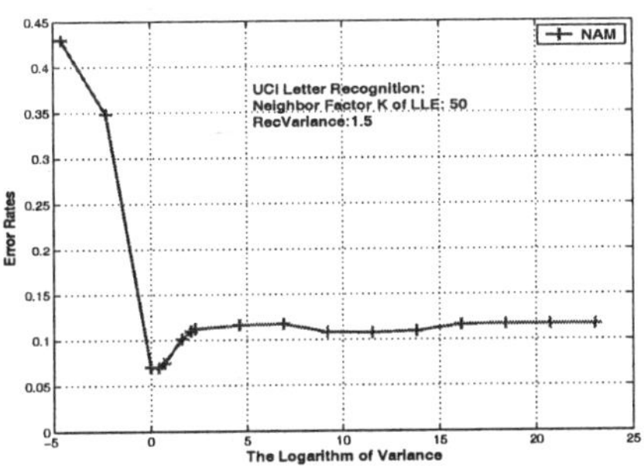

(a) Variance Influence of NAMs for UCI Database

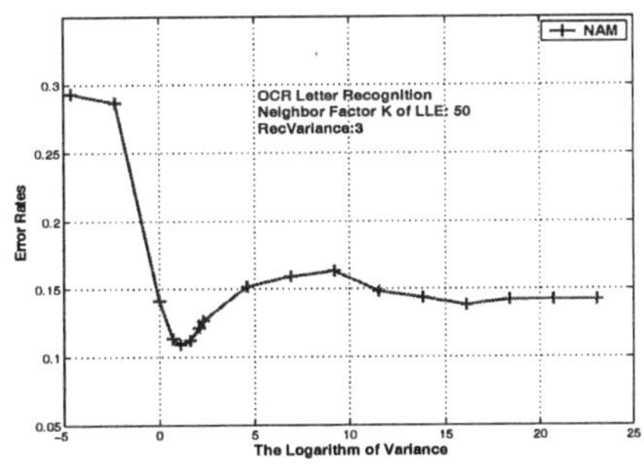

(b) Variance Influence of NAMs for OCR Database

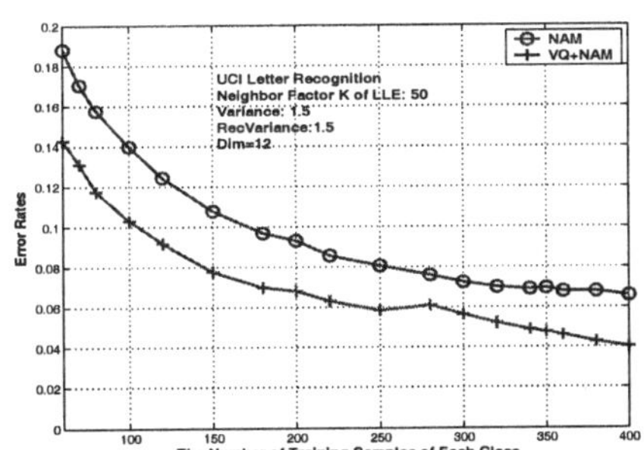

(c) Influence of Training samples for UCI Character Recognition

Fig. 11. Parameter Influences

And the influences of the number of training samples about recognition rates are investigated and the results for the UCI database are illustrated in Figure 11(c). From the Figure, it can be noted that there is remarkable improvement in the error rates of the recognition tasks as the number of training samples increases. Experiments on the influence on selecting Gaussian RBF centers of the proposed NAM through vector quantization techniques (VQ) are also carried out on UCI character databases as in Figure 11(c), it is not difficult to see that with the combination of NAM and VQ the error rate has remarkablely decreased, therefore NAM+VQ can obtain the same error rates as NAMs with fewer RBF centers and training samples.

6 Conclusions

In this paper, we propose two recognition approaches (MLA+LDA and NAM) based on manifold learning. If data to be classified belong to the same or similar cognitive category such as face, MLA+LDA is employed. Otherwise, NAM approach is implemented.

Assuming that object manifolds of different classes lie on the same feature subspace, object manifolds of different classes are first reduced into the intrinsic principal feature subspace with proposed MLA. And then the within-classes distances are further enlarged and the between-classes distances are decreased with LDA. The final classification task is completed based on the reduced dimensions of MLA+LDA.

If data to be classified are from remarkable different categories (for example, character 'a' and 'b'), recognition achieved under the common feature subspace seems to be unreasonable. And the proposed nonlinear dimension reduction method MLA+LDA is not effective in this case. We therefore propose a new constructive nonlinear auto-associative modeling based on manifold learning. Based on the proposed NAM, the intrinsical principal features are extracted for preserving the principal structure of each manifold, and then reconstruction is achieved. With auto-associative mechanism, the reconstructed data through NAM having the same cognitive concept than through NAMs having the different cognitive concept will have less deviation. Therefore, the probability metric for recognition is naturally established. Our propped NAM has several obvious merits: Firstly, it avoids problems with local minimum and convergence. Secondly, it is constructive, and geometrically intuitive. Meanwhile, the nonlinear auto-associative modeling can be used for the construction of both mapping and inverse mapping relationship between the observation spaces and corresponding feature spaces without dimensionality limitation.

Some potential problems remain. First, several parameters influence the experimental results. How to select parameters automatically deserves research profoundly. Second, the number of intrinsical principal features of manifold is related to the error rates of recognition. In the future work, it is necessary to find a more effective approach which can estimate the number of principal features. The proposed NAM has semi-supervised learning characteristics which can find unlabelled sample through predefined threshold and can facilitate adding new NAMs without redesigning original NAMs.

Moreover, how to utilize these properties for modelling unknown concepts and designing new algorithms is also the future work.

Acknowledgement

The authors are very grateful to the reviewers for their valuable comments.

References

1. T. Hastie, and W. Stuetzle (1988) Principla Curves. Journal of the American Statistical Association, 84(406), pp. 502-516
2. B. Kégl, A. Krzyzak, T. Linder, and K. Zeger (2000) Learning and design of principal curves. IEEE Transactions on Pattern Analysis and Machine Intelligence, vol. 22, no. 3, pp. 281-297.
3. C.M. Bishop, M. Sevensen, and C.K.I. Williams (1998) GTM: The generative topographic mapping. Neural Computation,10, pp. 215-234
4. K. Chang and J. Ghosh (2001) A unified model for probabilistic principal surfaces. IEEE transactions on Pattern Analysis and Machine Intelligence, 23(1), pp. 22-41
5. A.J. Smola, S.Mika, et al (1999) Regularized Principal Manifolds. In Computational Learning Theory: 4th European Conference, Vol 1572 of Lecture Notes in Artificial Intelligence, New York: Springer, pp. 251-256
6. J. B. Tenenbaum, de Silva, V. & Langford, J.C (2000) A global geometric framework for nonlinear dimensionality reduction. Science, 290, pp. 2319-2323
7. V. S.Silva, J. B. Tenenbaum (2002) Unsupervised learning of curved manifolds. Nonlinear Estimation and Classification, Springer-Verlag, New York
8. S. T. Roweis, and K. S. Lawrance (2000) Nonlinear Dimensionality reduction by locally linear embedding. Science, 290, pp. 2323-2326
9. Mikhail Belkin, and Partha Niyogi (2003) Laplacian Eigenmaps for Dimensionality Reduction and Data Representation Neural Computation, 15(6), 1373 - 1396.
10. G. Hinton and S. Roweis (2002) Stochastic Neighbor Embedding. Neural Information Proceeding Systems:Natural and Synthetic, Vancouver, Canada, December 9-14
11. M. Brand, MERL (2002) Charting a manifold. Neural Information Proceeding Systems: Natural and Synthetic, Vancouver, Canada, December 9-14
12. Dick de Ridder, Robert P.W. Duin (2002) Locally Linear Embedding for Classification. Technical Reports, Delft University of Technology, The Netherlands
13. Daniel L. Swets and John (Juyang) Weng (1996) Using Discriminant Eigenfeatures for Image Retrieval. IEEE Transactions on Pattern Analysis and Machine Intelligences, Vol. 18, No. 8, pp.831-836
14. F. S. Samaria (1994) Face Recognition Using Hidden Markov Models. PhD thesis, University of Cambridge
15. H. Wechsler, P. J. Phillips, V. Bruce, F. Fogelman-Soulie and T. S. Huang (1998) Characterizing virtual Eigensignatures for General Purpose Face Recognition. Daniel B Graham and Nigel M Allinson. In Face Recognition: From Theory to Applications; NATO ASI Series F, Computer and Systems Sciences, Vol. 163, pp. 446-456

16. Michael J. Lyons, Julien Budynek, and Shigeru Akamatsu (1999) Automatic classification of Single Facial Images. IEEE Transactions on Pattern Analysis and Machine Intelligence, vol.21, no. 12, pp. 1357-1362
17. Frey, P. W., Slate, D. J. (1991). Letter recognition using holland-style adaptive classifiers. Machine Learning, 6, 161–182
18. Kumar, S., Ghosh, J., Crawford, M. (2000) A Bayesian Pairwise Classifier for Character Recognition. Cognitive and Neural Models for Word Recognition and Document Processing. Nabeel Mursheed (Ed), World Scientific Press
19. Steve Lawrence, C. Lee Giles, A. C. Tsoi, and A. D. Back (1997) Face recognition: A convolutional neural network approach. IEEE Transactions on Neural Networks, vol. 8, no. 1, pp. 98-113
20. Y. Moses, Y. Adini, and S. Ullman (1994) Face Recognition: The Problem of compensating for changes in illumination direction. in Proceedings of the European Conference on Computer Vision, vol. A, pp: 286-296
21. M. Turk, and A. Pentland (1991) Eigenfaces for Recognition. Journal of Cognitive Neuroscience, vol 3, no.1, pp.71-86
22. Junping Zhang, Stan Z. Li, Jue Wang (2004) Nearest Manifold Approach for Face Recognition. The 6th IEEE International Conference on Automatic Face and Gesture Recognition, May 17-19, Seoul, Korea, 2004.
23. Junping Zhang (2003) Manifold Learning and Applications. PhD Thesis, Institute of Automation, Chinese Academy of Sciences, Beijing, China.

Face Recognition Using Discrete Cosine Transform and RBF Neural Networks

Weilong Chen[1], Meng Joo Er[2], and Shiqian Wu[3]

[1] School of Electrical and Electronic Engineering, Nanyang Technological University, 50 Nanyang Avenue, Singapore 639798

[2] Intelligent Systems Centre, 50 Nanyang Drive, 7th Storey Research TechnoPlaza, BorderX Block, Singapore 637533

[3] Institute for Infocomm Research, 21 Heng Mui Keng Terrace, Singapore 119613

Abstract. In this chapter, an efficient method for face recognition based on the Discrete Cosine Transform (DCT), the Fisher's Linear Discriminant (FLD) and Radial Basis Function (RBF) neural networks is presented. First, the dimensionality of the original face image is reduced by using the DCT and large area illumination variations are alleviated by discarding the first few low-frequency DCT coefficients. Next, the truncated DCT coefficient vectors are clustered using the proposed clustering algorithm. This process makes the subsequent FLD more efficient. After implementing the FLD, the most discriminating and invariant facial features are maintained and the training samples are clustered well. As a consequence, further parameter estimation for the RBF neural networks is fulfilled easily which facilitates fast training in the RBF neural networks. Simulation results show that the proposed system achieves excellent performance with high training and recognition speed and recognition rate as well as very good illumination robustness.

Keywords: face recognition, discrete cosine transform, fisher's linear discriminant, RBF neural networks

1 Introduction

Human face recognition has become a very active research area in recent years mainly due to increasing security demands and its potential commercial and law enforcement applications. Numerous approaches have been proposed for face recognition and considerable successes have been reported in [1]. However, it is still a difficult task for a machine to recognize human faces accurately in real-time, especially under variable circumstances such as variations in illumination, pose, facial expression, makeup, etc. The similarity of human faces and the unpredictable variations are the greatest obstacles in face recognition.

Generally speaking, research on face recognition can be grouped into two categories, namely, feature-based and holistic (also called template matching)

approaches [1], [2]. Feature-based approaches are based on the shapes and geometrical relationships of individual facial features including eyes, mouth, nose and chin. On the other hand, holistic approaches handle the input face images globally and extract important facial features based on the high-dimensional intensity values of face images automatically. Although feature-based schemes are more robust against rotation, scale, and illumination variations, they greatly rely on the accuracy of facial feature detection methods and it has been argued that existing feature-based techniques are not reliable enough for extracting individual facial features. Holistic face recognition has attracted more attention since the well-known statistical method, the Principal Component Analysis (PCA)(also known as Karhunen-Loeve Transform (KLT)) was applied in face recognition [3], [4]. Another well-known approach is the Fisherfaces in which the Fisher's Linear Discriminant (FLD) is employed after the PCA is used for dimensionality reduction [5]. Compared with the Eigenface (PCA) approach, the fisherface approach is more insensitive to large variations in lighting direction and facial expression. However, the computational requirements of the two approaches are greatly related to the dimensionality of the original data and the number of training samples. When the face database becomes larger, the training time and the memory requirement will significantly increase. Moreover, the system based on the PCA should be retrained when new classes are added. As a consequence, it is impractical to apply the PCA in systems with a large database. More recently, the Discrete Cosine Transform (DCT) has been employed in face recognition [7]-[10]. The DCT has several advantages over the PCA: (1) The DCT is data independent; (2) The DCT can be implemented using a fast algorithm. In [7], the DCT is applied for dimensionality reduction and then the selected low-frequency DCT coefficient vectors are fed into a multi-layer perceptron (MLP) classifier. It is well-known that the problems arising from the *curse of dimensionality* should be considered in pattern recognition. It has been suggested that as the dimensionality increases, the sample size needs to increase exponentially in order to have an effective estimate of multivariate densities [12]. In face recognition applications, the original input data are usually of high dimension, whereas only limited training samples are available. Therefore, dimensionality reduction is a very important step which will greatly improve the performance of the face recognition system. However, if only the DCT is employed for dimensionality reduction, we cannot keep sufficient frequency components for important facial features in order to compromise the problem of *curse of dimensionality.* Besides, some variable features exist in the low-dimensional features extracted by the DCT. Hence, in our proposed system, the FLD is also employed in the DCT domain to extract the most discriminating feature of face images. With the combination of the DCT and the FLD, we can keep more DCT coefficients and the most discriminating feature can be extracted at high speed.

In [17], the clustering process is implemented after the FLD is employed. However, the FLD is a linear projection method and the results are globally optimal only for linearly separable data. There are lots of nonlinear variations in human faces such as pose and expression. Once the faces with different poses are put into the same class, they will actually smear the optimal projection such that we cannot get the most discriminating feature and good generalization. For this reason, we should ensure that the face images in each class should not have large nonlinear variations. Instead of regarding each individual as one class, we propose a sub-clustering method to split one class into several subclasses before implementing the FLD. Moreover, the sub-clustering process is very crucial to structure determination of the following RBF neural networks. In fact, the number of clusters is simply the number of hidden neurons in the RBF neural networks.

Neural networks have been widely applied in pattern recognition for the reason that neural-networks-based classifiers can incorporate both statistical and structural information and achieve better performance than the simple minimum distance classifiers [1]. Multilayered networks (MLNs), usually employing the backpropagation (BP) algorithm, are widely used in face recognition [16]. Recently, RBF neural networks have been applied in many engineering and scientific applications including face recognition [17]. The RBF neural networks possess the following salient features: 1) They are universal approximators; 2) They have a simple topological structure; 3) The learning algorithm is fast because of locally tuned neurons. Based on the advantages of RBF neural networks and the efficient feature extraction method, a high-speed RBF neural networks classifier whereby near-optimal parameters can be estimated according to the properties of the feature space, rather than using the gradient descent training algorithm, is proposed. As a consequence, our system is able to achieve high training and recognition speed which facilitates real-time applications of the proposed face recognition system. The block diagram of our proposed face recognition system is shown in Fig. 1.

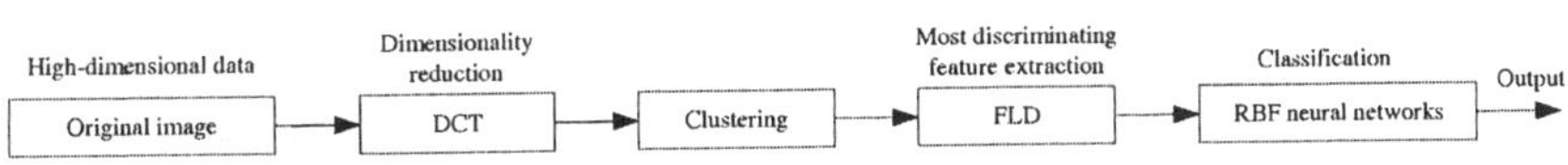

Fig. 1. Block diagram of face recognition based on DCT and RBF neural networks

The organization of the chapter is as follows: In Section 2, we first present the DCT-based feature extraction method together with its relevant properties against illumination variations. Then, the proposed clustering algorithm and the FLD method implemented in the DCT domain are presented. Section 3 describes the architecture of RBF neural networks and the parameter estimation approach, which is based on the properties of previously extracted feature vectors. Experimental results are presented and discussed in Section 4. Finally, conclusions are drawn in Section 5.

2 Feature Extraction

2.1 Discrete Cosine Transform (DCT)

The Discrete Cosine Transform (DCT) has been widely applied to solve numerous problems in the digital signal processing community. In particular, many data compression techniques employ the DCT, which has been found to be asymptotically equivalent to the optimal Karhunen-Loeve Transform (KLT) for signal decorrelation. The formula of DCT and its inverse transform can be found in [11].

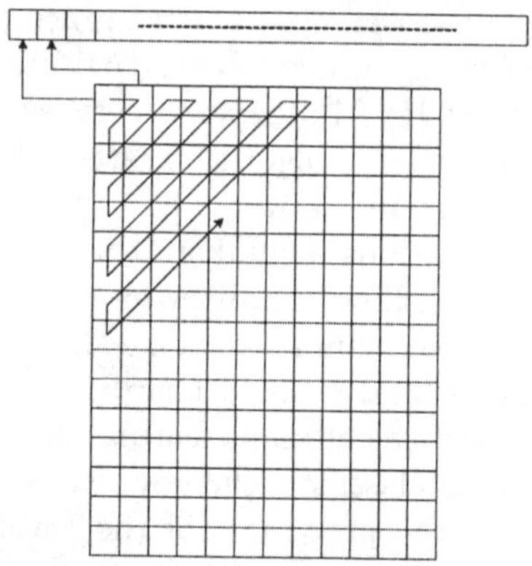

Fig. 2. Scheme of scanning 2D DCT coefficients to a one-dimensional vector

In the JPEG image compression standard, the original images are initially partitioned into rectangular non-overlapping blocks (8×8 blocks) and then the DCT is performed independently on the subimage blocks [11]. In our proposed system, we simply apply the DCT on the entire face image. If the DCT is only applied on the subimage independently, some relationship information between subimages cannot be obtained. However, we can obtain all frequency components of a face image by applying the DCT on the entire face image. In addition, some low-frequency components are only related to illumination variations which can be discarded.

For an $M \times N$ image, we have an $M \times N$ DCT coefficient matrix covering all the spatial frequency components of the image. The DCT coefficients with great magnitude are mainly located in the upper-left corner of the DCT matrix. Accordingly, as illustrated in Fig. 2, we scan the DCT coefficient matrix in a zig-zag manner starting from the upper-left corner and subsequently convert it to a one-dimensional vector. Detailed discussions about image reconstruction errors using only a few significant DCT coefficients can be found in [7]. As a holistic feature extraction method, the DCT converts high-dimensional face images into low-dimensional spaces in which the most significant facial features such as outline of hair and face, position of eyes, nose and mouth are maintained. These facial features are more stable than the variable high-frequency facial features. As a matter of fact, the human visual system is more sensitive to variations in the low-frequency band.

Illumination variations are still an unsolved problem in face recognition, particularly for the holistic approach. For the PCA (Eigenface) method, it has been suggested that by discarding the three most significant principal components, variations due to lighting can be reduced. In [5], experimental results showed that the PCA method performs better under variable lighting conditions after removing the first three principal components. However, the first several components not only correspond to illumination variations, but also some useful information for dicrimination [5]. Besides, since the PCA method is highly dependent on the training samples, different components are obtained with different training samples. Therefore, it is not guaranteed that the first three principal components are definitely related to illumination variations. In this chapter, we investigate the illumination invariant property of the DCT by discarding its several low-frequency coefficients. It is well-known that the first DCT coefficient represents the DC component of the image which is solely related to the brightness of the image. Therefore, it becomes *DC-free* (i.e., zero mean) and invariant against uniform brightness change by simply removing the first DCT coefficient. Fig. 3 illustrates the robustness of the *DC-free* DCT against uniform brightness variation.

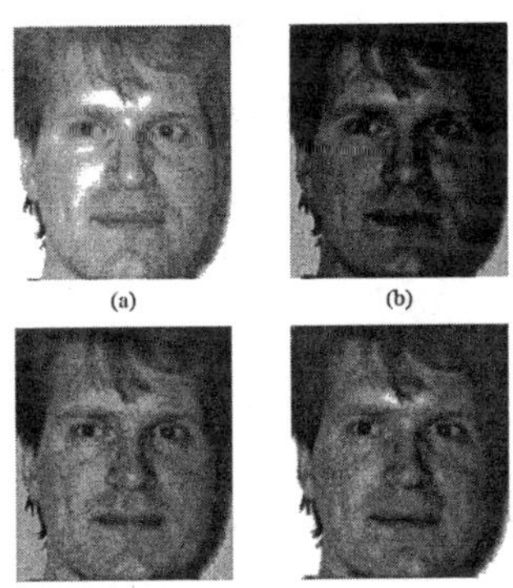

Fig. 3. Illustration of the brightness invariance of the *DC-free* DCT: (a), (b) are the same images with different brightness; (c), (d) are respectively obtained from the inverse DCT transform of (a) and (b) after setting the first coefficients to the same value. (Since the first coefficient represents the DC component of the image, after inverse DCT transform, some of the image intensity values will become negative if the first coefficient is set to zero. Therefore, in order to display the images correctly after taking the inverse DCT transform, we choose a median value between the first DCT coefficients of (a) and (b).)

It should be noted that the two reconstructed images (c) and (d) in Fig. 3 are slightly different. This is because in adjusting the original image to different levels of brightness, some intensity values of the image reach the maximum or minimum value (for an 8-bit grayscale intensity image, the maximum and minimum intensity value is 255 and 0 respectively) and some information is lost. In addition, the *DC-free* DCT is only invariant against linear brightness variations. In other words, it is not robust against varying contrast.

Some of the low-frequency components of DCT also account for the large area of non-uniform illumination variations. Consequently, the non-uniform illumination effect can be reduced by discarding several low-frequency DCT coefficients. Face images under different lighting conditions and their corresponding reconstructed images after discarding the first three coefficients are illustrated in Fig. 4. In the proposed system, the truncated DCT works like a band-pass filter which inhibits high-frequency irrelevant information and low-frequency illumination variations.

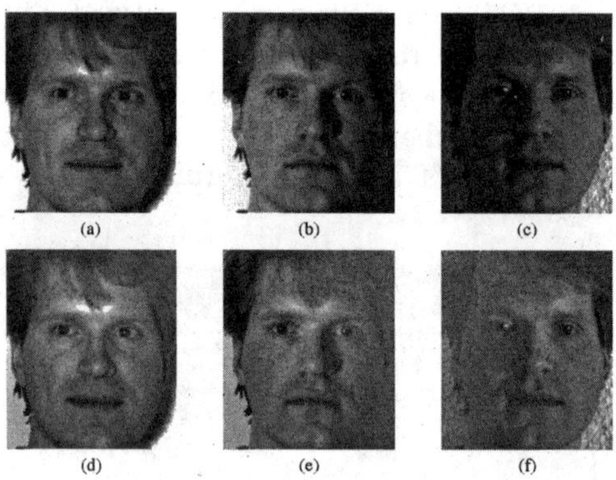

Fig. 4. Effect of non-uniform illumination reduction of DCT after discarding the first three coefficients: (a), (b) and (c) is under different lighting condition(center-light, left-light, right-light); (d), (e) and (f) are obtained from the inverse DCT transform after setting the first coefficient to the same appropriate value, the second and the third coefficients to zero.

2.2 Clustering

Several well-known clustering algorithms such as k-means clustering and fuzzy k-means clustering are widely used in RBF neural networks [20], [21]. However, these clustering approaches are unsupervised learning algorithms and no category information about patterns is used. On the contrary, in face recognition, the category information of training samples is previously known. Accordingly, we can simply cluster the training samples in each class. As depicted in Fig. 5, it is impossible for a purely unsupervised clustering algorithm to separate each class accurately.

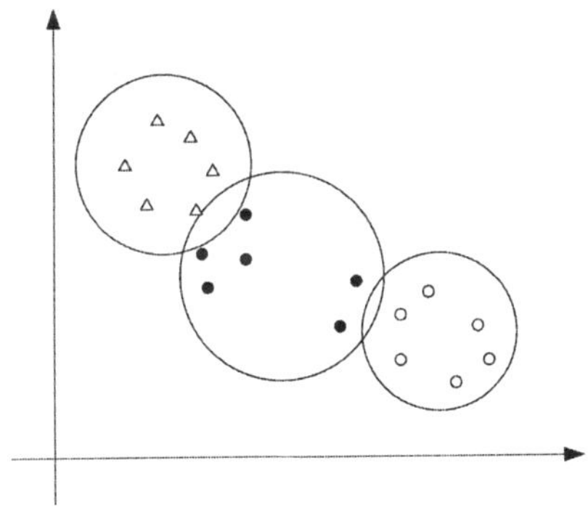

Fig. 5. Clustering with category information

In the proposed system, the classes are split in terms of their Euclidean distances. It is unreasonable to split the classes according to the degree of overlap because there are still great overlaps between classes after performing the DCT. Moreover, the following FLD will reduce the within-class scatter and thus make the sparsely distributed training samples in each subclass tighter. Hence, we only need to prevent the samples with large variations from being clustered in the same subclass. The proposed clustering algorithm is as follows:

1) Let u be the total number of clusters and s be the number of classes. Initially, set each class to be one cluster, i.e. $u = s$.
2) Find two training samples $x^k(f)$, $x^k(g)$ with the largest Euclidean distance $d^k(f,g)$ in class k, $k = 1, 2, \ldots, s$. These two samples are called clustering reference sample (CRS).
3) Compute the Euclidean distances from the two samples to the samples $x^j(i)$ in other classes j, $j = 1, 2, \ldots, s$, $j \neq k$, denoted as $d^{kj}(f,i)$ and $d^{kj}(g,i)$, $i = 1, 2, \ldots, n^{\bar{k}}$, where $n^{\bar{k}}$ is the number of samples not belonging to class k, respectively

$$d^{kj}(f,i) = \| x^j(i) - x^k(f) \|, \quad j \neq k \tag{1}$$

$$d^{kj}(g,i) = \| x^j(i) - x^k(g) \|, \quad j \neq k \tag{2}$$

where $\| \cdot \|$ denotes the Euclidean norm.
4) Compute the mean value and the standard deviation of $d^{kj}(f,i)$, $d^{kj}(g,i)$ as follows:

$$\bar{d^k}(f) = \frac{1}{n^{\bar{k}}} \sum_{i=1}^{n^{\bar{k}}} d^{kj}(f,i) \tag{3}$$

$$v^k(f) = \left[\frac{1}{n^{\bar{k}}}\sum_{i=1}^{n^{\bar{k}}}(d^{kj}(f,i) - \bar{d^k}(f))^2\right]^{\frac{1}{2}} \tag{4}$$

$$\bar{d^k}(g) = \frac{1}{n^{\bar{k}}}\sum_{i=1}^{n^{\bar{k}}} d^{kj}(g,i) \tag{5}$$

$$v^k(g) = \left[\frac{1}{n^{\bar{k}}}\sum_{i=1}^{n^{\bar{k}}}(d^{kj}(g,i) - \bar{d^k}(g))^2\right]^{\frac{1}{2}} \tag{6}$$

5) Define the scope radius of the two CRSes $r^k(f)$, $r^k(g)$ as follows:

$$r^k(f) = \bar{d^k}(f) - \alpha v^k(f) \tag{7}$$

$$r^k(g) = \bar{d^k}(g) - \alpha v^k(g) \tag{8}$$

where α is a positive constant clustering factor. If $d^k(f,g) > \max\{r^k(g),\ r^k(f)\}$, then split the cluster into two clusters with CRSes $x^k(f)$ and $x^k(g)$ respectively and set $u = u + 1$.

6) There are three scenarios for any sample $x^k(h)$ in class k ($x^k(h)$ is not CRS). These scenarios as depicted in Fig. 6 will be handled as follows:
   i) If only one CRS's scope comprises $x^k(h)$, then $x^k(h)$ will be merged with the cluster to which this CRS belongs.
   ii) If more than one CRS's scope comprise $x^k(h)$, then $x^k(h)$ will be merged into the cluster to which the CRS with the shortest distance to $x^k(h)$ belongs.
   iii) If no CRS's scope comprise $x^k(h)$, then $x^k(h)$ is regarded as another CRS belonging to a new cluster. Set $u = u + 1$ and compute the radius $r^k(h)$ according to (4)-(5). Repeat (6), until u dose not change.
7) Apply (2)-(6) to all classes.

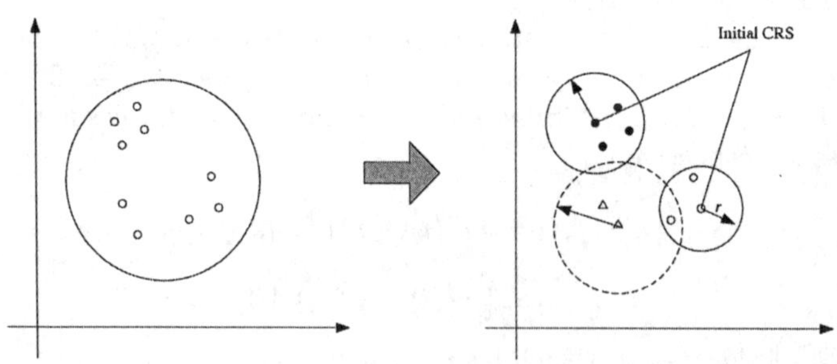

Fig. 6. Illustration of one class split into three subclasses

It follows from (7) and (8) that the radius of the CRS is chosen according to the mean distance and standard deviation from this CRS to the training samples belonging to other classes. The clustering factor α controls the clustering extent. The larger the value of α, the more clusters there are. Therefore, α should be chosen carefully so that the FLD will work efficiently. After the clustering algorithm and the FLD are implemented, the sparsely distributed training samples cluster more tightly which simplifies parameter estimation of the RBF neural networks in the sequel.

2.3 Fisher's Linear Discriminant (FLD)

In order to obtain the most salient and invariant features of human faces, the FLD is applied in the truncated DCT domain. The FLD is one of the most popular linear projection methods for feature extraction. It is used to find a linear projection of the original vectors from a high-dimensional space to an optimal low-dimensional subspace in which the ratio of the between-class scatter and the within-class scatter is maximized. We apply the FLD to discount the variation such as illumination and expression. The details about the FLD can be found in [2]. It should be noted that we apply the FLD after clustering such that the most discriminating facial feature can be effectively extracted. The discriminating feature vectors P projected from the truncated DCT domain to the optimal subspace can be calculated as follows:

$$P = E_{optimal}^{T} \cdot X \tag{9}$$

where X are truncated DCT coefficient vectors, and $E_{optimal}$ is the FLD optimal projection matrix.

3 Classification Using RBF Neural Networks

3.1 Structure Determination and Parameter Estimation of RBF Neural Networks

The traditional three-layer RBF neural networks is employed for classification in the proposed system. The architecture is identical to the one used in [17]. We employ the most frequently used Gaussian function as the radial basis function since it best approximates the distribution of data in each subset. In face recognition applications, the RBF neural networks are regarded as a mapping from the feature hyperspace to the classes. Therefore, the number of inputs to the RBF neural networks is determined by the dimension of input vectors. In the proposed system, the truncated DCT vectors after implementing the FLD are fed to the input layer of the RBF neural networks. The number of outputs is equal to the class number. The hidden neurons are very crucial to the RBF neural networks, which represent the subset of the input data. After the clustering algorithm is implemented, the FLD projects the training samples into the subspace in which the training samples are clustered more tightly. Our experimental results show that the training samples are separated well and there are no overlaps between subclasses after the FLD is performed. Consequently, in our system, the number of subclasses (i.e. the number of hidden neurons of the RBF neural networks) is determined by the previous clustering process.

In the proposed system, we simplify the estimation of the RBF parameters according to the data properties instead of supervised learning since the non-linear supervised method often suffers from a long training time and the possibility of being trapped in local minima. Two important parameters are associated with each RBF unit, the center C_i and the width σ_i. Each center should well represent each subclass because the classification is actually based on the distances between the input samples and the centers of each subclass. There are different strategies in selecting RBF centers with respect to different applications [18]. Here, as the FLD keeps the most discriminating feature for each sample in each subclass, it is reasonable to choose the mean value of the training samples in every subclass as the RBF center as follows:

$$C_i = \frac{1}{n^i} \sum_{j=1}^{n^i} P_j^i \tag{10}$$

where P_i^j is the jth sample in the ith subclass and n^i is the number of training samples in the ith subclass.

Width Estimation

To our knowledge, every subclass has its own features which lead to different scopes for each subclass. The width of an RBF unit describes the properties of a subclass because the width of a Gaussian function represents the standard deviation of the function. Besides, the width controls the amount of overlapping of different Gaussian functions. If the widths are too large, there will be great overlaps between classes so that the RBF units cannot represent the subclasses well and the output belonging to the class will not be so significant which will lead to great misclassifications. On the contrary, too small a width will result in rapid reduction in the value of a Gaussian function and thus poor generalization. Accordingly, our goal is to select the width that minimizes the overlaps between different classes so as to preserve local properties, as well as maximizes the generalization ability of the networks.

As foreshadowed earlier, the FLD enables the subclasses to be separated well. However, it has been indicated that the FLD method achieves the best performance on the training data, but generalizes poorly to new individuals, particularly when the training data set is small [19]. The distribution of training samples cannot represent the new inputs well. Hence, in this special case, the width of each subclass cannot be estimated merely according to the small number of training samples in each subclass. Our studies show that the distances from the centers of RBF units to the new input samples belonging to other classes are similar to the distances to the training samples in other classes. These distances can be used to estimate the widths of RBF units since they generally reflect the range of RBF units. In [22], it was indicated that the patterns which are not consistent with data statistics (noisy patterns) should be rejected rather than used for training. Accordingly, the following method for width estimation is proposed:

$$dcc(j,i) = \| C_j^l - C_i^k \| \tag{11}$$

$$d_{med}(i) = \text{med}\{dcc(j,i)\} \tag{12}$$

$$i,j = 1,2,\ldots,u \ i \neq j \quad k,l = 1,2,\ldots,s, \ k \neq l$$

where C_i^k is the center of the ith cluster belonging to the kth class and C_j^l is the center of the jth cluster belonging to the lth class and $d_{med}(i)$ is the median distance from the ith center to the centers belonging to other classes. In the proposed system, since the centers of RBF units well represent the training samples in each cluster, we estimate the width of one cluster by calculating the distances from this center to the centers belonging to other classes instead of the individual training samples so as to avoid excessive computational complexity. Hence, the width σ_i of the ith cluster is estimated as follows:

$$\sigma_i = \frac{d_{med}(i)}{\sqrt{|\ln \gamma|}} \tag{13}$$

where γ is a factor that controls the overlap of this cluster with other clusters belonging to different classes. Equation (13) is derived from the Gaussian function. It should be noted that $d_{med}(i)$ is determined by the distances to the cluster centers belonging to other classes (not other clusters) because one class can be split into several clusters and the overlaps between clusters from the same class are allowed to be great. The median distance $d_{med}(i)$ well measures the relative scope of RBF units. Furthermore, by selecting a proper factor γ, suitable overlaps between different classes can be guaranteed.

Weight Adjustment

In the first stage, we estimate the parameters of the RBF units by using unsupervised training methods. The second phase of training is to optimize the second-layer weights of the RBF neural networks. Since the output of the RBF neural networks is a linear model, we can apply linear supervised learning to minimize a suitable error function. The sum-of-squares error function is given by

$$E = \frac{1}{2}\sum_{i=1}^{n}\sum_{j=1}^{s}(t_i^j - y^j(P_i))^2 \tag{14}$$

where t_i^j is the target value for output unit j when the ith training sample P_i is fed to the network, $y^j(P_i) = \sum_{k=1}^{u} w(j,k)R_k$, R_k is the kth output of the RBF unit, u is the number of RBF units generated according to the clustering algorithm in Section 2.2 and n is the total number of training samples. This problem can be solved by the linear least square (LLS) paradigm [12].

Let r and s be the number of input and output neurons respectively. Furthermore, let $R \in \Re^{u \times n}$ be the RBF unit matrix and $T = (T_1, T_2, \dots, T_n)^T \in \Re^{s \times n}$ be the target matrix consisting of "1's" and "0's" with exactly one per column that identifies the processing unit to which a given exemplar belongs. Find an optimal weight matrix $W^* \in \Re^{s \times u}$ such that the error function (14) is minimized as follows:

$$W^* = (TR^\dagger)^T \tag{15}$$

where $R^\dagger$ is the pseudoinverse of R and is given by

$$R^\dagger = (R^T R)^{-1} R^T \tag{16}$$

In the proposed system, however, direct solution of (16) can lead to numerical difficulties due to the possibility of $R^T R$ being singular or near singular. This problem can be best solved by using the technique of singular value decomposition (SVD) [23].

4 Experimental Results and Discussions

In order to evaluate the proposed face recognition system, our experiments are performed on three benchmark face databases: 1) The ORL database; 2) The FERET database; 3) The Yale database. Besides, for each database, we use three different evaluation methods which are mostly used in each database respectively. In this way, the experiment results can be compared with other face recognition approaches fairly.

4.1 Testing on the ORL Database

First, our face recognition system is tested on the ORL database. There are 400 images of 40 subjects. In the following experiments, 5 images are randomly selected as the training samples and another 5 images as test images. Therefore, a total of 200 images are used for training and another 200 for testing and there are no overlaps between the training and testing sets. Here, we verify our system based on the average error rate, E_{ave}, which is defined as

$$E_{ave} = \frac{\sum_{i=1}^{q} n_{mis}^i}{q n_t} \tag{17}$$

where q is the number of simulation runs. (The proposed system is evaluated on ten runs, $q = 10$.), n_{mis}^i is the number of misclassifications for the ith run and n_t is the total number of testing samples for each run. We also denote the maximum and minimum misclassification rates for the ten runs as E_{max} and E_{min} respectively.

The dimension of feature vectors fed into the RBF neural networks is essential for accurate recognition. In [17], experimental results showed that the best results are achieved when the feature dimension is 25-30. If the feature dimension is too small, the feature vectors do not contain sufficient information for recognition. However, it does not mean that more information will result in higher recognition rate. It has been indicated that if the dimension of the network input is comparable to the size of the training set, the system is liable to overfitting and result in poor generalization [24]. Moreover, the addition of some unimportant information may become noise and degrade the performance. Our experiments also showed that the best recognition rates are achieved when the feature dimension is about 30. Hence, the feature dimension of 30 will be adopted in the following simulation studies.

Parameter Selection

Two parameters, namely the clustering factor α and the overlapping factor γ need to be determined. As foreshadowed in Section 2.2, the sub-clustering process is based on the mean value and standard deviation of the distances from the CRS to the samples in other classes. Normally, we can choose $\alpha = 1$ as the initial value since the difference between the mean distance and standard deviation approximately implies the scope of CRS. Nevertheless, with different databases and applications, an appropriate value of α can be obtained by proper adjustment. For the ORL database, the following experimental results show that the proper value of α lies in the range of $1 \leq \alpha \leq 2$.

Since the overlapping factor γ is not related to α, we can fix the value for α when estimating γ. The value of α is set to 1 for the following parameter estimation process. It follows from (13) that the factor γ actually represents the output of the RBF unit when the distance between the input and the RBF center is equal to d_{med}. As a result, γ should be a small value. We can initially assume that γ lies in the range of $0 < \gamma < 0.3$. More optimal and precise γ can be further estimated by finding the minimum value of the root mean square error (RMSE). The RMSE curves for five different training sets are depicted in Fig. 7. It is evident that there is only one minimum value in each RMSE curve and it usually lies in the range of $0.05 \leq \gamma \leq 0.1$. We should not choose the exact minimum value of γ because the FLD makes the training samples in each cluster tighter in comparison with the testing samples. Accordingly, in order to obtain better generalization, we choose a slightly larger value of γ. In the following experiments, we choose the value of 0.1 for the overlapping factor γ which is shown to be a proper value for the RBF width estimation in our system.

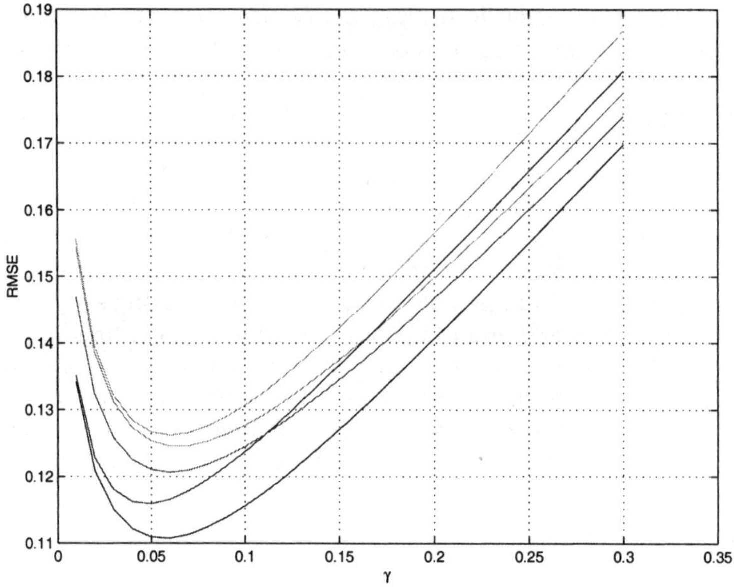

Fig. 7. RMSE curve

Number of DCT Coefficients

In order to determine how many DCT coefficients should be chosen, we evaluate the recognition performance with different numbers of DCT coefficients. Simulation results are summarized in Table 1. Here, the clustering coefficient α is set to 1. We can see from Table 1 that more DCT coefficients do not necessarily mean better recognition performance because high-frequency components are related to unstable facial features such as expression. There will be more variable information for recognition when the DCT coefficients increase. According to Table 1, the best performance is obtained when 50-60 DCT coefficients are used in our recognition system. In addition, Table 1 shows that the performance of our system is relatively stable when the number of DCT coefficients changes significantly. This is mainly due to the FLD algorithm which discounts the irrelevant information as well as keeps the most invariant and discriminating information for recognition.

Effect of Clustering

As mentioned in Section 2, the FLD is a linear projection paradigm and it cannot handle nonlinear variations in each class. Therefore, the proposed subclustering algorithm is applied before taking the FLD. The clustering factor α controls the extent of clustering as well as determines the number of RBF units. Small number of clusters may lead to great overlap between classes and

Table 1. Recognition performance versus number of DCT coefficients ($\alpha = 1$ $\gamma = 0.1$)

No. of DCT coefficients	Feature dimension	$E_{min}(\%)$	$E_{max}(\%)$	$E_{ave}(\%)$
35	30	1.5	10.0	4.55
40	30	1.5	7.0	3.90
45	30	1.5	8.5	3.85
50	30	2.0	7.5	3.60
55	30	1.0	6.5	3.20
60	30	1.5	8.0	3.30
70	30	2.5	9.0	4.05
80	30	1.5	8.0	3.80
90	30	2.0	9.0	4.90
100	30	3.5	10.0	5.50

cannot obtain the optimal FLD projection direction. On the other hand, an increase of clusters may result in poor generalization because of overfitting. Moreover, since the training samples in each class are limited, the increase of clusters leads to reduction of training samples in each cluster so that the FLD will work inefficiently. Table 2 shows one run of the recognition results with different numbers of clusters where E denotes the misclassification rate. The best performance is obtained when α lies in the range of 1.0-2.0. The results show that sub-clustering will improve the performance even when the FLD is applied on small clusters. Without the clustering process, face images with large nonlinear variations will be in the same cluster. The FLD will discount some important facial features instead of extracting them since the FLD is a kind of linear global projection method. Therefore, for face images with large variations such as pose, scale etc., sub-clustering is necessary before implementing the FLD. This process will be more effective if there are more training samples for each cluster.

Table 2. Recognition performance versus clustering factor α ($\gamma = 0.1$)

No. of DCT coefficients	Feature dimension	No. of clusters	α	$E(\%)$
55	30	40	0.0	4.0
55	30	42	0.5	3.0
55	30	44	1.0	3.0
55	30	46	1.2	3.0
55	30	50	1.5	2.5
55	30	55	1.8	3.0
55	30	58	2.0	3.0
55	30	74	2.5	4.0
55	30	107	3.0	4.5

By setting the optimal parameters in the proposed system, we obtain high recognition performance based on ten simulation studies whose results are shown in Table 3.

Table 3. Performance on 10 simulations

No. of DCT coefficients	Feature dimension	α	γ	$E_{min}(\%)$	$E_{max}(\%)$	$E_{ave}(\%)$
55	30	1.5	0.1	0.0	4.5	2.45

Comparisons with Other Approaches

Many face recognition approaches have been performed on the ORL database. In order to compare the recognition performance, we choose some recent approaches tested under similar conditions for comparison. Approaches are evaluated on recognition rate, training time and recognition time. Comparative results of different approaches are shown in Table 4. Our experiments are performed on a Pentium II 350MHz computer, using Windows 2000 and Matlab 6.1. It is hard to compare the speed of different algorithms which are implemented on different computing platforms. Nevertheless, according to the information of different computing systems as listed in Table 4, we can approximately compare their relative speeds. It is evident from the Table that our proposed approach achieves high recognition rate as well as high training and recognition speed.

Table 4. Recognition performance comparison of different approaches

Approach	Error rate(%)		Training time	Recognition time	Platform
	Best	Mean			
Pseudo-2D HMM [25]	5.0	n/a	n/a	4 min.	Sun Sparc II
SOM+CN [14]	1.5	3.8	4 hr.	0.5 sec.	SGI Indy 100M
PDBNN [15]	n/a	4.0	20 min.	0.1 sec.	SGI Indy 100M
DCT+HMM [9]	0.5	n/a	23.5 sec.	3.5 sec.	Pentium 200M
Pseudo-2D HMM+DCT [10]	0.0	n/a	n/a	1.5 sec.	Pentium 400M
LVQ+RBF+FEC [26]	0.5	n/a	n/a	0.777 sec.	Intel 200M
DCT+MLP [7]	3.0	5.8	1 min.	0.0002 sec.*	IBM 450M
FND [27]	n/a	1.75	61 sec.	3.23 sec.	Pentium II 400M
NFA-II+NFL [28]	n/a	4.05	n/a	0.16 sec.	IBM 1700M
Our proposed approach	0.0	2.45	14 sec.	0.055 sec.	Pentium II 350M

* It is not clear if the computational time for the DCT is counted in because the DCT takes about 0.046 seconds per image in our system. The time for classification is only about 0.009 seconds.

Computational Complexity

In this section, in order to provide more information about the computational efficiency of the proposed system, the approximate complexity of each part is analyzed and the results are summarized in Table 5.

Table 5. Computational Complexity

Part	Complexity
DCT	$O(N^2 \log N N_{tr})$
Clustering	$O(N_{DCT} N_{tr}^2)$
FLD	$O(N_u N_{DCT} + N_r^3 + N_{DCT} N_r N_{tr})$
RBF parameter estimation	$O(N_u^3)$
LLS	$O(N_s N_u N_n + N_n^2 N_s + N_{tr}^2 \log N_{tr} + N_n N_s^2)$
Classification	$O(N^2 \log N + N_{DCT} N_r + N_u N_s)$

N The dimension of an $N \times N$ face image (N is a power of 2)
N_{tr} The number of training samples
N_{DCT} The number of truncated DCT coefficients
N_r The number of input neurons (The dimension of the FLD feature vectors)
N_u The number of clusters (The number of RBF units)
N_s The number of output neurons (The number of classes)

In face recognition applications, the dimensionality of an original face image is usually considerably greater than the number of training samples. Therefore, the computational complexity mostly lies in the dimensionality reduction stage. The training and recognition speed are greatly improved because the fast DCT reduces the computational complexity from $O(N^4)$ to $O(N^2 \log N)$ for an $N \times N$ image where N is a power of 2. Moreover, the proposed parameter estimation method is much faster than the gradient descent training algorithm which will take up to hundreds of epochs.

Performances with Different Numbers of Training Samples

Since the FLD is a kind of statistical method for feature extraction, the choice of training samples will affect its performance. In [6], the authors indicate that the FLD works efficiently only when the number of training samples is large and representative for each class. Moreover, a small number of training samples will result in poor generalization for each RBF unit. Simulation results with different numbers of training samples are shown in Fig. 8. Our approach is promising if more training samples are available.

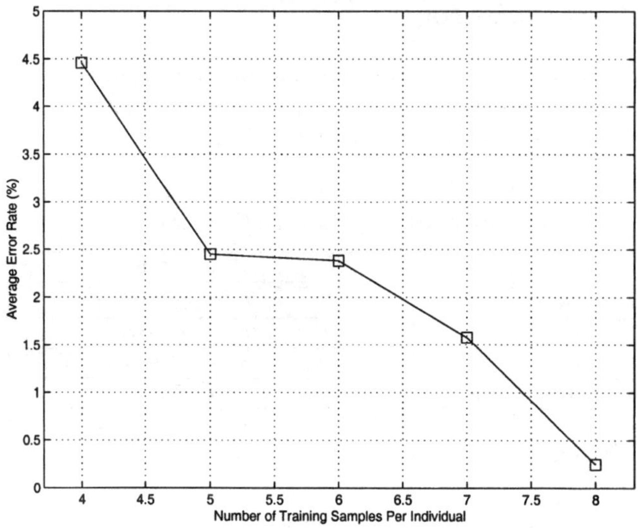

Fig. 8. Performances with different numbers of training samples (Results are based on ten runs)

Performances after Discarding Several DCT Coefficients

As illustrated in Section 2, the *DC-free* DCT has the robustness against linear brightness variations. The truncated DCT also alleviates the effect of the large area non-uniform illumination by discarding several low-frequency components. However, there are no such large illumination variations in the ORL database. Therefore, discarding the first three DCT coefficients will not get better performance. On the contrary, the performance will get worse (see Table 8). The reason is that some holistic facial features, for example, the relative intensity of the hair and the face skin, will be more or less ruined since they are low-frequency components (see Fig. 9). In fact, this kind of influence is slight compared to large area illumination variations. We can see from Fig. 9 that the main facial features such as face outline, eyes, nose and mouth are well maintained after discarding several low-frequency DCT coefficients. Furthermore, in many face recognition applications, only faces without hair are used for recognition for the reason that the human's hair is a kind of unstable feature which will change greatly with time. In this case, discarding the first several low-frequency DCT coefficients will mainly reduce large area illumination variations.

4.2 Testing on the FERET Database

The proposed feature extraction method is also tested on the FERET database which contains more subjects with different variations [29]. We employ the

Table 6. Performances after discarding several DCT coefficients

No. of discarded coefficients	0	1	3
$E_{ave}(\%)$	2.45	3.35	4.55

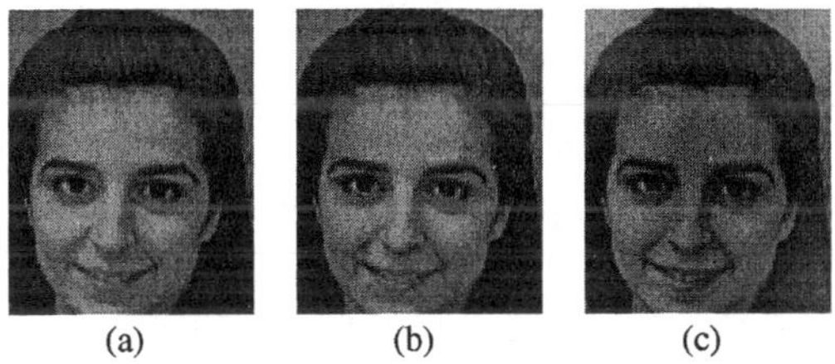

Fig. 9. Reconstructed images after discarding several low-frequency DCT coefficients: (a) Original image; (b) Reconstructed image after discarding the first three DCT coefficients; (c) Reconstructed image after discarding the first six DCT coefficients; (In order to display the image, the first coefficient is actually retained.)

CSU Face Identification Evaluation System to evaluate our feature extraction method [30]. The original face images are first normalized by using the preprocessing program provided in the CSU evaluation system. An example of a normalized image is shown in Fig. 10. Four testing probe subsets with different evaluation tasks are used (See Table 7). We only compare our proposed feature extraction method with the baseline PCA method with or without the first three principal components. To generate the cumulative match curve, the Euclidean distance measure is used. Here, we can only evaluate our proposed feature extraction method but not the classifier. Since only normalized frontal face images are used in this experiment and the training samples for each class are limited, the sub-clustering process is skipped. The cumulative match curves for four probe sets are respectively shown in Fig. 11, Fig. 12, Fig. 13 and Fig. 14. (For the PCA approach, 50 components are used. For the DCT + FLD approach, 70 DCT coefficients are used and the dimensionality of the feature vectors is also 50 after implementing the FLD).

From the cumulative match curves of the four different probe sets, we can see that the performance is improved by discarding the first three DCT low-frequency coefficients because illumination variations are reduced. The histogram equalization in the preprocessing procedure can only deal with the uniform illumination. However, by discarding several low-frequency DCT coefficients, both uniform and nonuniform illumination variations can be reduced. We can see from Fig. 14 that the performance of PCA is greatly improved by discarding the first three components. However, in other probe sets, the performance becomes even worse without the first three components. Because the PCA is a kind of statistical approach which is data dependent, the first three components are not necessarily related to illumination variations. It depends

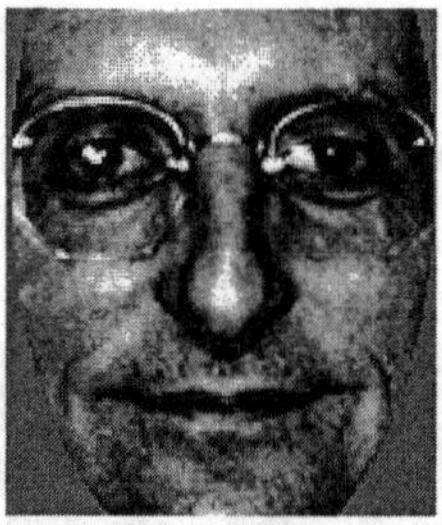

Fig. 10. Example of a normalized FERET face image

Table 7. Four probe subsets and their evaluation task

Probe subsets	Evaluation task
Dup 1	Aging of subjects
Dup 2	Aging of subjects
Fafb	Facial expression
Fafc	Illumination

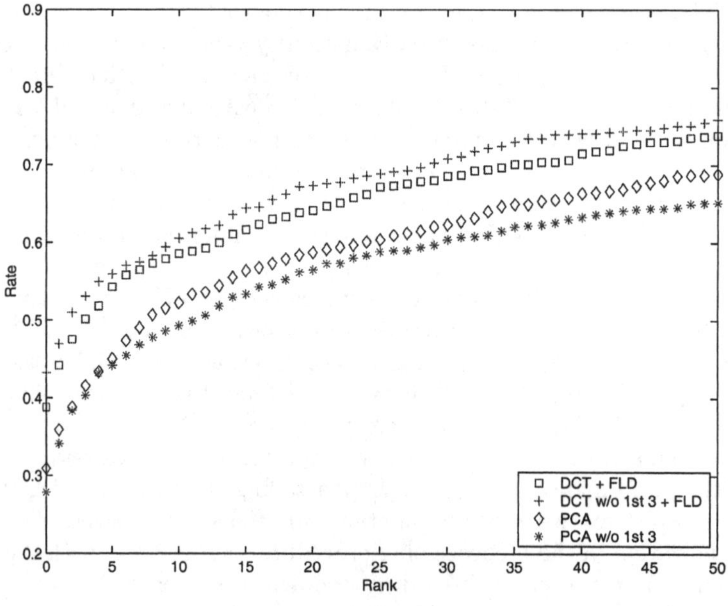

Fig. 11. Cumulative match curves: FERET dup 1 probe set

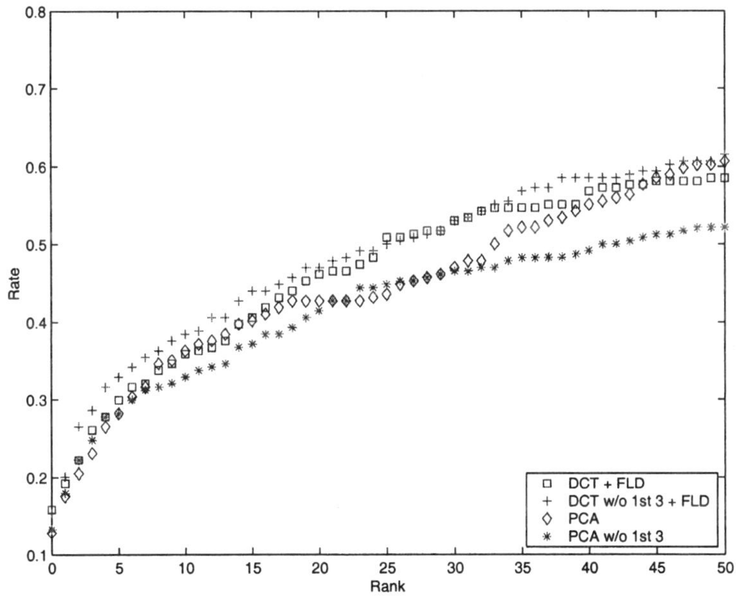

Fig. 12. Cumulative match curves: FERET dup 2 probe set

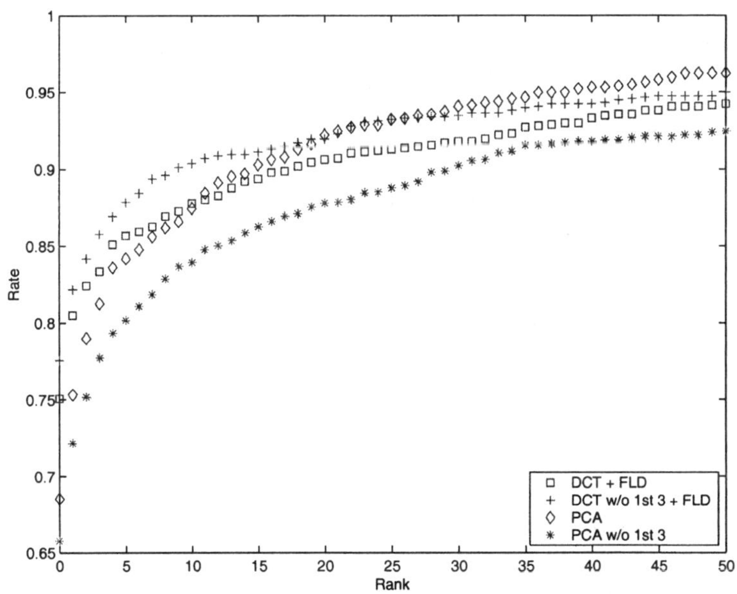

Fig. 13. Cumulative match curves: FERET fafb probe set

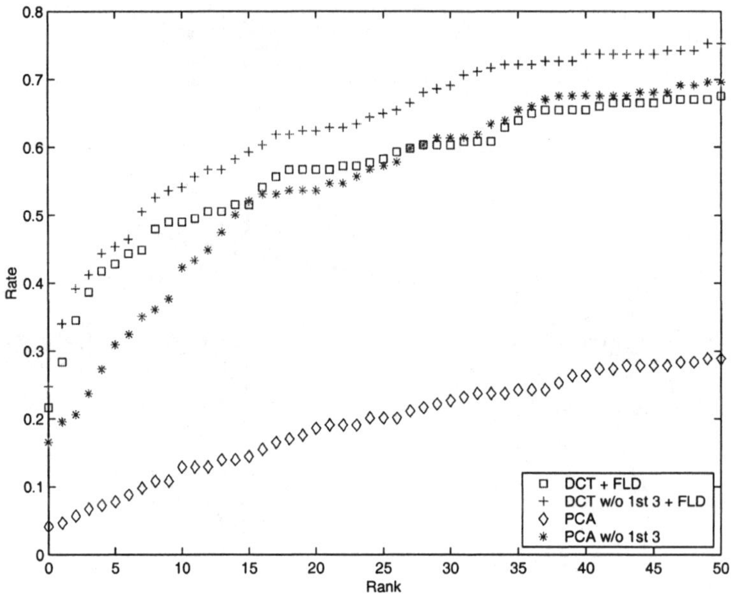

Fig. 14. Cumulative match curves: FERET fafc probe set

on the training and testing sets. We can see from the experimental results that only the probe set Fafc with large illumination changes will get better performance by discarding the first three components. It should be highlighted that the low-frequency DCT coefficients are mainly associated with the illumination variations for the face image without hair. Therefore, discarding several low-frequency coefficients will only reduce illumination variations but not ruin some facial features. It should be noted that we do not compare our feature extraction approach with all other available approaches tested on the FERET database and we do not claim that our approach achieve the best performance on the FERET database. The main objective of this experiment is to show that the performance is indeed improved by discarding the first several low-frequency DCT coefficients. Moreover, compared with the baseline PCA approach, our approach performs better on the four probe sets and the computational load is greatly reduced.

4.3 Testing on the Yale Database

We further test our proposed approach on the Yale database which contains 165 frontal face images covering 15 individuals taken under 11 different conditions. Each individual has different facial expressions (happy, sad, winking, sleepy, and surprised), illumination conditions (center-light, left-light, right-light) and small occlusion (with glasses). In order to be consistent with the experiments of [5], the centered face images of the normalized Yale face database and their closely cropped images are used in our experiment.[§] Examples of the centered Yale images and the closely cropped Yale images are shown in Fig. 15 and Fig. 16 respectively.

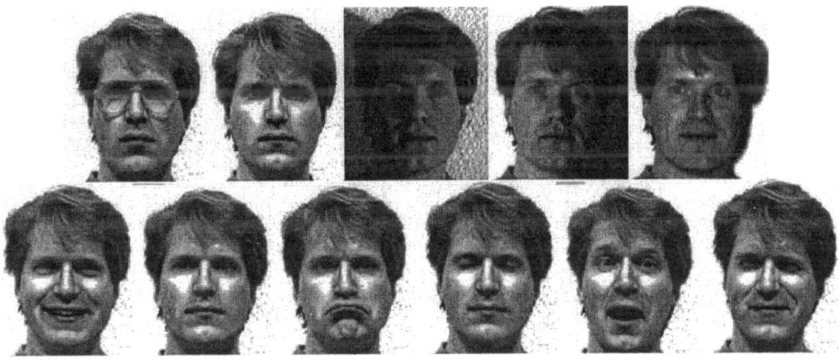

Fig. 15. Examples of the centered Yale images

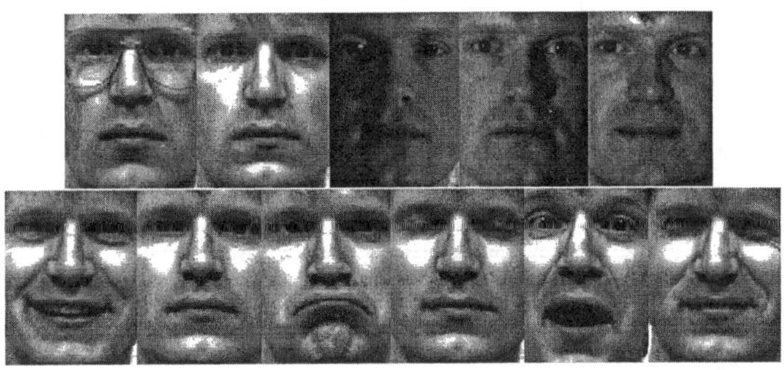

Fig. 16. Examples of the closely cropped Yale images

For the Yale face database, our system is also tested by using the "leaving-one-out" strategy which was used in [5]. In order to fairly evaluate different feature extraction methods, the nearest neighbor classifier was used for classification. We also skip the sub-clustering process since only frontal normalized face images are used. Comparative results are shown in Table 8. The results of the Eigenface (PCA) and Fisherface in our experiment are not identical to the results shown in [5]. This is mainly due to a slightly different cropping size and normalization. Nevertheless, the results are very close. By discarding the first three coefficients, the DCT achieves better performance because the variations due to lighting is reduced. However, if the FLD is further applied

[§]The normalized Yale face database can be obtained from http://www-white.media.mit.edu/vismod/classes/mas622-00/datasets/

to the DCT feature vectors, discarding the first three coefficients will not improve the performance significantly because the FLD also discounts illumination variations. We can see from Table 8 that our feature extraction method achieves similar performance compared to the Fisherface method. However, the main advantage of our method is its low computational load which is crucial for high-speed face recognition in large databases. If we use the proposed RBF neural networks for classification, our system gets better performance. (See Table 9).

Table 8. Comparison on the Yale database

Approach	Reduced space	Error rate (%) Close crop	Error rate (%) Full face
Eigenface	30	25.5	17.6
Eigenface w/o 1st 3	30	17.6	12.1
Fisherface	15	6.1	3.0
DCT	55	26.1	20.0
DCT w/o 1st 3	55	20.6	13.9
DCT + FLD	15	6.7	3.6
DCT w/o 1st 3 + FLD	15	7.3	3.0

Table 9. Performance on the Yale database ($\gamma = 0.1$)

Approach	Error rate (%) Close crop	Error rate (%) Full face
DCT + FLD + RBF	4.8	1.8

5 Conclusions

This chapter presents a face recognition method based on the techniques of DCT, FLD and RBF neural networks. Facial features are first extracted by the DCT which greatly reduces dimensionality of the original face image as well as maintains the main facial features. Compared with the well-known PCA approach, the DCT has the advantages of data independency and fast computational speed. Besides, we have explored another property of DCT. It turns out that by simply discarding the first DCT coefficient, the proposed system is robust against the uniform brightness variations of images. Furthermore, by discarding the first few low-frequency DCT coefficients, the effect of non-uniform illumination can be alleviated. In order to obtain the most invariant and discriminating feature of faces, the FLD, a linear projection method, is further applied to the feature vectors. Before implementing the

FLD, we propose a clustering algorithm to prevent the training samples with large variations from being clustered in the same class. This process guarantees the optimal projection direction for the FLD as well as determines the number of hidden neurons of the RBF neural networks for classification. After the FLD is applied, there are no overlaps between classes and the architecture and parameters of RBF neural networks are determined according to the distribution properties of the training samples. Simulation results on three benchmark face databases show that our system achieves high training and recognition speed, as well as high recognition rate. More importantly, it is insensitive to illumination variations.

References

1. R. Chellappa, C. L. Wilson and S. Sirohey (1995) Human and Machine Recognition of Faces: A Survey. Proc. IEEE 83:705–740.
2. R. Brunelli and T. Poggio (1993) Face Recognition: Features Versus Templates. IEEE Trans. on Pattern Analysis and Machine Intelligence 15:1042–1053.
3. M. Kirby and L. Sirvoich (1990) Application of The Karhunen-Loeve Procedure For The Characterization of Human Faces. IEEE Trans. Pattern Analysis and Machine Intelligence 12:103–108.
4. M. A. Turk and A. P. Pentland (1991) Eigenfaces for Recognition. J. Cognitive Neuroscience 3:71–86.
5. P. N. Belhumeur, J. P. Hespanha and D.J. Kriegman (1997) Eigenfaces Versus Fisherfaces: Recognition Using Class Specific Linear Projection. IEEE Trans. Pattern Analysis and Machine Intelligence 19:711–720
6. A. Martinez and A. Kak (2001) PCA versus LDA. IEEE Trans. on Pattern Analysis and Machine Intelligence 23(2):228–233.
7. Z. Pan, R. Adams and H. Bolouri (2000) Image Redundancy Reduction for Neural Network Classification using Discrete Cosine Transforms. Proc. of The IEEE-INNS-ENNS International Joint Conf. on Neural Networks, Como, Italy 3:149-154.
8. Z. M. Hafed and M. D. Levine (2001) Face Recognition Using the Discrete Cosine Transform. International Journal of Computer Vision 43(3):167–188.
9. V. V. Kohir and U. B. Desai (1998) Face Recognition Using Face Recogntion Using DCT-HMM Approach. In Workshop on Advances in Facila Image Analysis and Recognition Technology (AFIAER), Freibureg, Germany.
10. S. Eickeler, S. Müller, and G. Rigoll (1999) High Quality Face Recognition in JPEG Compressed Images. In Proceedings IEEE Intern. Conference on Image Processing (ICIP), Kobe, Japan 672–676.
11. W. Pennebaker and J. Mitchell (1993) JPEG Still Image Data Compression Standard. Van Nostrand Reinhold, New York.
12. C. M. Bishop (1995) Neural Networks for Pattern Recognition. Oxford University Press Inc, New York.
13. J. Mao and A. K. Jain (1995) Artificial Neural Networks for Feature Extraction and Multivariate Data Projection. IEEE Trans. Neural Networks 6:296–317.
14. S. Lawrence, C. L. Giles, A. C. Tsoi and A. D. Back (1997) Face Recognition: A Convolutional Neural-Network Approach. IEEE Trans. Neural Networks, Special Issue on Neural Networks and Pattern Recognition 8(1):98–113

15. S.-H. Lin, S.-Y. Kung, and L.-J. Lin (1997) Face Recognition/Detection by Probabilistic Decision-Based Neural Network. IEEE Trans. Neural Networks 8:114–132.
16. D. Valentin, H. Abdi, A. J. O'Toole and G. W. Cottrell (1994) Connectionist Models of Face Processing: a Survey. Pattern Recognition 27:1209–1230.
17. M. J. Er, S. Wu, J. Lu and H. L. Toh (2002) Face Recognition With Radial Basis Function (RBF) Neural Networks. IEEE Trans. on Neural Networks 13(3):697–710.
18. S. Haykin (1994) Neural Networks, A Comprehensive Foundation. New York: Macmillan
19. G. Donato, M. S. Bartlett, J. C. Hager, P. Ekman, and T. J. Sejnowski (1999) Classifying Facial Actions. IEEE Trans. Pattern Analysis and Machine Intelligence 21:974–989
20. W. Pedrycz (1998) Conditional Fuzzy Clustering in the Design of Radial Basis Function Neural Networks. IEEE Trans. Neural Networks 9:601–612
21. J. Moody and C. J. Darken (1989) Fast Learning in Network of Locally-Tuned Processing Units. Neural computation 1:281–294.
22. A. G. Bors and I. Pitas (1996) Median Radial Basis Function Neural Network. IEEE Trans. Neural Networks 7:1351–1364.
23. W. H. Press, S. A. Teukolsky, W. T. Vetterling, B. P. Flannery (1992): Numerical Recipes in C: The Art of Scienti.c Computing, Cambridge University Press.
24. J. L. Yuan and T. L. Fine (1998) Neural-Network Design for Small Training Sets of High Dimension. IEEE Trans. Neural Networks 9:266–280.
25. F. Samaria (1994) Face Recognition Using Hidden Markov Models. PhD thesis, Trinity College, University of Cambridge, Cambridge.
26. A. S. Tolba, and A. N. Abu-Rezq (1999) Combined Classifiers For Invariant Face Recognition. in Proc. Int. Conf. Information Intelligence and Systems 350–359.
27. T. Tan and H. Yan (2001) Object Recognition Based on Fractal Neighbor Distance. Signal Processing 81:2105–2129.
28. Y.-S. Ryu and S.-Y. Oh (2002) Simple hybrid classifier for face recognition with adaptively generated virtual data. Pattern Recognition Letters 23:833–841.
29. P. J. Phillips, H. Wechsler, J. Huang, and P. Rauss (1998) The FERET Database and Evaluation Procedure for Face Recognition Algorithms. Image and Vision Computing J 16(5):295–306.
30. R. Beveridge, D. Bolme, M. Teixerira and B. Draper (2003) The CSU Face Identification Evaluation System User's Guide: Version 5.0. Colorado State University.

Probabilistic Reasoning for Closed-Room People Monitoring

Ji Tao and Yap-Peng Tan

School of Electrical and Electronic Engineering
Nanyang Technological University
50 Nanyang Avenue, Singapore 639798

Abstract. In this chapter, we present a probabilistic reasoning approach to recognizing people entering and leaving a closed room by exploiting low-level visual features and high-level domain-specific knowledge. Specifically, people in the view of a monitoring camera are first detected and tracked so that their color and facial features can be extracted and analyzed. Then, recognition of people is carried out using a mapped feature similarity measure and exploiting the temporal correlation and constraints among each sequence of observations. The optimality of recognition is achieved in the sense of maximizing the joint posterior probability of the multiple observations. Experimental results of real and synthetic data are reported to show the effectiveness of the proposed approach.

Keywords: people monitoring, probabilistic reasoning, Viterbi algorithm, domain knowledge, HMM

1 Introduction

With the increased concern for physical security in the face of global terrorism and outbreaks of infectious viruses, automated video surveillance for enhanced security in human living and work places has received unprecedented attention from industries, research institutes, and governmental agencies over the past few years [1, 2]. One main task of many video surveillance systems is to associate each person with an identity or to correspond a same person observed at different time instances. The results allow the derivation of such useful information as how long a person has stayed in a site, how many people are in the room during a certain period of concern, and who they are. Potential applications of such a system include, for example, understanding human activities in a monitored work place [8, 9], keeping aware of user identities in an intelligent room [3], and identifying who could possibly be infected with a newly identified victim of Severe Acute Respiratory Syndrome (SARS) [10].

A number of related solutions have been proposed in the literature for people access control and monitoring. For example, biometrics have been increasingly used for identity recognition and obtained satisfactory results. Representative work in biometric-based recognition ranges from fingerprint and iris identification to face and gait recognition [11–14, 16]. However, many of these methods require intrusive data collection, e.g., demanding human proactive action and collaboration during the course of identification, and thus, work mainly in well-controlled environments. Although gait recognition can partly address this limitation by exploring human motion dynamics, gait feature, by itself, has limited discriminating power and only works for people whose motion patterns have been well characterized and pre-stored in a database for matching.

Regardless of the type of features used, most existing approaches accomplish the recognition task based on some maximum likelihood classification rule [15], where a definite decision is made based on features observed at a single time instance/duration. The temporal correlation and constraints among the observations obtained over time, however, are seldom utilized even they exist in some specific contexts; for example, in the case of closed-room monitoring, a person currently inside the room cannot enter the room again without first leaving it, and vice versa.

On the other hand, dynamic Bayesian networks (DBNs) [30, 31] are becoming popular in probabilistic inference due to their ability in incorporating various prior constraints and dealing with uncertainties in a systematic manner. In particular, hidden Markov models (HMMs), a specific form of DBNs, are well suited for modeling and identifying an event, represented as a state sequence, which can best explain a series of observations, for at least two reasons [24–26]. First, the topology among the hidden states, i.e., their interdependencies, can encode prior knowledge about how the event evolves. Second, the forward-backward and Viterbi algorithms [29], which are developed based on HMM's lattice structure, allow one to evaluate the probabilities of different state sequences efficiently, and thus to identify the most likely state sequence.

In this chapter, we present a video-based system using probabilistic reasoning and based on the Viterbi algorithm for monitoring people entering and leaving a closed room (i.e., a room with only a single entrance/exit; e.g., a lab, class room, or meeting room). The system consists of two modules: a feature extraction module to detect/track people entering or leaving the only entrance/exit of the closed room and extract their low-level features for recognition in an unintrusive manner, and a people recognition module to correspond each observed person with a person previously entering the room or to identify him/her as a new person unseen before. Figure 1 depicts the architecture of the proposed system. Rather than using only a single observation, we perform recognition by exploiting the temporal correlation and constraints among multiple people observations acquired at different time instances. Consequently, our method can effectively enhance the limited discriminating power of low-level features, such as color histograms and face features acquired using a camera from a distance. Experimental results demonstrate that the proposed system can achieve superior recognition accuracy as compared with the existing systems using maximum likelihood approaches.

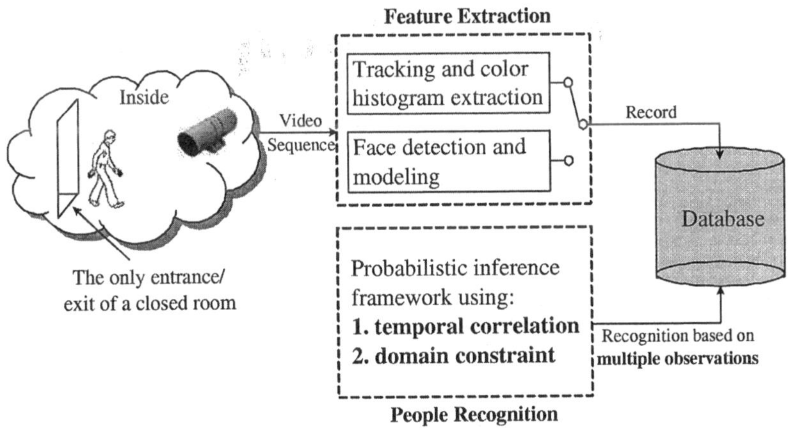

Fig. 1. Overview of the proposed closed-room people monitoring system

2 Viterbi Algorithm

In this section, we briefly review preliminaries of HMM and the Viterbi algorithm, based on which our proposed system is constructed.

In general, an HMM can be characterized by a set of parameters $\Lambda = \{A, B, \pi\}$, where $A = \{a_{ij} | a_{ij} = P[q_{t+1} = S_j | q_t = S_i]\}$ denotes the transition probabilities from state S_i at time t to state S_j at time $t+1$, $B = \{b_j | b_j(O_t) = P([O_t | q_t = S_j]\}$ the observation probabilities of state S_j, and $\pi = \{\pi_i | \pi_i = P[q_1 = S_i]\}$ the initial state probabilities. An example of a three-state HMM is shown in Fig. 2.

With these probabilities, three basic problems can generally be addressed with an HMM [27]: 1) Evaluate $P[O|\Lambda]$, the probability of an observation sequence O given the model Λ; 2) Find the most likely state sequence given the model and an observation sequence; and 3) Find the model $\Lambda = \{A, B, \pi\}$ that maximizes $P[O|\Lambda]$ for a given observation sequence. The first and third problems are known as model evaluation and training, respectively, and can be solved by forward-backward algorithm and Balm-Welch method [27]. Of relevance to our application is the second problem, in which the Viterbi algorithm plays an important role.

Consider a discrete-time dynamical system which is governed by a Markov chain and generates a sequence of observable outputs (observations) according to a number of hidden (unobservable) states. Our objective is to infer the most probable state sequence from the observation sequence. Straightforwardly, one

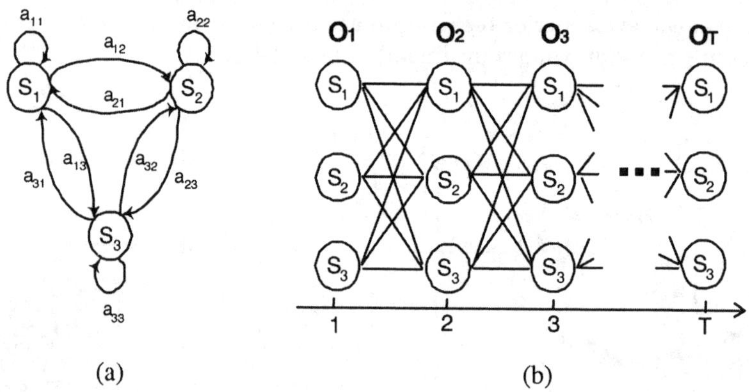

Fig. 2. Structure of a 3-state HMM: (a) transition diagram and (b) temporal view

can find the most probable state sequence by enumerating all possible state sequences and evaluating the probability of the observation sequence due to each possible state sequence. While viable, this exhaustive approach is computationally intensive even for a small number of states and observations. For example, with five observations (i.e. $T = 5$), the 3-state HMM shown in Fig. 2 will have 243 possible state sequences.

Using the Viterbi algorithm, one can exploit the dynamic programming technique to simplify the computation substantially. To see this, let us first define the quantity

$$\delta_t(i) = \max_{q_1, q_2, \cdots, q_{t-1}} P[q_1 q_2 \cdots q_t = S_i, O_1 O_2 \cdots O_t | \Lambda], \tag{1}$$

which is the highest probability of a state sequence which accounts for the first t observations and ends in state S_i at time t. By induction, it is easy to see that

$$\delta_{t+1}(j) = [\max_i \delta_t(i) a_{ij}] \cdot b_j(O_{t+1}). \tag{2}$$

Hence, for each state S_i at time t, one can find one state sequence ending in it and assuming the highest probability $\delta_t(i)$. We shall refer to this state sequence as the partial best state sequence. Once we have determined the hidden state corresponding to the observation obtained at time t, the uncertainties up to t can be resolved. For an HMM with N states, there are N partial best state sequences due to each observation. At the end of the observation (i.e., time T), the Viterbi algorithm can find the most probable state sequence with probability $\max_i \delta_T(i)$. We shall refer to this state sequence as the *best state sequence.*

The procedure for finding the most probable state sequence can be summarized as follows [27]:

1) Initialization:

$$\delta_1(i) = \pi_i b_i(O_1), \qquad 1 \le i \le N \tag{3a}$$

$$\psi_1(i) = 0. \tag{3b}$$

2) Recursion:

$$\delta_t(j) = \max_{1 \le i \le N} [\delta_{t-1}(i) a_{ij}(t-1)] b_j(O_t), \qquad 2 \le t \le T, 1 \le j \le N, \tag{4a}$$

$$\psi_t(j) = \arg\max_{1 \le i \le N} [\delta_{t-1}(i) a_{ij}(t-1)], \qquad 2 \le t \le T, 1 \le j \le N. \tag{4b}$$

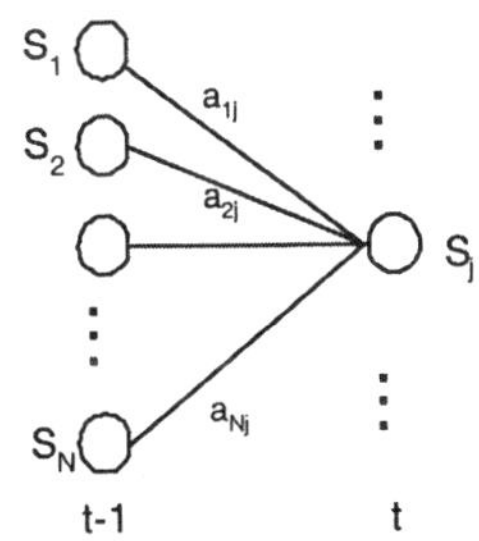

Fig. 3. Illustration of recursive computation of the Viterbi algorithm

3) Termination:

$$p^* = \max_{1 \le i \le N} [\delta_T(i)], \tag{5a}$$

$$q_T^* = \arg\max_{1 \le i \le N} [\delta_T(i)]. \tag{5b}$$

4) Path (state sequence) backtracking:

$$q_t^* = \psi_{t+1}(q_{t+1}^*), \qquad t = T-1, T-2, \cdots, 1. \tag{6}$$

The array ψ is introduced to keep track of the argument that maximizes (2) for each t and j, indicating all the preceding states along each partial best state sequence. With ψ, one can retrieve the *best state sequence* of the whole process as well as the partial best state sequence ending at a given state at any time. The latter is particularly useful in our people monitoring application as we shall show later.

From Fig. 3, we can see that the recursion computation of the Viterbi algorithm can be derived based on the temporal view structure of an HMM as shown in Fig. 2(b). The key point of its efficiency is that since there are only N possible states at each observation time, all the possible state sequences will end in these N states no matter how long the observation sequences are.

Apart from its tractability in computation, the Viterbi algorithm bears another important property: it does not make any maximum likelihood decision at each intermediate observation time, but obtains an overall decision by taking into account the whole sequence of observations. Ambiguity and/or misjudgement based on partial observations can be corrected later when more observations become available. This is well suited for our application, as it can exploit the temporal correlation among the observation sequence and recognize people based on multiple observations, reducing the chance of error due to making hard decision based on features with low discriminating power.

3 Low-Level Features

The feature extraction module of our proposed system currently makes use of two types of low-level features as illustrated in Fig. 4: color histograms and low-resolution human faces. These features are described in detail below.

Color histogram is a popular color feature for content-based image and video analysis [20–22]. It is easy to compute and rather invariant to change in shape or size [19]. Our system detects and tracks each moving person as a foreground region and counts the color distribution of pixels within the region (i.e. color histogram) as the appearance feature of the person. The feature similarity of two observed people c_i and c_j can be measured by their color histogram intersection, defined as $\sum_{k=1}^{K} \min(H_i(k),\ H_j(k))$, where H_i and H_j are the normalized color histograms of the two people, respectively, and K is the total number of color bins in the histogram. For the details of a color histogram based people tracking and recognition system, see our previous work [17,18].

For facial feature, we make use of two functions provided in Intel Open Source Computer Vision Library (OpenCV) [4], HarrFaceDetection and HMMFaceRecognition, to automatically detect and model human faces in video sequences. The face detector was originally proposed by Viola [5] and further improved by Lienhart [6], while the embedded HMM (EHMM) face recognizer was developed by Nefian *et al.* [7]. It has been shown that the EHMM recognizer can exploit the natural structure of frontal faces and achieve outstanding performance. With a number of face images of a same person, say c_i, we train his/her EHMM feature using a set of observation vectors obtained from the corresponding 2D-DCT coefficients. The likelihood of an unknown face observation c_j with respect to person c_i can be calculated by a doubly embedded Viterbi algorithm [7].

Direct application of the color histogram and face similar measures as defined above poses some potential problems. For example, the color histogram intersection of two different people is generally larger than zero for the reason that some of their appearance features, such as hair and skin, could share similar colors. On the other hand, the same person observed at different times may not have identical color histograms due to difference in lighting conditions, camera view angles, and segmentation results. The low-resolution face features are also subject to similar problems. Moreover, owing to successive multiplications of values less than one, the likelihood of faces calculated by

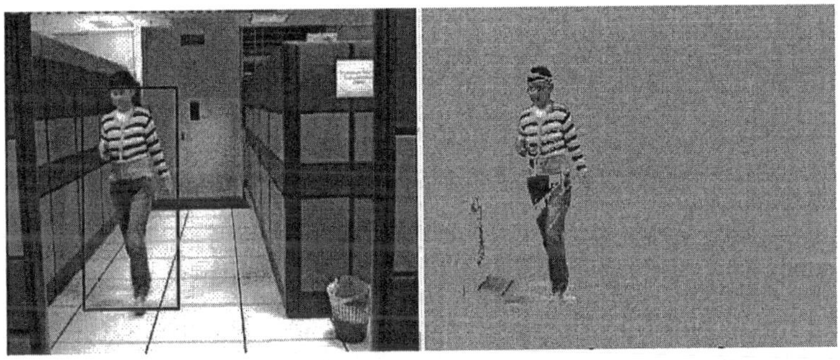

(a)

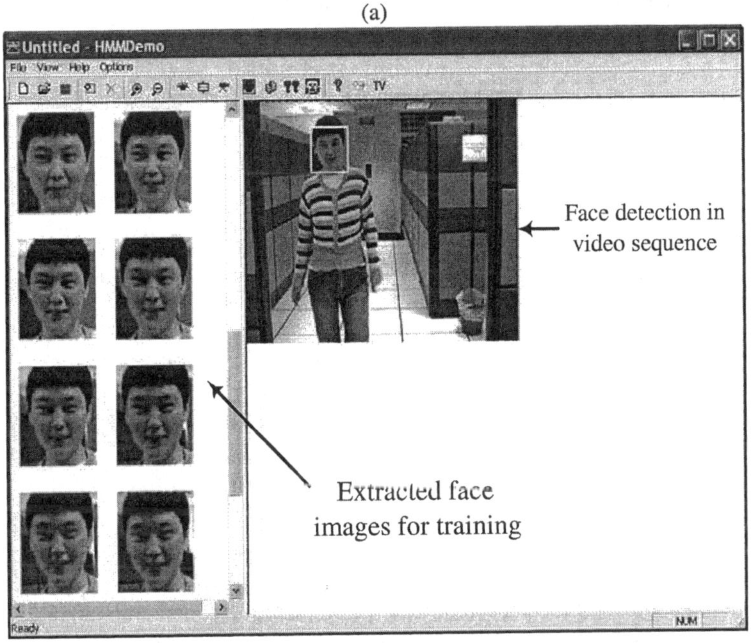

(b)

Fig. 4. Two types of low-level features considered: (a) the color histogram of segmented foreground region and (b) the EHMM feature of detected face

the doubly embedded Viterbi algorithm is numerically very small and subject to round-off errors. A function is therefore required to map the value of similarity measure based on color histograms or face features of two observed people c_i and c_j, denoted as $S(c_i, c_j)$, onto a similarity probability $P(c_i \sim c_j)$, which indicates how likely c_i and c_j correspond to the same person.

Conceivably, the mapping function needs to have the following properties: 1) it should be non-decreasing; 2) it should be approaching 0 or 1 as $S(c_i, c_j)$ takes values near its lower or upper limit; and 3) the transition from low to high mapped values should take place at where the value of $S(c_i, c_j)$ becomes evident to support that the two observed people are likely the same. After some subjective studies and comparisons, we select the *sigmoid* function [23] to perform the mapping, which can be expressed as follows:

$$P[c_i \sim c_j] = \frac{1}{1 + \exp[-\alpha(S(c_i, c_j) - \beta)]}, \tag{7}$$

where α and β are two parameters determining the shape of a sigmoid curve with α controlling the steepness of the transition and β defining the center of transition point. By experiments, we have determined the proper values of these two parameters for the similarity measures based on color histogram and face features, respectively.

It should be noted that many other features/attributes (e.g., fingerprint, iris pattern, voice, gait, etc.) for which a similarity measure is defined can be used in our proposed people monitoring system. To make the system less intrusive, we have only made use of color histogram and face features in the work reported here.

4 Probabilistic Reasoning Framework

4.1 Problem Formulation

Our first attempt is to develop a suitable HMM for the recognition task in a closed room by making use of the Viterbi algorithm. However, the parameters of HMMs need to be pre-learned from a set of representative data based on a fixed number of states. This situation, however, is not applicable to our case as the number of people as well as their activity patterns, i.e., the frequencies of entering and leaving the room, are generally different from place to place or time to time, and hard to be estimated from prior data.

To construct a framework that is well suited for the problem of our concern, we employ the lattice structure and parameter setting of HMMs, and formulate the problem of people recognition as follows. Assume that the closed room is empty when the system is first activated. When a person is entering the room, we append a new state to the state set (database) to represent his/her identity; when a person leaves at time t, he/she will be recorded as a new observation O_t. Thus the states in the state set at time t, denoted as $\mathbf{S}(t) = \{S_1 \cdots S_{N_t}\}$, correspond to the people identities in the database (i.e., people that possibly stay in the room at time t). When an observation sequence $O = \{O_1 \cdots O_T\}$ has been obtained over a period of time, the identities of the people leaving the room can be recognized from the state sets, $\mathbf{S}(1), \mathbf{S}(2), \cdots$, and $\mathbf{S}(T)$, recorded over the same period. By characterizing this inference framework with a time-variant parameter set $\Lambda(t) = \{A(t), B(t), \pi(t)\}$, we can use the Viterbi algorithm to find an optimal state sequence $Q = \{q_1 \cdots q_T\}$ associated with the observation sequence to maximize a joint posterior probability $P(Q, O|\Lambda(t))$. In this way, each leaving person can correspond to one of those who are judged still inside the room.

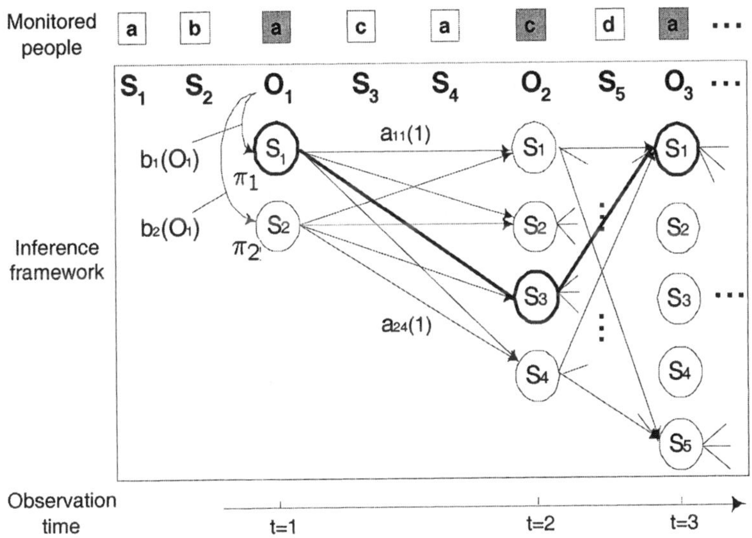

Fig. 5. Recognition example of the proposed probabilistic reasoning framework. The squares in the top row represent the observed people with their real identities manually labeled. The filled and unfilled squares denote the people leaving and entering, respectively

Fig. 5 illustrates a recognition example of the proposed framework, where the optimal state sequence obtained is shown in bold lines. From this sequence, we can identify O_1 as S_1, O_2 as S_3, O_3 as S_1, etc. We can see that the framework has a lattice structure similar to HMMs; however, there are several key differences that distinguish our framework from conventional HMMs. First, the parameter set $\Lambda(t)$ is time variant and needs to be derived at each observation time instance based on all the previous possible states and current observations rather than from some training data. Second, the number of states in our model is not fixed but can increase over time before a decision is made. Third, the states can be indefinite because more than one states could be associated with the same person, e.g., both states S_1 and S_4 in Fig. 5 represent the person 'a'. It can be seen that when 'a' leaves again at $t = 3$, the framework recognizes him/her as S_1 rather than S_4, which is consistent with his/her identity (state) recognized at $t = 1$ in his/her first exit.

It should be noted that in our framework a state could represent the feature model or the identity of a person. For clarity, we shall use $\mathbf{s}_i$ to denote a person's identity and S_i his/her feature model.

4.2 Framework Construction

From the problem formulation, it can be seen that the main task in constructing the proposed framework lies in the estimation of the time-variant parameter set $\Lambda(t)$. Once $\Lambda(t)$ is known, we can find the optimal path indicating the recognized people by a "turn-the-crank" procedure given by the Viterbi algorithm [28]. Our solutions are given as follows.

• **Initial state distribution, π:**

According to the definition of the state set $\mathbf{S}(t) = \{S_1 \cdots S_{N_t}\}$, there are N_1 states (people) in the database when the first observation of exit is obtained at $t = 1$. Without any other prior knowledge, we assume that everyone inside the room has an equal probability of leaving the room. Hence,

$$\pi_i = \frac{1}{N_1}, \ 1 \leq i \leq N_1. \tag{8}$$

• **Output probability of state i at time t, $b_i(O_t)$:**

In analogy with the definition in HMMs, let $b_i(O_t)$ be the probability of observation O_t generated by state i. We regard this probability as how likely an observed O_t is due to person $\mathbf{s}_i$, and simply approximate it by Eq. (7) using their feature similarity as

$$b_i(O_t) = P[O_t \sim S_i], \ 1 \leq i \leq N_t. \tag{9}$$

• **State transition probability, $a_{ij}(t)$:**

Before proceeding to the next step, we define a set of probabilities between observation times t and $t+1$ as shown in Fig. 6. For conciseness, we shall refer to "observation time" as "time" hereafter when there is no confusion. Let $P[\mathbf{s}_{i,t^{+/-}} = 1]$ be the probability of person $\mathbf{s}_i$ staying in the room at time instance $t^{+/-}$, where t^+ and t^- denote the times right after and before the observation O_t being made. (Straightforwardly, we have $P[\mathbf{s}_{i,t^{+/-}} = 0] = 1 - P[\mathbf{s}_{i,t^{+/-}} = 1]$). Let M be a likelihood matrix characterizing the similarities between people entering between times t and $t+1$ (i.e., $S_{N_t+1} \cdots S_{N_{t+1}}$) and the people staying in the room at time t (i.e., $S_1 \cdots S_{N_t}$), defined as

$$M = \{m_{uv} | m_{uv} = P[S_{N_t+v} \sim S_u]\}, \ 1 \leq u \leq N_t, 1 \leq v \leq N_t^{t+1}, \tag{10}$$

where N_t is the number of states (people who possibly stay in the room) at time t and $N_t^{t+1} = N_{t+1} - N_t$ is the number of people entering between times t and $t+1$. With these auxiliary probabilities, we can now derive the transition probability using the following three steps.

i) *Transition probability, $a_{ij}(t)$:*

The transition probability $a_{ij}(t)$ measures the odds that person $\mathbf{s}_i$ leaves the room at time t and person $\mathbf{s}_j$ leaves at time $t+1$ (i.e., $q_t = \mathbf{s}_i$ and $q_{t+1} = \mathbf{s}_j$). Lacking other knowledge, it is reasonable to assume that the probability for $\mathbf{s}_j$ to leave at time $t+1$ is proportional to his/her existence odds in the room at time $t+1^-$. Conceivably, a person cannot leave a room if he/she is not in the room at all. Hence, we compute the transition probability as

$$a_{ij}(t) = \frac{P[\mathbf{s}_{j,t+1^-} = 1 | q_t = \mathbf{s}_i]}{\sum_j P[\mathbf{s}_{j,t+1^-} = 1 | q_t = \mathbf{s}_i]}, \ 1 \leq i \leq N_t, 1 \leq j \leq N_{t+1}, \tag{11}$$

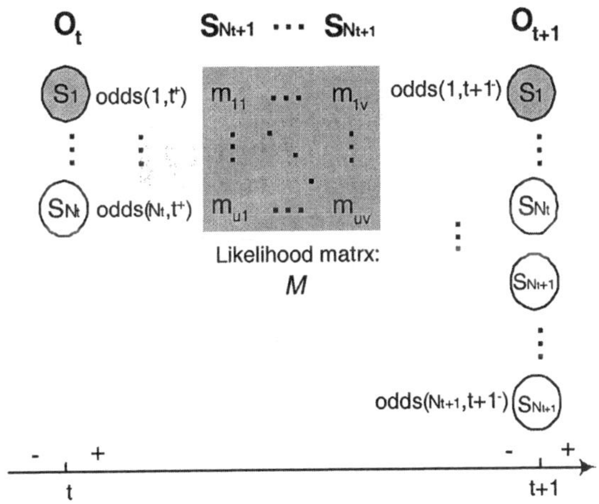

Fig. 6. The likelihood matrix M between times t and $t+1$ and the existence odds of a person associated with a certain state at times t^+ and $t+1^-$, where $odds(i,t^+) = P[\mathbf{s}_{i,t^+} = 1]$ and $odds(j,t+1^-) = P[\mathbf{s}_{j,t+1^-} = 1]$

where the denominator is a normalization factor so that $\sum_j a_{ij}(t) = 1$ for each i. The numerator in Eq. (11) can be further expanded for each particular state $\mathbf{s}_{\hat{i}}$ as

$$P[\mathbf{s}_{j,t+1^-} = 1|q_t = \mathbf{s}_{\hat{i}}] = \sum_{\text{all } cond} P[\mathbf{s}_{j,t+1^-} = 1|cond] \cdot P[cond|q_t = \mathbf{s}_{\hat{i}}], \quad (12)$$

where $cond = \{\mathbf{s}_{1,t^+} = \theta_1 \cdots \mathbf{s}_{N_t,t^+} = \theta_{N_t}\}$ is one of the possible realizations of $\{\mathbf{s}_{1,t^+} \cdots \mathbf{s}_{N_t,t^+}\}$ over all $\boldsymbol{\theta}$, and $\theta_i = 1$ *or* 0 designates that the *status* of person $\mathbf{s}_i$ is in or out of the room. By assuming that the status of each person is independent of the others, we can express the second term on the right hand side of Eq. (12) as

$$P[cond|q_t = \mathbf{s}_{\hat{i}}] = \prod_{i=1}^{N_t} P[\mathbf{s}_{i,t^+} = \theta_i|q_t = \mathbf{s}_{\hat{i}}]. \quad (13)$$

From Eqs. (11)–(13), we can see that the transition probability $a_{\hat{i}j}(t)$ depends on two probabilities: $P[\mathbf{s}_{j,t+1^-} = 1|cond]$ and $P[\mathbf{s}_{i,t^+} = \theta_i|q_t = \mathbf{s}_{\hat{i}}]$; the former is the conditional odds of person $\mathbf{s}_j$ existing in the room at time $t+1^-$ given the status of people observed up to time t^+, and the latter is the probability of person $\mathbf{s}_i$ assuming status θ_i at time t^+ given that person $\mathbf{s}_{\hat{i}}$ leaves the room at time t. These two probabilities can be calculated as follows.

ii) *Conditional probability*, $P[\mathbf{s}_{j,t+1^-} = 1|cond]$:

We compute this conditional probability with the aid of the likelihood matrix M defined in Eq. (10). The calculation is given by

$$P[\mathbf{s}_{j,t+1^-} = 1|cond] = \begin{cases} \theta_j + \sum_v \widetilde{m}_{jv} & 1 \le j \le N_t \\ 1 - \sum_u \widetilde{m}_{u(j-N_t)} & N_t \le j \le N_{t+1}, \end{cases} \tag{14}$$

where $\widetilde{m}_{uv}$ is the entry of a modified matrix $\widetilde{M}$ which is derived from M to indicate how likely person $\mathbf{s}_{N_t+v}$ is in fact person $\mathbf{s}_u$ re-entering the room under a given *cond*. We introduce matrix $\widetilde{M}$ in order to incorporate the domain knowledge in the context of the *cond*, making our estimation more accurate. In particular, the value $\sum_v \widetilde{m}_{jv}$ can be considered as the gain of the existence odds for person $\mathbf{s}_j$ due to newly entered people between times t and $t+1$. This gain, along with the existence odds of person $\mathbf{s}_j$ at time t^+, which is the binary value of θ_j, constitutes his/her existence odds at time $t+1^-$. For those newly added states $\mathbf{s}_j$, where $N_t \le j \le N_{t+1}$, the value $1 - \sum_u \widetilde{m}_{u(j-N_t)}$ can therefore be considered as the odds for person $\mathbf{s}_j$ being a new person. Note that in this framework we attempt to estimate these odds in an approximate manner, which has been found to be effective for improving the recognition rates.

Specifically, $\widetilde{m}_{uv}$ is derived from m_{uv} as

$$\widetilde{m}_{uv} = \eta^{2D}[\varepsilon(\theta_u)\rho(S_u)m_{uv}], \tag{15}$$

In (15), η^{2D} is a 2-D normalization operation which will be explained later;

$$\varepsilon(\theta_u) = \begin{cases} 0 & \text{if } \theta_u = 1 \text{ in } cond \\ 1 & \text{otherwise,} \end{cases} \tag{16}$$

and

$$\rho(S_u) = \begin{cases} 0 & \text{if } S_u \notin PT(S_k, t) \\ 1 & \text{otherwise,} \end{cases} \tag{17}$$

are two indication factors which incorporate the domain knowledge of a particular *cond*. Specifically, $\varepsilon(\theta_u)$ shows that it is impossible for one to enter a closed room if he/she is currently inside, while $\rho(S_u)$ accounts for the fact that an existing person could not enter the room again if he/she has not been observed leaving the room. S_k is the state for which the transition probability is to be calculated at time t and $PT(S_k, t)$ is the partial best state sequence ending in state S_k at time t, i.e., the highest probable state sequence that is retrieved by array ψ and includes all the people who have been observed leaving the room up to time t.

To illustrate the calculation in detail, we provide in the following a numerical example, in which five people enter and three leave a closed room, forming a process of three observations as shown in Fig. 7.

For time pair {t, t+1} shown in Fig. 7, suppose that the likelihood matrix obtained by Eq. (10) is equal to

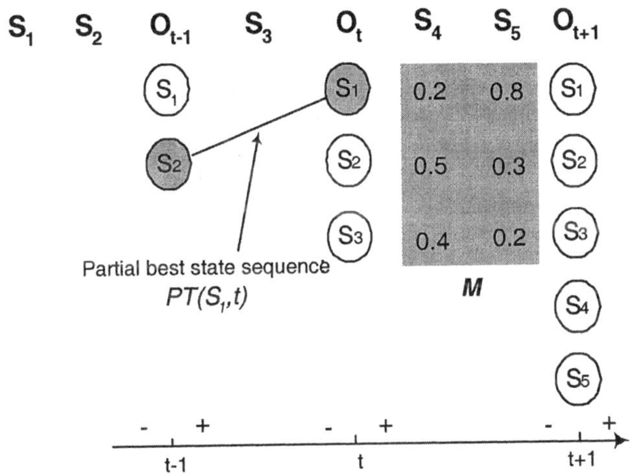

Fig. 7. Estimation of conditional probabitliy

$$M = \begin{array}{ccc} & s_4 & s_5 \\ s_1 & 0.2 & 0.8 \\ s_2 & 0.5 & 0.3 \\ s_3 & 0.4 & 0.2 \end{array}.$$

Consider one possible realization of people's status at time t^+: $cond^* = \{s_{1,t^+} = 0, s_{2,t^+} = 0, s_{3,t^+} = 1\}$; that is, $\{\theta_1 = 0, \theta_2 = 0, \theta_3 = 1\}$ and all people are outside the room at time t^+ except for person s_3. The conditional probabilities that need to be computed are $P[s_{j,t+1^-} = 1|cond^*], 1 \le j \le 5$.

First, we incorporate the knowledge of the people status into the likelihood matrix M by using the two indication factors. From Eq. (16), $\varepsilon(\theta_3) = 0$ and the third row of M will be set to zero. This is because if s_3 is known to be inside the room, then neither s_4 nor s_5 can be s_3 regardless of their similarities. The second indication factor relies on the partial best state sequence ending in the state for which the transition probability is to be calculated. Assume that S_1 at time t is the state and the partial best state sequence $PT(S_1, t)$ is as shown in Fig. 7. Since S_3 is not on this path, it means that person s_3 has not left the room since he/she entered. So none of s_4 and s_5 could be s_3 and $\rho(S_3) = 0$ according to Eq. (17). With this domain knowledge, the original likelihood matrix M can be modified as

$$M' = \begin{array}{ccc} & s_4 & s_5 \\ s_1 & 0.2 & 0.8 \\ s_2 & 0.5 & 0.3 \\ s_3 & 0 & 0 \end{array}.$$

In this example, the two indication factors affect the same row of the likelihood matrix M. In general, the adjustment could be made on different rows depending on the *cond* as well as the state chosen for evaluating the transition probability.

Next, the likelihood matrix M' is normalized so that the summations of the likelihoods corresponding to all possible circumstances are equal to one. To do this, we introduce a normalization operation, referred to as the correlated normalization operation and denoted as η, which works as follows. Consider a person $\mathcal{T}$ and a group of candidates $\boldsymbol{\mathcal{C}}$ consisting of N people, and define the similarity measure $w_n = P[\mathcal{C}_n \sim \mathcal{T}]$, $\mathcal{C}_n \in \boldsymbol{\mathcal{C}}$. Under the constraint that at most one person (or none) of $\boldsymbol{\mathcal{C}}$ could be $\mathcal{T}$, we can obtain the following new similarity measures

$$P[\mathcal{C}_n \sim \mathcal{T}|constr] \propto w_n \cdot \prod_{j \neq n}(1 - w_j), \; 1 \leq n \leq N, \tag{18}$$

$$P[\mathcal{T} \notin \boldsymbol{\mathcal{C}}|constr] \propto \prod_{i=1}^{N}(1 - w_i). \tag{19}$$

To make the probabilities corresponding to all possible circumstances sum up to one, the η operation is defined to normalize the new similarity measures as

$$\eta[w_n] = \frac{w_n \cdot \prod_{j \neq n}(1 - w_j)}{\sum_{i=1}^{N} w_i \prod_{j \neq i}(1 - w_j) + \prod_{i=1}^{N}(1 - w_i)}, 1 \leq n \leq N. \tag{20}$$

This normalization operation aims to correlate likelihoods that are measured independently by imposing the above-mentioned constraint. It should be noted that this constraint can be applied to the adjusted likelihood matrix M' both row-wise and column-wise. For instance, at most one of $\mathbf{s}_4$ and $\mathbf{s}_5$ (or none of them) could be $\mathbf{s}_1$, while $\mathbf{s}_4$ could be at most one of $\mathbf{s}_1$, $\mathbf{s}_2$ and $\mathbf{s}_3$ (or none of them, i.e., $\mathbf{s}_4$ is a new person) in the example shown in Fig. 7. For simplicity, we apply a 2-D η operation (η^{2D}), a row-wise normalization followed by a column-wise normalization, to normalize the likelihood matrix M' and obtain

$$\widetilde{M} = \begin{array}{ccc} & \mathbf{s}_4 & \mathbf{s}_5 \\ \mathbf{s}_1 & 0.05 & 0.72 \\ \mathbf{s}_2 & 0.40 & 0.05 \\ \mathbf{s}_3 & 0 & 0 \end{array}.$$

From this normalized likelihood matrix $\widetilde{M}$, we can obtain useful information such as the existence odds of $\mathbf{s}_1$ is increased by $0.05 + 0.72 = 0.77$, the odds that $\mathbf{s}_4$ is a new person is $1 - 0.05 - 0.40 - 0 = 0.55$, etc. Consequently, the existence odds at time $t+1^-$ under *cond** can be obtained using Eq. (14) as

$$P[\mathbf{s}_{1,t+1^-} = 1|cond^*] = 0 + 0.05 + 0.72 = 0.77$$
$$P[\mathbf{s}_{2,t+1^-} = 1|cond^*] = 0 + 0.40 + 0.05 = 0.45$$
$$P[\mathbf{s}_{3,t+1^-} = 1|cond^*] = 1 + 0 + 0 = 1$$
$$P[\mathbf{s}_{4,t+1^-} = 1|cond^*] = 1 - 0.05 - 0.40 - 0 = 0.55$$
$$P[\mathbf{s}_{5,t+1^-} = 1|cond^*] = 1 - 0.72 - 0.05 - 0 = 0.23$$

Applying the same procedure to all possible *cond*'s, we can obtain all the conditional probabilities $P[\mathbf{s}_{j,t+1^-} = 1|cond]$ needed in Eq. (12).

iii) *Probability* $P[\mathbf{s}_{i,t^+} = 1|q_t = \mathbf{s}_{\hat{i}}]$:

The remaining unknown for calculating the transition probability $a_{\hat{i}j}(t)$ is $P[\mathbf{s}_{i,t^+} = 1|q_t = \mathbf{s}_{\hat{i}}]$, which is the existence odds of person $\mathbf{s}_i$ at time t^+ given that the person leaving at time t is $\mathbf{s}_{\hat{i}}$. To illustrate how to compute this unknown, we shall extend the example of Fig. 7 to time $t+1$ and show instead how to compute $P[\mathbf{s}_{j,t+1^+} = 1|q_{t+1} = \mathbf{s}_{\hat{j}}]$ by making use of the probabilities obtained so far and assuming the full knowledge of $P[\mathbf{s}_{i,t^+} = 1|q_t = \mathbf{s}_{\hat{j}\_}]$, where $S_{\hat{j}\_}$ is the previous state of $S_{\hat{j}}$ in the partial best state sequence $PT(S_{\hat{j}}, t+1)$. By the same procedure, $P[\mathbf{s}_{i,t^+} = 1|q_t = \mathbf{s}_{\hat{i}}]$ can be similarly estimated based on $P[\mathbf{s}_{h,t-1^+} = 1|q_{t-1} = \mathbf{s}_{\hat{i}\_}]$. Note that, h, i, and j are indices of the states at times $t-1$, t and $t+1$, respectively.

As shown in Fig. 8, assume that person $\mathbf{s}_1$ leaves the room at times t and $t+1$, i.e., $\hat{j}_- = 1$ and $\hat{j} = 1$ (denoted by the shaded circles in Fig. 8). We indicate the values of $P[\mathbf{s}_{i,t^+} = 1|q_t = \mathbf{s}_1]$, which are assumed to be known, on the right hand side of the observation made at time t, and the computed values of $P[\mathbf{s}_{j,t+1^-} = 1|q_t = \mathbf{s}_1]$ on the left hand side of the observation made at time $t+1$. The estimation for the probabilities on the right hand side of observation O_{t+1} and the results are shown in Table 1.

We first examine the gain of existence odds for each person from time t^+ to $t+1^-$: $\gamma(j) = P[\mathbf{s}_{j,t+1^-} = 1|q_t = \mathbf{s}_1] - P[\mathbf{s}_{j,t^+} = 1|q_t = \mathbf{s}_1]$. Clearly, $\sum_j \gamma(j) = 2$ because the gain in existence odds is due to the two newly entered persons. However, if we know for sure that $\mathbf{s}_1$ leaves the room at time $t+1$, then he/she must be in the room at time $t+1^-$, and thus, $\gamma(1)$ should be equal to 1 rather than 0.77. In other words, the gain for each person needs to be re-adjusted ($\tilde{\gamma}$ in the table) to incorporate the knowledge of this new assumption to ensure that $\tilde{\gamma}(1) = 1$. That $\tilde{\gamma}(1)$ is equal to one can also be explained as follows: since $\mathbf{s}_1$ leaves at time t and time $t+1$ successively, one of the entered persons $\mathbf{s}_4$ and $\mathbf{s}_5$ must be $\mathbf{s}_1$. As there is no reason to favor any person other than $\mathbf{s}_1$, our approach is to increase $\mathbf{s}_1$'s existence odds from 0.77 to 1 and decrease the others' proportionally. This is sensible as once we know that the person who leaves the room at time $t+1$ is $\mathbf{s}_1$, then $\mathbf{s}_4$ and $\mathbf{s}_5$ should be more likely to be $\mathbf{s}_1$ than what we originally estimate, and consequently, less likely to be other people. At time $t+1^+$, the existence odds of $\mathbf{s}_1$ becomes zero due to his exit, and the others' can be obtained as the summation of their existence odds at time t^+ and the re-adjusted gain, i.e., $P[\mathbf{s}_{j,t^+} = 1|q_t = \mathbf{s}_1]$ and $\tilde{\gamma}(j)$.

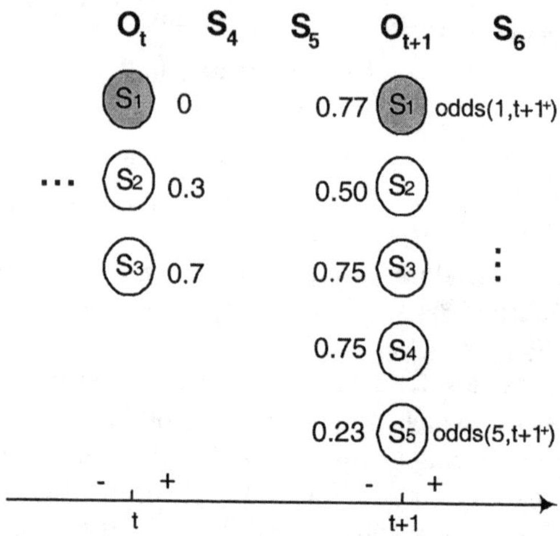

Fig. 8. Estimation of existence odds, where $odds(j, t+1^+) = P[\mathbf{s}_{j,t+1^+} = 1 | q_{t+1} = \mathbf{s}_1]$

Table 1. Estimation of the existence odds

	$P[\mathbf{s}_{j,t^+} = 1 \vert q_t = \mathbf{s}_1]$	$P[\mathbf{s}_{j,t+1^-} = 1 \vert q_t = \mathbf{s}_1]$	γ	$\widetilde{\gamma}$	$P[\mathbf{s}_{j,t+1^+} = 1 \vert q_{t+1} = \mathbf{s}_1]$
$\mathbf{s}_1$	0	0.77	0.77	1	0
$\mathbf{s}_2$	0.30	0.50	0.20	0.16	0.46
$\mathbf{s}_3$	0.70	0.75	0.05	0.04	0.74
$\mathbf{s}_4$	n.a.	0.75	0.75	0.61	0.61
$\mathbf{s}_5$	n.a.	0.23	0.23	0.19	0.19

The above analysis and calculation can be summarized into the general formulas below

$$P[S_{j,t+1^+} = 1 | q_{t+1} = S_{\hat{j}}] = \begin{cases} 0 & \text{if } j = \hat{j} \\ P[S_{j,t^+} = 1 | q_t = S_{\hat{j}\_}] + \widetilde{\gamma}(j) & \text{otherwise,} \end{cases} \quad (21)$$

$$\widetilde{\gamma}(j) = \begin{cases} 1 & \text{if } j = \hat{j} \\ \gamma(j)\left(1 - \frac{1 - P[S_{\hat{j},t+1^-} = 1 | q_t = S_{\hat{j}\_}]}{\sum_{j \neq \hat{j}} \gamma(j)}\right) & \text{otherwise,} \end{cases} \quad (22)$$

$$\gamma(j) = P[S_{j,t+1^-} = 1 | q_t = S_{\hat{j}\_}] - P[S_{j,t^+} = 1 | q_t = S_{\hat{j}\_}]. \quad (23)$$

It can be seen from these formulas that the estimation of existence odds is recursive; that is, one's existence odds at time $t+1^+$ depends on that at t^+. To initialize the estimation, we set $P[\mathbf{s}_{i,1^+} = 1 | q_1 = \mathbf{s}_{\hat{i}}] = 1$ for all $i \neq \hat{i}$ and $P[\mathbf{s}_{\hat{i},1^+} = 1 | q_1 = \mathbf{s}_{\hat{i}}] = 0$ if $\mathbf{s}_{\hat{i}}$ is the first person leaving the room (i.e. $q_1 = \mathbf{s}_{\hat{i}}$), since all the people who have entered the room, except for $\mathbf{s}_{\hat{i}}$, should be inside at time 1^+.

It should also be noted that although the above derivation may appear somewhat complex, it leads to an important underlying property of the proposed framework: the summation of the existence odds of all states at any time instance $t^{+/-}$ (i.e., $\sum_i P[\mathbf{s}_{i,t^{+/-}} = 1|q_t = \mathbf{s}_j])$ for any t and j is always equal to the number of people who really stay in the room at that time.

Batch recognition of observations (people who have left the room) can be performed at any time when necessary by retrieving the state sequence with the maximum score of joint posterior probability as the *best state sequence.*

To use the proposed framework for recognizing people re-entering the room is equivalent to finding and merging those states associated with a same person in the *best state sequence.* This can be accomplished by the following local maximum likelihood scheme. Let $q_t = S_i$ and search backward in the *best state sequence* for $q_{t'} = S_i$, where $t' \in \{1, \cdots, t-1\}$ and $t - t'$ is minimized. If such $q_{t'}$ exists, person $\mathbf{s}_{\widehat{j}}$ can be assumed as person $\mathbf{s}_i$ re-entering, where $\widehat{j}$ is obtained as

$$\widehat{j} = \arg\max_{j \in \mathbf{S}(t) \backslash \mathbf{S}(t')} P[S_j \sim S_i], \tag{24}$$

and $\mathbf{S}(t)$ is the state set at time t. Then, $S_{\widehat{j}}$ should be merged into S_i and removed from all the state sets containing it thereafter. The backward search is performed from $t = 2$ to the end of the *best state sequence* until all the states possibly representing a same person are identified and merged.

5 Experimental Results

To test the proposed people monitoring system, we have captured two videos in a research laboratory using a low-cost PC camera monitoring the lab's only entrance. During an one-hour monitoring period, video-I recorded eleven people who were unaware of the experiment, of which four entered and left twice, another four entered and left only once, and three entered without leaving. Video-II simulated the process of people entering and leaving with the help of eight students, among whom seven entered and left the lab for three times and another one for two times. In video-II, the volunteers were asked to approach the camera so that their faces could be recorded by the camera from a reasonable distance.

In our experiments described below, color histogram is tested on Video-I and Video-II while face is tested on Video-II and the face database of Olivetti Research (400 images of 40 individuals, 10 images per individual at the resolution of 92×112 pixels). A synthetic process generator is also designed to randomly re-arrange the entries and exits from the two videos and synthesize processes from the face database according to the rule that one cannot enter unless he/she is outside the lab, and vice versa. This generator allows us to simulate a large combinations of entries and exits over time from the same group of people.

For comparison, we also implement a recognition approach based on maximum likelihood (ML) classification [32, 33] as follows. When a person is detected entering a closed room, he/she is compared with people who are in the system's database and currently labeled as 'out'. If the maximum likelihood with respect to an 'out' person is larger than a threshold T_m, they are considered the same person. Then, the observed person is labeled as 'in' and his/her corresponding feature template in the database is updated with the latest one. Otherwise, the person is assumed to be new and then labeled as 'in' with a new identity label. When there are multiple exits without entries among them, the leaving people are recognized from the people with label 'in' by maximizing a joint likelihood.

We now use an example of the synthesized entry/exit process to illustrate the superiority of our approach against the maximum likelihood approach. The process is obtained based on the eight people ($P1$–$P8$) recorded in video-II as shown in Table 2, where 'I' and 'O' represent in (entry) and out (exit), respectively. A total of 44 entries and exits are observed, among them 22 are entering while the other 22 are exiting. Note that in this example we take color histogram as the low-level feature .

Table 2. A sequence of entries and exits obtained from the synthetic generator using the eight people observed in Video-II

Person	P6	P2	P6	P6	P1	P1	P3	P2	P1	P8	P2	P1	P7	P5	P3
In/Out	I	I	O	I	I	O	I	O	I	I	I	O	I	I	O
Person	P5	P1	P8	P7	P3	P5	P2	P6	P4	P6	P8	P5	P8	P7	P2
Cont'd	O	I	O	O	I	I	O	O	I	I	I	O	O	I	I
Person	P7	P2	P6	P5	P7	P4	P4	P4	P7	P1	P3	P8	P8	P5	
Cont'd	O	O	O	I	I	O	I	O	O	O	O	I	O	O	

Table 3. Comparison of the recognition results obtained by the maximum likelihood (ML) approach and our proposed approach

Obs. time	1	2	3	4	5	6	7	8	9	10	11
Ground truth	S_1	S_4	S_2	S_4	S_5	S_{10}	S_7	S_9	S_2	S_1	S_{10}
Proposed approach	S_1	S_4	S_2	S_4	S_5	S_{10}	S_7	S_9	S_2	S_1	S_{10}
ML approach	S_1	S_4	S_2	S_4	S_5	S_{10}	S_4	S_9	S_2	S_3	S_{10}
cont'd	12	13	14	15	16	17	18	19	20	21	22
Ground truth	S_7	S_9	S_2	S_1	S_{14}	S_{14}	S_9	S_4	S_5	S_7	S_{10}
Proposed approach	S_7	S_9	S_2	S_1	S_{14}	S_{14}	S_9	S_4	S_5	S_7	S_{10}
ML approach	S_7	S_{17}	S_2	S_3	S_{14}	S_{14}	S_{12}	S_{16}	S_9	S_7	S_{10}

The recognition results of the eight people (at observation time) are given in Table 3. The results obtained by our proposed approach and the ML approach are compared against the ground truth. In this particular example, our approach achieves 100% recognition rate, outperforming the ML approach. On the other hand, the ML approach wrongly recognizes $P8$ as $P1$ at time 7 and the other way around at time 19. Furthermore, $P7$ is incorrectly identified as $P3$ at time 18 and reversely at time 20. These recognition errors are mainly due to that the similarity measures between these different people exceed the preset threshold T_m. On the contrary, the errors at times 10, 13 and 15, where $P6$ and $P7$ are wrongly identified as new people when they are just re-entering, are due to that the similarities of their features observed at different times are lower than T_m. In other words, the ML approach is rather sensitive to the threshold T_m, inappropriate selection of which often results in false recognitions. In comparison, our proposed approach benefits from the threshold-free scheme; therefore, it is more robust to variations in feature extractions as well as changes in lighting conditions or view angles.

Recall that at each observation time there is a partial best state sequence ending in each individual state with the probability score of $\delta_t(i)$. To make a recognition decision at time t is thus to choose from all the partial best state sequence the one with the largest value of $\delta_t(i)$. Consequently, a confidence index can be defined in the range $[0, 1]$ to evaluate the reliability of a decision that is made at each time

$$Conf(t) = \frac{\max(\delta_t(i))}{\sum_i \delta_t(i)}. \tag{25}$$

Fig. 9 shows the variation of the confidence index over time for the above example.

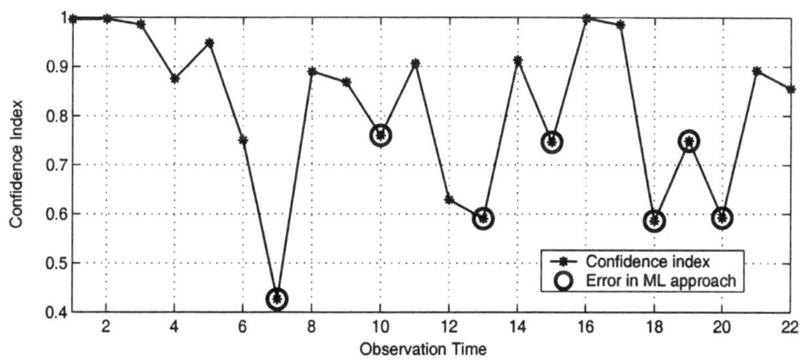

Fig. 9. The confidence index over observation time

In the early stage of monitoring, the system has only few choices for making decision (few people are observed); therefore, the confidence index is usually high. With the increase of the state number, i.e., more possible paths to choose from, the reliability of a decision may decrease. However, the advantage of our approach lies in that it is capable of maintaining the decision reliability at a later observation time by collectively considering all the available observations—a merit of the Viterbi algorithm as described in Sec. 2. In Fig. 9, when the confidence index is lower than 0.8, the ML approach is likely to make a wrong decision at the corresponding time (as indicated by the circles). Meanwhile, the proposed approach can still make the right choice since the probabilities (or scores) of the other paths are even lower.

It should be noted that the computational complexity of our framework increases rapidly when more states are generated. However, when the confidence index is sufficiently high, the total number of states can be reduced by making a definite decision to merge the states associated with the same person (e.g., at time 16 in Fig. 9). We consider this a promising topic for future investigation.

Table 4 summarizes the recognition performances of the experimental results, where 20 synthesized processes of entries and exits are generated for each test data set and for each feature type considered. It is evident from the table that our proposed approach can notably improve the recognition accuracies as compared with that of the ML approach.

Table 4. Recognition accuracies obtained by the maximum likelihood (ML) approach and our proposed approach for two types of low-level features

	Color histogram		Face feature	
Data	ML	Proposed	ML	Proposed
Video-I	83.3%	99.6%	—	—
Video-II	75.0%	97.5%	82.3%	98.5%
ORL Database	—	—	85.0%	100%

6 Conclusion

We have presented in this chapter a novel probabilistic reasoning framework for monitoring people in a closed room. Rather than identifying each single observation from a database, the framework is devised to recognize people based on multiple observations by exploiting the temporal correlations and constraints imposed by the application domain. In addition, the proposed framework permits its parameters to be estimated and updated at each observation instance by combing low-level features and domain-specific knowledge. Experimental results demonstrate that the proposed approach outperforms the existing maximum-likelihood approach when using the same features and being tested with the same test videos.

It should be noted that the proposed system can be readily extended to monitor multiple entrances or adjacent areas with the use of an array of cameras, all being interconnected and sharing the results obtained by each own analysis unit.

References

1. Sage, K., Young, S. (1999) Security applications of computer vision. IEEE Aerospace and Electronic Systems Magazine, **14**, 19-29
2. Foresti, G.L. (1999) Object recognition and tracking for remote video surveillance. IEEE Trans. Circuits and Systems for Video Technology, **9**, 1045-1062
3. http://research.microsoft.com/easyliving/
4. Open source computer vision library reference manual. Intel Corporation
5. Viola, P., Jones, M. (2001) Robust real-time object detection. Technical Report, Compaq CRL
6. Lienhart, R., Maydt, J. (2002) An extended set of Haar-like features for rapid object detection. Proc. IEEE International Conf. on Image Processing (ICIP 2002), **1**, 900-903
7. Nefian, A.V., Hayes III, M.H. (1999) An embedded HMM based approach for face detection and recognition. Proc. IEEE International Conf. on Acoustics, Speech, and Signal Processing (ICASSP 1999), **6**, 3553-3556
8. Oliver, N.M., Rosario, B., Pentland, A.P. (2000) A Bayesian computer vision system for modeling human interactions. IEEE Trans. Pattern Analysis and Machine Intelligence, **22**, 831-843
9. Haritaoglu, I., Harwood, D., Davis, L.S. (2000) W^4: Real time surveillance of people and their activities. IEEE Trans. Pattern Analysis and Machine Intelligence, **22**, 809-830
10. CDC SARS Investigative Team, Fleischauer, A.T. (2003) Outbreak of Severe Acute Respiratory Syndrome – Worldwide. Morbidity and Mortality Weekly Report, **52**, 269-272
11. Shen, W., Surette, M., Khanna, R. (1997) Evaluation of automated biometrics-based identification and verification systems. Proc. IEEE, **85**, 1464-1478
12. Chellappa, R., Wilson, C.L., Sirohey, S. (1995) Human and machine recognition of faces: a survey. Proc. IEEE, **83**, 705-741
13. Kale, A., Rajagopalan, A., Cuntoor, N., Kruger, V. (2002) Gait-based recognition of humans using continuous HMMs. Proc. of the IEEE International Conf. on Automatic Face and Gesture Recognition, 321-326
14. Bhanu, B., Han, J. (2002) Bayesian-based performance prediction for gait recognition. Workshop on Motion and Video Computing, 145–150
15. Duda, R., Hart, P., Stork, D. (2001) Pattern classification, second edition. Wiley-Interscience
16. Vega, I.R., Sarkar, S. (2003) Statistical motion model based on the change of feature relationships: human gait-based recognition. IEEE Trans. Pattern Analysis and Machine Intelligence, **25**, 1323-1328
17. Lu, W., Tan, Y.-P. (2001) A color histogram based people tracking system. Proc. IEEE International Symposium on Circuits and Systems (ISCAS 2001), **2**, 137-140

18. Tao, J., Tan, Y.-P. (2003) Color appearance-based approach to robust tracking and recognition of multiple people. the Fourth International Conference on Information, Communications & Signal Processing and Fourth Pacific-Rim Conference on Multimedia, **1**, 95-99
19. Swain, M., Ballard, D. (1991) Color Indexing. Intl. Journal of Computer Vision, **7**, 11-22
20. Deng, Y., Manjunath, B.S., Kenney, C., Moore, M.S., Shin, H. (2001) An efficient color representation for image retrieval. IEEE Trans. Image Processing, **10**, 140-147
21. Ferman, A.M., Tekalp, A.M., Mehrotra, R. (2002) Robust color histogram descriptors for video segment retrieval and identification. IEEE Trans. Image Processing, **11**, 497-508
22. Moreno, F., Tarrida, A., Andrade-Cetto, J., Sanfeliu, A. (2002) 3D real-time head tracking using color histograms and stereovision. Proc. 16th International Conference on Pattern Recognition, 368-371
23. Kalman, B.L., Kwasny, S.C., (1992) Why tanh: choosing a sigmoidal function., Proc. International Joint Conference on Neural Networks, **4**, 7-11
24. Yang, J., Xu, Y., Chen, S.C. (1997) Human action learning via hidden Markov model. IEEE Trans. Systems, Man, and Cybernetics, **27**, 34-44
25. Starner, T.E., Pentland, A.P. (1995) Visual recognition of American sign language using hidden Markov models. Proc. International Workshop on Automatic Face- and Gesture-Recognition, 189-194
26. Nair, V., Clark, J.J. (2002) Automated visual surveillance using hidden Markov models. Proc. the 15th Vision Interface Conference, 88-92
27. Rabiner, L.R. (1989) A tutorial on hidden Markov models and selected applications in speech recognition. Proc. IEEE, **77**, 257-285
28. Church, K. (1992) Comments on Computational Learning Model for Metrical Phonology. R. Levine, (ed.), Formal Grammar: Theory and Implementation, Vancouver Studies in Cognitive Science Series, UBC Press, **2**
29. Forney, G.D. (1973) The Viterbi algorithm. Proc. IEEE, **61**, 268-278
30. Heckerman, D. (1995) A tutorial on learning with Bayesian networks, Microsoft Research. Technical Report
31. Murphy, K. (1998) A brief introduction to graphical models and Bayesian networks. available at http://www.ai.mit.edu/~murphyk/Bayes/bnintro.html
32. Siskind, J.M., Morris, Q. (1996) A maximum-likelihood approach to visual event classification. Proc. the 4th European Conference on Computer Vision, 347-360
33. McKenna, S.J., Jabri, S., Duric, Z., Rosenfeld, A., Wechsler, H. (2000) Tracking groups of people. Computer Vision and Image Understanding, **80**, 42-56

Human-Machine Communication by Audio-Visual Integration

Satoshi Nakamura, Tatsuo Yotsukura[1] and Shigeo Morishima[12]

[1] ATR Spoken Language Translation Research Labs.
2-2-2, "Keihanna-science city", Kyoto 619-0288 Japan
satoshi.nakamura@atr.jp, tatsuo.yotsukura@atr.jp

[2] Department of Applied Physics School of Science and Engineering, Waseda University
3-4-1 Okubo Shinjuku Tokyo 169-8555 Japan shigeo@waseda.jp

Abstract The use of audio-visual information is inevitable in human communication. Complementary usage of audio-visual information enables more accurate, robust, natural, and friendly human communication in real environments. These types of information are also required for computers to realize natural and friendly interfaces, which are currently unreliable and unfriendly.

In this chapter, we focus on synchronous multi-modalities, specifically audio information of speech and image information of a face for audio-visual speech recognition, synthesis and translation. Human audio speech and visual speech information both originate from movements of the speech organs triggered by motor commands from the brain. Accordingly, such speech signals represent the information of an utterance in different ways. Therefore, these audio and visual speech modalities have strong correlations and complementary relationships. There is indeed a very strong demand to improve current speech recognition performance. The performance in real environments drastically degrades when speech is exposed to acoustic noise, reverberation and speaking style differences. The integration of audio and visual information is expected to make the system robust and reliable and improve the performance. On the other hand, there is also a demand to improve speech synthesis intelligibility as well. The multi-modal speech synthesis of audio speech and lip-synchronized talking face images can improve intelligibility and naturalness. This chapter first describes audio-visual speech detection and recognition which aim to improve the robustness of speech recognition performance in actual noisy environments in Section 1. Second, a talking face synthesis system based on a 3-D mesh model and an audio-visual speech translation system are introduced. The audio-visual speech translation system recognizes input speech in an original language, translates it into a target language and synthesizes output speech in a target language in Section 2.

Keywords: speech recognition, voice detection, lip-reading, audio-visual speech recognition, speech translation, audio-visual speech translation, talking head, lip-synchronization, face model

1 Audio-Visual Speech Detection and Recognition

It is well known that speech recognition performance seriously degrades in acoustically noisy environments. Audio-visual ASR [1, 2, 3] systems offer the possibility of improving conventional speech recognition performance by incorporating visual information, since the speech recognition performance always degrades in acoustically noisy environments whereas visual information does not [1].

First, detection of the target speaker's speech is very important for maintaining speech recognition performance. However, this is very difficult especially in the noisy environments. Thus, a "push-to-talk" scenario is sometime used for this situation. On the other hand, a perceptual study has suggested that human beings are also sensitive to visual mouth movement information for communication [1]. This section describes how to automatically extract audio and visual information and integrate them in an efficient way.

Second, audio and visual phonetic features are correlated with each other while uttering speech, since they are produced by the same speech organ. However, the durations of the events in each modality are usually different by nature. In other words, there is loose synchronicity between them. For instance, a speaker opens his or her mouth before making an utterance, and closes it after making the utterance. Furthermore, the time lag between the movement of the mouth and the voice might be dependent on the speaker or context.

In this section, audio-visual speech detection and audio-visual speech recognition are described in subsection 1.1 and subsection 1.2, respectively.

1.1 Audio-Visual Speech Detection

A "push-to-talk" scenario is often used for recognizing speech in noisy environments, since it can easily indicate the speech section. However, the "push-to-talk" scenario should be replaced by robust automatic speech section detection for better human-machine interface. Our research aims to improve the usability and performance of real-time speech recognition systems by extracting and fusing information from audio and video modalities, i.e., *face-to-talk*, which consists of a facial orientation based switch and audio-visual speech section detection (Fig.1).

For visual information, the most important thing is to find speech-related face features, such as facial orientation, and speech-related motions proposed in [4, 5]. We have also proposed a face detection method [6], where both color and spatial features are used to reduce the candidates to be searched, and then spatial feature template matching is applied for accurate and automatic face detection. The face orientation is also detected by spatial features. We limit the problem to finding the location and scale of only one frontal face within each frame of the image sequence. The algorithm finds a location (x, y) and a scale (scale) that maximize the frontal face function F(x, y; scale) in the following.

[Step1] The candidates for the face are pruned by color.
[Step2] A spatial filter is applied to reduce lighting differences and emphasize the horizontal component.
[Step3] The (x, y; scale) is estimated for the candidates selected in step 1 to maximize the F(x, y; scale) by template matching for the filtered input image.

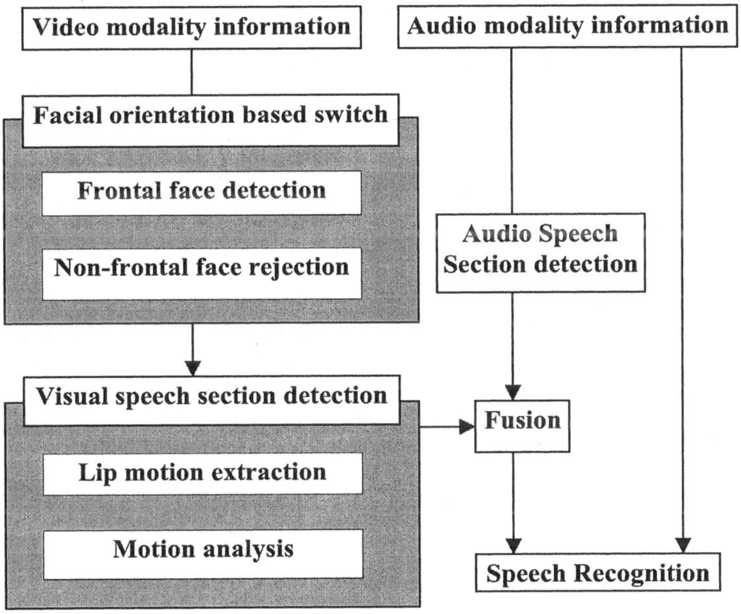

Fig. 1. Procedure Overview

[Step4] The face orientation is calculated to reject non-frontal faces by matching them with the oriented face templates.

We calculate a scale by the distance between the center of the irises in the image (in pixels) and a location (x, y) by the midpoint of the irises in the facial layout mask in Fig.2.

Detecting the cross section of the lips

The speaker's frontal face can be detected by locating the two irises. To detect speech, the time history of a cross-section image of the lips is used. To enhance robustness against the facial yaw, a one-pixel line image on the perpendicular bisector of the two irises is extracted as the cross section. The mouth opening and closing information can be detected by taking a look at this cross section line image which always spans the mouth region. We recorded a one-pixel line image along the cross section per frame. We call this image a "Liprogram". Furthermore, to reduce shift variance in the image caused by eye blinks and detection errors, this cross-section image is shifted up to +/-25 pixels upward and downward along the perpendicular bisector to minimize the difference between subsequent frames. This cross-section image is recorded as L,a,b(f, i), where f is the number of frames and i is the vertical pixel location along the line. Figure 3 shows a 5.5s Liprogram example. Although there are shifts of the face caused by the speaker's motion and eyes, the detected Liprogram is practically unaffected.

Visual speech detection

As seen in Fig.3, it should be easy to detect speech motion. To do this, we define inter-frame energy $E(f)$: where $L_{f,j}, a_{f,i}, b_{f,j}$, are $L*, a*, b*$ values of frame f, vertical position i respectively.

$$E(f) = \sum_i \{(L_{f,i} - L_{f-1,i})^2 + (a_{f,i} - a_{f-1,i})^2 + (b_{f,i} - b_{f-1,i})^2\}^{\frac{1}{2}} \quad (1)$$

Figure 4 shows $E(f)$ of the cross-section record seen in Fig.3. Because $Lab(f,i)$ is recorded to minimize the color difference, $E(f)$ reflects the transformation of the image. It is clear that the value of $E(f)$ is higher during speech. Although it seems quite easy to detect speech from $E(f)$ with a previously determined threshold, there are also non-speech motions as described in the previous section that give a higher $E(f)$ value. To identify the speech, we must therefore evaluate the duration of the motion, which can clearly distinguish speech from non-speech motions, as seen in Fig.4. We carried out experiments using 520 Japanese isolated words. In the experiments the speech section is detected if the detected section exceeds one second.

Audio speech detection and fusion

As described earlier, a visually detected section is longer than an audio detected section. To reduce the excess length, which may cause insertion errors, audio modality speech detection is applied to the visually detected section. We apply a power-based speech section detection algorithm ATR-EPD (ATR-EPD: speech detection module of ATR SPREC [7].

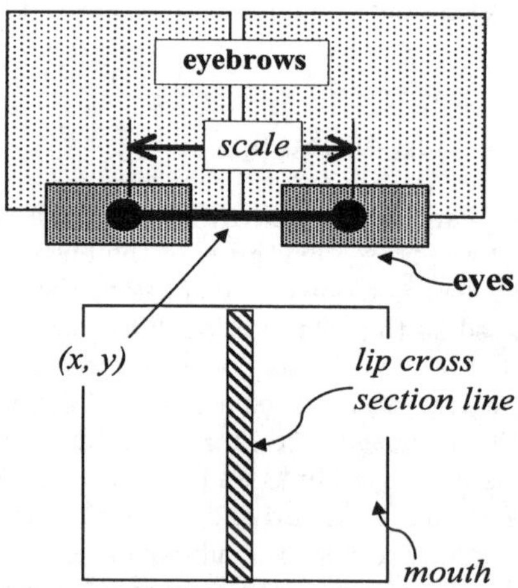

Fig. 2. Layout Mask

Because the objective of applying audio modality speech detection is to truncate the excess section, we simply evaluate the intersection of the speech sections of two modalities.

Two Japanese native-speaking males utter 56 sentences sitting on a fixed chair in a soundproof room and facing a camera. The domain is travel related. Incandescent light powered by 60-Hz AC illuminates the examinee. The speech of the subjects was recorded by an NTSC digital video camera (720 x 480 pixels, 29.97 fps, fixed on a stable tripod) and a close-talk microphone (48 kHz 16-bit sampling).

To compare the speech section detection performance of the proposed method with that of conventional methods, the word accuracy and insertion count are evaluated. The proposed method and conventional (audio or video single modality) methods are applied to the test data. Table 1 shows word accuracy and Table 2 shows the insertion count. These results confirmed that the proposed method outperforms single modality methods in all cases.

Table 1. Word accuracy (%) of each method

Word acc.	Proposed method	Audio only	Video only
Clean	92.3	90.4	86.2
SNR10dB	70.2	66.8	52.6

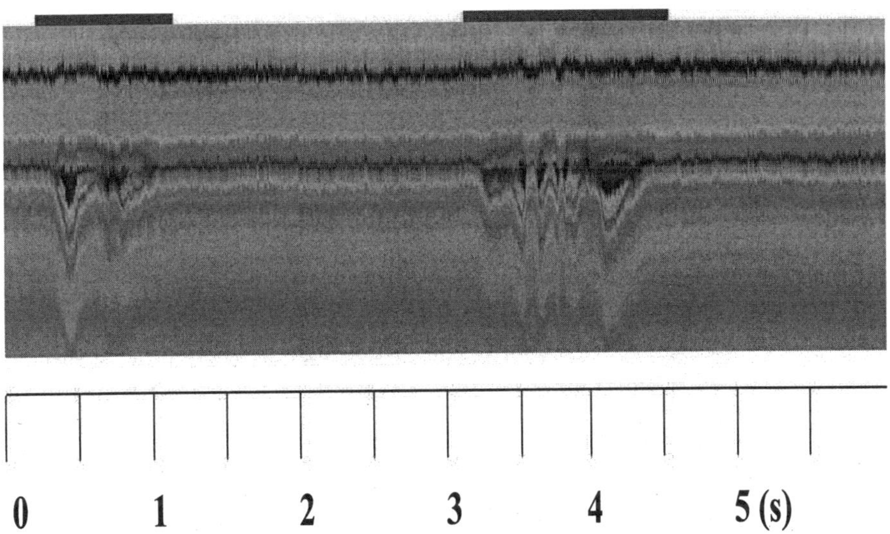

Fig. 3. Liprogram(Time sequence of lip cross section)

Table 2. Word insertion count of each method

Insertions	Proposed method	Audio only	Video only
Clean	41	71	91
SNR10dB	126	190	273

1.2 Audio-Visual Speech Recognition Based on Asynchronicity Modeling

Recently, the demand for Audio-visual Speech Recognition (AVSR) has increased in order to make speech recognition systems robust to acoustic noise. There are two kinds of research issues in audio-visual speech recognition, i.e., modeling of different modalities considering asynchronicity, and adaptive information weighting on the modalities according to information reliability. This paper describes our attempts to effectively integrate audio and visual information for robust speech recognition [8, 9, 10].

Figure 5 shows an overview of the audio-visual speech recognition procedure. Figure 6 shows the proposed HMM topology. First, in order to create the audio and visual phoneme HMMs independently, audio features and visual features are extracted from audio data and visual data, respectively. Then the audio and visual features are modeled individually by two HMMs using the EM algorithm. Finally, an audio-visual phoneme HMM is composed as the product of these two HMMs based on HMM composition. The output probability at state ij of the audio-visual HMM is,

$$b_{ij}(O_t) = b_i^A(O_t^A)^{\alpha_A} \times b_j^V(O_t^V)^{\alpha_V} \tag{2}$$

Here, $b_i^A(O_t^A)^{\alpha_A}$ is the output probability of the audio feature vector at time instance t in state i, $b_j^V(O_t^V)^{\alpha_V}$ is the output probability of the visual feature vector at time

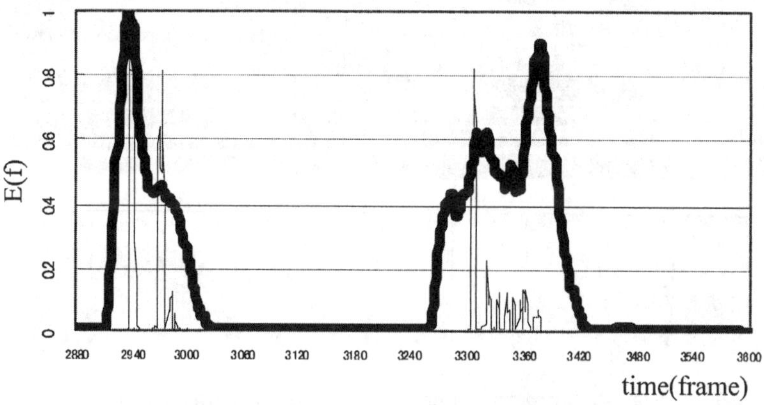

Fig. 4. Audio power and interframe energy

instance t in state j, and α_A and α_V are the audio stream weight and visual stream weight, respectively. We set $\alpha_A + \alpha_V = 1$ in this paper. In evaluation experiments performance is investigated by only changing α_A. In a similar manner, the transition probability from state ij to state kl in the audio-visual HMM is defined as follows,

$$p_{ij,kl} = p_{a_{i,k}} \times p_{v_{j,l}} \tag{3}$$

where $p_{a_{i,k}}$ is the transition probability from state i to state k in the audio HMM, and $p_{v_{j,l}}$ is the transition probability from state j to state l in the visual HMM. This composition is performed for all phonemes. In the method proposed by [3], a similar composition is used for the audio and visual HMMs. However, because the audio and visual HMMs are trained individually, the dependencies between the audio and visual features are ignored.

Loose Synchronicity Modeling

The first problem is the inability of the conventional product HMMs to represent loose state synchronicity within a phoneme. This problem is caused by the independence assumption of two HMMs. We propose new product HMMs whose parameters are re-estimated using audio-visual synchronous adaptation data [8, 9]. The re-estimation is able to introduce the loose state synchronicity of the states of two modalities into the product HMM. Figure 7 shows results comparing audio HMMs, visual HMMs, early integration, late integration, and product HMMs with and without re-estimation [9] with regard to audio stream weights in equation 2.

The second problem is that the conventional product HMMs force a strict synchronization on every phoneme boundary. This is because the speech organs normally move earlier than the speech to be produced. Sometimes, the speech organs are already articulated in the previous audio phoneme utterance. Accordingly, we

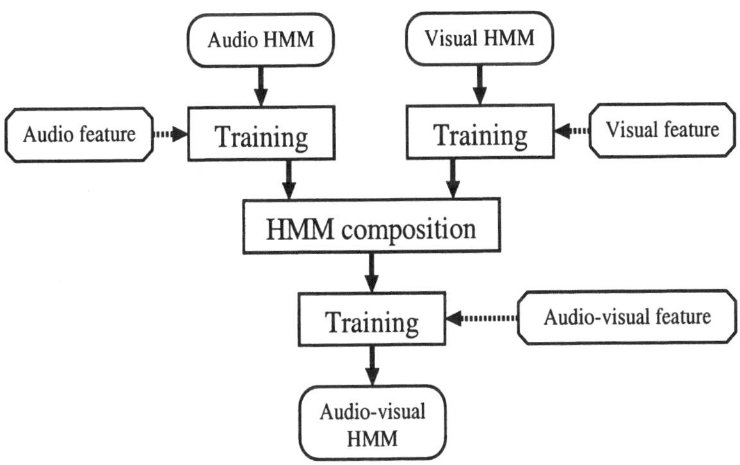

Fig. 5. Procedure Overview

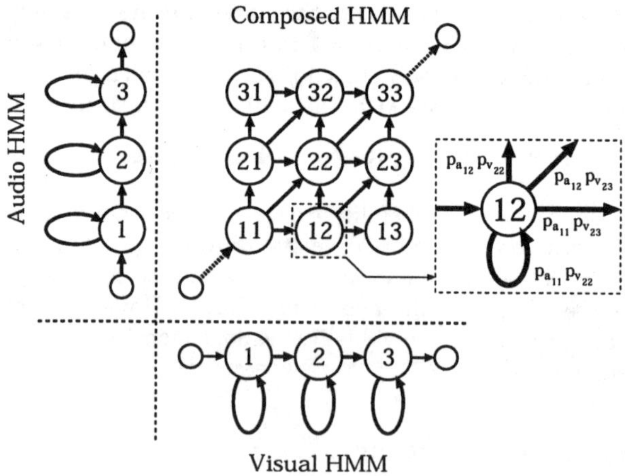

Fig. 6. Product HMM

have to consider state synchronous modeling beyond the phoneme boundary. We propose new product HMMs that include extra asynchronous states on phoneme boundaries as indicated in Fig. 8. The core states of the phoneme HMMs are the same as those of context independent phoneme product HMMs. In addition, the new product HMMs have two extra HMM states that aim to work in a manner that is similar to the word HMMs. Since these extra states are dependent on the preceding phoneme, they can only be re-estimated in a manner similar to the bi-

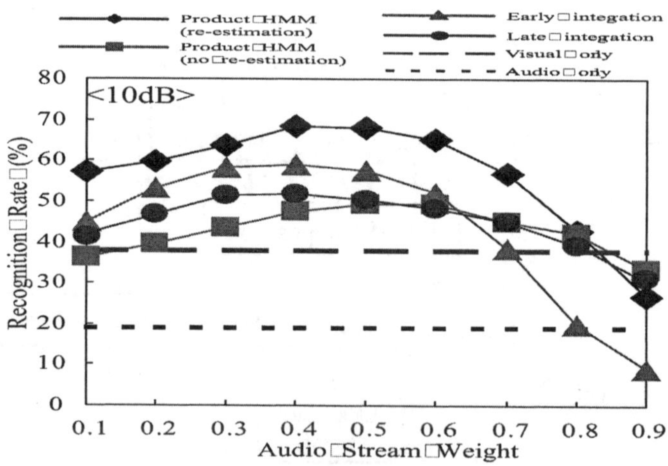

Fig. 7. Results of Product HMMs

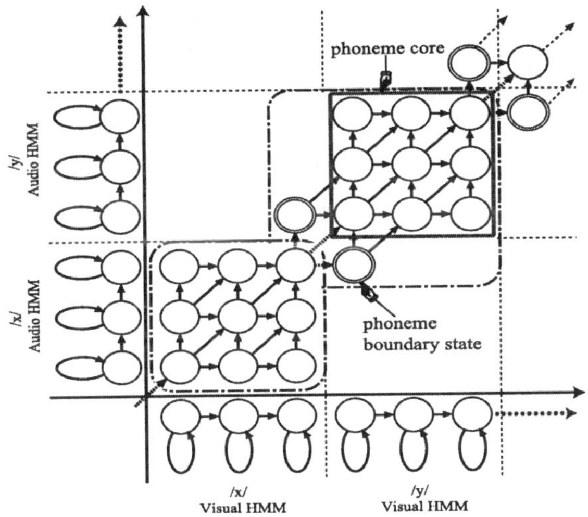

Fig. 8. Pseudo-biphone product HMMs

phone HMMs. Therefore, we call them HMM pseudo-biphone product HMMs. The proposed HMMs can tolerate one state asynchronicity beyond a phoneme boundary.

Evaluation Experiments

The audio signal is sampled at 12 kHz (down-sampled) and analyzed with a frame length of 32 msec every 8 msec. The audio features are 16-dimensional MFCC(Mel Frequency Cepstral Coefficient) and 16-dimensional delta MFCC. On the other hand, the visual image signal is sampled at 30 Hz with 256 gray scale levels from RGB. Then, the image level and location are normalized by a histogram and template matching. Next, the normalized images are analyzed by two-dimensional FFT to extract 6x6 log power 2-D spectra for audio-visual ASR. Finally, 35-dimensional 2D log power spectra and their delta features are extracted. These two parameters are used to build audio-HMMs and visual-HMMs. We use 4,740 words for HMM training and two sets of 500 words for testing. These 500 words are different from the words used in the training. The context of the data for the adaptation differs from that of the test data. The GPD(Generalized Probabilistic Decent) algorithm is used to estimate the weight using 25 words for each modality [10].

We compared the processed product HMMs without re-estimation (Product-HMM(W/O Re-est.)), the proposed product HMMs with re-estimation (Product-HMM(W Re-est.)), the proposed pseudo-biphone product HMMs without re-estimation (Pseudo-Biphone(W/O Re-nest.)), the proposed pseudo-biphone product HMMs with re-estimation (Pseudo-Biphone(W Re-est.)), and GMM for GPD-based stream weight optimization for acoustic SNR=15, 0, and -5dB. White noise was used to reduce the acoustic SNR in this experiment. The audio HMMs were trained using the SNR=15dB data. The results indicate that the re-estimation of the product HMMs is quite effective for improving performance. The re-estimation is able to

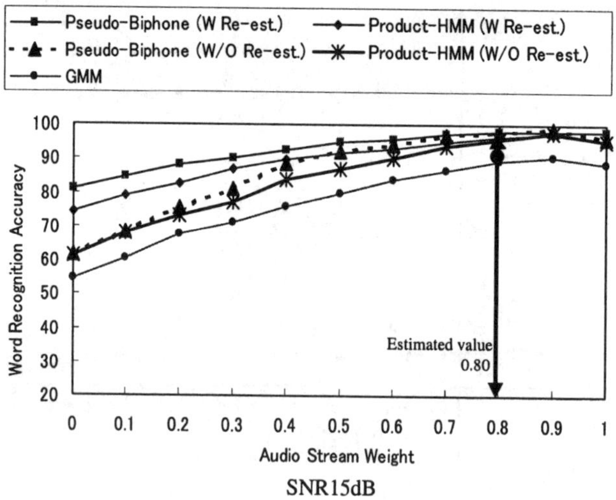

Fig. 9. Word Accuracy (SNR=15dB)

introduce the loose state synchronicity of the states of two modalities into the product HMMs. The state synchronous modeling beyond the phoneme boundary by a pseudo-biphone product HMM also results in significant improvements to the product HMMs. It is confirmed that the re-estimation further improves the performance of pseudo-biphone product HMMs. The figures show that optimal stream weights for the maximum performance vary according to each method and acoustic SNR. The solid arrows show the results by simplified GPD-based stream weight estimation using 25 adaptation words [10]. The proposed GPD-based simplified stream weight optimization algorithm successfully estimated stream weight with almost the best performance.

2 Multi-modal Speech Translation

A speech translation system has been investigated to realize natural human communication beyond language barriers. Toward more natural audio-visual communication, visual information such as face and lip movements will be necessary. The system has been studied mainly for verbal information. However, both verbal and nonverbal information is indispensable for natural human communication. In particular, lip movements transmit speech information with audio speech. For example, stand-in speech in movies has the problem that it does not match the lip movements. Face movements are also necessary to transmit nonverbal information of the speaker. If we could develop a technology that could translate facial speaking motion synchronized to the translated speech, a natural multilingual audio-visual speech translation could be realized. There have been some studies [11, 12] on facial image generation

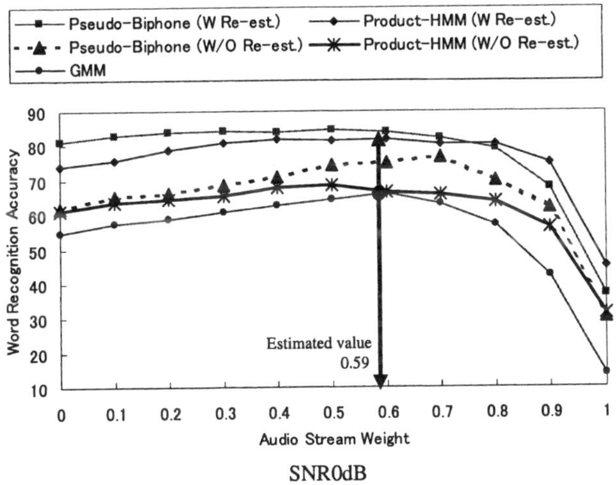

Fig. 10. Word Accuracy (SNR=0dB)

to transform lip-shape based on concatenating variable units from a large database. However, since images generally contain much more information than sounds, it is difficult to prepare large image databases. Thus, conventional systems need to limit the number of speakers.

In this section, we propose a method to generate a 3D personal face model with an actual personal face shape, and to track face motion-like movement and rotation automatically in a video sequence for audio-visual speech translation. We also describe a spoken language translation system which is based on a speech-to-speech translation system developed by ATR [13]. Finally we will show the subjective evaluation result by connected-digit discrimination using data with and without audio-visual lip-synchronization (lip-sync).

2.1 System Overview

Figure 12 shows an overview of the audio-visual translation system. The system is divided broadly into two parts. One is the *Speech-Translation Part* and the other is the *Image-Translation Part*. The Speech-Translation Part is composed of ATR-MATRIX (ATR's Multi-lingual Automatic Translation System for Information Exchange) [13]. ATR-MATRIX is composed of ATR-SPREC to execute speech recognition, TDMT to handle text-to-text translation [17], and CHATR [14, 15] to generate synthesized speech. The two parameters of phoneme notation and duration information, which are outputs from CHATR, are used for the facial image translation. The first step of the image-translation part is to make a 3D object of the mouth region for each speaker by fitting a standard facial wire-frame model to an input frontal face image. Because of the differences in facial bone structures, it is necessary to prepare

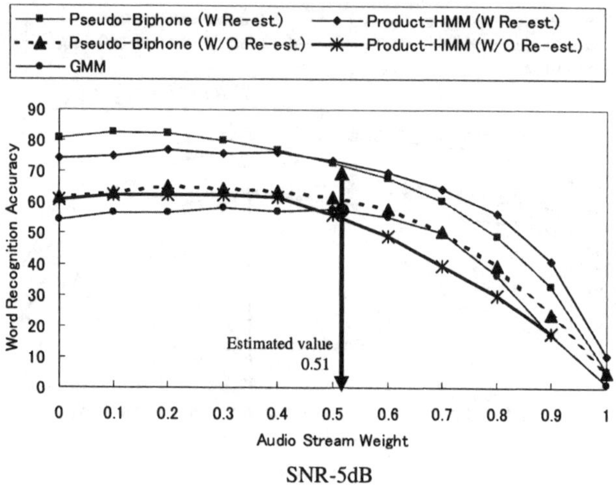

Fig. 11. Word Accuracy (SNR=-5dB)

a personal model for each speaker, but this process is required only once for each speaker, manually. Next, we track the face in the video sequence to create a personal face object preserving natural head movements using an automatic face-tracking algorithm. The third step of the Image-Translation Part is to generate lip movements for the corresponding utterance. The 3D object is transformed by controlling the acquired lip-shape parameters so that they correspond to the phoneme notations from the database used at the speech synthesis stage. Duration information is also applied and interpolated by linear interpolation for smooth lip movement. Here, the lip-shape parameters are defined by a momentum vector derived from the natural face at the nodes of a polygon on a wire-frame for each phoneme. Therefore, this database does not need speaker adaptation. In the final step, the translated synthetic mouth region's 3D object is embedded into an input video sequence. In this step, the 3D object's color and scale are adjusted to the input images. Even if an input video sequence is moving during an utterance, we can acquire natural synthetic images because the 3D object has geometry information. Consequently, the system outputs a lip-synchronized face movie to the translated synthetic speech and image sequence at 30 frames/sec.

2.2 Speech Translation System

This system is based on a speech-to-speech translation system developed at ATR [13]. This system is called ATR-MATRIX. The system consists of speech recognition, language translation, and speech synthesis modules. The speech recognition module is able to recognize naturally spoken utterances in the source language. The language translation module is able to translate the recognized utterances to sentences of

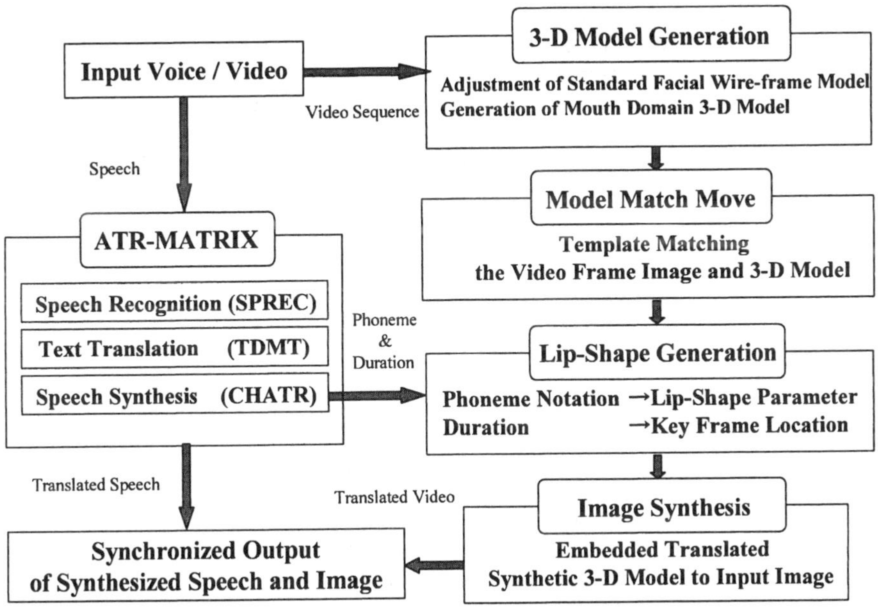

Fig. 12. Overview of the audio-visual translation system

the target language. Finally the text-to-speech synthesis module synthesizes the translated sentences. In the following subsection, each of the modules is described.

Speech Recognition System

The long research history and continuous efforts of data collection at ATR have made a statistical model-based speech recognition module possible. The module is speaker-independent and able to recognize naturally spoken utterances. In particular, the system drives multiple acoustic models in parallel in order to handle differences in gender and speaking styles. Speech recognition is achieved by the maximum a posterior (MAP) decoder, which maximizes the probability using the two parameters: *acoustic model probability* and *language model probability*. We devised a method called Hmnet (Hidden Markov Net-work), which is a data-driven automatic state network generation algorithm. This algorithm iteratively increases the state network by splitting one state into two states by considering the phonetic contexts so as to increase likelihood [16].

For the language model, a statistical approach called the *N-gram language model* is also widely used. The length of N should be determined by considering the trade-off between the number of parameters and the amount of training data. Once we get a text corpus, the N-gram language model can be easily estimated. For the word triplets that infrequently occur probability smoothing is applied. In our system, a word-class-based N-gram model is used.

Finally, the speech recognition system searches for the optimal word sequence using the acoustic models and the language models. The search is a time-synchronous two-pass search after converting the word vocabulary into a tree lexicon. The multiple acoustic models can be used in the search but get pruned by considering likelihoods. The performance of speaker-independent recognition in the travel arrangement domain was evaluated. The word error rates for face-to-face dialog speech, bilingual speech, and machine-friendly speech are 13.4%, 10.1% and 5.2%.

Speech Synthesis System

The speech synthesis system generates natural speech from the translated texts. The system developed at ATR is called *CHATR* [14, 15]. The CHATR synthesis relies on the fact that a speech segment can be uniquely described by the joint specification of its phonemic and prosodic environmental characteristics. The synthesizer performs a retrieval function, first predicting the information that is needed to complete a specification from an arbitrary level of input and then indicating the database segments that best match the predicted target specifications. The basic requirement for input is a sequence of phone labels, with associated fundamental frequency, amplitudes, and durations for each. If only words are specified in the input, then their component phones will be generated from a lexicon or by rule; if no prosodic specification is given, then a default intonation will be predicted from the information available.

Language Translation System

The translation subsystem uses an example-based approach to handle spoken-language [17]. Spoken-language translation faces problems different from those of written-language translation. The main requirements are 1) techniques for handling ungrammatical expressions, 2) a means for processing contextual expressions, 3) robust methods for speech recognition errors, and 4) real-time speed for smooth communication.

The backbone of ATR's approach is the translation model called TDMT (Transfer-Driven Machine Translation) [18], which was developed within an example-based paradigm. TDMT's Constituent Boundary parsing [19] provides efficiency and robustness. We have also explored the processing of contextual phenomena and a method for dealing with recognition errors and have made much progress in these explorations.

2.3 Image Translation System

Personal Face Modeling

It is necessary to create an accurate face object that has the target person's features for the face recreation by computer graphics. Furthermore, there is demand for a face object that doesn't need heavy calculation. In our research, we used a 3D face model [20] (Fig.13 (b)) and tried to make a 3D object of the mouth region. This 3D face model is composed of around 750 polygons.

A face fitting tool developed by the Galatea project [20, 21] is part of an open-source toolkit to generate a 3D face object using one's frontal photograph. But the manual-fitting algorithm of this tool is slightly difficult and requires around 10 minutes for users to generate a face object with a real personal face image, although it is able to generate a model with a nearly real personal shape with many photographs. Fig.13(a) is an original face image, Fig. 13(b) shows the fitting result of a generic face model and Fig.13(c) is a mouth part model constructed by a personal model used for mouth synthesis in lip synchronization.

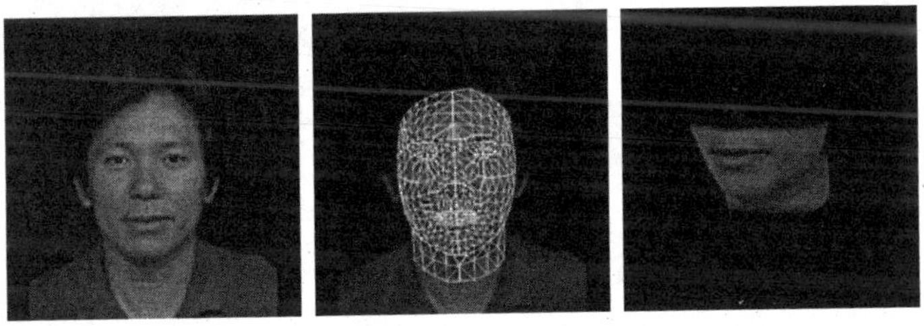

Fig. 13. 3-D face object generation process. From left to right, (a) an original face image, (b)a fitting result of generic face model, and (c) a mouth part model constructed by a personal model used for mouth synthesis for lip synchronization.

Automatic Face Tracking

Next, we describe an automatic face-tracking algorithm using a 3D face object. The tracking process using template matching can be divided into three steps. First, texture mapping of one of the video frame images is applied to the 3D individual face shape object model created as previously mentioned. Here, a frontal face image is chosen out of video frames for the texture mapping. Next, we make a 2D template image for translation and rotation using the 3D object shown in Fig.14. Resolutions are one pixel for translation, 0.25 degree for rotation, and 0.01 for scaling. Here, in order to reduce the matching error, the mouth region is excluded in a template image. Therefore, even while the person in a video image is speaking something, tracking can be carried out more stably. Approximation is used because not very much expression change happens in all video sequences. Finally, we carry out template matching between the template images and an input video frame image and estimate translation and rotation values so that the matching error becomes minimum. An example of a face model match-move into video frame is shown in Fig.15. The top row is an original video frame chosen from sequences randomly. The second row is a synthetic face according to estimated position and rotation angle information by our algorithm. The third row is an image generated by replacing the original face with the synthetic one.

Lip Shape in Utterance

When a person says something, the lips and jaw move simultaneously. In particular, the movements of the lips are closely related to the phonological process, so the 3D

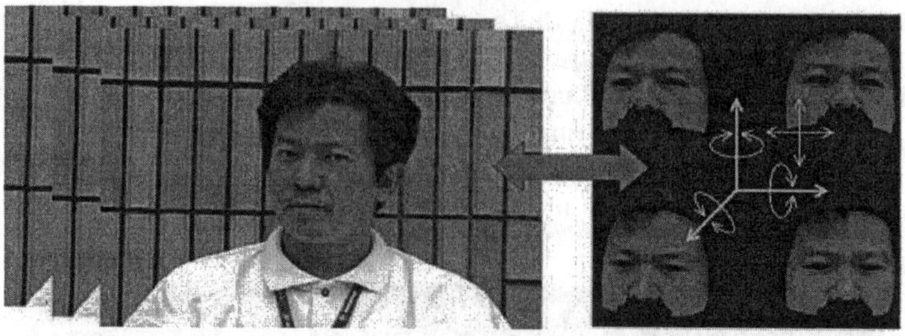

Fig. 14. Template matching using face object

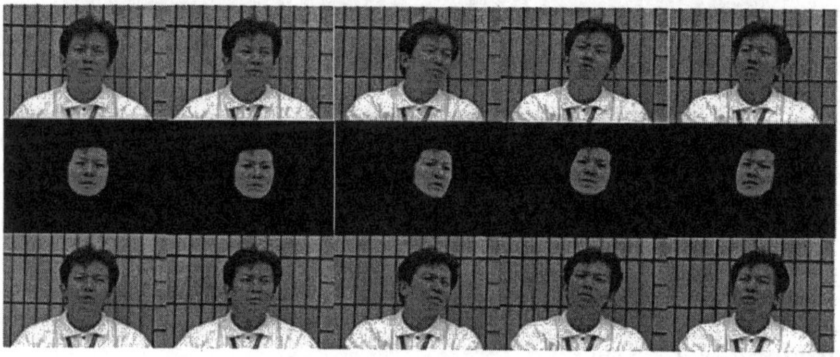

Fig. 15. Example of face object match-move

model must be controlled accurately. For accurate control of the mouth region a 3D face model developed by [20] that defines seven control points on the model is adopted. These points could be controlled by geometric movement rules based on the bone and muscle structure. In this research, we prepared reference lip-shape images from the front and side. Then, we transformed the wire-frame model to approximate the reference images. In this process, we acquired momentum vectors of nodes on the wire-frame model. Then, we stored these momentum vectors in the lip-shape database. This database is normalized by the mouth region's size, so we do not need speaker adaptation. Thus, this system has realized talking face generation with a small database. We create 22 kinds of lip-shapes in a database based on VISEMEs, which are generally defined for lip movement information like [au] and [ei] of the phonetic alphabet like phonemes in speech. The database is defined only by the momentum vector of nodes on a wire-frame. However, there are no transient data among the standard lip-shapes. The system must have momentum vectors of the node data on the wire-frame model while phonemes are being uttered. Therefore, we defined that the 3D model configures a standard lip-shape when a phoneme is uttered at any point in time. This point is normally the starting point of phoneme utterance and we defined key-frame at the starting point of each phoneme segment and interpolated it by a linear or sinusoidal curve between key-frames. Although this method is not directly connected with kinesiology, we believe that it provides a realistic lip-shape image.

2.4 Evaluation of Lip-sync Animation

We performed subjective experiments to evaluate the effectiveness of the proposed image synthesis algorithm. In order to verify the effectiveness of the proposed system, we carried out a subjective digit discrimination perception test when synthesized talking face animations were represented to subjects under an acoustically noisy environment. Audio-visual samples for testing are composed of 4 digits.

We tested this using original speech, original speech without face movie (voice only), and synthesized talking face animations in speech. Talking face animations are interpolated by either linear key-frame interpolation or sinusoidal key-frame interpolation. The audio SNRs of the original speech are 0, -6, -20, and -30dB using white Gaussian noise. The total number of subject is 13 and all subjects' gender is male. In each test, a test sequence is selected randomly and played back over a headphone. This test is performed using a web page. Fig.16 shows the results.

In every case, according to the low audio SNR, the subjective discrimination rates degrade. In the case of less than -20dB, by adding a face movie or synthesis face animation the rate is increased. *Original* is a combination of an original voice and a video-captured natural face image. In this case, even in -30dB a high discrimination rate can be achieved. Note that voice only digit discrimination in audio SNR=-30dB was 0% in the experiments. As a result, the combination of voice and face animation provides better scoring than voice only. We also compare the original movie and synthesized face animations; the original movie is slightly better in discrimination on average.

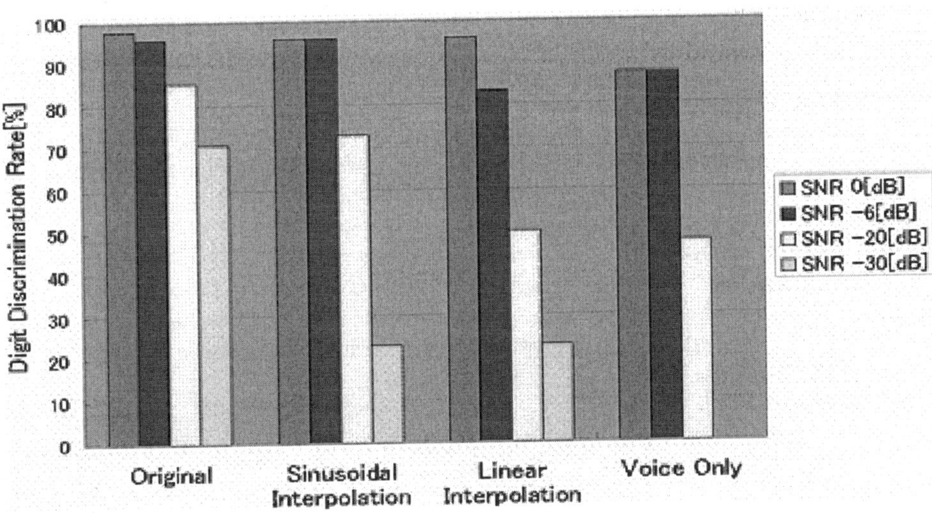

Fig. 16. Evaluation of subjective digit discrimination perception test

3 Conclusion

This chapter first described audio-visual speech detection and recognition algorithms which improve the robustness of speech recognition performance in actual noisy environments. Second, a talking face synthesis system based on a 3-D mesh model and its application to audio-visual speech translation system were introduced.

A proposed audio-visual speech section detection algorithm was proved to be very robust to acoustically noisy environments in word accuracy and word insertion count for the speech recognition. An audio-visual speech recognition algorithm based on the pseudo-biphone product HMM structure was proposed and its effectiveness was verified. Both results showed that the method integrating audio and visual modalities outperformed single modality methods in all cases. Audio-visual integration has further potential to improve speech recognition performance in adverse environments.

We also described a system that can create any lip-shape with an extremely small database, and is also speaker-independent. It preserves the speaker's original facial expression by using input images other than the mouth region. Furthermore, this facial-image synthesis system was applied to an audio-visual speech translation system, which is capable of audio-visual multi-lingual translation. For the time being, this system only works off-line. To operate the system on-line in real time, more effort is needed to reduce the computation amount while improving performance.

Multi-modal information integration is the essential mechanism for human beings to interact and communicate with each other more reliably. The integration methods considered in this chapter can deal with multiple modalities with only slight time asynchronicity. However, human beings in reality utilize much more information adaptively in the type and time delay of asynchronicity. Understanding human beings to a greater degree through psycho-physical audio-visual research will give clues for further development of sophisticated statistical multi-modal integration models.

Acknowledgments
The research reported here was supported in part by a contract with the National Institute of Information and Communications Technology entitled "A study of speech dialogue translation technology based on a large corpus".

References

1. Stork D G, Hennecke M E (1996) Speechreading by humans and machines, Springer, Berlin
2. Nakamura S, Nagai R, Shikano K (1997), Improved bimodal speech recognition using tied-mixture HMMs and 5000 word audio-visual synchronous database. Proceedings of Eurospeech: 1623–1626
3. Tomlinson M J, Russell M J, Brooke N M (1996), Integrating audio and visual information to provide highly robust speech recognition"', Proceedings of ICASSP, Vol.2: 821–824
4. de Cuetos P, Neti C, Senio A (2000), Audio-visual intent to speak detection for human-computer interaction, Proceedings of ICASSP: 1325–1328

5. Iyengar G, Neti C (2001), A vision-based microphone switch for speech intent detection, Proceedings of IEEE Workshop on Real-Time Analysis of Face and Gesture
6. Murai K, Kumatani K, Nakamura S (2001), A robust end point detection by speaker's facial motion, Proceedings of International Workshop of Hands-free speech communication(HSC2001): 199–202
7. Naito M, Singer H, Yamamoto H, Nakajima H, Matsui T, Tsukada H, Nakamura A, Sagisaka Y (1999), Evaluation of ATRSPREC for travel arrangement task, Proceedings of Fall Meeting of Acoustic Society of Japan: 113–114
8. Nakamura S (2001), Fusion of audio-visual information for integrated speech processing, Proceedings on Third International Conference on Audio- and Video-based Biometric Person Authentication, LNCS2091, Springer, : 127–143
9. Kumatani K, Nakamura S, Shikano K (2001), An adaptive integration method based on product HMM for bi-modal speech recognition, Proceedings of International Workshop of Hands-free Speech Communication(HSC2001) : 195–198
10. Nakamura S, Kumatani K, Tamura S (2002), State synchronous modeling of audio-visnual information for bi-modal speech recognition, Proceedigns of IEEE Workshop of Automatic Speech Recognition and Understanding
11. Breglar C, Covell M, Slaney T (1997), Video rewrite: driving visual speech with audio. Proceedings of ACM SIGGRAPH: 353–360
12. Ezzat T, Geiger G, Poggio T (2002), Trainable videorealistic speech pnimation. Proceedings of ACM SIGGRAPH 2002: 388–398
13. Takezawa T, Morimoto T, Sagisaka Y, Campbell N, Iida, Sugaya F, Yokoo A, Ya-mamoto S (1998), Japanese-to-english speech translation system: ATR-MATRIX. Proceedings of International Conference of Spoken Language Processing, ICSLP: 957–960
14. Campbell N, Black AW (1995), Chatr: a multi-lingual speech re-sequencing synthesis system. Proceedings of IEICE Technical Report, sp96-7: 45–72
15. Campbell N (1996) CHATR: A high definition speech re-sequencing system. Proceedings of ASA/ASJ Joint meeting: 1223–1228
16. Ostendorf M, Singer H (1997) HMM topology design using maximum likelihood suc-cessive state splitting. Proceedings of Computer Speech and Language, vol 11, no 1: 17–41
17. Sumita E, Yamada S, Yamamoto K, Paul M, Kashioka H, Ishikawa K, Shirai S (1999), Solutions to problems inherent in spoken-language translation: The ATR-MATRIX approach. Proceedings of MT Summit VII: 229–235
18. Furuse O, Kawai J, Iida H, Akamine S, Kim D (1995), Multi-lingual spoken-language translation utilizing translation examples. Proceedings of NLPRS5: 544–549
19. Furuse O, Iida H (1996), Incremental translation utilizing constituent boundary pat-terns. Proceedings of Coling '96: 412–417
20. Yotsukura T, Morishima S (2002), An open source development tool for anthropomor-phic dialog agent - face image synthesis and lip synchronization-. Proceedings of IEEE Fifth Workshop on Multimedia Signal Processing, 03_01_05.pdf
21. Kawamoto S et al (2002) Open-source software for developing anthropomorphic spo-ken dialog agent. Proceedings of International

Workshop on Lifelike Animated Agents - Tools, Affective Functions and Applications: 64–69

Probabilistic Fusion of Sorted Score Sequences for Robust Speaker Verification

Ming-Cheung Cheung[1], Man-Wai Mak[1], and Sun-Yuan Kung[2]

[1] Center for Multimedia Signal Processing,
Dept. of Electronic and Information Engineering,
The Hong Kong Polytechnic University, Hong Kong
[2] Department of Electrical Engineering, Princeton University, USA

Abstract. Fusion techniques have been widely used in multi-modal biometric authentication systems. While these techniques are mainly applied to combine the outputs of modality-dependent classifiers, they can also be applied to fuse the decisions or scores from a single modality. The idea is to consider the multiple samples extracted from a single modality as independent but coming from the same source. In this chapter, we propose a single-source, multi-sample data-dependent fusion algorithm for speaker verification. The algorithm is data-dependent in that the fusion weights are dependent on the verification scores and the prior score statistics of claimed speakers and background speakers. To obtain the best out of the speaker's scores, scores from multiple utterances are sorted before they are probabilistically combined. Evaluations based on 150 speakers from a GSM-transcoded corpus are presented. Results show that data-dependent fusion of speaker's scores is significantly better than the conventional score averaging approach. It was also found that the proposed fusion algorithm can be further enhanced by sorting the score sequences before they are probabilistically combined.

Keywords: decision fusion, speaker verification, feature transformation, GSM-transcoded speech

1 Introduction

In recent years, research has focused on using fusion techniques to improve the performance of speaker verification systems. One popular approach is to fuse the scores obtained from modality-specific classifiers. For example, in [1][2] the scores from a lip recognizer are fused with those from a speaker recognizer, and in [3] a face classifier is combined with a voice classifier using a variety of combination rules. These types of systems, however, require multiple sensors, which tend to increase system costs and require extra cooperation from users, e.g. users may need to present their faces as well as to utter a sentence to support their claim. While this requirement can be alleviated by fusing different speech features from the same utterance [4], the effectiveness of this approach relies on the degree of independence among these features.

This chapter investigates the fusion of scores from multiple utterances to improve the performance of speaker verification from GSM-transcoded speech. The simplest way to achieve this goal is to average the scores obtained from multiple utterances, as in [5]. While score averaging is a reasonable approach to combining the scores, the approach weighs the contribution of speech patterns from multiple utterances equally, which may not produce optimal fused scores. In our previous work [6][7], we computed the optimal fusion weights based on the score distribution of the utterances and on the prior score statistics determined from enrollment data. To further enhance the fusion algorithm, we propose in this chapter to sort the score sequences before fusion takes place. With this arrangement, the contribution of some erroneous scores of one utterance can be compensated by the scores of another utterance. Compared with the conventional equal-weight approach, the new algorithm is able to reduce the equal error rate by 23%.

The remainder of the chapter is organized as follows. In Section 2, the data-dependent decision fusion algorithm proposed in [6] is briefly reviewed and the proposed score sorting approach is introduced. This is followed by a theoretical analysis demonstrating the benefit of the proposed score sorting approach. The proposed method is further evaluated in Section 3 via a speaker verification experiment using GSM-transcoded speech. Finally, in Section 4, concluding remarks are provided.

2 Data-Dependent Decision Fusion Model

2.1 Architecture

Assume that K streams of features vectors (e.g. MFCCs) can be extracted from K independent utterances $\mathcal{U} = \{\mathcal{U}_1, \ldots, \mathcal{U}_K\}$. Let us denote the observation sequence corresponding to utterance $\mathcal{U}_k$ by

$$\mathcal{O}^{(k)} = \{\mathbf{o}_t^{(k)} \in \Re^D; t = 1, \ldots, T_k\} \qquad k = 1, \ldots, K \tag{1}$$

where D and T_k are respectively the dimensionality of $\mathbf{o}_t^{(k)}$ and the number of observations in $\mathcal{O}^{(k)}$. We further define a normalized score function

$$s(\mathbf{o}_t^{(k)}; \Lambda) \equiv \log p(\mathbf{o}_t^{(k)} | \Lambda_{\omega_c}) - \log p(\mathbf{o}_t^{(k)} | \Lambda_{\omega_b}) \tag{2}$$

where $\Lambda = \{\Lambda_{\omega_c}, \Lambda_{\omega_b}\}$ contains the Gaussian mixture models (GMMs) characterizing the client speaker (ω_c) and the background speakers (ω_b), and $\log p(\mathbf{o}_t^{(k)} | \Lambda_\omega)$ is the output of Λ_ω, $\omega \in \{\omega_c, \omega_b\}$, given observation $\mathbf{o}_t^{(k)}$.

In [6], frame-level fused scores are computed as

$$s(\mathbf{o}_t^{(1)},\ldots,\mathbf{o}_t^{(K)};\Lambda) = s(\mathbf{O}_t;\Lambda) = \sum_{k=1}^{K} \alpha_t^{(k)} s(\mathbf{o}_t^{(k)};\Lambda) \tag{3}$$

$$\alpha_t^{(k)} \in [0,1] \text{ and } \sum_{k=1}^{K} \alpha_t^{(k)} = 1,$$

where $\mathbf{O}_t = \{\mathbf{o}_t^{(1)},\ldots,\mathbf{o}_t^{(K)}\}$ contains the K observations from the K utterances at time t and $\alpha_t^{(k)}$ represents the confidence (reliability) of the observation $\mathbf{o}_t^{(k)}$.

During enrollment, the mean score of each client speaker ($\tilde{\mu}_c$) and of the background speakers ($\tilde{\mu}_b$) are determined. Then, the prior score and prior variance are respectively computed as follows:

$$\tilde{\mu}_p = \frac{K_c\tilde{\mu}_c + K_b\tilde{\mu}_b}{K_c + K_b} \qquad \text{and} \qquad \tilde{\sigma}_p^2 = \frac{1}{K_c + K_b} \sum_{n=1}^{K_c+K_b} \left[s(\tilde{\mathcal{O}}^{(n)};\Lambda) - \tilde{\mu}_p \right]^2 \tag{4}$$

where $s(\tilde{\mathcal{O}}^{(n)};\Lambda) = \frac{1}{T_n}\sum_{t=1}^{T_n} s(\tilde{\mathbf{o}}_t^{(n)};\Lambda)$ is the mean score of the n-th training utterance and K_c and K_b are respectively the numbers of client speaker's utterances and background speakers' utterances. Then, during verification, the claimant is asked to utter K utterances, and the data-dependent fusion weights are computed as:

$$\alpha_t^{(k)} = \frac{\exp\left\{[s_t^{(k)} - \tilde{\mu}_p]^2 \big/ 2\tilde{\sigma}_p^2\right\}}{\sum_{l=1}^{K} \exp\left\{[s_t^{(l)} - \tilde{\mu}_p]^2 \big/ 2\tilde{\sigma}_p^2\right\}} \qquad k = 1,\ldots,K. \tag{5}$$

where for ease of presentation, we have defined $s_t^{(k)} \equiv s(\mathbf{o}_t^{(k)};\Lambda)$. The mean fused score

$$s(\mathcal{U};\Lambda) = \frac{1}{T}\sum_{t=1}^{T} s(\mathbf{O}_t;\Lambda) \tag{6}$$

is compared against a decision threshold for decision making. Fig. 1 depicts the architecture of the fusion model.

Note that this method requires the K utterances to contain the same number of feature vectors, i.e. $T_k = T \; \forall \; k = 1,\ldots,K$. If it is not the case, we may move some of the vectors from the tail of the longer utterances to the tail of the shorter utterances to make the number of vectors in all utterance equal.[3]

[3] As it is likely that the utterances are obtained from the same speaker under the same environment in a verification session, moving feature vectors from utterances to utterances will have the same effect as partitioning a long utterance into a number of equal-length short utterances.

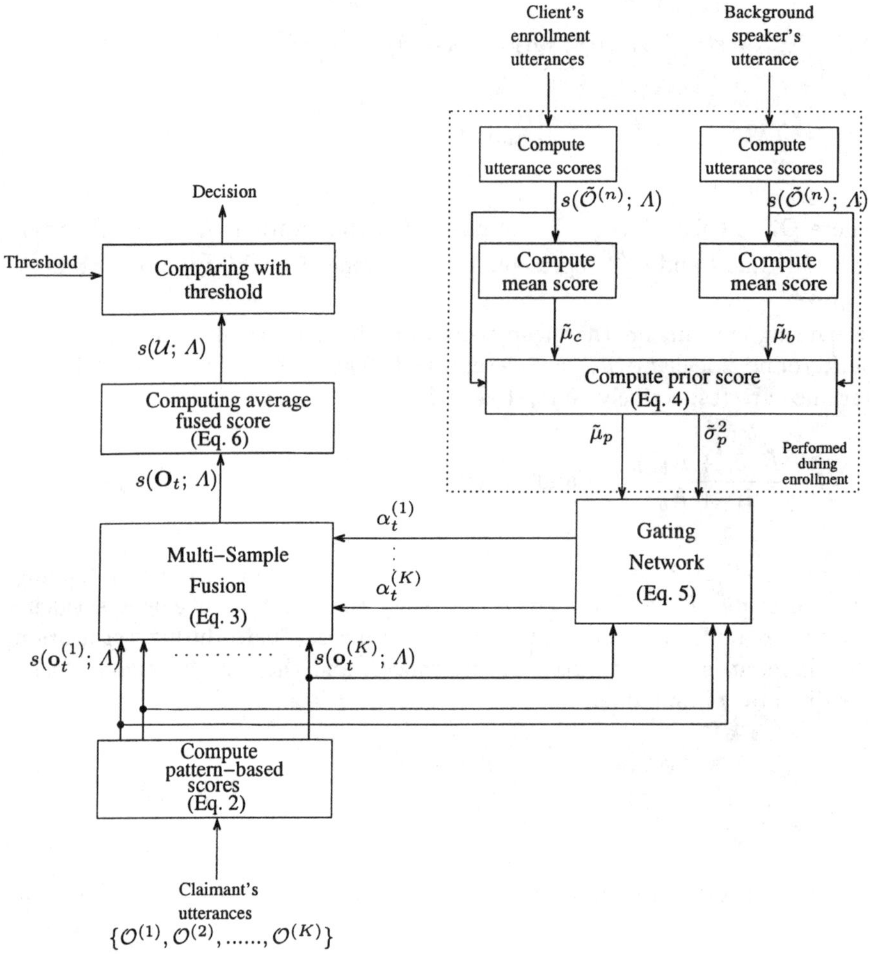

Fig. 1. Architecture of the multi-sample decision fusion model.

2.2 Gaussian Example

Fig. 2 illustrates an example where the distributions of the client speaker scores and the impostor scores are assumed to be Gaussian. It is also assumed that both the client and impostor utter two utterances. The client speaker's mean scores for the first and second utterances are equal to 1.2 and 0.8 respectively. Likewise, the impostor's mean scores for the two utterances are equal to -1.3 and -0.7. Obviously, equal-weight fusion will produce a mean speaker score of 1.0 and a mean impostor score of -1.0, resulting in a score dispersion of 2.0. These two mean scores (-1.0 and 1.0) are indicated by the two vertical lines in Fig. 2(b). We can see from Fig. 2(b) and Fig. 2(c) that when the prior score $\tilde{\mu}_p$ is set to a value between these two means (i.e. between the vertical lines), the scores dispersion can be larger than 2.0.

2.3 Theoretical Analysis

Here we provide a theoretical analysis of the fusion algorithm. Through this analysis, we will be able to explain how and why the fusion algorithm achieves better performance as compared to the equal-weight fusion approach. The reason behind the increase in the score dispersion in Fig. 2 can also be explained.

We consider the case where the score sequences of two independent utterances are fused, i.e. $K = 2$ in (3). The extension to multiple sequences is trivial. As the two utterances are independent, their scores $s_t^{(1)}$ and $s_t^{(2)}$ are also independent. Differentiating both side of (5) with respect to $s_t^{(k)}$ and using the independence between $s_t^{(1)}$ and $s_t^{(2)}$, we obtain

$$\frac{\partial \alpha_t^{(k)}}{\partial s_t^{(k)}} = \frac{C(s_t^{(k)} - \tilde{\mu}_p)}{\tilde{\sigma}_p^2} \left[\frac{e^{\{(s_t^{(k)} - \tilde{\mu}_p)^2 / 2\tilde{\sigma}_p^2\}}}{\left(\sum_{l=1}^{2} e^{\{(s_t^{(l)} - \tilde{\mu}_p)^2 / 2\tilde{\sigma}_p^2\}}\right)^2} \right] \qquad k = 1, 2. \quad (7)$$

where $C = \sum_{l \neq k} e^{\{(s_t^{(l)} - \tilde{\mu}_p)^2 / 2\tilde{\sigma}_p^2\}} > 0$. Equation (7) suggests that when $s_t^{(k)} > \tilde{\mu}_p$, $\partial \alpha_t^{(k)} / \partial s_t^{(k)} > 0$, and vice versa for $s_t^{(k)} < \tilde{\mu}_p$.

Let us consider two scenarios:

Scenario A: $\tilde{\mu}_p < \mu$, where μ is the mean score of the two utterances. For example, $\mu = 1$ for the two client utterances in Fig. 2(a). In this scenario, the claimant is more likely to be a client speaker than an impostor because the two utterances produce many large pattern-based scores to make $\mu > \tilde{\mu}_p$. Since the majority of the pattern-based scores ($s_t^{(k)}$ and $s_t^{(l)}$) are large, we have the following conditions (see Fig. 3 for an illustration):

Condition A-1: $P(s_t^{(k)} > \tilde{\mu}_p) > P(s_t^{(k)} < \tilde{\mu}_p) \quad k \in \{1, 2\}$

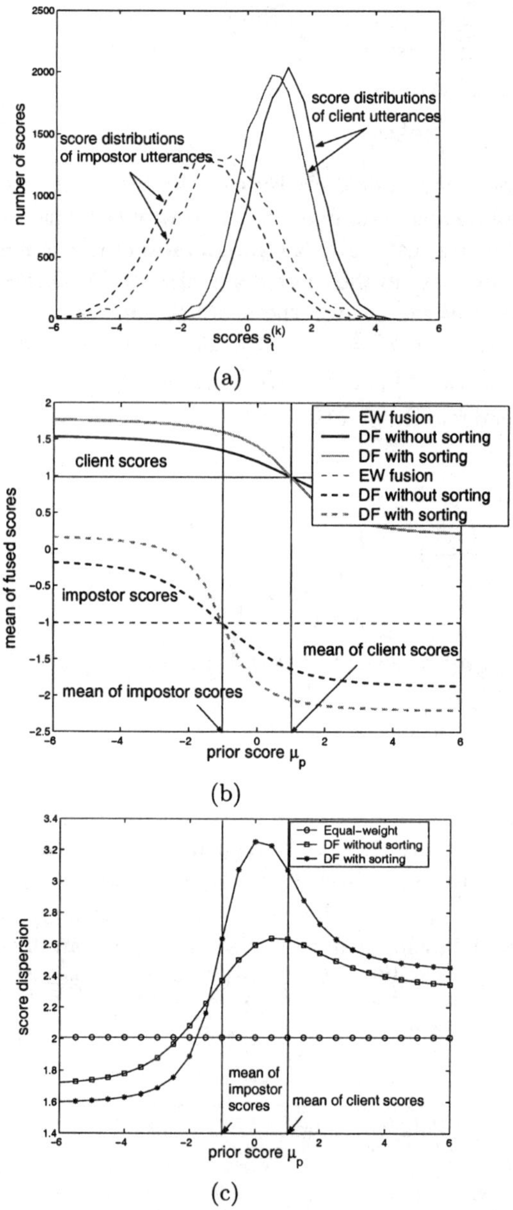

Fig. 2. (a) Distributions of client scores and impostor scores as a result of two utterances: one from a client speaker and another from an impostor. The means of client scores are 0.8 and 1.2, and the means of impostor scores are −1.3 and −0.7. (b) The mean of fused client scores and the mean of fused impostor scores versus the prior score $\tilde{\mu}_p$. (c) Difference between the mean of fused client scores and the mean of fused impostor scores under different values of prior scores $\tilde{\mu}_p$'s based on equal-weight fusion and data-dependent fusion (DF) with and without score sorting.

Condition A-2:

$$\begin{aligned}
& P(\text{emphasizing large scores}) \\
&= P(\mathcal{S}1 \cup \mathcal{S}2 \cup \mathcal{S}3) \\
&= P(\{(s_t^{(k)} > \tilde{\mu}_p) \cap (s_t^{(l)} > \tilde{\mu}_p)\} \cup \\
&\quad \{(s_t^{(k)} > \tilde{\mu}_p) \cap (s_t^{(l)} < \tilde{\mu}_p) \cap (s_t^{(k)} - \tilde{\mu}_p > \tilde{\mu}_p - s_t^{(l)})\} \cup \\
&\quad \{(s_t^{(k)} < \tilde{\mu}_p) \cap (s_t^{(l)} > \tilde{\mu}_p) \cap (\tilde{\mu}_p - s_t^{(k)} < s_t^{(l)} - \tilde{\mu}_p)\}) \\
&= P(\{(s_t^{(k)} > \tilde{\mu}_p) \cap (s_t^{(l)} > \tilde{\mu}_p)\} \cup \\
&\quad \{(s_t^{(k)} > \tilde{\mu}_p) \cap (s_t^{(l)} < \tilde{\mu}_p) \cap (s_t^{(k)} + s_t^{(l)} > 2\tilde{\mu}_p)\} \cup \\
&\quad \{(s_t^{(k)} < \tilde{\mu}_p) \cap (s_t^{(l)} > \tilde{\mu}_p) \cap (2\tilde{\mu}_p < s_t^{(k)} + s_t^{(l)})\}) \\
&> P(\{(s_t^{(k)} < \tilde{\mu}_p) \cap (s_t^{(l)} < \tilde{\mu}_p)\} \cup \\
&\quad \{(s_t^{(k)} > \tilde{\mu}_p) \cap (s_t^{(l)} < \tilde{\mu}_p) \cap (s_t^{(k)} + s_t^{(l)} < 2\tilde{\mu}_p)\} \cup \\
&\quad \{(s_t^{(k)} < \tilde{\mu}_p) \cap (s_t^{(l)} > \tilde{\mu}_p) \cap (2\tilde{\mu}_p > s_t^{(k)} + s_t^{(l)})\}) \\
&\quad \text{from Condition A-1} \\
&= P(\{(s_t^{(k)} < \tilde{\mu}_p) \cap (s_t^{(l)} < \tilde{\mu}_p)\} \cup \\
&\quad \{(s_t^{(k)} > \tilde{\mu}_p) \cap (s_t^{(l)} < \tilde{\mu}_p) \cap (s_t^{(k)} - \tilde{\mu}_p < \tilde{\mu}_p - s_t^{(l)})\} \cup \\
&\quad \{(s_t^{(k)} < \tilde{\mu}_p) \cap (s_t^{(l)} > \tilde{\mu}_p) \cap (\tilde{\mu}_p - s_t^{(k)} > s_t^{(l)} - \tilde{\mu}_p)\}) \\
&= P(\mathcal{S}4 \cup \mathcal{S}5 \cup \mathcal{S}6) \\
&= P(\text{emphasizing small scores})
\end{aligned}$$

where $P(\mathcal{S})$ stands for the probability of having the scores fall on the set $\mathcal{S}$, and its value can be obtained by integrating the 2-D Gaussian density function over the region defined by $\mathcal{S}$. As the peak of the 2-D density function falls on $\mathcal{S}1$ (see Fig. 3(b)), the volume under $\mathcal{S}1 \cup \mathcal{S}2 \cup \mathcal{S}3$ should be larger than that under $\mathcal{S}4 \cup \mathcal{S}5 \cup \mathcal{S}6$. This observation agrees with the inequality in Condition A-2.
The above argument shows that $P(\mathcal{S}1 \cup \mathcal{S}2 \cup \mathcal{S}3) > P(\mathcal{S}4 \cup \mathcal{S}5 \cup \mathcal{S}6)$. Here, we explain why $P(\mathcal{S}1 \cup \mathcal{S}2 \cup \mathcal{S}3)$ is the probability of emphasizing large scores and $P(\mathcal{S}4 \cup \mathcal{S}5 \cup \mathcal{S}6)$ is the probability of emphasizing small scores. In $\mathcal{S}1$, since both $s_t^{(k)}$ and $s_t^{(l)}$ are larger than the prior score $\tilde{\mu}_p$, (5) will emphasize the larger score only. In $\mathcal{S}2$, although $s_t^{(l)}$ is smaller than the prior score $\tilde{\mu}_p$, (5) will still emphasize the larger score (i.e. $s_t^{(k)}$ in this set) as the difference between $s_t^{(k)}$ and $\tilde{\mu}_p$ is larger than that between $s_t^{(l)}$ and $\tilde{\mu}_p$. The situation in $\mathcal{S}3$ is similar to that in $\mathcal{S}2$, except the large score is $s_t^{(l)}$ and the small score is $s_t^{(k)}$; again the larger score $s_t^{(l)}$ is emphasized because it is further away from $\tilde{\mu}_p$ than $s_t^{(k)}$ is. Therefore, by merging these three sets together, we can obtain

the probability of emphasizing large scores. Similar arguments can be applied to $\mathcal{S}4$, $\mathcal{S}5$ and $\mathcal{S}6$ to obtain the probability of emphasizing the small scores.

Scenario A suggests that when the majority of scores are greater than the prior score $\tilde{\mu}_p$, the fusion algorithm has a higher chance of emphasizing large scores. Meanwhile (7) suggests that if $s_t^{(k)}$ increases, the fusion weight $\alpha_t^{(k)}$ for the corresponding score will also increase (because $\partial\alpha_t^{(k)}/\partial s_t^{(k)} > 0$). Putting these two observations together suggests that the mean fused score should be larger than the mean scores of the two utterances.

Scenario B: $\tilde{\mu}_p > \mu$, where μ is the mean score of the two utterances. For example, $\mu = -1$ for the two impostor utterances in Fig. 2(a). In this scenario, the claimant is more likely to be an impostor because the two utterances produce many small pattern-based scores to make $\mu < \tilde{\mu}_p$. Since the majority of the pattern-based scores ($s_t^{(k)}$ and $s_t^{(l)}$) are small, we have the following conditions (see Fig. 4 for an illustration):

Condition B-1: $P(s_t^{(k)} < \tilde{\mu}_p) > P(s_t^{(k)} > \tilde{\mu}_p) \quad k \in \{1, 2\}$

Condition B-2:

$$
\begin{aligned}
& P(\text{emphasizing small scores}) \\
&= P(\mathcal{S}4 \cup \mathcal{S}5 \cup \mathcal{S}6) \\
&= P(\{(s_t^{(k)} < \tilde{\mu}_p) \cap (s_t^{(l)} < \tilde{\mu}_p)\} \cup \\
&\qquad \{(s_t^{(k)} > \tilde{\mu}_p) \cap (s_t^{(l)} < \tilde{\mu}_p) \cap (s_t^{(k)} - \tilde{\mu}_p < \tilde{\mu}_p - s_t^{(l)})\} \cup \\
&\qquad \{(s_t^{(k)} < \tilde{\mu}_p) \cap (s_t^{(l)} > \tilde{\mu}_p) \cap (\tilde{\mu}_p - s_t^{(k)} > s_t^{(l)} - \tilde{\mu}_p)\}) \\
&> P(\{(s_t^{(k)} > \tilde{\mu}_p) \cap (s_t^{(l)} > \tilde{\mu}_p)\} \cup \\
&\qquad \{(s_t^{(k)} > \tilde{\mu}_p) \cap (s_t^{(l)} < \tilde{\mu}_p) \cap (s_t^{(k)} - \tilde{\mu}_p > \tilde{\mu}_p - s_t^{(l)})\} \cup \\
&\qquad \{(s_t^{(k)} < \tilde{\mu}_p) \cap (s_t^{(l)} > \tilde{\mu}_p) \cap (\tilde{\mu}_p - s_t^{(k)} < s_t^{(l)} - \tilde{\mu}_p)\}) \\
&\qquad \text{from Condition B-1} \\
&= P(\mathcal{S}1 \cup \mathcal{S}2 \cup \mathcal{S}3) \\
&= P(\text{emphasizing large scores})
\end{aligned}
$$

where $P(\mathcal{S})$ stands for the probability of having the scores fall on the set $\mathcal{S}$, and its value can be obtained by integrating the 2-D Gaussian density function over the region defined by $\mathcal{S}$. As the peak of the 2-D density function falls on $\mathcal{S}4$ (see Fig. 4(b)), the volume under $\mathcal{S}4 \cup \mathcal{S}5 \cup \mathcal{S}6$ should be larger than that under $\mathcal{S}1 \cup \mathcal{S}2 \cup \mathcal{S}3$. This observation agrees with the inequality in Condition B-2.

Scenario B suggests that when the majority of scores are smaller than the prior score $\tilde{\mu}_p$, the fusion algorithm has a higher chance of emphasizing small scores. At the same time, we can observe from (7) that when $s_t^{(k)}$ decreases, the fusion weight $\alpha_t^{(k)}$ for the corresponding score will also increases (because $\partial\alpha_t^{(k)}/\partial s_t^{(k)} < 0$). These two observations lead to the conclusion that the mean fused score of the two utterances should be smaller than the utterances' mean score.

Based on the above analysis, we can see that if the claimant is more likely to be a client speaker, the fusion algorithm will increase his/her mean fused score and vice versa if he/she is an impostor. This has the effect of increasing the score dispersion, as demonstrated in Fig. 2(c).

2.4 Fusion of Sorted Scores

As the proposed fusion algorithm depends on the pattern-based scores of individual utterances, the positions of scores in the score sequence also affect the final fused scores. Moreover, as illustrated in Section 2.3, the emphasis of large speaker scores under Scenario A and the de-emphasis of small impostor scores under Scenario B are probabilistic, i.e. there is no guarantee that these situations will always occur. In order to overcome this limitation, we have proposed to sort scores before fusion so that small scores will always be fused with large scores [8].

Here, we provide a theoretical analysis to explain the benefit of sorting the scores before fusion. We assume that there are two sorted score sequences with equal mean (μ), one being arranged in ascending order and the other in descending order. We further assume that the scores in the sequences follow a Gaussian distribution. If the numbers of scores in the sequences are sufficiently large, we can obtain the following relationship:

$$\mu - s_t^{(1)} \approx s_t^{(2)} - \mu, \text{ i.e., } s_t^{(2)} \approx 2\mu - s_t^{(1)} \tag{8}$$

where $s_t^{(1)}$ and $s_t^{(2)}$ respectively represent the scores less than and greater than the score mean μ. Without loss of generality, we denote the smaller score as $s_t^{(1)}$ and the larger one as $s_t^{(2)}$, i.e. $s_t^{(1)} < s_t^{(2)}$. Substituting (8) into (5), the fusion weight for the small scores $s_t^{(1)}$ can be expressed as

$$\begin{aligned}\alpha_t^{(1)} &= \frac{\exp\{(s_t^{(1)} - \tilde{\mu}_p)^2/2\tilde{\sigma}_p^2\}}{\sum_{l=1}^{2}\exp\{(s_t^{(l)} - \tilde{\mu}_p)^2/2\tilde{\sigma}_p^2\}} \\ &= \frac{\exp\{(s_t^{(1)} - \tilde{\mu}_p)^2/2\tilde{\sigma}_p^2\}}{\exp\{(s_t^{(1)} - \tilde{\mu}_p)^2/2\tilde{\sigma}_p^2\} + \exp\{(2\mu - s_t^{(1)} - \tilde{\mu}_p)^2/2\tilde{\sigma}_p^2\}}.\end{aligned} \tag{9}$$

Differentiate both side of (9) with respect to $s_t^{(1)}$, we obtain

$$\frac{\partial\alpha_t^{(1)}}{\partial s_t^{(1)}} = \frac{\frac{2(\mu-\tilde{\mu}_p)}{\tilde{\sigma}_p^2} e^{\{(s_t^{(1)}-\tilde{\mu}_p)^2/2\tilde{\sigma}_p^2\}} e^{\{(2\mu-s_t^{(1)}-\tilde{\mu}_p)^2/2\tilde{\sigma}_p^2\}}}{\left[e^{\{(s_t^{(1)}-\tilde{\mu}_p)^2/2\tilde{\sigma}_p^2\}} + e^{\{(2\mu-s_t^{(1)}-\tilde{\mu}_p)^2/2\tilde{\sigma}_p^2\}}\right]^2}.$$

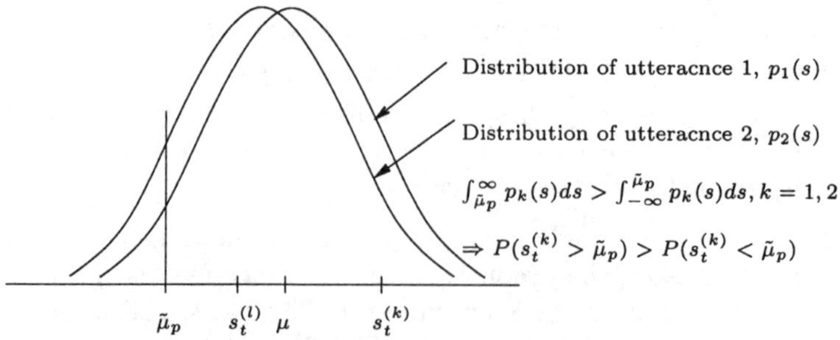

(a) Condition A-1

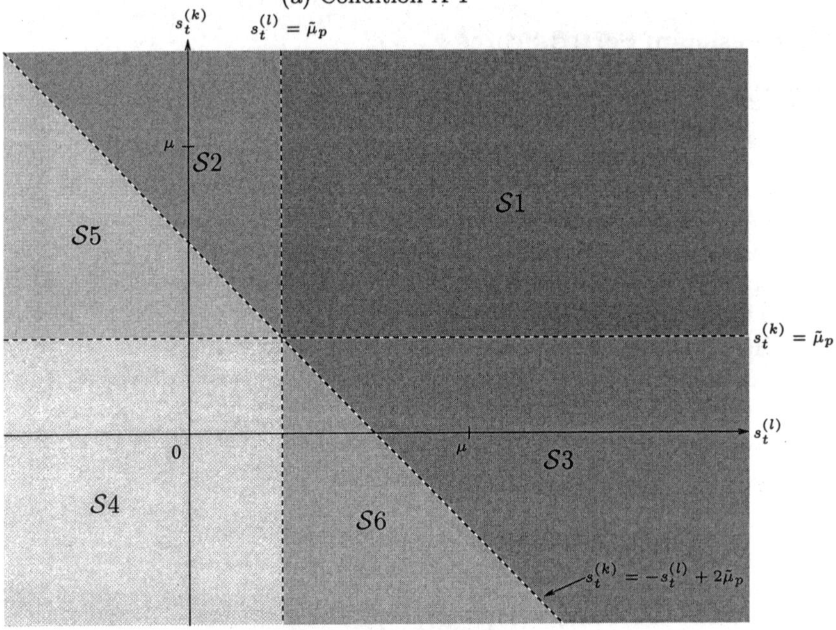

$$\mathcal{S}1 = \{(s_t^{(k)} > \tilde{\mu}_p) \cap (s_t^{(l)} > \tilde{\mu}_p)\}$$
$$\mathcal{S}2 = \{(s_t^{(k)} > \tilde{\mu}_p) \cap (s_t^{(l)} < \tilde{\mu}_p) \cap (s_t^{(k)} - \tilde{\mu}_p > \tilde{\mu}_p - s_t^{(l)})\}$$
$$\mathcal{S}3 = \{(s_t^{(k)} < \tilde{\mu}_p) \cap (s_t^{(l)} > \tilde{\mu}_p) \cap (\tilde{\mu}_p - s_t^{(k)} < s_t^{(l)} - \tilde{\mu}_p)\}$$
$$\mathcal{S}4 = \{(s_t^{(k)} < \tilde{\mu}_p) \cap (s_t^{(l)} < \tilde{\mu}_p)\}$$
$$\mathcal{S}5 = \{(s_t^{(k)} > \tilde{\mu}_p) \cap (s_t^{(l)} < \tilde{\mu}_p) \cap (s_t^{(k)} - \tilde{\mu}_p < \tilde{\mu}_p - s_t^{(l)})\}$$
$$\mathcal{S}6 = \{(s_t^{(k)} < \tilde{\mu}_p) \cap (s_t^{(l)} > \tilde{\mu}_p) \cap (\tilde{\mu}_p - s_t^{(k)} > s_t^{(l)} - \tilde{\mu}_p)\}$$

(b) Condition A-2

Fig. 3. Illustration of the two conditions in Scenario A ($\tilde{\mu}_p < \mu$). (a)$P(s_t^{(k)} > \tilde{\mu}_p) > P(s_t^{(k)} < \tilde{\mu}_p)$; (b)$P$(emphasizing large scores) $> P$(emphasizing small scores).

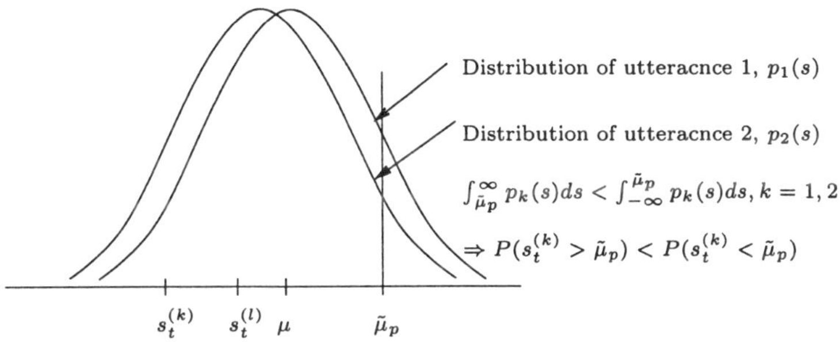

(a) Condition B-1

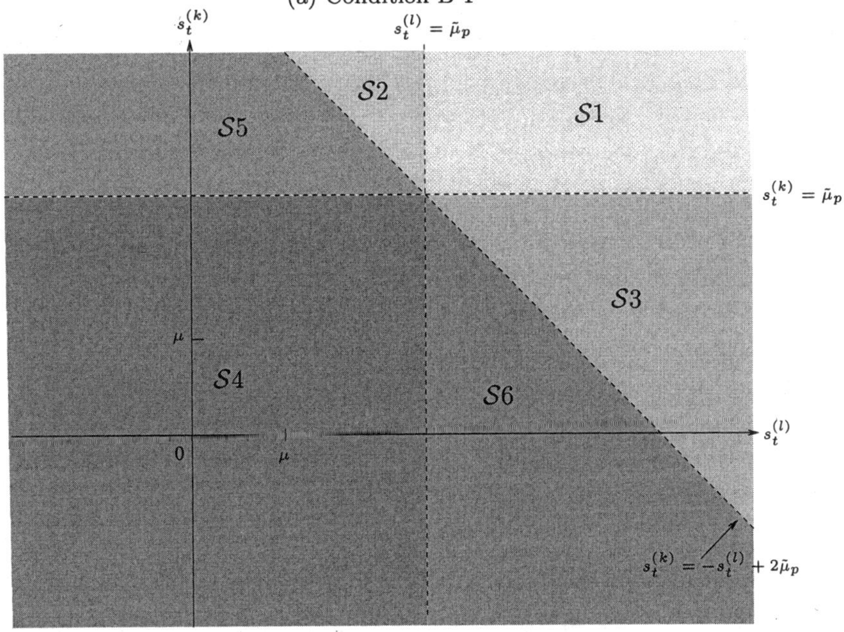

$$\mathcal{S}1 = \{(s_t^{(k)} > \tilde{\mu}_p) \cap (s_t^{(l)} > \tilde{\mu}_p)\}$$
$$\mathcal{S}2 = \{(s_t^{(k)} > \tilde{\mu}_p) \cap (s_t^{(l)} < \tilde{\mu}_p) \cap (s_t^{(k)} - \tilde{\mu}_p > \tilde{\mu}_p - s_t^{(l)})\}$$
$$\mathcal{S}3 = \{(s_t^{(k)} < \tilde{\mu}_p) \cap (s_t^{(l)} > \tilde{\mu}_p) \cap (\tilde{\mu}_p - s_t^{(k)} < s_t^{(l)} - \tilde{\mu}_p)\}$$
$$\mathcal{S}4 = \{(s_t^{(k)} < \tilde{\mu}_p) \cap (s_t^{(l)} < \tilde{\mu}_p)\}$$
$$\mathcal{S}5 = \{(s_t^{(k)} > \tilde{\mu}_p) \cap (s_t^{(l)} < \tilde{\mu}_p) \cap (s_t^{(k)} - \tilde{\mu}_p < \tilde{\mu}_p - s_t^{(l)})\}$$
$$\mathcal{S}6 = \{(s_t^{(k)} < \tilde{\mu}_p) \cap (s_t^{(l)} > \tilde{\mu}_p) \cap (\tilde{\mu}_p - s_t^{(k)} > s_t^{(l)} - \tilde{\mu}_p)\}$$

(b) Condition B-2

Fig. 4. Illustration of the two conditions in Scenario B ($\tilde{\mu}_p > \mu$). (a)$P(s_t^{(k)} > \tilde{\mu}_p) < P(s_t^{(k)} < \tilde{\mu}_p)$; (b)$P(\text{emphasizing large scores}) < P(\text{emphasizing small scores})$.

Therefore, we have

$$\frac{\partial \alpha_t^{(1)}}{\partial s_t^{(1)}} \begin{cases} < 0 \text{ when } \mu < \tilde{\mu}_p \ , \\ = 0 \text{ when } \mu = \tilde{\mu}_p \ , \\ > 0 \text{ when } \mu > \tilde{\mu}_p \ . \end{cases} \quad (10)$$

Similarly, we can show that

$$\frac{\partial \alpha_t^{(2)}}{\partial s_t^{(2)}} \begin{cases} < 0 \text{ when } \mu < \tilde{\mu}_p \ , \\ = 0 \text{ when } \mu = \tilde{\mu}_p \ , \\ > 0 \text{ when } \mu > \tilde{\mu}_p \ . \end{cases} \quad (11)$$

Equations (10) and (11) suggest that when $\mu < \tilde{\mu}_p$ (i.e. most of the scores are smaller than the prior score $\tilde{\mu}_p$), the fusion weights for small scores $\alpha_t^{(1)}$ increase when $s_t^{(1)}$ decreases, and the fusion weights for large scores $\alpha_t^{(2)}$ decrease when $s_t^{(2)}$ increases. This implies that (3) and (5) will emphasize small scores and thus decrease the mean fused score. In Fig. 2(b), the right vertical line represents the mean of client scores and the left vertical line the mean of impostor scores. We can notice that both the mean of the fused client scores and that of the fused imposter scores decrease when the prior score $\tilde{\mu}_p$ is greater than the respective mean, i.e. $\tilde{\mu}_p > 1.0$ for the client and $\tilde{\mu}_p > -1.0$ for the impostor. Similarly, when $\mu > \tilde{\mu}_p$ (i.e. most of the scores are larger than the prior score $\tilde{\mu}_p$), the fusion weights for small scores $\alpha_t^{(1)}$ decrease when $s_t^{(1)}$ decreases and the fusion weights for large scores $\alpha_t^{(2)}$ increase when $s_t^{(2)}$ increases. As a result, the proposed fusion algorithm ((3) and (5)) favors larger scores only when $\mu > \tilde{\mu}_p$, which has the effect of increasing the mean fused scores. We can also notice from Fig. 2(b) that both the mean of the fused client scores and that of the fused imposter scores increase when the prior score $\tilde{\mu}_p$ is smaller than the respective mean, i.e. $\tilde{\mu}_p < 1.0$ for the client and $\tilde{\mu}_p < -1.0$ for the impostor. Finally, when $\mu = \tilde{\mu}_p$, the proposed fusion approach will be equivalent to equal-weight fusion. This can be observed from Fig. 2(b) where the fused mean scores are equal to $\tilde{\mu}_p$'s, i.e. $\tilde{\mu}_p = 1.0$ for the client and $\tilde{\mu}_p = -1.0$ for the impostor. The curves intersect each other when the prior score $\tilde{\mu}_p$ is equal to the mean of impostor scores. This suggests that the mean of fused scores is equal regardless of the fusion algorithm used.

To conclude, our fusion algorithm will either increase or decrease the mean of fused scores depending on the value of the prior score $\tilde{\mu}_p$ and the score mean μ before fusion. We can observe from Fig. 2(b) that when the prior score is set between the means of client scores and impostor scores (i.e. between the two vertical lines), theoretically the mean of fused client scores increases and the mean of fused impostor scores decreases. This has the effect of increasing the difference between the means of fused client scores and that of the fused impostor scores, as demonstrated in Fig. 2(c). As the mean of fused scores is used to make the final decision, increasing the score dispersion can decrease the speaker verification error rate.

2.5 Comparison between Fusion of Sorted and Unsorted Scores

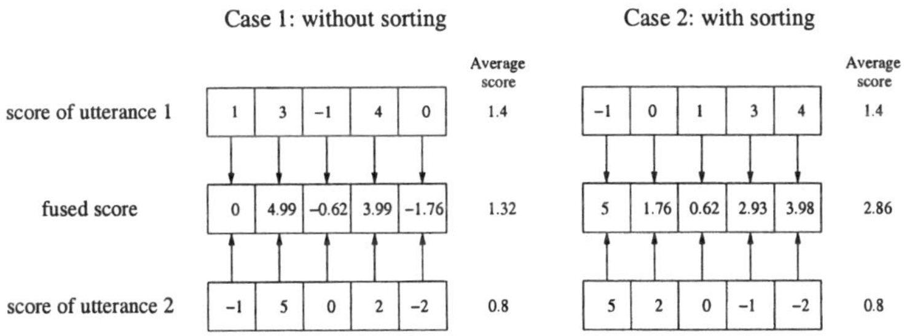

Fig. 5. Fused scores derived from unsorted (left figure) and sorted (right figure) score sequences obtained from a client speaker. Here we assume $\tilde{\mu}_p = 0$ and $\tilde{\sigma}_p^2 = 1$ in (5).

In the previous subsection, we have argued that the fusion of sorted score sequences increases the score dispersion. Here, we compare the fusion of unsorted scores with the fusion of sorted scores in terms of verification performance. Fig. 5 shows a hypothetical situation in which the scores were obtained from two client utterances. For client utterances, we would prefer (5) to favor large scores and de-emphasize small scores. However, Case 1 in Fig. 5 clearly shows that the fifth score (-2, which is very small) in utterance 2 is emphasized by a relatively larger score in utterance 1. This is because the fifth score of utterance 1 is identical to the prior score ($\tilde{\mu}_p = 0$), which makes the fused score dominated by the fifth score of utterance 2. The influence of these extremely small client scores on the final mean fused score can be reduced by sorting the scores of the two utterances in opposite order before fusion such that small scores will always be fused with large scores. With this arrangement, the contribution of some extremely small client scores in one utterance can be compensated by the large scores of another utterance. As a result, the mean of the fused client scores will be increased. Fig. 5 shows that the mean of fused scores increases from 1.32 to 2.86 after sorting the scores. Likewise, if this sorting approach is applied to the scores of impostor utterances with a proper prior score $\tilde{\mu}_p$ (i.e. greater than the mean of impostor scores, see Fig. 2(b)), the contribution of some extremely large impostor scores in one utterance can be greatly reduced by the small scores in another utterance, which has the net effect of minimizing the mean of the fused impostor scores. Therefore, this score sorting approach can further increase the dispersion between client scores and impostor scores, resulting in a lower error rate. This is demonstrated in Fig. 2(c) where the score dispersion achieved by data-dependent fusion with score sorting is significantly larger than that without score sorting.

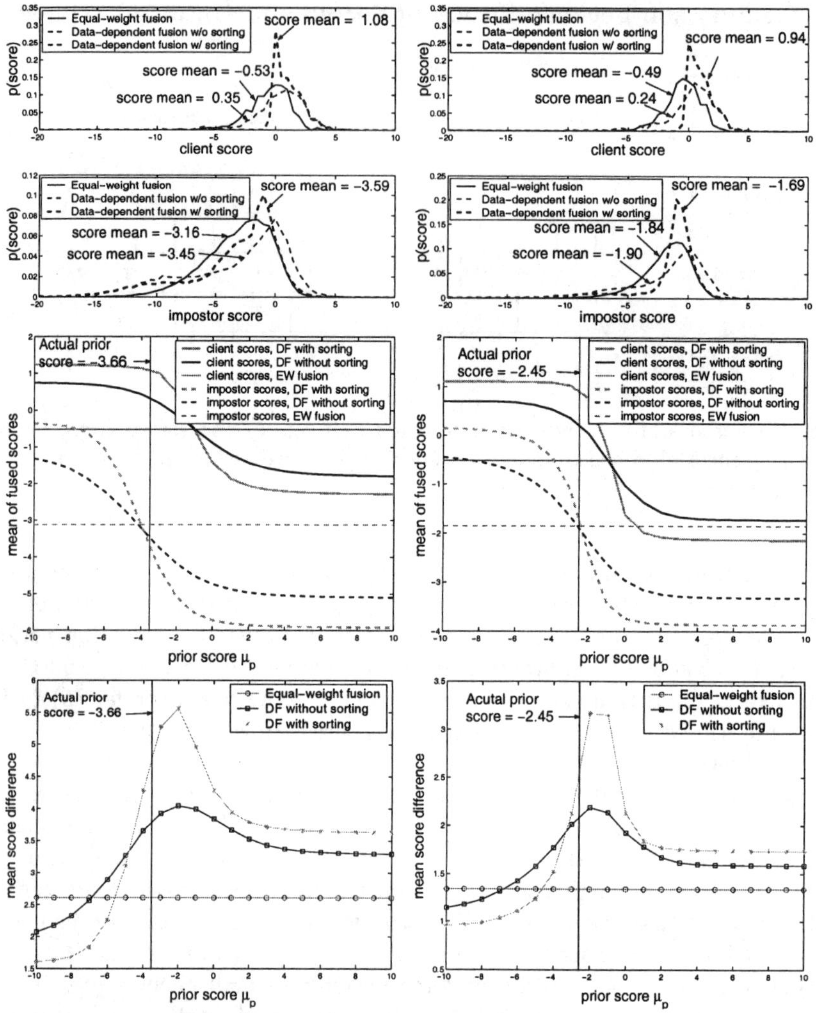

(a) From client speaker "mdac0" (b) From client speaker "faem0"

Fig. 6. Distributions of pattern-by-pattern client scores (figures in the first row) and impostor scores (figures in the second row), the mean of fused client scores and the mean of fused impostor scores (figures in the third row), and difference between the mean of fused client scores and the mean of fused impostor scores (figures in the fourth row) based on equal-weight fusion (score averaging) and data-dependent fusion with and without score sorting. The means of speaker scores and impostor scores obtained by both fusion approaches are also shown.

To further demonstrate this phenomenon, we select two client speakers (faem0 and mdac0) from the HTIMIT corpus [9] and plot the distributions of the fused speaker scores and fused impostor scores in Fig. 6. In (4), we use the overall mean $\tilde{\mu}_p$ as the prior score. However, as the number of background speakers' utterances is usually much larger than that of client speaker's utterances during the training phase, the overall mean is very close to the mean score of background speakers, i.e. $\tilde{\mu}_p \approx \tilde{\mu}_b$. According to Fig. 2(b) and the third row of Fig. 6, when $\tilde{\mu}_p \approx \tilde{\mu}_b$, the mean of fused impostor scores are almost identical regardless of the fusion algorithm used. However, the same $\tilde{\mu}_p$ will increase the mean of fused client scores significantly, especially when the client scores were sorted before fusion.

Fig. 6(a) shows that the mean of client scores increases from 0.35 to 1.08 and the mean of impostor scores decreases from -3.45 to -3.59 after sorting the score sequences.[4] Therefore, the dispersion between the mean client score and the mean impostor score increases from 3.80 to 4.67. We can notice from Fig. 6(b) that both the mean of client scores and the mean of impostor scores increase. This is because the means of impostor scores obtained from verification utterances are greater than the prior score $\tilde{\mu}_p$. This results in the increase of the mean of fused impostor scores. However, as the increase in the mean client scores is still greater than the increase in the mean impostor scores, there is still a net increase in the score dispersion. Specifically, the dispersion in Fig. 6(b) increases from $2.14 (= 0.24 - (-1.90))$ to $2.63 (= 0.94 - (-1.69))$. As verification decision is based on the mean scores, the wider the dispersion between the mean client scores and the mean impostor scores, the lower the error rate.

3 Speaker Verification Experiments

The proposed fusion algorithm was applied to telephone-based speaker verification. We used a GSM speech codec to transcode the HTIMIT corpus [9] and applied the resulting transcoded speech in a speaker verification experiment similar to [10] and [11]. HTIMIT was obtained by playing a subset of the TIMIT corpus through 9 different telephone handsets and one Sennheizer head-mounted microphone. Speakers in the corpus were divided into a speaker set (50 male and 50 female) and an impostor set (25 male and 25 female).

Sequences of 12th order MFCCs were extracted from 28ms speech frames of uncoded and GSM-transcoded utterances at a frame rate of 71 Hz. During enrollment, we used the SA and SX utterances from handset "senh" of the uncoded HTIMIT to create a 32-center GMM for each speaker. A 64-center universal background GMM [12] was also created based on the speech of 100

---

[4]The decrease in the mean of fused impostor scores is due to the fact that the prior score $\tilde{\mu}_p$ is greater than the mean of the un-fused impostor scores, see fourth row of Fig. 6(a).

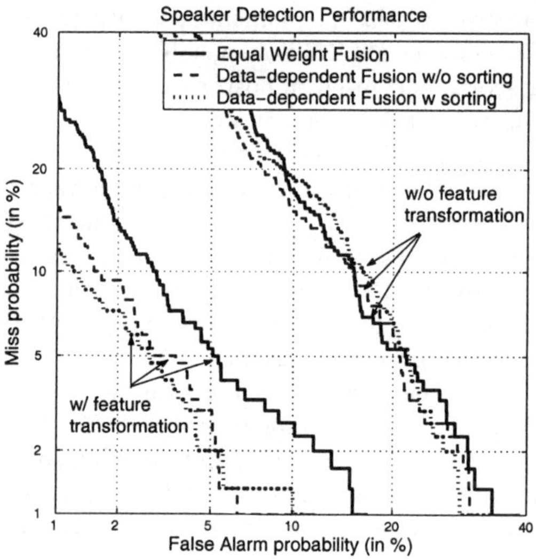

Fig. 7. DET curves for equal-weight fusion (score averaging) and data-dependent fusion with and without score sorting. The curves were obtained by using the utterances of handset "cb1" as verification speech.

client speakers recorded from handset "senh". The background model was shared among all client speakers in all verification sessions.

For verification, we used the GSM-transcoded speech from all ten handsets in HTIMIT. As a result, there were handset- and coder- mismatches between speaker models and verification utterances. We used stochastic feature transformation with handset identification [10][13] to compensate the mismatches. We assumed that a claimant will be asked to utter two sentences during a verification session. Therefore, for each client speaker and each impostor, we applied the proposed fusion algorithm to fuse two independent streams of scores obtained from his/her SI sentences. As the fusion algorithm requires the two utterances to have an identical number of feature vectors (length), we computed the average length of the two utterances and appended the extra patterns in the longer utterance to the end of the shorter utterance. Then, we sorted the score sequences in opposite order and fused the sorted scores according to (3) and (5).

Fig. 7 depicts the detection error trade-off curves [14] based on 100 client speakers and 50 impostors using utterances from handset "cb1" for verification. Fig. 7 clearly shows that with feature transformation, data-dependent fusion is able to reduce the error rate significantly, and sorting the scores before fusion can reduce the error rate further. However, without feature transformation, the performance of data-dependent fusion with score sorting is not significantly better than that of equal-weight fusion. This is caused by the mismatch between the prior scores $\tilde{\mu}_p$'s in (5) and the scores of the distorted features. Therefore, it is very important to use feature transformation to reduce the mismatch between the enrollment data and verification data.

Fig. 8 shows the detection error trade-off curves based on 100 client speakers and 50 impostors using all the scores from ten handsets. It shows that data-dependent fusion with score sorting outperforms equal-weight fusion for all operating points and by 23% in terms of equal error rate.

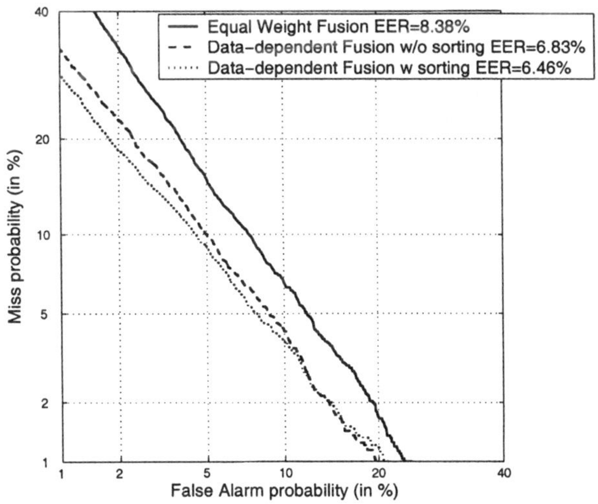

Fig. 8. DET curves for equal-weight fusion (score averaging) and data-dependent fusion with and without score sorting. The curves were obtained by concatenating the scores from ten handsets.

Table 1 shows the speaker detection performance of 100 speakers and 50 impostors for the equal-weight fusion approach and the proposed fusion approach with and without sorting the score sequences. Table 1 clearly shows that our proposed fusion approach outperforms the equal-weight fusion. In particular, after the score sequences have been sorted, the equal error rate is further reduced.

4 Conclusions

We have presented a decision fusion algorithm that makes use of prior score statistics and the distribution of the recognition data. The fusion algorithm was combined with feature transformation for speaker verification using GSM-transcoded speech. Results show that the proposed fusion algorithm outperforms equal-weight fusion. It was also found that performance can be further improved by the fusion of sorted scores.

Table 1. Equal error rates achieved by different fusion approaches, using utterances from 10 different handsets for verification. Each figure is based on the average of 100 speakers, each impersonated by 50 impostors. DF stands for data-dependent fusion. "No fusion" means the verification results were obtained from using single utterance per verification session. "average" is the average EER of 10 handsets.

	Equal Error Rate (%)										
Fusion Method	cb1	cb2	cb3	cb4	el1	el2	el3	el4	pt1	senh	**average**
No fusion	6.31	6.36	19.96	15.35	5.89	10.83	11.79	8.18	9.38	4.90	**9.90**
Equal-weight fusion	5.11	4.33	19.15	12.89	4.42	8.31	9.96	6.29	7.57	2.99	**8.10**
DF w/o sorting	4.01	3.27	15.92	10.55	3.04	6.51	8.67	4.75	7.51	2.32	**6.67**
DF w/ sorting	3.60	2.86	15.30	9.91	3.49	4.65	6.81	4.02	6.59	1.99	**5.92**

5 Acknowledgement

This work was supported by the Hong Kong Polytechnic University Grant No. G-T860 and HKSAR RGC Project No. PolyU 5131/02E.

References

1. Wark, T., Sridharan, S. (2001) Adaptive fusion of speech and lip information for robust speaker identification. Digital Signal Processing, vol. 11, pp. 169–186
2. Jourlin, P., Luettin, J., Genoud, D., Wassner, H. (1997) Acoustic-labial speaker verification. Pattern recognition letters, vol. 18, no. 9, pp. 853–858
3. Kittler, J., Hatef, M., Duin, R.P.W., Matas, J. (1998) On combining classifiers. IEEE Trans. on Pattern Anal. Machine Intell., vol. 20, no. 3, pp. 226–239
4. Sanderson, C., Paliwal, K. K. (2001) Joint cohort normalization in a multi-feature speaker verification system. The 10th IEEE International Conference on Fuzzy Systems 2001, vol. 1, pp. 232–235
5. Poh, N., Bengio, S., Korczak, J. (2002) A multi-sample multi-source model for biometric authentication. Proc. IEEE 12th Workshop on Neural Networks for Signal Processing, pp. 375–384
6. Mak, M.W., Cheung, M.C., Kung, S.Y. (2003) Robust speaker verification from GSM-transcoded speech based on decision fusion and feature transformation. Proc. IEEE ICASSP'03, pp. II745–II748
7. Cheung, M.C., Mak, M.W., Kung, S.Y. (2003) Adaptive decision fusion for multi-sample speaker verification over GSM networks. Eurospeech'03, pp. 1681–1684
8. Cheung, M.C., Mak, M.W., Kung, S.Y. (2004) Multi-sample data-dependent fusion of sorted score sequences for biometric verification. Proc. IEEE ICASSP04, pp. V681–V684
9. Reynolds, D.A. (1997) HTIMIT and LLHDB: speech corpora for the study of handset transducer effects. Proc. IEEE ICASSP'97, pp. II1535–II1538
10. Mak, M.W., Kung, S.Y. (2002) Combining stochastic feature transformation and handset identification for telephone-based speaker verification. Proc. IEEE ICASSP'2002, pp. I701–I704

11. Yu, W.M., Mak, M.W., Kung, S.Y. (2002) Speaker verification from coded telephone speech using stochastic feature transformation and handset identification. The 3rd IEEE Pacific-Rim Conference on Multimedia 2002, pp. 598–606.
12. Reynolds, D.A., Quatieri, T.F., Dunn, R.B. (2000) Speaker verification using adapted gaussian mixture models. Digital Signal Processing, vol. 10, pp. 19–41
13. Tsang, C.L., Mak, M.W., Kung, S.Y. (2002) Divergence-based out-of-class rejection for telephone handset identification. Proc. ICSLP'02, pp. 2329–2332
14. Martin, A., Doddington, G., Kamm, T., Ordowski, M., Przybocki, M. (1997) The DET curve in assessment of detection task performance. Proc. Eurospeech '97, pp. 1895–1898

Adaptive Noise Cancellation Using Online Self-Enhanced Fuzzy Filters with Applications to Multimedia Processing

Meng Joo Er[1] and Zhengrong Li[2]

[1] Intelligent Systems Centre, 50, Nanyang Drive, 7th Storey, Research TechnoPlaza, BorderX Block, Singapore 637533
Email: emjer@ntu.edu.sg
[2] Computer Control Laboratory, School of of Electrical and Electronic Engineering, Block S1, Nanyang Avenue 50, Nanyang Technological University, Singapore 639798
Email: lizhengrong@pmail.ntu.edu.sg

Abstract. Adaptive noise cancellation is a significant research issue in multimedia signal processing, which is a widely used technique in teleconference systems, hands-free mobile communications, acoustical echo and feedback cancellation and so on. For the purpose of implementing real-time applications in nonlinear environments, an online self-enhanced fuzzy filter for solving adaptive noise cancellation is proposed. The proposed online self-enhanced fuzzy filter is based on radial-basis-function networks and functionally is equivalent to the Takagi-Sugeno-Kang fuzzy system. As a prominent feature of the online self-enhanced fuzzy filter, the system is hierarchically constructed and self-enhanced during the training process using a novel online clustering strategy for structure identification. In the process of system construction, instead of selecting the centers and widths of membership functions arbitrarily, an online clustering method is applied to ensure reasonable representation of input terms. It not only ensures proper feature representation, but also optimizes the structure of the filter by reducing the number of fuzzy rules. Moreover, the filter is adaptively tuned to be optimal by the proposed hybrid sequential algorithm for parameters determination. Due to online self-enhanced system construction and hybrid learning algorithm, low computation load and less memory requirements are achieved. This is beneficial for applications in real-time multimedia signal processing.

Keywords: adaptive noise cancellation, self-enhanced, fuzzy filter

1 Introduction

Signals are usually corrupted by noise in the real world. How to extract the true information signal from its corrupted signal or reduce the influence of noise is one of the challenging problems in the research area of signal processing.

One of the common and frequently used methods is to pass the noisy signal to a filter which is used to suppress the noise and to recover the original signal. There are many approaches to achieve the objective of noise cancellation or noise suppression. In the context of filters, frequency-selective filters such as band-pass and band-limited filters with fixed structure and parameters are widely employed. In the aforementioned cases, the signal and noise occupy fixed and separate frequency bands so that the conventional frequency-selective filters can work well. However, in the case where the spectrum of the noise overlaps with the original signal, or in the situation where there is no *a priori* knowledge about the noise, the frequency-selective filters with fixed structure and parameters can no longer be employed.

Adaptive filtering is an effective way of solving the aforementioned problems which the conventional filter cannot handle. It has achieved widespread applications and success in many areas such as control, image processing, and communications [1]. Among various adaptive filters, adaptive linear filters are the most widely used and can be easily analyzed and implemented due to low hardware requirements and their inherent properties, like convergence, global minimum, misadjustment errors and simple training algorithms [2]. There is no doubt that adaptive filters can be employed to track and cancel nonlinear noise distortion but only for the cases where the nonlinearity is mild or the operating point changes relatively slowly [3]. These restrictions make it difficult to apply adaptive linear filters in highly nonlinear environments. Otherwise, the system performance is degraded. Therefore, the development of adaptive nonlinear filters is necessary and desirable.

With the development of neural networks and fuzzy systems, a lot of attention has been focused on employing them in signal processing. Actually, neural networks and fuzzy systems share lots of features and characteristics in common [4]. Those include distributed representation of knowledge, model-free estimators, fault tolerance capability and handling of uncertainties and imprecision. Also, neural networks and fuzzy systems are universal nonlinear approximators [5, 6]. They can approximate any linear or nonlinear function to any prescribed accuracy if sufficient hidden neurons or fuzzy rules are available. As a matter of fact, introducing neural networks and fuzzy systems into signal processing brings about a new way of designing adaptive nonlinear filters.

The key idea of fusing neural networks and fuzzy systems is that an neural networks-based filter can be made adaptive by virtue of the learning ability of neural networks. As a matter of fact, many common points exist in the methods used by adaptive noise filtering and neural networks. One significant common point is that both of them have the property of adaptive linear combiners. Also, the most widely used backpropagation algorithm for neural networks training is essentially a generalized Widrow's Least Mean Square (LMS) algorithm and can be contrasted with the LMS algorithm usually used in adaptive filtering. Thanks to the powerful learning and generalization abilities, neural networks have become an attractive approach in adaptive signal processing [7, 8]. However, it is not easy to determine the structure of neural networks because the internal layers of neural networks are opaque to users. Another shortcoming of neural networks-based filters is that repeated backpropagation or backpropagation-like learning cycles must be performed and the computation time will be very long. At the same time, practical applications of expert knowledge, which is normally expressed by linguistic information to solve real-world problems, has received increasing attention. To utilize those information expressed in linguistic terms, fuzzy logic was developed as an essential approach to represent, manipulate and process uncertain information.

A promising approach of reaping both the benefits of neural networks and fuzzy systems and solving their respective problems is to combine them into an integrated system termed fuzzy neural networks. With the synergy of neural networks and fuzzy systems, the fuzzy neural networks inherit the advantages of neural networks and fuzzy systems such as global approximation and nonlinear mapping. Recently, many fuzzy neural networks have been developed for applications in system identification, prediction and function approximation. Actually, it can be employed as a powerful approach of designing nonlinear filters.

The initial concept of adaptive noise cancellation is investigated in [9] by B. Widrow and et al. Up to now, many techniques based on the principle of adaptive noise cancellation have been investigated for applications in multimedia signal processing such as speech enhancement in communications, hands-free mobile communications, acoustical echo and feedback cancellation, etc. The principle of adaptive noise cancellation is concerned with the enhancement of noise-corrupted signals and is based upon the availability of a primary input source and an auxiliary (reference) input source located in the noise field. Fig. 1 illustrates the schematic diagram of an adaptive noise cancellation system.

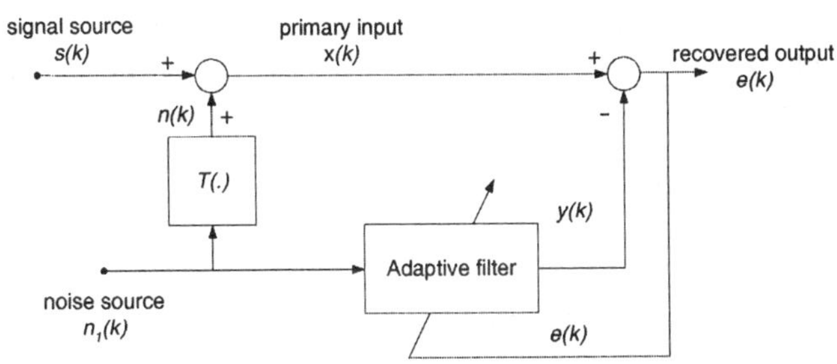

Fig. 1. Adaptive noise cancellation system

In Fig. 1, the primary input source contains the desired signal s, which is corrupted by the noise n generated from the noise source n_1. The received signal is thus given by

$$x(k) = s(k) + n(k) \tag{1}$$

The secondary or auxiliary (reference) input source receives the noise n_1, which is correlated with the corrupting noise n. The transfer function $T(.)$ represents the nonlinear dynamics of the channel between n and n_1. The principle of adaptive noise cancellation is to adaptively process (by adjusting the filter's weights) the reference noise n_1 to generate a replica of n and then subtract the replica of n from the primary input x to recover the desired signal s. The adaptive filter output, which is the replica of n, is denoted by the process y. It is assumed that s, n and n_1 are stationary zero-mean processes, s is uncorrelated with n and n_1, and n and n_1 are correlated. From Fig. 1, we have

$$e(k) = s(k) + n(k) - y(k) \tag{2}$$

Squaring and taking expectation on both sides gives

$$E[e^2(k)] = E[s^2(k)] + E[(n(k) - y(k))^2] \tag{3}$$

The objective of adaptive noise cancellation is to minimize $E[(n(k) - y(k))^2]$. From Eq.(3), it is obvious that the objective is equivalent to minimizing $E[e^2(k)]$ and when $E[(n(k) - y(k))^2] = E[(n(k) - F(n_1(k)))^2]$ approaches zero, the remaining error $e(k)$ is, in fact, the desired signal $s(k)$, where $F(.)$ represents the dynamics of the nonlinear adaptive filter.

Essentially, adaptive noise cancellation can be considered as a system identification problem [10], that is, identifying the channel dynamics $T(.)$ by using an adaptive filter that is characterized by $F(.)$. Obviously, adaptive linear filters are not feasible if the characteristics of the transmission path, $T(.)$, are highly nonlinear. Otherwise, the slightest error could result in increased output noise power which will lead to performance degradation. Therefore, adaptive nonlinear filters are desirable in this case. Based on the fact that the fuzzy neural networks-based approaches are global and nonlinear, we investigated some fuzzy neural networks-based approaches to solve the adaptive noise cancellation problem with high performance.

2 Online Self-enhanced Fuzzy Filters

2.1 Background

To design an adaptive nonlinear filter, online processing ability and nonlinearity, which are widely investigated problems in the research area of signal processing, are significant for real-time applications such as control, image processing, and communications [1], [2].

With the development of neural networks and fuzzy systems and based on the fact that both of them are global nonlinear approximators, many new approaches of designing adaptive nonlinear filters have been proposed. Thanks to the powerful learning and generalization abilities, neural networks have become an attractive approach in adaptive signal processing [11–13]. However, it is not easy to determine the structure of neural networks because the internal layers of neural networks are opaque to users. fuzzy systems provide an approach of representing the systems to be nonlinear approximators so that they can be understood by users because the rule base is constructed by linguistic IF-THEN rules. However, the difficulty of extracting fuzzy rules from numerical input-output pairs limits its applications. A promising approach of reaping both the benefits of neural networks and fuzzy systems and solving their respective problems is to combine them into an integrated system termed fuzzy neural networks. The technical basis and the integration of fuzzy neural networks are discussed in [4] and [14] in details. Many fuzzy neural networks approaches have been developed for applications in system identification, prediction and function approximation [15–17].

Two central issues of the fuzzy neural networks-based approaches are structure identification and parameters determination (optimization). For most fuzzy neural networks-based approaches, pre-clustering of the data space and backpropagation or backpropagation-like algorithms are employed for structure identification and parameters determination respectively. It needs to collect the training data in advance so that batch training mode is possible. This makes real-time applications difficult. In [14], an adaptive-network-based fuzzy inference system is investigated. This approach implements structure identification by fuzzy pre-clustering of the data space which means *a priori* knowledge about input signals is a prerequisite. A recurrent self-organizing neural fuzzy inference network is investigated in [18]. In the approach, data space is partitioned by an aligned clustering method and fuzzy rules are constructed during online learning. The aligned clustering method reduces the number of membership functions, but cannot ensure the aligned clusters coincide with real data distribution. Moreover, the centers are allocated initially and optimized by a Gradient-Descent(GD)-based algorithm when a new fuzzy rule is generated. Usually, the arbitrarily allocated centers, although optimized during the training process, are not the final centers of clusters in the sense of data distribution. Similar methods, whose main idea is to generate the system structure hierarchically and fix it after training, are proposed in [16,19,20]. Recently, many fuzzy neural networks systems based on Radial-Basis-Function Networks (RBFN) have been proposed in [21–23]. In [21], a modified hierarchical method, which is based on the hierarchically self-organizing learning algorithm proposed in [22] for RBFN, is developed for adaptive fuzzy systems. Unfortunately, the algorithm is essentially offline and all parameters are trained by the GD algorithm that leads to heavy computation load and slow convergence. Recurrent Radial Basis Function Networks (RRBFN) are proposed for adaptive noise cancellation in [3]. In [3], the k-means clustering algorithm, which is only suitable for batch learning, is employed to allocate the centers for structure identification. In [23], a sequential algorithm to implement the Minimal Resource Allocation Networks (M-RAN) is discussed. The sequential algorithm is capable of dealing with real-time applications, but the past observations over a sliding window must be stored in order to generate the hidden neurons. This violates the principle of parallel computation. Its performance is evaluated in [24] and [25]. In [26] and [27], an approach of dynamic fuzzy neural networks with adjustable structure are proposed for applications in function approximation, system identification and prediction. However, in order to determine free parameters in the consequent parts and adjust the structure dynamically, all past training data must be stored and heavy memory and computation load are unavoidable. It will be a problem to apply this approach in real-time applications and realize online filtering. In summary, there are two main types of training algorithm to optimize free parameters for the RBFN-based systems. One is to optimize all free parameters in premise and consequent parts by the GD or GD-like algorithms. Its disadvantage is that it needs heavy and repeated computation and is not suitable for online learning. In other words, it can work with deterministic problems well, but not stochastic problems. Another typical algorithm employs a forward pass to train parameters in the consequent parts by some linear regression methods and a backward pass to tune parameters in the premise parts by the GD-like methods. In this case, the change of second-order statistics of linear regression models in consequent parts, which is caused by the change of free parameters in hidden neurons in the premise parts, will lead to slow convergence and performance degradation.

In order to facilitate online implementation and realize real-time applications under the constraint of low system resource requirements, an online self-enhanced fuzzy filter, which is functionally equivalent to the Takagi-Sugeno-Kang (TSK) inference system, is proposed in this chapter. A prominent feature of the online self-enhanced fuzzy filter is that the system is hierarchically constructed and self-enhanced employing a novel online clustering strategy for structure identification during the training process. Moreover, the filter is adaptively tuned to be optimal by the proposed hybrid sequential algorithm for parameters determination. In detail, the proposed algorithm has the following salient features: (1) Hierarchical structure for self-construction. There is no predetermination initially for the online self-enhanced fuzzy filter, i.e., it is not necessary to determine the initial number of fuzzy rules and input space clustering in advance. The fuzzy rules, i.e., the Radial Basis Function (RBF) neurons are generated automatically during the training process using the minimum firing strength criterion. (2) Online clustering. Instead of selecting the centers and widths of membership functions arbitrarily, an online clustering method is applied to ensure reasonable representation of an input variable. It not only ensures proper feature representation, but also optimizes the structure of the filter by reducing the number of fuzzy rules. (3) All free parameters in the premise and consequent parts are determined online by a hybrid sequential algorithm without repeated computation so as to facilitate real-time applications. The centers and widths of membership functions of an input variable are allocated initially in the scheme of structure identification and optimized in the scheme of parameters determination. The parameters in the consequent parts of the online self enhanced fuzzy filter are updated in each iteration by a sequential recursive algorithm. Due to the hybrid sequential algorithm, low computation and less memory are required. Simulation results, compared with other similar approaches for some benchmark problems, show that the proposed adaptive filter can tackle these problems with fewer fuzzy rules and achieve better or similar accuracy with lower system resource requirements.

2.2 Structure of Online Self-enhanced Fuzzy Filters

The adaptive RBFN-based filter which is functionally equivalent to a TSK inference system is depicted in Fig. 2.

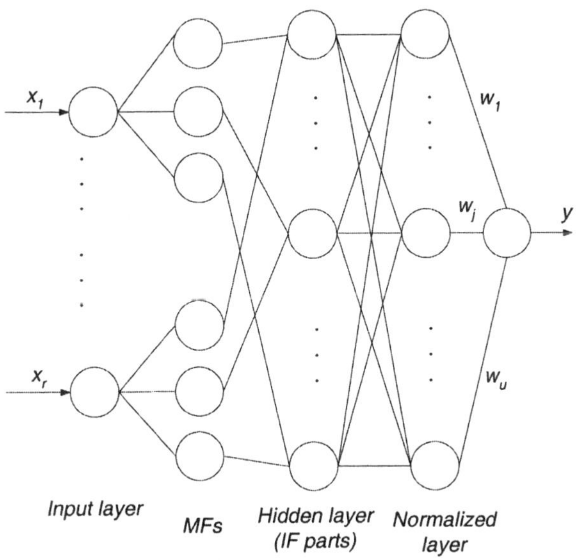

Fig. 2. Structure of the adaptive RBFN-based filter

The functions of the various nodes in each of the five layers are described here:

Layer 1: Each node in layer 1 is an input node. These nodes simply transmit input signals to the next layer directly. In this layer, we have:

$$X = [x_1, x_2, ..., x_r]^T \tag{4}$$

where r is the number of input variables in the RBFN-based filter.

Layer 2: Nodes in this layer stand for input terms of the input variables. In this layer, each input variable is characterized by

$$A_i = [a_{i1}, a_{i2}, ..., a_{iu}] \quad i = 1, 2, ...r \tag{5}$$

where A_i is the term set of the ith input variable, and a_{ij} is a fuzzy number with a one-dimensional membership function which is a Gaussian function of the following form:

$$\mu_{ij}(x_i) = exp[-\frac{(x_i - c_{ij})^2}{\sigma_j^2}] \quad j = 1, 2, ...u \tag{6}$$

where u is the number of input terms of each input variable, c_{ij} is the center of the jth Gaussian membership function of x_i and σ_j is the width of the jth Gaussian membership function of x_i.

Layer 3: Each node in layer 3 represents a possible IF-part for a fuzzy IF-THEN rule. The number of fuzzy rules in this system is exactly the number of RBF neurons. For the jth fuzzy rule R_j, its firing strength is given by

$$\begin{aligned} \phi_j &= \prod_{i=1}^{r} \mu_{ij}(x_i) \\ &= exp[-\frac{\sum_{i=1}^{r}(x_i - c_{ij})^2}{\sigma_j^2}] \\ &= exp[-\frac{\| X - C_j \|^2}{\sigma_j^2}] \end{aligned} \tag{7}$$

where $C_j = [c_{1j}, c_{2j}, ..., c_{rj}]$.

Layer 4: Nodes in this layer are called normalized nodes. The number of normalized nodes is equal to that of RBF neurons. The output of the normalized nodes is given by

$$\begin{aligned} \psi_j &= \frac{\phi_j}{\sum_{j=1}^{u} \phi_j} \\ &= \frac{exp[-\frac{\|X - C_j\|^2}{\sigma_j^2}]}{\sum_{j=1}^{u} exp[-\frac{\|X - C_j\|^2}{\sigma_j^2}]} \end{aligned} \tag{8}$$

The nodes in layer 4 are fully connected with the nodes in layer 3 for normalization.

Layer 5: Each node in this layer represents an output variable which is the summation of incoming signals from layer 4. Its output is given by

$$y = \sum_{j=1}^{u} w_j.\psi_j$$
$$= \frac{\sum_{j=1}^{u} w_j exp[-\frac{\|X-C_j\|]^2}{\sigma_j^2}]}{\sum_{j=1}^{u} exp[-\frac{\|X-C_j\|^2}{\sigma_j^2}]} \tag{9}$$

where y is the value of the output variable and w_k is essentially the consequent part of each rule.

In a TSK fuzzy inference system implemented by the online self-enhanced fuzzy filter, the fuzzy rule base contains a set of fuzzy logic rules R. For the jth fuzzy rule R_j, we have

$$R_j : IF\ (x_1\ is\ a_{1j}\ and\ x_2\ is\ a_{2j}\ ...\ x_r\ is\ a_{rj})\ \ THEN\ (y\ is\ w_j)$$

For the consequent part, the inferred output of the jth fuzzy rule is given by

$$w_j = t_{j0} + t_{j1}x_1 + ... + t_{jr}x_r \tag{10}$$

where $j = 1, 2, ...u$. The parameters $t_{j0}, t_{j1}, ...t_{jr}$ are free parameters of the jth fuzzy rule.

We rewrite Eqs.(9) and (10) in the following matrix form:

$$y = \sum_{j=1}^{u} w_j(t_{j0}, t_{j1}, ..., t_{jr}; X)\psi_j(C_j, \sigma_j, X) \tag{11}$$

From Eq.(11), it is apparent that the output of the RBFN-based online self-enhanced fuzzy filter y is a nonlinear function of the input X and the filter works as a nonlinear Finite Impulse Response (FIR) filter which means it is inherently stable and can tackle the nonlinear filtering problem. Moreover, the filter is a TSK fuzzy system and the fuzzy rules can be extracted from numerical input/output pairs after training.

From Fig. 2 and the detailed functions of the nodes, it can be deduced that the following conditions hold in order to make the online self-enhanced fuzzy filter equivalent to a TSK fuzzy inference system.

1. From the viewpoint of a TSK fuzzy system, the number of linguistic terms of each input variable, i.e., the number of membership functions, is equal to the number of RBF neurons.
2. Every RBF neuron stands for a fuzzy logic rule.
3. For the RBF neurons, no bias is considered.
4. The inferred output of each fuzzy rule is a first-order linear function, i.e., the fuzzy inference system is Sugeno type of [28].

2.3 Hybrid Algorithm for Structure Identification and Parameters Determination

The online learning algorithm consists of two main parts, namely structure identification and parameters determination. In structure identification, new RBF neurons are generated under the criterion of minimum firing strength and the input space is automatically partitioned into the receptive fields of the corresponding RBF units. Furthermore, online clustering, which is a kind of fuzzy clustering method, is utilized to adjust the centers and widths of membership functions and to partition the input space according to data distribution. Parameters determination involves optimization of parameters in the premise parts and determination of free parameters in the consequent parts.

Generation of RBF Neurons

Many fuzzy neural networks-based approaches implement structure identification (construction) under the criterion of system errors. In essence, new hidden neurons (RBF neurons for those RBFN-based approaches) will be generated when the system error exceeds a predefined threshold. However, the system error cannot be used to evaluate whether new hidden neurons are needed in some cases such as adaptive noise cancellation. Based on the fact that the hidden neurons of neural networks essentially perform nonlinear mapping for input signals, a new criterion is proposed here to generate new hidden neurons (or fuzzy rules in the sense of fuzzy inference systems). Geometrically, in RBFN, an RBF neuron corresponds to a cluster in the input space with C_j and σ_j representing the centers and variance of those clusters. For each incoming pattern X, the firing strength $\phi_j(\phi_j \in [0,1])$, which is computed by Eq.(7), can be interpreted as the degree that the incoming pattern belongs to the corresponding receptive field. From the viewpoint of fuzzy rules, a fuzzy rule is a local representation over a region defined in the input space. It is reasonable to use the firing strength as a criterion to generate new rules to make sure that every pattern can be represented in sufficient match degree by one rule or a few rules. In view of this, the minimum firing strength criterion is proposed here.

The main idea of the minimum firing strength criterion is the following: For any input in the operating range, there exists at least one RBF neuron (fuzzy rule) so that the match degree (firing strength) is greater than a predefined constant, that is, the value of the minimum firing strength. Superior to the other model selection approaches such as Akaike information criteria and Bayesian information criteria, it is no necessary to provide the number of parameters estimated in the model in advance when applying the proposed minimum firing strength criterion.

Using the firing strength measure, the following criterion of generating RBF neurons is obtained. For any newly arrived patterns, the firing strengths of existing RBF neurons (fuzzy rules) are calculated by Eq.(7) and we find

$$J = arg(\ max(\phi_j)) \tag{12}$$

where $j = 1...u$, and u is the number of existing rules. If $\phi_J \leq F_{gen}$, which means that there are no rules to meet the minimum firing strength criterion, a new RBF neuron is generated, where $F_{gen}(F_{gen} \in [0,1])$ is a prespecified threshold whose value increases during the learning process. This is the concept of "Hierarchical Learning" [22]. The main idea is that F_{gen}, which underpins the criterion of rules generation, is not fixed but adjusted dynamically. Initially, F_{gen} is set small for achieving rough but global representation. Then, it gradually increases for fine learning. It is given by

$$F_{gen} = min[F_{min} \times \delta^{-j}, F_{max}] \tag{13}$$

where $\delta(\delta \in (0,1))$ is the decay constant, and j is the number of existing RBF neurons.

Allocation of RBF Units and Online Clustering

The centers and widths for a new RBF neuron are allocated after it is generated. In contrast with other fuzzy neural networks-based approaches where the centers and widths are allocated arbitrarily and optimized by the GD method, in our proposed online self-enhanced fuzzy filter, the centers and widths are allocated initially to construct the system, adjusted using the scheme of online clustering to partition the input space and then optimized using the scheme of parameters determination.

Allocation of RBF Units

In the sense of neural networks, the width of an RBF unit is significant for its generalization. If the width is less than the distance between adjacent inputs which means underlapping, the RBF neuron does not generalize well. However, if the width is too large, the output of the RBF neuron may always be large (near 1.0) irrespective of inputs and the partition will make no sense in this case.Therefore, the width must be carefully selected so as to ensure proper and sufficient degree of overlapping.

Due to the fact that the centers will be adjusted by online clustering and optimized using the scheme of parameters determination, when a new RBF neuron is generated, the centers are initially allocated as follows:

$$C_{new} = X \tag{14}$$

Following the minimum firing strength criterion for rule generation, i.e., to ensure sufficient match degree for any pattern in the input space, the width of the newly generated RBF neuron can be computed as follows:

$$\sigma_j = \frac{max\{\parallel X - C_a \parallel, \parallel X - C_b \parallel\}}{\sqrt{ln(1/F_{gen})}} \tag{15}$$

where C_a and C_b are the two "nearest" neighboring centers of the clusters adjacent to the receptive field where the newly arrived pattern is located, in the sense of Euclidean distance. After the centers and widths are allocated by the aforementioned method, the next arrived pattern which is represented by the newly generated RBF neuron or the existing RBF neurons will meet the minimum firing strength criterion so that the match degree (firing strength) will be greater than F_{gen}.

Online Clustering

Proper clustering is not only necessary for feature extraction, but also reduction of the number of fuzzy rules when constructing a fuzzy inference system. Either hard clustering method or fuzzy clustering method needs to collect the training data and stipulate the number of clusters in advance which does not comply with online learning. The method of subtractive clustering, which is based on a measure of the density of data points in the feature space (see [29] for more details), can make clusters without determining the number of clusters. However, all data points in the data space must be processed to find the points with the highest number of neighbors as the centers of clusters. As a consequence, it violates the principle of practical real-time applications, i.e., low computation load and less memory requirement. In our proposed online self-enhanced fuzzy filter, the number of clusters is determined by automatically generating RBF neurons based on the fact that the receptive field of each RBF neuron is a cluster characterized by the corresponding centers and widths. However, the partition implemented by generating RBF neurons is coarse and cannot coincide with data distribution. Therefore, an online clustering method to adjust the centers and widths in the training process so that the receptive fields of RBF neurons can represent the data space reasonably well is proposed here. Moreover, the centers and widths will be optimized according to the scheme of parameters determination.

The main idea of online clustering is the following: Based on the coarse partition produced by the generation of RBF neurons under the minimum firing strength criterion, the centers are adjusted to move toward the direction of the area with high-density data points. For each incoming sample, it will influence the data distribution represented by the current clusters. The input terms of each input variable will be adjusted individually due to the feature of local representation of RBF neurons. Therefore, for each input variable, only the input term which provides the biggest degree of representation for incoming sample will be tuned online according to data representation. To prevent the fluctuation caused by those training samples which are far away from the centers and bring little information, a threshold is set to check whether online clustering should be operated. Only those samples which are sufficiently "close" to the centers are employed to tune the clusters.

Therefore, for the ith input variable, find

$$K = arg(min\|x_i - c_{ij}\|) \quad j = 1, 2, ..., u \tag{16}$$

If $\|x_i - c_{iK}\| < c_{thres}$, the corresponding center is tuned as follows:

$$c'_{iK} = c_{iK} + \alpha'(x_i - c_{iK}) \tag{17}$$

$$\alpha' = \alpha\mu_{iK}(x_i) \tag{18}$$

where c_{thres} is the threshold, α is a constant learning rate and α' is a varying learning rate related to the value of the membership function μ_{iK} computed by Eq.(6). Eq.(18) shows that the incoming sample which is nearer to the center c_{iK} will lead to bigger learning rate and vice versa.

After the centers are adjusted, all the widths should be re-checked adaptively to ensure that the criterion of minimum firing strength is fulfilled. For the jth RBF neuron, we have

$$\sigma_j = \frac{max(\|C_j - C_{j-1}\|, \|C_j - C_{j+1}\|,)}{\sqrt{ln(1/F_{gen})}} \tag{19}$$

where C_{j-1} and C_{j+1} are the two "nearest" neighboring centers to C_j in the sense of Euclidean distance.

Figs. 3 and 4 show the partition and the distribution of membership function on one dimension (x_1) without online clustering. Figs. 5 and 6 show the partition and the distribution of membership functions on x_1 dimension with online clustering for the same training set. It can be observed that, instead of allocating the centers and widths of membership functions, the proposed online clustering technique can ensure reasonable partition and reduction of the number of RBF neurons. This means that the structure of the filter is simplified.

The scheme of structure identification, including generation of new RBF neurons, allocation of precondition parameters and online clustering, is shown in Fig. 7.

Optimization of Free Parameters

Contrary to the conventional fuzzy neural networks-based approaches, the parameters in the consequent part of the RBFN-based online self-enhanced fuzzy filter can be computed without the backpropagation-based algorithm. This is possible because an RBF network can be regarded as a two-layer forward network which is linear after the corresponding centers and widths are allocated. Therefore, the scheme of parameters determination consists of two passes, i.e., the forward pass which determines free parameters of the linear regression model and the backward pass which optimizes parameters of the membership function. During the forward pass, the centers and widths of membership functions are assumed to be fixed and only the free parameters in multiple linear models need to be determined. During the backward pass, the centers and widths will be optimized by a gradient descent method. It is basically a sequential (online) hybrid algorithm from the view point of stochastic signal processing.

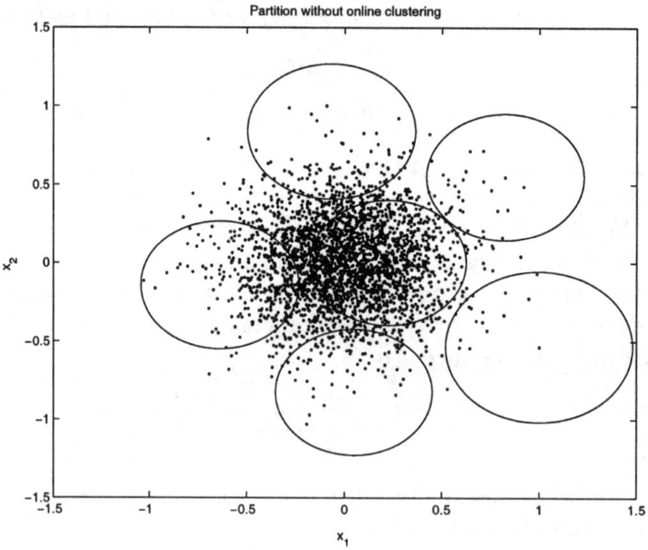

Fig. 3. The partition without online clustering

To optimize free parameters in the RBFN-based online self-enhanced fuzzy filter, we adopt the following cost function

$$E = \sum_{k=1}^{N} e^2(k) = \sum_{k=1}^{N} [d(k) - y(k)]^2 \tag{20}$$

where $d(k)$ is the desired output.

From Eq.(10), we define the free parameters of each fuzzy rule as follows:

$$T_j = [t_{j0}, t_{j1}, ..., t_{jr}] \tag{21}$$

and the free parameters of all fuzzy rules are written as follows:

$$T = [T_1, T_2, ..., T_u] \tag{22}$$

Therefore, Eq.(11) can be rewritten as follows:

$$\begin{aligned} y &= \sum_{j=1}^{u} T_j X'(k) \psi_j(C_j, \sigma_j, X(k)) \\ &= \sum_{j=1}^{u} T_j \theta_j(C_j, \sigma_j, X(k)) \\ &= T\Theta \end{aligned} \tag{23}$$

where $X'(k) = [1, x(k), x(k-1), ..., x(k-r+1)]^T = [1, X(k)^T]^T$ and $\theta_j = X'(k)\psi_j(C_j, \sigma_j, X(k))$.

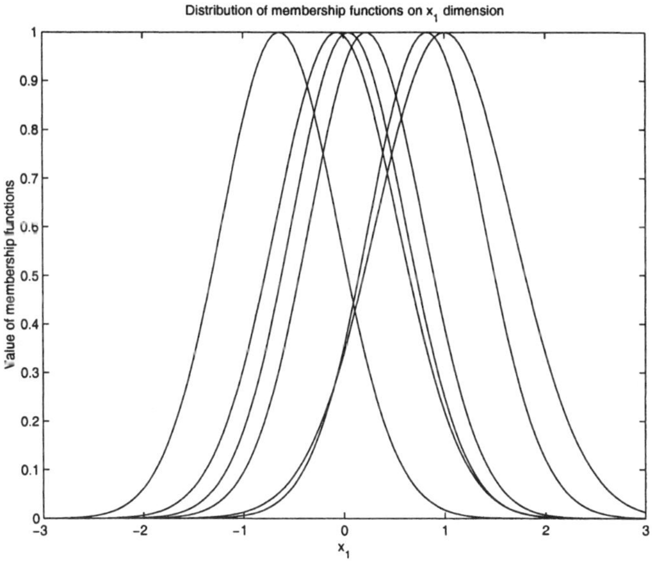

Fig. 4. The distribution of membership function on x_1 dimension without online clustering

Eqs.(20) and (23) show that the problem of determining free parameters is equivalent to a linear fitting problem which is essentially a linear least square problem and is feasible to be solved by some linear methods such as LMS, Recursive Least Square (RLS) and normalized LMS etc (see [2] for more details). For simplicity, we adopt the RLS algorithm to determine free parameters T.

The solution of the problem is given by

$$T^* = \Phi_{cov}^{-1} Z \tag{24}$$

where Φ_{cov}, the correlation matrix and Z, the cross-correlation vectors are respectively given by:

$$\Phi_{cov} = \Theta \Theta^T \tag{25}$$

$$Z = \Theta d(k) \tag{26}$$

The free parameters T can be updated in each iteration by the following recursive algorithm. The recursive algorithm is initialized by setting:

$$\Phi_{cov}^{-1}(0) = \gamma I \quad \gamma \textit{ is a large positive constant}$$
$$T(0) = 0$$

For each instant of time, $k = 1, 2, ..., N$, T is updated as follows:

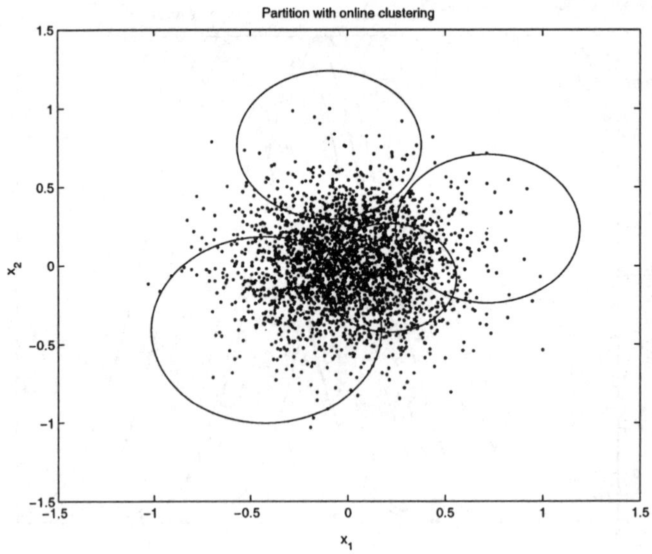

Fig. 5. The partition with online clustering

$$l(k) = \frac{\Phi_{cov}^{-1}(k-1)\Theta(k)}{\lambda + \Theta(k)^T \Phi_{cov}^{-1}(k-1)\Theta(k)} \tag{27}$$

$$\xi(k) = d(k) - T(k-1)\Theta(k) \tag{28}$$

$$T(k) = T(k-1) + l(k)\xi(k) \tag{29}$$

$$\Phi_{cov}^{-1}(k) = \lambda^{-1}(\Phi_{cov}^{-1}(k-1) - l(k)\Theta(k)^T \Phi_{cov}^{-1}(k-1)) \tag{30}$$

where $\lambda \in (0,1)$ is a forgetting factor. Normally, it is set to 0.99.

After the forward pass is finished, parameters of the membership function will be updated by the following gradient descent algorithm.

The centers will be updated as follows:

$$c'_{ij} = c_{ij} + \mu_c \triangle c_{ij} \tag{31}$$

where

$$\triangle c_{ij} = -\frac{\partial E}{\partial c_{ij}} = -\frac{\partial E}{\partial y}\frac{\partial y}{\partial \psi_j}\frac{\partial \psi_j}{\partial c_{ij}} \tag{32}$$

$$= 4(d(k) - y(k))(w_j - y(k))\psi_j \frac{x_i - c_{ij}}{\sigma_j^2} \tag{33}$$

and the widths will be updated as follows:

$$\sigma'_j = \sigma_j + \mu_\sigma \triangle \sigma_j \tag{34}$$

where

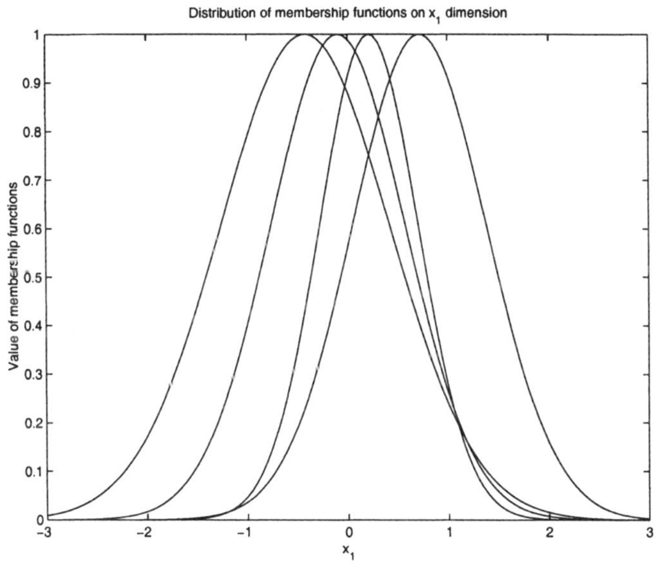

Fig. 6. The distribution of membership function on x_1 dimension with online clustering

$$\triangle\sigma_j = -\frac{\partial E}{\partial \sigma_j} = -\frac{\partial E}{\partial y}\frac{\partial y}{\partial \psi_j}\frac{\partial \psi_j}{\partial \sigma_j} \tag{35}$$

$$= 4(d(k) - y(k))(w_j - y(k))\psi_j \frac{\|X(k) - C_j\|^2}{\sigma_j^3} \tag{36}$$

where μ_c and μ_σ are the learning rate of centers and widths respectively.

For the linear regression model in the consequent parts, the second-order statistics of the input signals Θ in Eq.(23) is not only decided by the filter's input X, but also by the nonlinear mapping which depends on the shape of the membership functions. In other words, the inputs of the linear regression model are non-stationary which is made possible by adjusting the centers and widths of membership functions. To optimize the filter, the recursive algorithm has to seek the optimal weight T^* and keep track of the changing position of the optimal point. To prevent deteriorating the performance, although the hybrid algorithm consists of forward pass and backward pass, the forward pass is executed in each iteration and the backward pass is executed in each P iteration which means the parameters in the membership function are not updated for each sample. Here, P is a constant which depends on the number of free parameters in the consequent part. Normally, P is set to $2\mu(r+1)$ because the RLS algorithm is convergent in the mean value for S time steps where $S \geq \mu(r+1)$ (if we consider the whole consequent part of the online self-enhanced fuzzy filter as a transversal FIR filter). Therefore, the centers and widths are updated as follows:

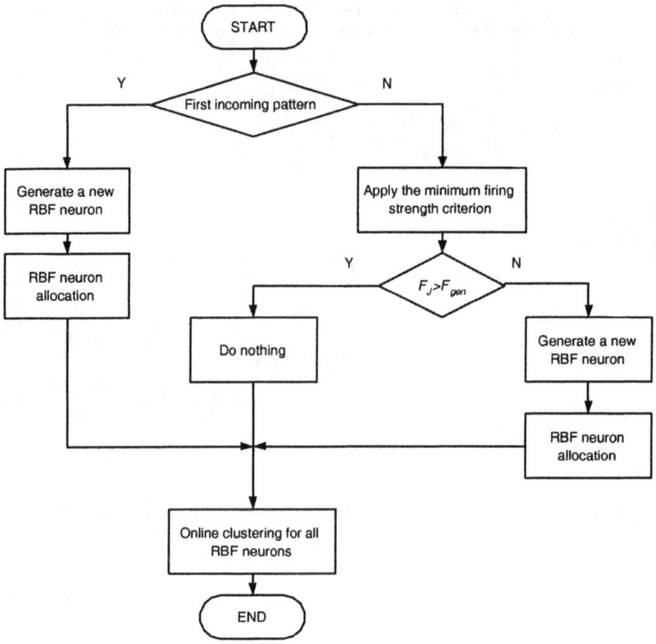

Fig. 7. Block diagram of structure identification

$$c'_{ij} = c_{ij} + \mu_c(-\frac{\partial E_P}{\partial c_{ij}}) \tag{37}$$

$$\sigma'_j = \sigma_j + \mu_\sigma(-\frac{\partial E_P}{\partial \sigma_j}) \tag{38}$$

where $E_P = \sum_{n=k}^{k+P-1}[d(n) - y(n)]^2$.

3 Simulation Results

In order to evaluate the effectiveness of the proposed Online Self-enhanced Fuzzy Filter (OSFF) in solving the nonlinear adaptive noise cancellation problem, simulation studies are carried out in this section. Firstly, we compare the proposed online self-enhanced fuzzy filter with other existing approaches via solving a nonlinear adaptive noise cancellation problem in order to show its salient features. Furthermore, the online self-enhanced fuzzy filter is applied for an audio noise cancellation problem in order to demonstrate its effectiveness in the context of multimedia processing.

3.1 Example 1

In this example, the proposed online self-enhanced fuzzy filter is applied as a transversal nonlinear filter to demonstrate its effectiveness for adaptive filtering. The original information signal $s(k)$ is a sawtooth signal of unit magnitude and a period of 50 samples as shown in Fig. 8. The noise $n(k)$ is generated by a uniformly distributed white noise sequence varying in the range of $[-2, 2]$. The noise source (reference noise) $n_1(k)$ was generated by a nonlinear autoregressive model with exogenous inputs of [30, 31] as follows:

$$\begin{aligned} n_1(k) = 0.25n_1(k-1) + 0.1n_1(k-2) + 0.5n(k-1) + 0.1n(k-2) \\ -0.2n(k-3) + 0.1n^2(k-2) + 0.08n(k-2)n_1(k-1) \end{aligned} \quad (39)$$

Optimal noise cancellation will be achieved if the noise cancellation filter $F(.)$ is implemented as a nonlinear IIR filter described as follows:

$$\begin{aligned} \hat{y}(k) = 2n_1(k) - 0.5n_1(k-1) - 0.2n_1(k-2) - 0.2\hat{y}(k-1) \\ +0.4\hat{y}(k-2) - 0.2\hat{y}^2(k-1) - 0.16n_1(k-1)\hat{y}(k-1) \end{aligned} \quad (40)$$

All assumptions for signals are the same with [3] and [25]. A total of 20000 samples are used and the first 2000 samples are discarded to avoid the transient process.

The optimal noise cancellation will be achieved if the online self-enhanced fuzzy filter can implement the dynamics of Eq.(40). Therefore, the input vector of the online self-enhanced fuzzy filter is defined as follows:

$$X = [n_1(k), n_1(k-1), n_1(k-2), \hat{y}(k-1), \hat{y}(k-2)]^T \quad (41)$$

Accordingly, the output of the nonlinear noise canceler is $\hat{y}(k)$.

The performance of noise cancellation is measured by the noise reduction factor NR which is defined as

$$NR = 10log\frac{E[n^2(k)]}{E[(s(k)-e(k))^2]} \quad (42)$$

This means that the larger the value of NR is, the better performance does the proposed noise cancellation approach achieve.

The generation of RBF neurons in the online self-enhanced fuzzy filter is shown in Fig. 9. There are only 4 RBF neurons employed in the online self-enhanced fuzzy filter, much less than M-RAN and RRBFN as shown in Table 1 respectively. It is due to the technique of online clustering that leads to reasonable data space partition. As a consequence, a parsimonious structure is obtained during online learning. The last 500 samples of the distorted signal and online recovered signal are shown in Fig. 10.

3.2 Example 2

In this example, in order to demonstrate the effectiveness of the online self-enhanced fuzzy filter in multimedia signal processing, real-world audio signals obtained from $MATLAB^{©}$ sound files *handel.mat* and *chirp.mat* are used as

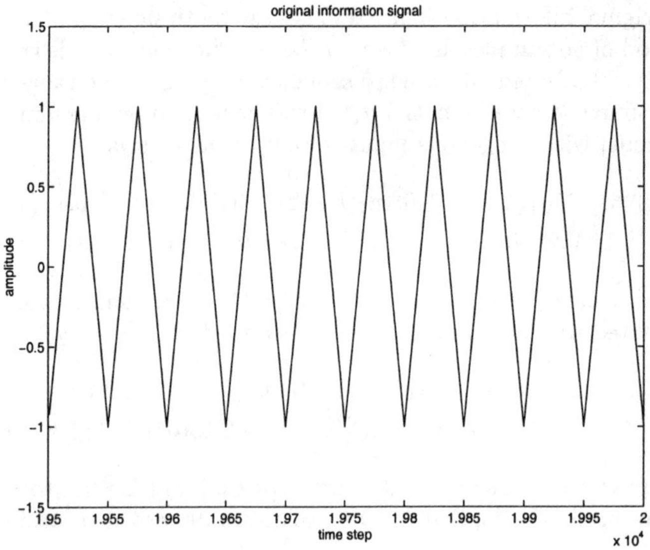

Fig. 8. Original information signal (signal of interest) $s(k)$

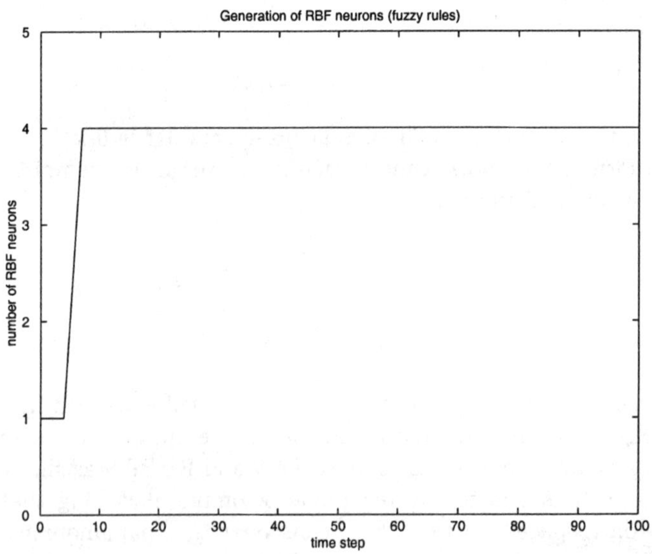

Fig. 9. Generation of RBF neurons (fuzzy rules) within 100 first samples

original information and noise signals respectively. The piece of audio signal in *handel.mat* is selected as the original information signal and the bird's chirping in *chirp.mat* is used as the noise source $n_1(k)$. The relation between the noise source and the corrupting noise is given by

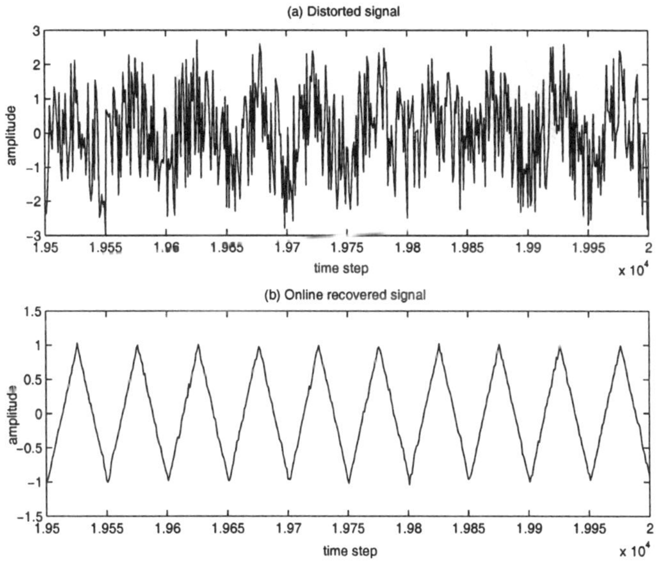

Fig. 10. (a) Distorted signal; (b) Online recovered signal

Table 1. Comparisons of OSFF with M-RAN and RRBFN

Approaches	Network size	NR(dB)
RRBFN	5-10-1	22.41
M-RAN	5-16-1	24.05
OSFF	5-4-1	30.23/41.67*

* 30.23 is the NR of the online training error; 41.67 is the NR of the testing error.

$$n(k) = \frac{8 \times sin(n_1(k) \times n_1(k-1) \times n_1(k-2))}{1 + [n_1(k-1)]^2 + [n_1(k-2)]^2} \tag{43}$$

The noise source and corrupting noise are shown in Fig. 11. In Figs. 12(a) and 12(b), the original information signal and the distorted signal are put together in order to illustrate that the original signal is heavily distorted by the corrupting noise.

To cancel the corrupting noise, the online self-enhanced fuzzy filter should emulate the dynamics of Eq.(43) for reproducing the noise. The input vector is defined as follows:

$$X = [n_1(k), n_1(k-1), n_1(k-2)]^T \tag{44}$$

The online self-enhanced fuzzy filter for noise cancellation is therefore based on the following nonlinear mapping

$$\hat{f} : \Re^X \rightarrow \Re^y \tag{45}$$

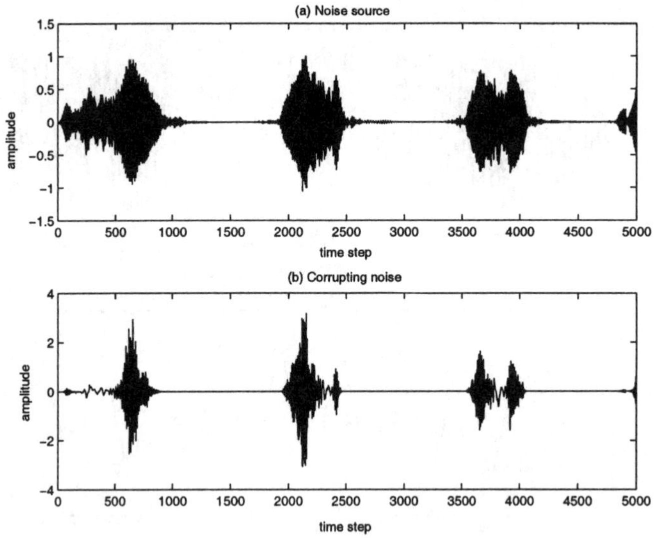

Fig. 11. (a) Noise source; (b) Corrupting noise

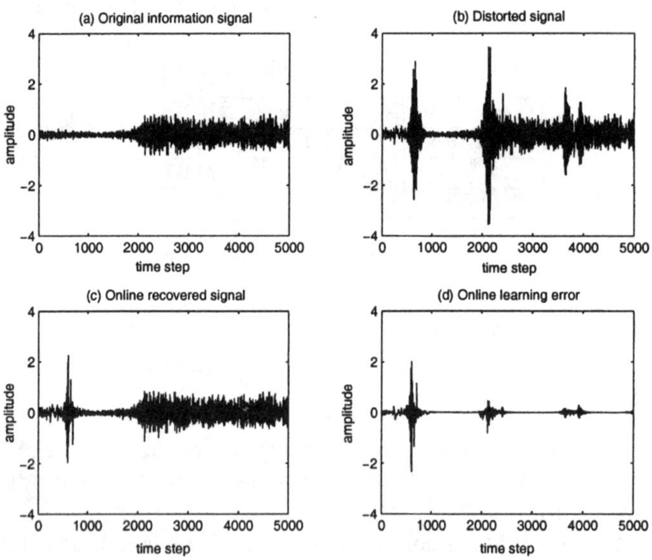

Fig. 12. (a) Original information signal; (b) Distorted signal; (c) Online recovered signal; (d) Online learning error

Figs. 12(c) and 12(d) show the online recovered signal and the online learning error respectively. The growth of fuzzy rules is depicted in Fig. 13 which shows that 6 fuzzy rules are generated during online learning. It is observed that the online self-enhanced fuzzy filter (noise canceler) is able to reproduce

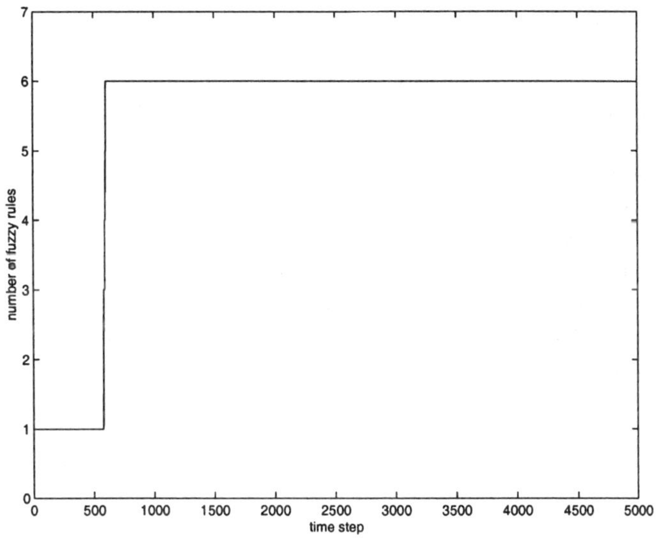

Fig. 13. The growth of fuzzy rules

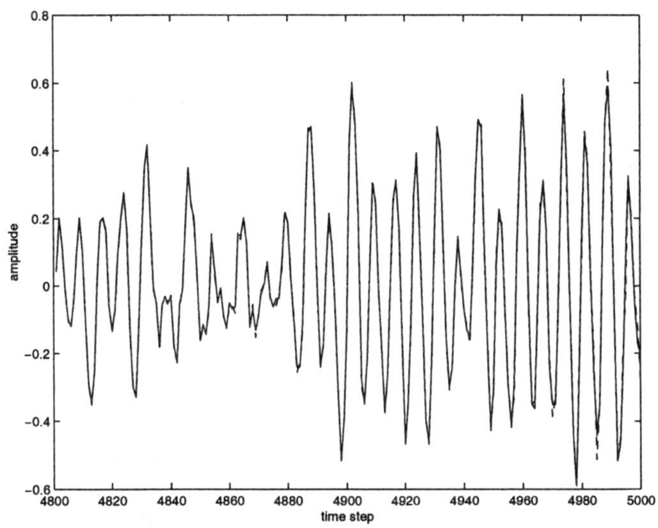

Fig. 14. The last 200 samples of original information signal and online recovered signal, '-' is the original information signal and '- -' is the recovered signal

the noise and cancel the interference successfully. In order to illustrate its performance clearly, the last 200 samples of the original information signal and the recovered signal are shown in Fig. 14.

4 Conclusions

In order to solve nonlinear noise cancellation in multimedia processing, a new online self-enhanced fuzzy filter with hybrid sequential algorithm is developed. The main feature of the proposed online self-enhanced fuzzy filter is that structure learning and parameters determination is adaptive and self-enhanced. For structure identification, the minimum firing strength criterion, based on the novelty of input signals in order to ensure proper nonlinear mapping, is proposed to generate new RBF neurons/fuzzy rules. Instead of selecting the centers and widths arbitrarily, online clustering will be carried out to make reasonable data representation. As a consequence, a parsimonious structure of fuzzy systems can be achieved. Furthermore, the hybrid sequential algorithm helps to tune free parameters optimally online.

In summary, the proposed online self-enhanced fuzzy filter has the following features: (1) Hierarchical structure for self-construction. There is no initial predetermination for the online self-enhanced fuzzy filter, i.e., it is not necessary to determine the initial number of fuzzy rules and input data space clustering in advance. The fuzzy rules, i.e., the RBF neurons are generated automatically during the training process using the minimum firing strength criterion. (2) Online clustering. Instead of selecting the centers and widths of membership functions arbitrarily, an online clustering method is applied to ensure reasonable representation of input terms of an input variable. It not only ensures proper feature representation, but also optimizes the structure of the filter by reducing the number of fuzzy rules. (3) All free parameters in the premise and consequent parts are determined online by the proposed hybrid sequential algorithm without repeated computation in order to facilitate real-time applications. The centers and widths of membership functions of an input variable are allocated initially in the scheme of structure identification and optimized in the scheme of parameters determination. The parameters in the consequent parts of the online self-enhanced fuzzy filter are updated in each iteration by a sequential recursive algorithm.

Simulation results show that the proposed online self-enhanced fuzzy filter can handle the nonlinear noise cancellation problem very well. In the online self-enhanced fuzzy filter, the attractive feature is the superb performance at the cost of economic system resources such as less memory storage and low computation load. Undoubtedly, the proposed online self-enhanced fuzzy filter has a great potential for multimedia signal processing.

References

1. B.Widrow and S.D.Stearnsa (1985) Adaptive Signal Processing. Englewood Cliffs, NJ:Prentice Hall
2. S. Haykin (1986) Adaptive filter theory. Englewood Cliffs, N.J, Prentice-Hall
3. S. A. Billings and C. F.Fung (1995) Recurrent radial basis function networks for adaptive noise cancellation. Neural Networks, **8**, 273–290

4. C.T.Lin (1994) Neural Fuzzy Control Systems with Structure and parameter Learning. World Scientific
5. K.Hornic, M.Stinchcombe, and H.White (1989) Multilayer feedforward networks are universal approximators. Neural Networks, **2**, 359–366
6. L.Wang (1992) Fuzzy systems are universial approximators. Proc. Int. Conf. Fuzzy Syst.
7. H. Leung, T. Lo, and S. Wang (2001) Prediction of noisy chaotic time series using an optimal radial basis function neural network. IEEE Trans. on Neural Networks, **12**, 1163–1172
8. S. A. Vorobyov and A. Cichocki (2001) Hyper radial basis function neural networks for interference cancellation with nonlinear processing of reference signal. Digital Signal Processing, **11**, 204–221
9. B. Widrow, J. Glover, and et al. (1975) Adaptive noise cancelling: Principles and applications. Proceedings of the IEEE, **63**, 1692–1716
10. B. Friedlander (1982) System identification techniques for adaptive noise cancellation. IEEE Trans. on Acoustics, Speech, and Signal Processing, **30**, 699–709
11. L.Yin, J.Astola, and Y.Neuvo (1993) A new class of nonlinear filters-neural filters. IEEE Trans. on Signal Processing, **41**, 1201–1222
12. W.G.Knecht, M.E.Schenkel, and G.S.Moschytz (1995) Neural network filters for speech enhancement. IEEE Trans. on Speech Audio Processing, **13**, 433–439
13. X.-P. Zhang (2001) Thresholding neural network for adaptive noise reduction. IEEE Trans. on Neural Networks, **12**, 567 –584
14. J.-S. R. Jang (1993) Anfis: Adaptive-network-based fuzzy inference system. IEEE Trans. on Systems, Man, and Cybernetics, **23**, 665–685
15. C.-F. Juang and C.-T. Lin (1998) An on-line self-constructing neural fuzzy inference network and its application. IEEE Trans. on Fuzzy Systems, **6**, 12–32
16. C.-F. Juang and C.-T. Lin (2001) Noisy speech processing by recurrently adaptive fuzzy filters. IEEE Trans. on Fuzzy Systems, **9**, 139–152
17. P. A.Mastorocostas and J. B.Theocharis (2002) A recurrent fuzzy-neural model for dynamic system identifation. IEEE Trans. on Systems, Man, and Cybernetics, **32**, 176–190
18. C.-F. Juang and X.-T. Lin (1999) A recurrent self-organizing neural fuzzy inference network. IEEE Trans. on Neural Networks, **10**, 828–845
19. C.T.Lin and C.F.Juang (1997) An adaptive neural fuzzy filter and its application. IEEE Trans. on Systems, Man, and Cybernetics, **27**, 635–656
20. C.-H. Lee and C.-C. Teng (2000) Identification and control of dynamic sy... using recurrent fuzzy neural networks. IEEE Trans. on Fuzzy System... 366
21. K. B. Cho and B. H. Wang (1996) Radial basis function b... systems and their applications to system identificatio... Sets and Systems, **83**, 325–339
22. S. Lee and R. M. Kil (1991) A gaussian poten... chically self-organizing learning. Neural N...
23. L. Yingwei, N. Sundararajan, and P. ... scheme for function approximat... networks. Neural Comput...
24. L. Yingwei, N. Sund... uation of a seque... algorithm. IEEE ...

25. S. Yonghong, P. Saratchandran, and N. Sundararajan (1999) Minimal resource allocation network for adaptive noise cancellation. ELECTRONICS LETTERS-IEE, **35**, 726–728
26. S. Wu, M. J. Er, and Y. Gao (2001) A fast approach for automatic generation of fuzzy rules by generalized dynamic fuzzy neural networks. IEEE Trans. on Fuzzy Systems, **9**, 578–594
27. S. Wu and M. J. Er (2000) Dynamic fuzzy neural networks-a novel approach to funtion approximation. IEEE Trans. on Systems, Man, and Cybernetics, **30**, 358–364
28. Sugeno. M. (1985) Industrial applications of fuzzy control. Elsevier Science Pub. Co.
29. J.-S. R. Jang, C.-T. Sun, and E. Mizutani. (1997) Neuro-fuzzy and soft computing. Prentice Hall
30. K. Narendra and K. Parthasarathy (1990) Identification and control of dynamical systems using neural network. IEEE Trans. on Neural Networks, 4–27
31. S. Chen, S. A. Billings, and P. M. Grant (1990) Nonlinear system identification using neural networks. Int. J. Contr., **51**, 1191–1214